Adaptation and Brain Function

Adaptation and Brain Function

Editor: Kylie Hill

AMERICAN
MEDICAL PUBLISHERS
www.americanmedicalpublishers.com

AMERICAN
MEDICAL PUBLISHERS
www.americanmedicalpublishers.com

Cataloging-in-Publication Data

Adaptation and brain function / edited by Kylie Hill.
p. cm.
Includes bibliographical references and index.
ISBN 978-1-63927-279-2
1. Brain. 2. Brain--Adaptation. 3. Brain--Physiology. I. Hill, Kylie.
QP376 .A33 2022
612.82--dc23

American Medical Publishers,
41 Flatbush Avenue,
1st Floor, New York,
NY 11217, USA

ISBN 978-1-63927-279-2 (Hardback)

Contents

Preface

The main aim of this book is to educate learners and enhance their research focus by presenting diverse topics covering this vast field. This is an advanced book which compiles significant studies by distinguished experts in the area of analysis. This book addresses successive solutions to the challenges arising in the area of application, along with it; the book provides scope for future developments.

Living organisms have to constantly change their body to adjust its behaviors and functions to adapt to the constantly changing environment. This continuous interaction between the organism and the environment is called adaptation. The brain is the command center of the nervous system. It receives information from the environment through the sensory organs and sends signals to the muscles and other parts of the body. Emotional and behavioral adaptations require the involvement of the entire brain. The feature of the brain which helps humans learn and adapt to their surroundings and situations is called plasticity. This book unravels the recent studies in adaptation and brain function. The topics covered herein are of utmost significance and bound to provide incredible insights to readers. Through this book, we attempt to further enlighten the readers about the new concepts in this field.

It was a great honour to edit this book, though there were challenges, as it involved a lot of communication and networking between me and the editorial team. However, the end result was this all-inclusive book covering diverse themes in the field.

Finally, it is important to acknowledge the efforts of the contributors for their excellent chapters, through which a wide variety of issues have been addressed. I would also like to thank my colleagues for their valuable feedback during the making of this book.

Editor

1

A reinterpretation of the cytoarchitectonics of the telencephalon of the Comoran coelacanth

R. Glenn Northcutt[1,2]* and Agustín González[3]

[1] Laboratory of Comparative Neurobiology, Scripps Institution of Oceanography, University of California San Diego, La Jolla, CA, USA
[2] Department of Neurosciences, School of Medicine, University of California San Diego, La Jolla, CA, USA
[3] Department of Cell Biology, Faculty of Biology, University of Complutense of Madrid, Madrid, Spain

Edited by:
Fernando Martinez-Garcia, Universidad de Valencia, Spain

Reviewed by:
Rudolf Nieuwenhuys, Netherlands Institute for Neuroscience, Netherlands
Ramon Anadon, Universidad de Santiago de Compostela, Spain

****Correspondence:***
R. Glenn Northcutt, Department of Neurosciences, University of California San Diego, 9500 Gilman Drive, La Jolla, CA 92093-0201, USA.
e-mail: rgnorthcutt@ucsd.edu

The cytoarchitecture of the telencephalon of the Comoran coelacanth, *Latimeria chalumnae*, was analyzed in the context of recent advances in our understanding of telencephalic organization in lungfishes and amphibians, which constitute the sister group to coelacanths. In coelacanths, the telencephalon is divided into pedunculated olfactory bulbs, paired hemispheres, and an unevaginated telencephalon impar. The hemispheres consist of a ventrally located subpallium and, dorsally, a greatly expanded pallium. Traditionally, the subpallium in coelacanths has been divided into a medial septal area and a lateral striatum. Re-examination of the lateral subpallial wall, however, suggests that the striatum is more restricted than previously believed, and it is replaced dorsally by a more scattered plate of cells, which appears to represent the ventral pallium. The putative ventral pallium is continuous with a ventromedial pallial formation, which appears to receive input from the lateral olfactory tract and should be considered a possible homolog of the lateral pallium in tetrapods. The putative lateral pallium is replaced by a more dorsomedial pallial formation, which may represent the dorsal pallium. This formation is replaced, in turn by an extensive lateral pallial formation, which appears to be homologous to the medial pallium of tetrapods. An expanded medial pallium in coelacanths, lepidosirenid lungfishes, and amphibians may be related to well developed spatial learning. Traditionally, the telencephalon impar of coelacanths, has been interpreted as an enlarged preoptic area, but reanalysis indicates that the so-called superior preoptic nucleus actually consists of the medial amygdalar nucleus.

Keywords: amygdala, *Latimeria*, lobe-finned fishes, medial pallium, ventral pallium

INTRODUCTION

During the Devonian, approximately 415 to 360 million years ago, the Sarcopterygii (lobe-finned fishes) constituted one of two major radiations of bony fishes. Today, only three groups of Sarcopterygii still exist: the coelacanths, the lungfishes, and the limbed vertebrates (Tetrapoda). All recent phylogenetic data indicate that lungfishes are the sister group of tetrapods, and that coelacanths are, in turn, the sister group of these taxa (Brinkmann et al., 2004; Takezaki et al., 2004). There are only two known living coelacanth species: the Comoran coelacanth, *Latimeria chalumnae*, and the Indonesian coelacanth, *L. menadoensis*. Both species are 1–2 m in length and weigh 65–100 kg. Both inhabit marine rocky slopes with caves at depths of 100–700 m. *L. chalumnae* was discovered in 1938, and over 100 specimens have been preserved in museums internationally. Their current population, however, is estimated to be less than 400 individuals (Hissmann et al., 1998). *L. menadoensis* was discovered only in 1997, and there are no estimates of their population size.

Although the anatomy of *L. menadoensis* has not been described, the general anatomy of *L. chalumnae* is known in detail (Millot and Anthony, 1958, 1965; Millot et al., 1978), and there are several descriptions of the brain, including detailed reports on cell groups and major pathways (Nieuwenhuys, 1965, 1998; Nieuwenhuys et al., 1977; Nieuwenhuys and Meek, 1990). However, recent molecular and connectional advances in the study of telencephalic organization in lungfishes (González and Northcutt, 2009; Northcutt, 2009) and amphibians (Marín et al., 1998; González et al., 2002; Brox et al., 2003, 2004; Moreno and González, 2004, 2005, 2006, 2007a,b) reveal that these taxa possess four, not three, pallial divisions and that the amygdalar complex consists of at least three distinct nuclei. For these reasons, the cytoarchitecture of the telencephalon of the Comoran coelacanth was reevaluated, with a particular focus on pallial and amygdalar organization.

MATERIALS AND METHODS

ANIMALS AND TISSUE PROCESSING

Two brains of *L. chalumnae* were dehydrated, paraffin embedded, and cut into 15 μm serial sections in the transverse plane. The first brain was donated by the Field Museum of Natural History, Chicago, IL, USA (CCC number 61 of Bruton and Coutouvidis, 1991). Unfortunately, the body of this coelacanth was frozen prior to fixation, and the brain histology is marginal. The second brain was dissected from specimen 80 (Bruton and Coutouvidis, 1991) and fixed in 4% paraformaldehyde shortly after death, and the brain histology is very good. The serial sections of this brain were divided into three series: One series was stained with the Bodian silver method to reveal myelinated and unmyelinated fiber tracts; A second series was stained with 1% cresyl violet to reveal neuronal cell bodies; The third series was stained with the Klüver–Barrera method to reveal myelinated tracts and neuronal cell bodies.

CYTOARCHITECTONIC CRITERIA

Six criteria are commonly used to recognize cell groups cytoarchitectonically: (1) differences in neuronal cell size; (2) differences in neuronal density; (3) relatively cell-free zones, which frequently indicate boundaries between cell groups; (4) differences in the distribution of genetic and immunohistochemical markers; (5) differences in the connectivity of the suspected cell groups; and (6) phylogenetic continuity of cellular groups and their molecular markers and connections within a clade. Frequently, when a brain region is first examined cytologically, the first three criteria are primarily used to generate hypotheses regarding the number of cell groups, their topology, and their possible homologs in other taxa. Ideally, these hypotheses are then tested using criteria 4 and 5. Criterion 6 is critical at both levels of analysis. Firstly, it has a predictive function at the first level of analysis, as brain organization within a clade is generally conserved, and cell groups that occur within members of a clade should be widely, if not universally, present (plesiomorphs) and can be predicted to occur in a member of the clade that has not yet been examined. Secondly, this criterion is critical in proposing homologies between cell groups in different members of a clade, as a cell group and its molecular and hodological characteristics should be widely, if not universally, present (plesiomorphs), or they should exhibit linear transformation (apomorphs) within the clade.

Unfortunately, in the case of the Comoran coelacanth, there are no molecular or hodological data to aid in proposing and evaluating hypotheses of the homology of neuronal cell groups. Thus, criteria 1–3, aided by the predictive power of criterion 6, are all that is presently available on which to base hypotheses regarding individual cell groups and their possible homology with cell groups in other taxa of lobe-finned fishes. For this reason, all statements regarding the recognition of cell groups in the telencephalon of the Comoran coelacanth, and their possible homologs in other taxa, can be only considered tentative. Hopefully they will be tested when molecular data becomes available, but given the rarity and endangered status of coelacanths, it may never be possible to undertake hodological experiments.

RESULTS

The olfactory bulbs were not collected with either of the brains so the cytoarchitecture of only the telencephalic hemispheres and the telencephalon impar is described. The olfactory bulbs lie immediately adjacent to the olfactory organs, so that the olfactory nerves are very short. The axons of the olfactory bulb collect as slender olfactory peduncles, which may be as long as 20 cm and can be traced caudally into the most rostral division of the telencephalic hemispheres, which form distinct lobes termed the rostral bodies (**Figures 1A,B and 2A,B**).

ROSTRAL BODIES

Each rostral body consists of a medial ependymal surface with scattered neurons that surround a dense core of secondary olfactory fibers (**Figures 2A,B**). These fibers arise from the olfactory peduncles, which divide into dorsally and ventrally situated tracts – i.e., the lateral and medial olfactory tracts (**Figure 2B**) – as each peduncle enters the ipsilateral rostral body along its lateral margin. Although the fibers of the olfactory peduncle initially divide into dorsal and ventral tracts as they course along the lateral margin of the rostral bodies (**Figures 2A,B**), these tracts are interpreted as homologous to the lateral and medial olfactory tracts of tetrapods, based on their subsequent trajectories in the telencephalic hemispheres. The fibers of both secondary olfactory tracts densely ramify within the rostral body, and it is clear that this body primarily receives olfactory input. The secondary olfactory tracts can be clearly distinguished from one another by their relative positions in the rostral body, and also by differences in fiber size, as fibers in the lateral olfactory tract are far more robust.

Many of the fibers of the medial olfactory tract terminate within the ventral half of the rostral body, but a number of these fibers continue more caudally and appear to innervate the subpallium of the rostral pole of the more caudal telencephalic hemisphere. The lateral olfactory tract, in addition to innervating the dorsal half of the rostral body, continues caudally as a distinct tract and enters the rostral pallium of the telencephalic hemisphere, where it can be traced medially into the core of the pallium (**Figure 2C**).

The rostral bodies appear to be pallial in origin, as caudally each rostral body is gradually replaced by the cell groups that form the rostral pallial telencephalon (**Figure 2C**). The cells of the dorsolateral rostral body are the first to be replaced by the larger cells of the medial pallium. Slightly more caudally the dorsomedial cells of the rostral body are replaced by the cells of the dorsal pallium, which at this level (**Figure 2C**) are embedded in a pale-staining neuropil. There is no distinct border between the ventral cells of the rostral body and those of the lateral pallium, only a gradual transition from one cell group to the other, marked by an expansion of the lateral olfactory tract.

TELENCEPHALIC HEMISPHERES

The telencephalic hemispheres of the Comoran coelacanth are clearly evaginated, with the subpallium consisting primarily of a distinct periventricular cellular plate, and the pallium comprising a massive lobe, which appears to have protruded into the lateral ventricle (**Figure 1D**). There is thus little evidence that the pallium participated in the extensive evagination that characterizes the subpallium.

A number of divisions of the subpallium can be recognized by differences in the thickness of its periventricular cellular plate. Medially, the periventricular plate lies very close to the ependymal lining of the ventricle and is approximately four to five cells in thickness, with the exception of a distinct cluster of neurons which occurs adjacent to the lamina terminalis (**Figure 1D**). The topology of the medial periventricular plate, and the migrated cell group at the border of the lamina terminalis, suggest that these cell groups are homologous to the lateral and medial septal nuclei, respectively, in other lobe-finned fishes.

As the subpallial periventricular plate is traced laterally, the plate becomes more distal to the ependymal layer of the lateral ventricle and thickens to approximately 10 cells (**Figures 1D and 2D**). It continues to thicken as it is traced laterally, as does the entire wall of the subpallium, so that the periventricular plate forms a distinct ventrolaterally directed cellular prominence with the deeper subpallial wall, bulging into the lateral ventricle (**Figures 1D,E**). This cellular prominence may mark the boundary

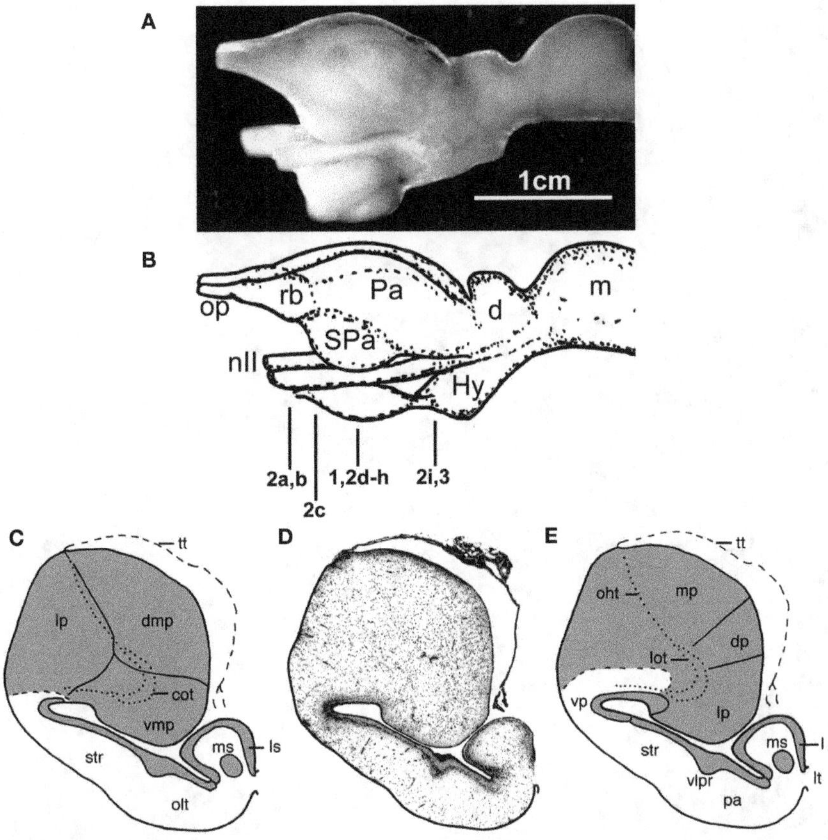

FIGURE 1 | The forebrain and midbrain the Comoran coelacanth. (A) Photograph of a lateral view of the forebrain and midbrain. **(B)** Line drawing of the lateral view, indicating the levels of the transverse section in **Figures 1–3. (C)** Line drawing of a transverse section through one telencephalic hemisphere showing the boundaries of cell groups interpreted by Nieuwenhuys (1965) and Nieuwenhuys and Meek (1990). **(D)** A Nissl-stained section from the present study, showing the actual histology. **(E)** Line drawing indicating the boundaries of the cell groups as interpreted in the present study. Dotted lines in **(C,E)** indicate the lateral olfactory and olfactohabenular tracts. Short, heavy dashed lines indicate the subpallial–pallial boundary **(C)** or the boundary between the neuropil of the ventral pallium and the medial pallium **(E)**. cot, Central olfactory tract; d, diencephalon; dmp, dorsomedial pallium; dp, dorsal pallium; Hy, hypothalamus; Hyp, hypophysis; lot, lateral olfactory tract; lp, lateral pallium; ls, lateral septum; lt, lamina terminalis; m, mesencephalon; mp, medial pallium; ms, medial septum; nII, optic nerve; oht, olfactohabenular tract; olt, olfactory tubercle; op, olfactory peduncle, Pa (in lateral view), pallium; pa (in transverse section), pallidum; rb, rostral body; SPa, subpallium; str, striatum; tt, telencephalic tela; vlpr, ventrolateral cellular prominence; vmp, ventromedial pallium; vp, ventral pallium.

between a dorsally situated striatum and a more ventrally situated pallidum, but this interpretation remains speculative without immunohistochemical data.

As the subpallial periventricular cellular plate is traced further laterally and dorsally, its characteristics again change. Near the extensive recess of the lateral ventricle, which appears to separate the subpallium and pallium, its cells become more scattered (**Figure 1D**), and they take on a typical pallial appearance dorsal to the lateral ventricular recess (**Figure 2E**). The topology and cellular organization of the subpallial periventricular plate suggest that this region is not part of the subpallium but is, rather, the ventral most division of the pallium, termed the ventral pallium in tetrapods.

The remaining three divisions of the pallium (the medial, dorsal, and lateral divisions) traditionally recognized in other lobed-finned fishes are clearly evident in the Comoran coelacanth. These divisions and their topology are most obvious in the rostral pole of the pallium (**Figure 2C**). The medial pallium is the most dorsally situated pallial division and, as in other lobe-finned fishes, it is continuous with the even more dorsally situated telencephalic tela (**Figure 2C**). At this level, the dorsal pallium appears to be a division of the pallium sandwiched between the more dorsolaterally situated medial pallium and the more ventrally situated lateral pallium. The cells of the dorsal pallium are smaller than those of either the medial or lateral pallial divisions and are surrounded by a paler staining neuropil (**Figure 2C**). At this level, the lateral pallium occupies the ventral half of the rostral pallial lobe, and its core consists of numerous fascicles of the lateral olfactory tract (**Figure 2C**), which appear to radiate into all three pallial divisions.

More caudally, the lateral pallium appears to be displaced from the lateral pial surface by the medial pallium (**Figures 1D,E**), but it is laterally continuous with the putative ventral pallium and is still bordered dorsally by the dorsal pallium. The lateral pallium at mid-hemispheric levels consists of a core of fascicles of the lateral olfactory tract and a neuropil surrounded by a more periventricularly located band of cells that is many times thicker than the central neuropil when seen in the transverse plane (**Figure 2F**). It has not been possible to trace fascicles of the lateral olfactory tract into the periventricular cellular band. Even at mid-hemispheric levels,

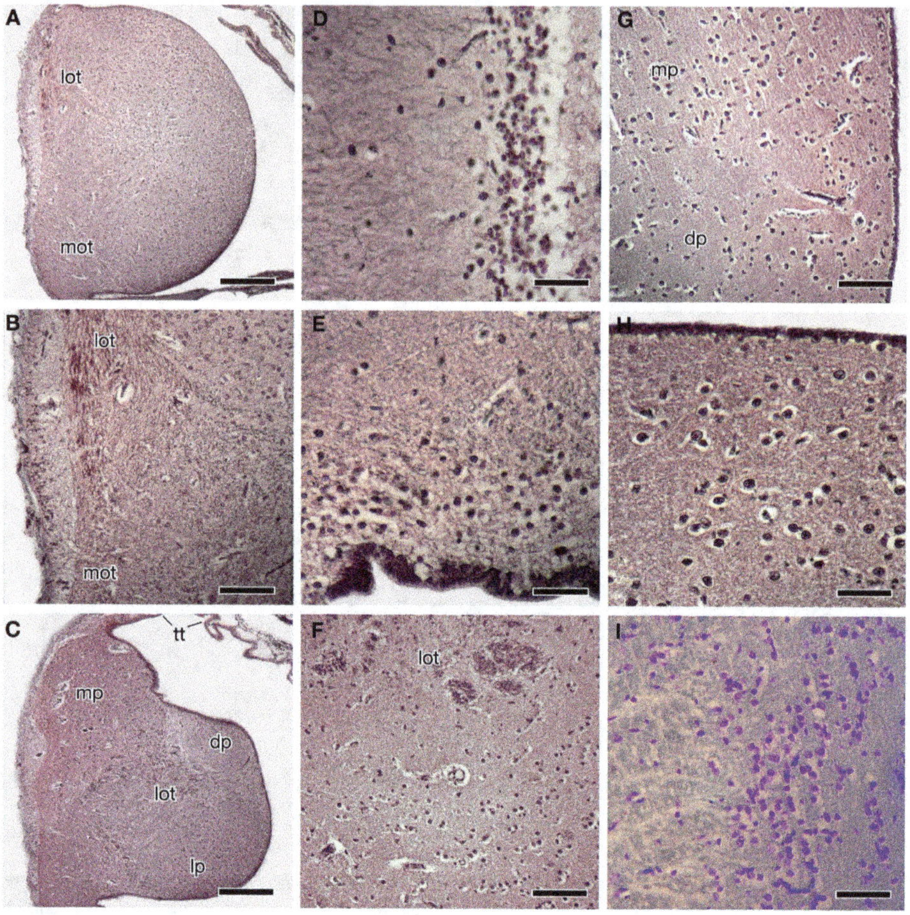

FIGURE 2 | Photomicrographs of transverse sections through the forebrain of the Comoran coelacanth showing various cell groups. (A,B) The rostral body. **(C)** The rostral pallium. **(D)** The striatum. **(E)** The ventral pallium. **(F)** The core and cellular band of the lateral pallium. **(G)** The medial border of the dorsal and medial pallia. **(H)** The cells of the medial pallium. **(I)** The cells of the central amygdalar nucleus. Sections in **(A–H)** are stained by the Bodian silver method; section I is stained with 1% cresyl violet. Scale bars = 100 µm **(D,E,H,I)**, 200 µm **(B,F,G)**, 500 µm **(A,C)**. dp, Dorsal pallium; lot, lateral olfactory tract; lp, lateral pallium; mot, medial olfactory tract, mp, medial pallium; tt telencephalic tela.

fascicles of the lateral olfactory tract can still be seen more laterally within the neuropil of the ventral pallium. The ventral pallium can be divided into a periventricularly located cell plate and a more superficial molecular layer (**Figures 1D,E**) which can be clearly distinguished from the adjacent neuropil of the medial pallium.

Throughout its rostrocaudal extent, the dorsal pallium can be distinguished from the lateral and medial pallia, because its cells are more scattered than those of the other two divisions (**Figure 2G**). Furthermore, even though the dorsal pallial cells are more scattered, their lamination is more distinct than that of cells in either the lateral pallium or the medial pallium. The cellular density of the medial pallium is at least twice that of the dorsal pallium (**Figure 2G**). The cells of the medial pallium also are larger and are embedded in a denser neuropil consisting of larger fibers (**Figure 2H**).

At caudal hemispheric levels, the pallial lobe has a deep horizontal sulcus along its medial edge, which clearly separates the dorsal and medial pallia from the lateral pallium. At this level, the periventricular cellular band of the lateral pallium decreases in cross-sectional thickness and forms a distinct periventricular cellular plate, which almost completely encircles the core of fascicles of the lateral olfactory tract. Lamination of the dorsal pallium also becomes more distinct, with the laminae being broader dorsally than ventrally as the caudal border of the dorsal pallium is reached. The medial pallium becomes narrower in cross-sectional thickness but appears to end more caudally in the telencephalon impar (**Figure 3B**).

TELENCEPHALON IMPAR

The telencephalon impar of the Comoran coelacanth is an unevaginated caudal part of the telencephalon, which forms a simple tube whose floor is formed rostrally by the optic chiasm and the walls of the preoptic recess of the third ventricle. Its lateral walls are slightly thickened, whereas its roof consists of a non-neural ependymal transverse velum (**Figure 3**). Unlike the situation in other vertebrates, the infundibulum of the hypothalamus and the hypophysis extend rostrally rather than caudally, apparently due to a general caudal shift of the rest of the brain during development. As a result, the infundibulum of the hypothalamus is located beneath the rostral most edge of the optic chiasm, and the ventral hypothalamus extends further rostral than in most vertebrates (**Figures 1A,B and 3**). Despite this distortion in the hypothalamus, the preoptic recess and adjacent preoptic nuclei

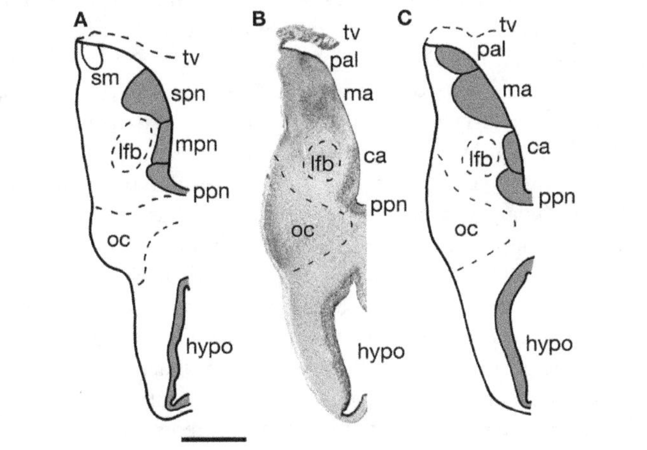

FIGURE 3 | A transverse section through one half of the telencephalon impar of the Comoran coelacanth. (A) Cell groups as interpreted by Nieuwenhuys (1965). **(B)** A Nissl-stained section from the present study showing the histology. **(C)** Cell groups as interpreted in the present study. Bar scale = 1 mm. ca, Central amygdalar nucleus; hypo, hypothalamus; lfb, lateral forebrain bundle; ma, medial amygdalar nucleus; mpn, magnocellular preoptic nucleus; oc, optic chiasm; pal, pallium; ppn, parvocellular preoptic nucleus; stria medullaris; spn, superior preoptic nucleus; tv, transverse velum.

appear unaffected. A parvocellular preoptic nucleus, composed of small densely packed neurons, can be traced dorsal to the optic chiasm, where it is replaced more caudally by the much larger cells of the magnocellular preoptic nucleus. More rostrally, a more scattered group of neurons (**Figures 2I and 3B**) occurs dorsal to the parvocellular preoptic nucleus. This cell group appears to be homologous to the central amygdalar nucleus of lungfishes and tetrapods (**Figures 3B,C**), which is also located adjacent to the lateral forebrain bundle and consists of the largest cells in the vicinity. More dorsally, the putative central amygdalar nucleus is replaced, in turn, by a group of smaller cells, which appears to be homologous to the medial amygdalar nucleus of lungfishes and tetrapods (**Figures 3B,C**). Although the topology and cytology of these nuclei in the Comoran coelacanth are consistent with the interpretation that they are homologs of amygdalar nuclei in other lobe-finned fishes, these hypotheses would be greatly supported by immunohistochemical data.

DISCUSSION

Our reinterpretation of the telencephalic cytoarchitectonics of the Comoran coelacanth generally agrees with the earlier studies of Nieuwenhuys and colleagues (Nieuwenhuys, 1965, 1998; Nieuwenhuys et al., 1977; Nieuwenhuys and Meek, 1990), but differs regarding four points: (1) the pallial–subpallial border and the recognition of a putative ventral pallium; (2) the organization of the striatum; (3) the borders of the medial pallium; and (4) the organization of the amygdala. Each of these points is discussed below.

PALLIAL–SUBPALLIAL BORDER

Nieuwenhuys and colleagues recognized the lateral pallial–subpallial border as occurring just dorsal to the lateral recess of the lateral ventricle (**Figure 1C**), and they interpreted the ventrolateral wall as homologous to the striatum of other lobe-finned fishes. Re-examination of the ventrolateral wall of the Comoran coelacanth suggests that the periventricular cellular plate that characterizes the striatum changes as it is traced dorsally and transforms to a cell group typical of the pallium, and we have therefore recognized it as a putative ventral pallium (**Figure 1E**). This interpretation is supported by new immunohistochemical data (Brox et al., 2003, 2004; Moreno et al., 2008; González and Northcutt, 2009) indicating that the pallium in the lobe-finned fish radiation (i.e., lobe-finned fishes and tetrapods) consists of not three but four pallial divisions, with the ventral pallium interposed between the lateral pallium and the striatum. As in other lobe-finned fishes, there is cytological evidence that the ventral pallium in the Comoran coelacanth may consist of dorsal and ventral subdivisions, which may be homologous to the dorsal ventricular ridge and lateral amygdalar nucleus, respectively, in amniotic vertebrates. This speculation, however, needs to be confirmed by molecular markers which have clearly delineated these cell groups in other lobe-finned fishes.

STRIATAL ORGANIZATION

The striatopallidal system of tetrapods is now believed to comprise a dorsal system, the dorsal striatum and dorsal pallidum, and a ventral system, the nucleus accumbens plus the olfactory tubercle and a ventral pallidum (Heimer et al., 1995; Marín et al., 1998). Similar systems have recently been recognized in lungfishes (González and Northcutt, 2009; Northcutt, 2009), but it is still unclear whether or not separate dorsal and ventral pallidal cell groups exist. In any case, the striatum recognized by Nieuwenhuys and colleagues, and in the present analysis of the Comoran coelacanth, appears to be homologous to the dorsal striatum of other lobe-finned fishes. However, the ventral striatum (olfactory tubercle) recognized by Nieuwenhuys and colleagues at mid-hemispheric levels (**Figure 1C**) appears to be far too caudal to represent the ventral striatum of other lobe-finned fishes. Based on the topology of the cell group, and the presence of a distinct ventrolateral cellular prominence dividing the ventrolateral hemispheric wall, this cell group is more parsimoniously interpreted as the pallidum (**Figure 1E**), although it is presently unclear whether it represents both pallidal cell groups or only the dorsal pallidum of other lobe-fined fishes (this situation is very similar to that observed in the subpallium of urodeles, Moreno and González, 2007a). Once again, there are molecular markers, such as DARPP-32, that could clarify these issues.

MEDIAL PALLIAL BORDERS

Nieuwenhuys (1965) recognized three pallial divisions in the Comoran coelacanth: his dorsomedial, ventromedial, and lateral pallia (**Figure 1C**). He noted that suspected secondary olfactory fibers, which he termed the central olfactory tract, penetrate the core of his ventromedial pallial division. Further, he concluded that the ventromedial pallium was probably homologous to the lateral pallium in other lobe-finned fishes (Nieuwenhuys, 1998). He concluded, however, that his dorsomedial and lateral pallial divisions could not be homologous to the dorsal and medial pallia in other vertebrates on topological grounds. We disagree with this conclusion. If the ependymal surface is followed dorsally, a second pallial division, which we interpret as a putative dorsal pallium, replaces the lateral pallium (**Figure 1E**). In turn, a putative dorsal pallium is replaced by a third pallial division, which we interpret as a putative medial pallium. As in other vertebrates, the telencephalic tela attaches at the pial–ependymal border (**Figures 1C–E**). Thus, topological relationships of the pallial divisions in the Comoran coelacanth are preserved along the ependymal surface. This is not the case, however, along the pial surface. In other vertebrates, the pallial divisions show a dorsoventral sequence from medial pallium, to dorsal pallium, to lateral pallium, to ventral pallium. In the Comoran coelacanth, the putative medial pallium borders the putative ventral and lateral pallia, as well as the putative dorsal pallium (**Figure 1E**). This topological distortion could have occurred by an outward bending (eversion) of the developing pallial wall, coupled with a secondary fusion of the closely opposed pial surfaces of the lateral and medial pallia, as a secondary fusion of the caudal telencephalic wall with the rostral wall of the diencephalon is known to occur in hagfishes (Wicht and Northcutt, 1992). There is no histological trace of such an eversion and secondary fusion of the pallial walls in the Comoran coelacanth, however, and the simplest explanation is that the developing medial pallium has expanded rostrally and medially, displacing the putative lateral pallium and secondarily contacting the putative ventral pallium. Where there is a distinct difference in the texture of the neuropils of the putative medial and ventral pallia (**Figure 1E**).

We also differ from Nieuwenhuys and colleagues concerning the boundary between the putative dorsal and medial pallia (**Figures 1C,E**). Nieuwenhuys (1965) indicated that this boundary was marked by a cell-free zone, whereas we believe it is marked by a sharp change in cellular density (**Figure 2G**). It appears that Nieuwenhuys focused on the position of the olfactohabenular tract to mark the border between his lateral and dorsomedial pallial divisions (**Figure 1C**), whereas we have focused on cell density as an indicator of the putative dorsal–medial pallial border (**Figure 1E**). In either case, however, the putative medial pallium of the Comoran coelacanth occupies an extensive segment of the pallium, equal to or much larger than the lateral pallium. Although few details are known about the general biology of the Comoran coelacanth, it is well documented that these fish return to marine caves during the day and that the same individuals have been identified in the same caves for several years (Fricke et al., 1991). Highly developed spatial learning is also documented in amphibians (Wells, 2007) as well, and also appears to be well developed in the lepidosirenid lungfish *Protopterus* (Greenwood, 1987). Thus it is possible that an expanded medial pallium and its associated circuitry mediates spatial learning in coelacanths as in other lobe-finned fishes.

AMYGDALAR ORGANIZATION

Following Rudebeck's (1945) description of the telencephalon impar in a lungfish, *Protopterus*, Nieuwenhuys (1965, 1998) divided the telencephalon impar of the Comoran coelacanth into an inferior preoptic nucleus and a superior preoptic nucleus. He further divided the inferior preoptic nucleus in a parvocellular nucleus and a magnocellular nucleus (**Figure 3A**). Like Rudebeck, Nieuwenhuys also concluded that the superior preoptic nucleus was probably homologous to the caudal part of the strio-amygdaloid complex in tetrapods. Studies of lungfishes (González and Northcutt, 2009; Northcutt, 2009; González et al., 2010) and tetrapods (Moreno and González, 2004, 2005, 2006, 2007a,b) have clearly established that the amygdalar complex consists of at least central, lateral, and medial nuclei.

The Comoran coelacanth also appears to exhibit this same pattern of amygdalar organization. As already noted, a putative ventral pallium can be recognized, and the ventral subdivision of this pallial division is most likely homologous to the lateral amygdalar nucleus in lungfishes and tetrapods. Based on cytology and topography, however, we believe that the nucleus identified as the magnocellular preoptic nucleus by Nieuwenhuys (**Figure 3A**) is actually homologous to the central amygdalar nucleus of lungfishes and tetrapods (**Figures 3B,C**). Another nucleus in the preoptic region of the Comoran coelacanth that is slightly more caudal and ventral appears to be a more likely candidate for a homolog of the magnocellular preoptic nucleus. This nucleus comprises larger, more compact cells that are located periventricularly, as in other lobe-finned fishes, and is thus a more likely homolog of the magnocellular preoptic nucleus than that recognized by Nieuwenhuys (1965, 1998).

We do agree with Rudebeck (1945) and Nieuwenhuys (1965, 1998) that the cell group recognized as a superior preoptic nucleus in lungfishes and the Comoran coelacanth is homologous to part of the amygdalar complex in tetrapods. Based on the topology of this nucleus in the Comoran coelacanth, it appears homologous to the medial amygdalar nucleus of lungfishes and tetrapods. It therefore appears that all extant lobe-finned fishes are characterized by the same pattern of amygdalar organization, which may have arisen even earlier in gnathostome phylogeny.

FUTURE DIRECTIONS

In spite of the relatively large numbers of coelacanths that have been captured, the quality of the brain histology presently available is clearly marginal. If the specimen on which this analysis is primarily based were captured today, rather than some 38 years ago, it would be possible to use the numerous molecular markers now available, and our knowledge of coelacanth brain organization and brain phylogeny in lobe-finned fishes would be greatly increased. Every attempt should be made by comparative neurobiologists to proselytize coelacanth researchers so that they understand the importance of properly fixing brain tissue from an available specimen. At the same time, preservation of coelacanth habitats and the protection of these fascinating fishes is uppermost. It would be criminal if humanity allowed these ancient fishes to become extinct in our lifetime.

ACKNOWLEDGMENTS

This work was supported by the U.S. National Science Foundation (IBN-0919077), by The Spanish Ministry of Sciences and Education (BFU2009-12315), and by private funding.

REFERENCES

Brinkmann, H., Venkatesh, B., Brenner, S., and Meyer, A. (2004). Nuclear protein-coding genes support lungfish and not the coelacanth as the closest living relatives of land vertebrates. *Proc. Natl. Acad. Sci. U.S.A.* 101, 4900–4905.

Brox, A., Puelles, L., Ferreiro, B., and Medina, L. (2003). Expression of the genes GAD67 and distal-less-4 in the forebrain of *Xenopus laevis* confirms a common pattern in tetrapods. *J. Comp. Neurol.* 461, 370–393.

Brox, A., Puelles, L., Ferreiro, B., and Medina, L. (2004). Expression of the genes Emxl, Tbr1 and Eomes (Tbr2) in the telencephalon of *Xenopus laevis* confirms the existence of four pallial divisions in tetrapods. *J. Comp. Neurol.* 474, 562–577.

Bruton, M. N., and Coutouvidis, S. E. (1991). An inventory of all known specimens of the coelacanth *Latimeria chalumnae*, with comments on trends in the catches. *Environ. Biol. Fishes* 32, 371–390.

Fricke, H., Hissmann, K., Schauer, J., Reinicke, O., Kasang, L., and Plante, R. (1991). Habitat and population size of the coelacanth *Latimeria chalumnae* at Grand Comoro. *Environ. Biol. Fishes* 32, 287–300.

González, A., López, J. M., Sánchez-Camacho, C., and Márin, O. (2002). Regional expression of the homeobox gene NKX2-1 defines pallidal and interneuronal populations in the basal ganglia of amphibians. *Neuroscience* 114, 567–575.

González, A., Morona, R., López, J. M., Moreno, N., and Northcutt, R. G. (2010). Lungfishes, like tetrapods, possess a vomeronasal system. *Front. Neuroanat.* 4:130. doi: 10.3389/fnana.2010.00130

González, A., and Northcutt, R. G. (2009). An immunohistochemical approach to lungfish telencephalic organization. *Brain Behav. Evol.* 74, 43–55.

Greenwood, H. (1987). "The natural history of African lungfishes," in *The Biology and Evolution of Lungfishes*, eds W. E. Bemis, W. W. Burggren, and N. E. Kemp (New York: Alan R. Liss, Inc.), 163–179.

Heimer, L., Zahm, D. S., and Alheid, G. F. (1995). "Basal ganglia," in *The Rat Nervous System*, ed. G. Paxinos (San Diego: Academic Press), 579–628.

Hissmann, K., Fricke, H., and Schauer, J. (1998). Population monitoring of the coelacanth (*Latimeria chalumnae*). *Conserv. Biol.* 12, 759–765.

Marín, O., Smeets, W. J. A. J., and González, A. (1998). Basal ganglia organization in amphibians: chemoarchitecture. *J. Comp. Neurol.* 392, 285–312.

Millot, J., and Anthony, J. (1958). *Anatomie de Latimeria chalumnae. Tome I. Squelette, Muscles et Formations de Soutien.* Paris: C.N.R.S., 122.

Millot, J., and Anthony, J. (1965). *Anatomie de Latimeria chalumnae. Tome II. Système Nerveux et Organes des Sens.* Paris: C.N.R.S., 131.

Millot, J., Anthony, J., and Robineau, D. (1978). *Anatomie de Latimeria chalumnae. Tome III. Appareil Digestif, Appareil Respiratoire, Appareil Urogenital, Glandes Endocrine, Appareil Circulatoire, Tégujments, Écailles, Conclusions Générales.* Paris: C.N.R.S., 198.

Moreno, N., Domínguez, L., Rétaux, S., and González, A. (2008). Islet 1 as a marker of subdivisions and cell types in the developing forebrain of *Xenopus*. *Neuroscience* 154, 1423–1439.

Moreno, N., and González, A. (2004). Localization and connectivity of the lateral amygdala in anuran amphibians. *J. Comp. Neurol.* 479, 130–148.

Moreno, N., and González, A. (2005). Central amygdala in anuran amphibians: neurochemical organization and connectivity. *J. Comp. Neurol.* 489, 69–91.

Moreno, N., and González, A. (2006). The common organization of the amygdaloid complex in tetrapods: new concepts based on developmental, hodological and neurochemical data in anuran amphibians. *Prog. Neurobiol.* 78, 61–90.

Moreno, N., and González, A. (2007a). Regionalization of the telencephalon in urodele amphibians and its bearing on the identification of amygdaloid complex. *Front. Neurosci.* 1:1. doi: 10.3389/neuro.05/001.2007

Moreno, N., and González, A. (2007b). Development of the vomeronasal amygdala in anuran amphibians: hodological, neurochemical, and gene expression characterization. *J. Comp. Neurol.* 5023, 815–831.

Nieuwenhuys, R. (1965). The forebrain of the crossopterygian *Latimeria chalumnae* Smith. *J. Morphol.* 117, 1–24.

Nieuwenhuys, R. (1998). "The coelacanth *Latimeria chalumnae*," in *The Central Nervous System of Vertebrates*, Vol. 2, eds R. Nieuwenhuys, H. J. ten Donkelaar, and C. Nicholson (Heidelberg: Springer-Verlag), 1007–1043.

Nieuwenhuys, R., Kremers, J. P. M., and van Huijzen, C. (1977). The brain of the crossopterygian fish *Latimeria chalumnae*: a survey of its gross structure. *Anat. Embryol.* 151, 157–169.

Nieuwenhuys, R., and Meek, J. (1990). "The telencephalon of sarcopterygian fishes," in *Cerebral Cortex, Vol. 8A, Comparative Structure and Evolution of Cerebral Cortex, Part 1*, eds E. G. Jones and A. Peters (New York: Plenum), 75–106.

Northcutt, R. G. (2009). Telencephalic organization in the spotted African lungfish, *Protopterus dolloi*: a new cytological model. *Brain Behav. Evol.* 73, 59–80.

Rudebeck, B. (1945). Contributions to forebrain morphology in Dipnoi. *Acta Zool.* 26, 9–157.

Takezaki, N., Figueroa, F., Zaleska-Rutczynska, Z., Takahata, N., and Klein, J. (2004). The phylogenetic relationship of tetrapod, coelacanth, and lungfish revealed by the sequences of forty-four nuclear genes. *Mol. Biol. Evol.* 21, 1512–1524.

Wells, K. D. (2007). *The Ecology and Behavior of Amphibians*. Chicago: The University of Chicago Press.

Wicht, H., and Northcutt, R. G. (1992). The forebrain of the Pacific hagfish: a cladistic reconstruction of the ancestral craniate forebrain. *Brain Behav. Evol.* 40, 25–64.

Conflict of Interest Statement: The authors declare that the research was conducted in the absence of any commercial or financial relationships that could be construed as a potential conflict of interest.

Received: 08 November 2010; paper pending published: 06 December 2010; accepted: 14 February 2011; published online: 24 February 2011.

Citation: Northcutt RG and González A (2011) A reinterpretation of the cytoarchitectonics of the telencephalon of the Comoran coelacanth. Front. Neuroanat. 5:9. doi: 10.3389/fnana.2011.00009

2

The non-evaginated secondary prosencephalon of vertebrates

Nerea Moreno* and Agustín González

Departamento de Biología Celular, Facultad de Biología, Universidad Complutense of Madrid, Madrid, Spain

Edited by:
Fernando Martinez-Garcia, Universidad de Valencia, Spain

Reviewed by:
Glenn R. Northcutt, University of California, USA
Sylvie Retaux, CNRS, France

****Correspondence:***
Nerea Moreno, Facultad de Biología, Departamento de Biología Celular, Universidad Complutense, Calle José Antonio Novais 2, 28040 Madrid, Spain.
e-mail: nerea@bio.ucm.es

The secondary prosencephalon (telencephalon plus hypothalamus) is probably the most complex area of the brain, with complicated patterning specifications. As yet, no prosomeric subdivisions have been reported and only distinct histogenetic territories have been recognized. In the present comparative study we analyzed cross-correlated expression maps in the non-evaginated territories of the secondary prosencephalon in different vertebrates throughout development, to assess the existence of comparable divisions and subdivisions in the different groups. Each division is characterized by expression of a unique combination of developmental regulatory genes, and each appears to represent a self-regulated and topologically constant histogenetic brain compartment that gives rise to a specific cell group. The non-evaginated area of the telencephalon corresponds to the preoptic region, whereas the hypothalamus, topologically rostral to the diencephalic prethalamus, includes basal (mammillary and tuberal) and alar (paraventricular and suprachiasmatic) parts. This complex area is specified by a cascade of transcription factors, among which the Dlx family members and Nkx2.1 are essential for the correct development. The only exception is found in the subdivision named termed the supraoptoparaventricular area, in which the transcription factor Orthopedia is essential in restricting the fate of multiple categories of neuroendocrine neurons, in the absence of the Dlx/Nkx2.1 combination. Our analysis, based on own data and published results by other researchers, suggests that common features are shared at least by all tetrapods and, therefore, they most likely were present in the stem tetrapods. The available data for agnathans (lampreys) and other fish groups indicate that not all subdivisions of the secondary prosencephalon were present at the origin of vertebrates, raising important questions about their evolution.

Keywords: preoptic area, hypothalamus, development, homology, tetrapods

THE NON-EVAGINATED SECONDARY PROSENCEPHALON

Developmental processes occurring from the neural plate stages and leading to the identification of all main brain regions entail dramatic changes, including a pronounced cephalic flexure. As the anterior neural tube closes, the embryonic brain subdivides into three primary vesicles: the rhombencephalon, the mesencephalon, and the prosencephalon, from caudal to rostral. Subsequently, the primary prosencephalon subdivides into two major components, the caudal diencephalon and the rostral secondary prosencephalon. The secondary prosencephalon constitutes the entire prechordal (rostralmost) portion of the neural tube, which gives rise to the hypothalamus ventrally, the eye vesicles dorsolaterally, the telencephalic vesicles dorsally, and a ventral telencephalic preoptic area (POA; reviewed in García-López et al., 2009; Vieira et al., 2010). Like the caudal vesicles, the secondary prosencephalon is formed by alar and basal derivatives. Thus, the hypothalamus includes alar and basal plate components, whereas the eye field and the telencephalon are completely derived from the alar region (**Figure 1**). The topological arrangement of these forebrain subdivisions is a consequence of the location of their primordia in the neural plate (Couly and Le Douarin, 1987; Eagleson and Harris, 1990; Rubenstein et al., 1998; Inoue et al., 2000; García-López et al., 2009; Vieira et al., 2010). The mechanisms leading to the formation of the prosencephalon and its subsequent patterning are highly conserved in evolution, especially the genetic codes that result in the production of forebrain subdivisions recognized along the rostrocaudal and dorsoventral axes in different vertebrates.

Apart from the evaginated telencephalic and eye vesicles, the rest of the secondary prosencephalon (here referred to as the non-evaginated secondary prosencephalon, regardless the diverse evaginations that may occur in the hypothalamus) has been traditionally considered as the ventral portion of the diencephalon. In particular, the term hypothalamus (hypo from the old Greek ÿpó: under) literally describes its topographical position beneath the thalamus. Thus, in the literature, frequent definitions describe the preoptic region (PO) and the hypothalamus proper as special regions of the ventral diencephalon that are involved in regulation of the endocrine system, the autonomic nervous system, and related brain systems (Bruce, 2008; Hodos, 2008). These definitions, older or current, treat the brain as a column, so that a transverse section of an adult brain shows the hypothalamus beneath the thalamus, and molecular and developmental data are not taken into account. However, detailed comparison of diverse developmental gene expression patterns gathered in the last decades led Puelles and Rubenstein to postulate in 1993 the prosomeric model, modified 10 years later (Puelles and Rubenstein, 1993, 2003) as a morphological framework (paradigm), which divides the forebrain into transverse segments (prosomeres) and longitudinal zones. In this prosomeric context, we refer in the present analysis to the non-evaginated portion of the secondary prosencephalon, only with the intention to use a short name that includes the hypothalamus and the PO of the telencephalon. Classically, the PO has been considered part of the hypothalamus (for review Butler and

Hodos, 2005), but in recent years this view has changed and the PO been considered part of the telencephalon, due to its topological position in the neural plate and its genetic specification (Flames et al., 2007; García-López et al., 2008; Sánchez-Arrones et al., 2009). Therefore, in the present analysis of the PO and hypothalamus we pay special attention to the boundaries between them in diverse vertebrate species in order to gain a better understanding of the evolution of these forebrain regions.

The regions under analysis are very complex in terms of genetic specification, morphological, hodological and neurochemical organization, and, especially, function (for review see ten Donkelaar, 1998; Butler and Hodos, 2005; Medina, 2008). However, it is interesting to note that in the last years, numerous data have shown conserved patterns in the evolution of vertebrates related to the embryological origin, cell types, neurochemical organization, hodology, and functional implications of the subregions in the secondary prosencephalon (reviewed in Medina, 2008; Moreno et al., 2009). In addition, it has been increasingly reported that in these regions many differences can also be observed among vertebrates, which may reflect not only the existence of divergent evolution in the different lineages but also secondary adaptations of each group. Moreover, to this complex evolutionary equation has to be added a high divergence of sizes, shapes, and complexity of centers related to sophisticated behaviors like human consciousness, songbird vocalization, electrical responses in some fishes, etc.

In this evolutionary context, when one accomplishes a comparative analysis the main aim is to establish homologous relationships. To this end, however, many different characteristics can be considered, which sometimes make this comparison extremely difficult and dense. At least in the last years, most comparative studies of the forebrain in different vertebrates have been framed within the prosomeric model as a paradigm to interpret the results (Puelles and Rubenstein, 2003). Those studies suggest that some characteristics are more important than others in this analysis, as they determine the topology of the neural plate, the genetic specification of a topographic domain in the neural tube, the histogenetic pattern, the neuronal differentiation, hodology and, finally, neuronal organization.

With these ideas in mind, the most convenient approach to establishing homologies is to assess the number of shared features, keeping in mind that homologous structures with common morphogenetic origin may have varied enormously in the course of evolution.

PATTERNING AND NEURAL SPECIFICATION

Substantial data reported in the last years have demonstrated that the combined expression of regulatory genes is very conserved in the evolution (Puelles and Rubenstein, 1993, 2003; Bachy et al., 2001, 2002; González et al., 2002a,b; Brox et al., 2003; Moreno et al., 2004, 2005, 2008a,b, 2010; Osorio et al., 2005, 2006; Flames et al., 2007; García-López et al., 2008; Abellán and Medina, 2009; González and Northcutt, 2009; Domínguez et al., 2010), suggesting that the molecular specifications unravel the morphogenetic field formation. When comparing across species, two main concepts are to be kept in mind, "developmental regulatory genes" and "basic histogenetic domains." Both concepts allow and help explain forebrain organization in the comparative approach.

In mammals, hypothalamic neurogenesis occurs in individual nuclei between embryonic day 10 (E10) and E16 in mice (Shimada and Nakamura, 1973; Shimogori et al., 2010). Numerous studies have identified many transcription factors that regulate the development of specific hypothalamic nuclei and neuronal subtypes (Schonemann et al., 1995; Labosky et al., 1997; Wehr et al., 1997; Michaud et al., 1998; Acampora et al., 1999; Davis et al., 2004; Goshu et al., 2004; Zhao et al., 2008; Szábo et al., 2009).

In general morphological terms, seeking terminological continuity, in the prosomeric model the hypothalamus constitutes the "rostral diencephalon" (Puelles and Rubenstein, 2003). It includes alar and basal components, while the eye field and the telencephalon are exclusively derived from the alar region. The alar portion, includes the suprachiasmatic (SC) and the supraopticparaventricular (SPV) regions, which will give rise their respective hypothalamic nuclei. The basal hypothalamus includes the tuberal hypothalamus, which contains among other structures, the ventromedial nucleus, the arcuate nucleus, and the mammillary hypothalamic region, which includes the subthalamic nucleus (reviewed in Medina, 2008).

In molecular terms, Shh is essential for the specification of the hypothalamus (Chiang et al., 1996; Szábo et al., 2009) through the action, among others, of the homeobox gene Nkx2.1, whose expression is triggered by prechordal Shh signals (Kimura et al., 1996). In addition, in mammalian forebrains, Nkx2.1 is expressed in the basal telencephalon– POA and the basal hypothalamus (Price et al., 1992), which is severely malformed and reduced in size in knockout mice (Kimura et al., 1996; Sussel et al., 1999; Marín et al., 2002). Specially, the neural Shh has a very important and specific role in the development of the lateral hypothalamus, possibly mediated by regulation of Dlx2, Dbx1, and FoxD. The lack of Shh expression in the hypothalamic neuroepithelium results in a very reduced lateral hypothalamus, in which some of the most functionally important and characteristic neuronal subpopulations are either very reduced or completely missing, whereas the POA and the SC nucleus show normal development (Szábo et al., 2009). The transcription factor Orthopedia (Otp) is expressed in the SPV of the alar hypothalamus, the arcuate nucleus, and the oblique perimammillary band (Simeone et al., 1994; Puelles and Rubenstein, 2003; Del Giacco et al., 2006; Bardet et al., 2008), where it operates in the proper differentiation of several neurohormone-secreting nuclei (Acampora et al., 1999; Wang and Lufkin, 2000; Michaud, 2001; Eaton and Glasgow, 2007; Blechman et al., 2007; Ryu et al., 2007; Eaton et al., 2008). Otp also contributes to progenitor cell proliferation, survival, and migration (Goshu et al., 2004). The transcription factor Sim1, in parallel to Otp, acts to differentiate a large population of neurohormone- containing cells (Michaud et al., 1998; Acampora et al., 1999; Wang and Lufkin, 2000; Goshu et al., 2004). In Otp, and Sim1 mutants, the prospective SPV cells are born and specified, but the cells do not terminally differentiate to express neuroendocrine hormone genes.

In terms of anatomical subdivisions the POA, which was previously believed to be derived from the ventral diencephalon, is currently regarded as derived from the Foxg1-positive telencephalic neuroepithelium (Zhao et al., 2008; Roth et al., 2010), whereas the hypothalamus can be subdivided into the Sim1-positive anterodorsal hypothalamic neuroepithelium, which contain the primordium of the paraventricular nucleus, and the Nkx2.1-positive posteroventral hypothalamic neuroepithelium, which contains the primordia of the arcuate nucleus and the ventromedial hypothalamic region, the premammillary neuroepithelium, and the mammillary neuroepithelium (reviewed in Medina, 2008; Zhao et al., 2008; Szábo et al., 2009; Shimogori et al., 2010). In terms of boundaries, the rostral hypothalamus correlates topographically with the early expression of Six3, which extends from the septum to the neurohypophysis. The boundary between the caudal hypothalamus and P3 is well defined by the expression of several genes. In the alar plate, it coincides with the sharp caudal limit of the Sim1, Otp, and Brn2 genes, which are expressed in the SPV, and with the sharp rostral limit of Arx, Dlx, and Pax6 transcripts in P3. Finally, a territorial boundary between the telencephalon and the hypothalamus has been recently defined and called the preoptohypothalamic boundary (POH; Bardet et al., 2006; Flames et al., 2007). It is delimited between the PO in the subpallium and the SPV of the hypothalamus and occupies the region just outside the Nkx2.1- and Shh-expressing POA and it also lies within the contiguous thin corridor, expressing only Dlx5 among the studied subpallial markers (Bardet et al., 2006).

To summarize, in mammals, Shh and Nkx2.1 are expressed in the entire non-evaginated prosencephalon, with the exception of the alar hypothalamus (reviewed in Medina, 2008). The absence of Nkx2.1 expression in the alar hypothalamus in mice correlates well with the absence of Lhx6 or Lhx7 expression in this area (Rétaux et al., 1999). In the alar hypothalamus, the SPV also contains an important population of Otp-expressing cells (Bardet et al., 2008).

EVOLUTIONARY TRAITS

In modern classification schemes, living vertebrates consist of two main groups, the jawless Agnatha (represented by hagfishes and lampreys) and the jawed Gnathostomata. Jawed vertebrates are divided again into two groups, the cartilaginous Chondrichthyes (represented by sharks, rays, and chimeras) and the bony Osteichthyes. The two main groups of bony vertebrates are the ray-finned fishes (Actinopterygii) and the lobe-limbed vertebrates (Sarcopterygii). The latter comprises three groups: coelacanths (Actinistia), lungfishes (Dipnoi), and limbed vertebrates, or Tetrapoda, encompassing amphibians, reptiles, birds, and mammals (Clack, 2002).

In recent years, evolutionary/developmental studies have revealed a segmentary pattern in the developing forebrain of all the vertebrates analyzed. In this kind of comparative analysis it is essential to consider the highest possible number of groups, especially those with crucial evolutionary positions. In particular, the phylogenetic position of reptiles, especially turtles, makes their study interesting because they are purported to be the most closely related to the extinct therapsids from which mammals arose (Northcutt, 1970) but, alternatively, they have been considered the sister group to crocodiles and birds (Zardoya and Meyer, 2001a,b). It is also essential to consider amphibians in analyzing ancestral brain organization, because they constitute the only group of tetrapod anamniotes and represent a key model in the anamniote/amniote transition, as they show shared features with other tetrapods (amniotes) and also shared features with fishes (anamniotes). In the context of this transition, the colonization of land by tetrapod ancestors is presumably one of the evolutionary events that could entail more neural changes. Molecular phylogenetic research addressing this transition and the most recent paleontological evidence, suggest that lungfishes are closest living relatives of tetrapods and that several of the features defining this group were highly conserved throughout the entire evolutionary history of land vertebrates (Meyer and Wilson, 1990; Meyer and Dolven, 1992; Hedges et al., 1993; Zardoya et al., 1998; Tohyama et al., 2000; Brinkmann et al., 2004a,b; Takezaki et al., 2004; Hallstrom and Janke, 2009), making this group of fishes of particular interest in comparative studies. And finally, lampreys are jawless vertebrates, belonging to the Agnatha, the sister group of gnathostome vertebrates. Their phylogenetic position makes them an invaluable model in the study of evolutionary developmental biology, as they allow us to gain new insights into ancestral characters in vertebrates, and they also help to reveal, but also to understand the emergence of novelties at important evolutionary transitions, such as the agnathan/gnathostome transition (Kuratani et al., 2002).

According to the rationale outlined above, the evolutionary analysis of transcription factors involved in the patterning of the non-evaginated secondary prosencephalon in key vertebrate groups would be of special interest for understanding its evolution (**Figures 2 and 3**). In recent years, cell groups and regions that were characterized according to gene expression patterns in the prosencephalon of mammals have been similarly analyzed in the brains of multiple vertebrates (**Figures 2 and 3**; Puelles and Rubenstein, 1993, 2003; Bachy et al., 2001, 2002; González et al., 2002a,b; Brox et al., 2003; Moreno et al., 2004, 2005, 2008a,b, 2010; Osorio et al., 2005, 2006; Flames et al., 2007; García-López et al., 2008; Abellán and Medina, 2009; Domínguez et al., 2010). These cell groups and regions in the secondary prosencephalon, and many of their neurochemical and connectional features, appear to be highly conserved in the evolution of tetrapods, since these features show similarities from amphibians through mammals (for review see Reiner et al., 1998; Marín et al., 1998; ten Donkelar, 1998; Moreno et al., 2009). Nevertheless, although many characteristics are shared, the degree of complexity increases during evolution from the common ancestor of tetrapods to birds and mammals.

Current theories regarding the organization of the forebrain in mammals consider that the subpallium encompasses the non-evaginated telencephalon, anterior (topologically dorsal) to the optic chiasm (see **Figure 1**; Flames et al., 2007; García-López et al., 2008). It is composed of the PO, which contains the commissural preoptic division (POC) and the POA proper, which is located at the base of (topologically rostral to) the former (for review see Moreno et al., 2009); both express Nkx2.1 and Shh in the ventricular layer during development. In chicks, the PO has been similarly recognized as a part of the subpallium and is characterized by the expression of both Nkx2.1 and Shh (Abellán and Medina, 2009). In addition to the distinct expression of Shh, the PO is also distinguished from the subpallial pallidal division (derived from the medial ganglionic eminence, MGE) by its expression of Islet1 (Abellán and Medina, 2009). The PO in birds is also said to contain the two major subdivisions: the commissural POA, comparable to the same-named subdivision in mice (pPO1 of Flames et al., 2007; POC of García-López et al., 2008) and characterized by strong expression of Shh and Lhx7 and by its relation to the anterior commissure; and a basal POA, comparable to the ventral preoptic subdivision (pPO2 of Flames et al. (2007; POv of García-López et al., 2008). In the vertebrates analyzed in our laboratory (**Figures 2A–F**), the situation in mice and chicks largely agrees with the results obtained in the PO of *Pseudemy scripta* (Moreno et al., 2010), *Xenopus laevis* (Moreno et al., 2008a; Domínguez et al., 2010), and the lungfishes *Protopterus dolloi* and *Neoceratodus forsteri* (unpublished observations). We identified the PO (**Figures 2A–C**) and the POC (**Figures 2D–E**) by the expression of Shh, Nkx2.1, Lhx7, and Isl1 and the absence of Tbr1 and Pax6 (Moreno et al., 2004, 2008a; 2010; Domínguez et al., 2010). In teleost fishes (including zebrafish), Shh is expressed in a small subdivision of the Nkx2.1-expressing domain of the basal telencephalon (Rohr et al., 2001; Scholpp et al., 2006; Menuet et al., 2007), suggesting that the subpallium of early jawed vertebrates likely included striatal, pallidal, and preoptic subdivisions. The existence of pallidal and preoptic domains in the subpallium

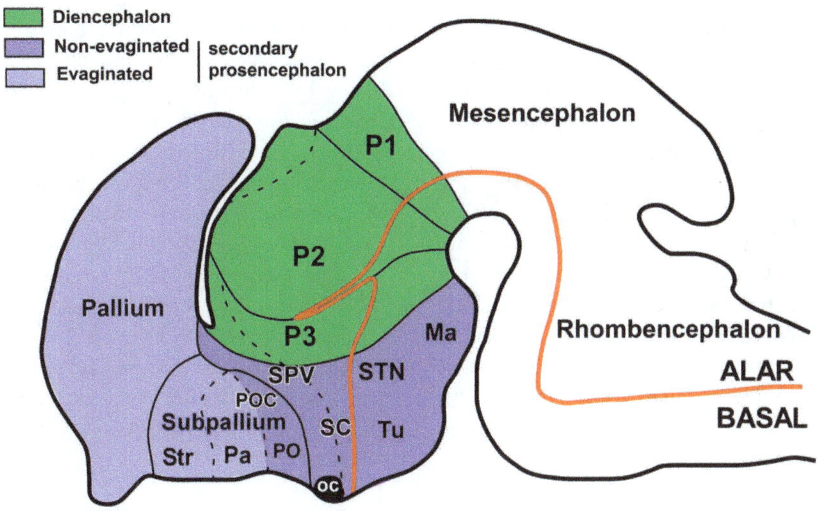

FIGURE 1 | The secondary prosencephalon in mammals. Schematic drawing of a lateral view of the brain showing the main subdivisions of the prosencephalon, as currently accepted. The dotted lines indicated subdivisions in the same domain. Ma, mammillary area; oc, optic chiasm; P1–3, prosomeres 1–3; Pa, pallidum; PO, preoptic region; POC, commissural preoptic area; SC, suprachiasmatic area; SPV, supraopticparaventricular area; STN, subthalamic nucleus; Str, striatum; Tu, tuberal hypothalamus. (Modified from Medina, 2008).

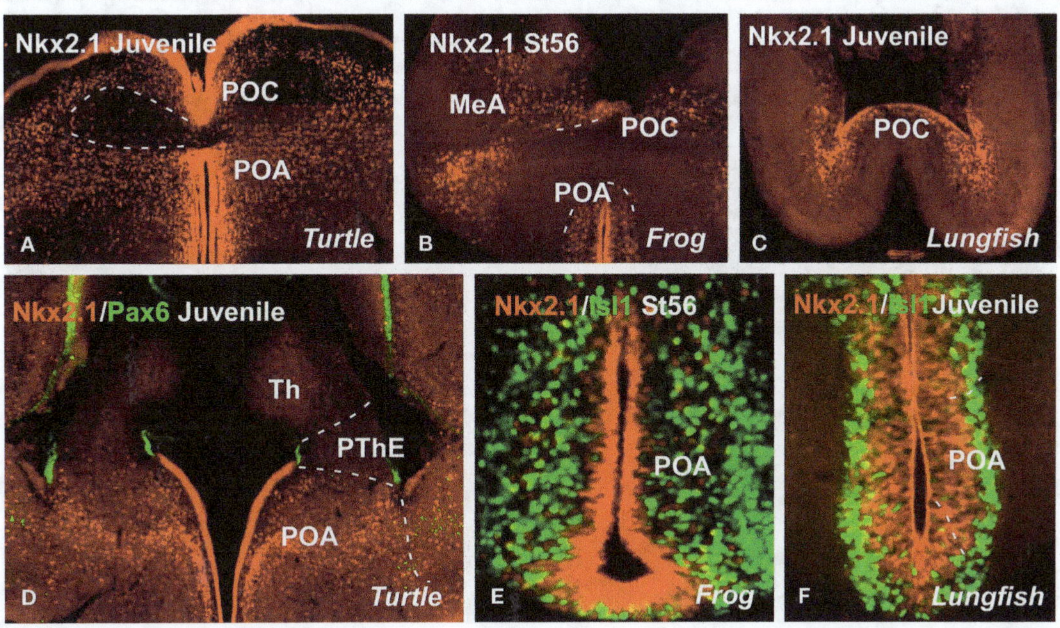

FIGURE 2 | Comparative aspects of the preoptic region. Photomicrographs of transverse sections through non-evaginated portion of the secondary prosencephalon of a turtle [*Pseudemys scripta*; **(A,D)**], a frog [*Xenopus laevis*; **(B,E)**], and a lungfish [*Neoceratodus forsteri*; **(C,F)**] illustrating by immunohistochemistry the developing expression of different transcription factors indicated in each figure. MeA, medial amygdala; POA, preoptic area; POC, commissural preoptic area; PThE, prethalamic eminence; Th, thalamus.

of teleost fishes expressing Nkx2.1 is correlated with expression of Lhx6 and/or Lhx7/8 in the same domains, and the presence of pallidal-like cell groups as well as cholinergic cells resembling those of the corticopetal system (Pérez et al., 2000; Mueller et al., 2004; Wullimann and Mueller, 2004; Menuet et al., 2007). However, more data are needed to determine whether the preoptic part of the subpallium in other jawed fishes (such as zebrafish) includes subdivisions similar to those of tetrapods. In a strikingly different situation, the homolog of Nkx2.1 in lampreys (LjNkx2.1, and a putative homolog of Sonic hedgehog (LfHh) in gnathostomes have no expression domain in the ventral telencephalon in lampreys(Ogasawara et al., 2001; Murakami et al., 2005; Osorio et al., 2005). The forebrain expression pattern of *LfHh* comprises two separate domains, a small hypothalamic domain and a large and robust coma-shaped domain in the diencephalon, showing continuity with floor plate expression all along the neural tube.

The alar part of the hypothalamus (**Figures 3A–F**) has been said to contain the SPV area and the SC region. The SPV is a component of the central neural circuitry that regulates several homeostatic variables through numerous connections among others with the posterior pituitary. The homeodomain transcription factor Otp is particularly expressed in this region in mice, chicks, amphibians, and lungfishes (**Figures 3A–C**), allowing it to be distinguished from the Shh- Nkx2.1- Dlx-expressing adjacent domains (Bardet et al., 2008; Moreno et al., 2010). Other shared features of this region, at least shared among amniotes, include Pax6 ventricular expression (Flames et al., 2007; Moreno et al., 2010). The SPV region in *Xenopus* could differ a little from that described in amniotes because, among other peculiarities, it does not include Pax6 expressing cells (Moreno et al., 2008b). The zebrafish genome contains two Otp orthologs, expressed in almost identical forebrain domains (Del Giacco et al., 2006), largely comparable to the Otp-expressing zones in mice (Simeone et al., 1994). In lampreys there are no detailed data on Otp expression, however it has been reported that its hypothalamic distribution resembles that of the Otp-positive neurons in zebrafish (Joly et al., 2007). However, Pax6 expression has not been described in the hypothalamic region (Murakami et al., 2001).

In the case of the SC region (**Figures 3D–F**), it has been shown to be *Dlx*-positive territory in all the vertebrates examined (Bachy et al., 2002; Brox et al., 2003; Flames et al., 2007; Domínguez et al., 2010). The expression of Nkx2.1, however, has been detected only in non-mammalian vertebrates (Bachy et al., 2002; Moreno et al., 2008a; van den Akker et al., 2008; Abellán and Medina, 2009; Domínguez et al., 2010; Moreno et al., 2010). This region of Nkx2.1 expression runs parallel to the hypothalamic zone of Shh expression, in a zone containing Arx- and Gad67-positive cells, and it is also defined by the expression of Lhx6, Lhx8, and Lhx1. In *Xenopus*,

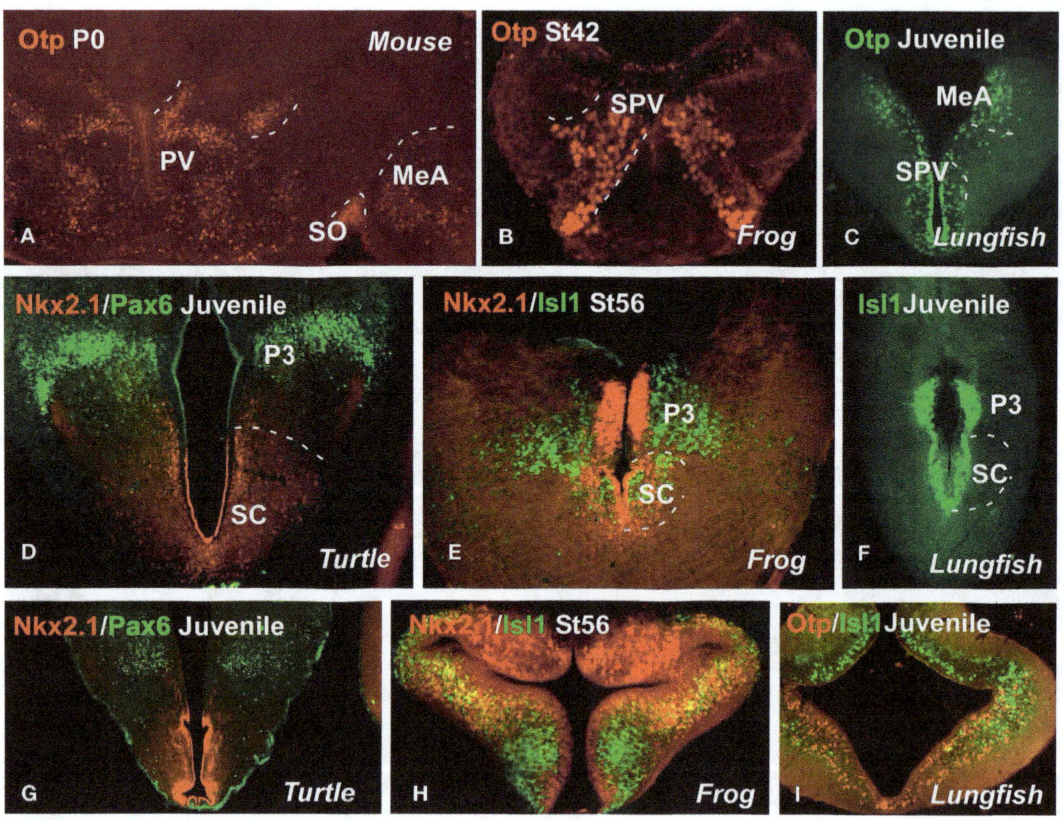

FIGURE 3 | Comparative aspects of the hypothalamus. Photomicrographs of transverse sections through non-evaginated portion of the secondary prosencephalon of a mouse **(A)**, a turtle [*Pseudemys scripta*; **(D,G)**], a frog [*Xenopus laevis*; **(B,E,H)**], and two lungfishes [*Neoceratodus forsteri*; **(C,F)** and *Protopterus dolloi*; **(I)**] illustrating by immunohistochemistry the developing expression of different transcription factors indicated in each figure. MeA, medial amygdala; P3, prosomere 3; PV, paraventricular nuclei; SO, supraoptic nuclei; SC, suprachiasmatic area; SPV, supraopticparaventricular area.

Isl1, xLhx1, and xLhx5 expression has been described as restricted to the SC area (Moreno et al., 2004, 2008a). Some distinction was noted in distribution, as the cells located just above and rostral to the optic chiasm only expressed xLhx1, whereas more caudally in the SC nucleus two regions could be distinguished: a dorsal portion that only expressed xLhx5 and a ventral portion that expressed both xLhx1 and xLhx5 (Moreno et al., 2004).

In regard to the basal hypothalamus, the ventral tuberomammillary cells in chick embryogenesis arise from a set of floor plate-like precursors that initially express Shh (Manning et al., 2006). The transcription factor Tbx2 is expressed only transiently in the mammillary region, for a slightly longer period in the tuberal region, and it is retained only at the junction of the retrochiasmic/tuberal hypothalamus (Manning et al., 2006). In the tuberal hypothalamus of *Pseudemy scripta* (Moreno et al., 2010), *X. laevis* (Moreno et al., 2008a; Domínguez et al., 2010), and the two lungfishes (unpublished observations) it was observed that the Nkx2.1 expression is strong in the vz of the tuberal area, whereas Isl1 is restricted to the svz; and the expression of Otp is restricted to the arcuate nucleus (**Figure 3I**). In *Xenopus*, xShh expression is strong in the basal hypothalamus, specifically in the mammillary band and the tuberal area. This expression is mainly restricted to the anterior levels, and xShh expression was not detected in the most posterior basal hypothalamic levels (Domínguez et al., 2010). The basal hypothalamus contains some populations of xGAD67- and xDll-4-expressing cells (Brox et al., 2003). The relatively few cells that express xLhx7 in the mammillary region in adults could be distinguished in the caudal hypothalamus from early premetamorphic stages (Moreno et al., 2004). The dorsomedial hypothalamic area and the superficial mammillary and mammillary nuclei contained a small to moderate number of xGAD67-expressing perikarya.

CONCLUDING REMARKS: EVOLUTIONARY HYPOTHESIS

The main conclusion of this comparative study is that major histogenetic processes thought to be a hallmark of so-called "higher vertebrates" actually existed early in vertebrate phylogeny (summarized in **Figure 4**).

At anterior levels in the PO, lampreys (jawless fish) lack expression of Nkx2.1 in the basal telencephalon (Murakami et al., 2001), and this is correlated with the absence of Shh expression (Osorio et al., 2005). This suggests that the subpallium of the first vertebrates not only lacked a pallidal domain (as noted above), but also appear to have lacked a subdivision comparable to the preoptic subpallium (for review see Osorio and Rétaux, 2008). This would correlate with the apparent lack of both pallidal-like cells (like those of the pallidal part of the basal ganglia) and basal forebrain cholinergic cells (Pombal et al., 1997a,b, 2001) in the telencephalon of lampreys. In teleosts, the detection of both Shh and Dlx expression shows that Shh expression can be localized in the basal telencephalon/POA at late developmental stages (Scholpp et al., 2006; Menuet et al., 2007). A pallidum expressing Nkx2.1 and a POC region comparable to that in amphibians have been demonstrated in the telencephalon of lungfishes (González and Northcutt, 2009), although the presence of Shh expression in the telencephalon needs to be investigated. Therefore, based on those lack of Nkx2.1 and Shh expression in lampreys (Osorio et al., 2005) and the organization of the POA demonstrated in amphibians (Moreno et al., 2008a; Domínguez et al., 2010) it can be postulated that the *de novo* expression of Shh and Nkx2.1 in the basal telencephalon of gnathostomes may be responsible for the emergence of new brain structures in the subpallium, the pallidum, and the PO, which probably emerged in the transition from agnathans to gnathostomes (see also Murakami et al., 2005; Osorio and Rétaux, 2008).

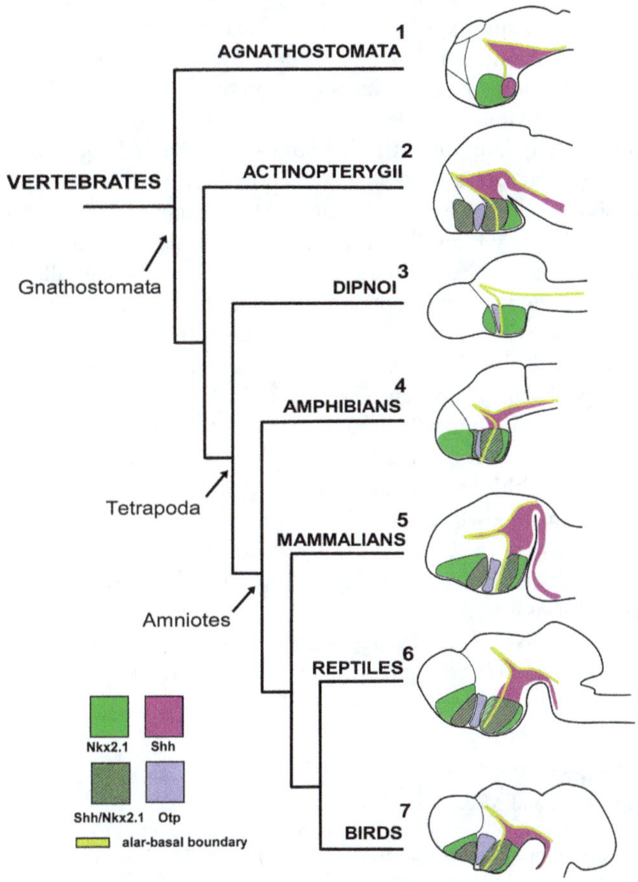

FIGURE 4 | The secondary prosencephalon in vertebrates. The expressions of different gene families during development in different vertebrates correspond to the conserved boundaries of the proliferative domains. Data from: [1]: Osorio et al. (2005); [2]: Scholpp et al. (2006), Menuet et al. (2007), Blechman et al. (2007), Del Giacco et al. (2008); [3]: González lab unpublished data; [4]: Domínguez et al. (2010); [5]: Flames et al. (2007), Bardet et al. (2008); [6]: Moreno et al. (2010); [7]: Abellán and Medina (2009); Bardet et al. (2010). No data are available for lungfish Shh developmental brain expression. The developmental stages showed are not comparable.

In the alar hypothalamus, the first thing to consider is the presence of the SPV throughout vertebrates. In all groups examined, this area expresses Otp and lacks Nkx2.1/Shh/Dlx, in a very conserved pattern (reviewed in Medina, 2008). In addition, the maintenance of Otp expression throughout development seems to be a conserved feature in vertebrates, as inferred from the cases in which late developmental stages or adult specimens were studied. It is noteworthy that Otp-expressing cells were consistently noted in some subdivisions of the amygdala (Bardet et al., 2008; Moreno et al., 2010), subdivisions whose cells most likely have a hypothalamic origin (Soma et al., 2009). At present, there are no anatomical data regarding possible Otp expression in the amygdala in teleosts or lampreys, but given the Otp expression found in the amygdala in adult lungfish (González and Northcutt, 2009) it will be an interesting aspect to investigate, in the context of evolution of the amygdaloid complex.

Finally, in amniotes the hypothalamic area lacking Nkx2.1 expresses Pax6. It is possible that the double Nkx2.1/Pax6 expression is an exclusive feature of the forebrain of anamniotes, not only present in the pallium but also in the hypothalamus. Consistent with this idea is the finding that, in mice, the absence of Nkx2.1 expression in the alar hypothalamus correlates with expression of Pax6 in the whole alar diencephalon, including the alar hypothalamus (Puelles et al., 2000; Marín et al., 2002). Thus, the mutually exclusive balance between Nkx2.1 and Pax6 in the telencephalon and diencephalon may be important for the relative size of pallial versus subpallial and thalamic versus hypothalamic territories. Any alteration of this balance, as occurs in Nkx2.1 knockout mice and Nkx2.1 knockdown *Xenopus* Sussel et al., 1999; Marín et al., 2002; van den Akker et al., 2008) or in Pax6 knockout mice (Stoykova et al., 2000; Yun et al., 2001), modifies the relative size of these subdivisions.

In the case of the SC region, the phylogenetic diagram in **Figure 4** shows the expression of the orthologous homeobox gene Nkx2.1 in several vertebrate species, including a jawless fish (a lamprey), a jawed fish (a zebrafish), an amphibian (a frog), a reptile (a turtle), a bird (a chicken), and a mammal (a mouse). This comparative representation highlights the peculiar lack of expression in this region only in the case of the forebrain of mammals. Considering the expression patterns observed in chicks and mice (Shimamura et al., 1995; Puelles et al., 2000), it appears that the alar hypothalamic expression of Nkx2.1 was either dramatically reduced or disappeared during the evolution to birds and mammals (Medina, 2008; van den Akker et al., 2008), a trend that perhaps started during the anamniote–amniote transition. Analysis of the xNkx2.1 knockdown *Xenopus* embryos indicates that xNkx2.1 controls the relative size of major regions in both the telencephalon (subpallium versus pallium) and the diencephalon (thalamus versus hypothalamus) of the forebrain (van den Akker et al., 2008). Changes in the regulation of Nkx2.1 expression have played an important role in the evolution of forebrain development, and they emphasize the potential of combined analysis of expression and function of master control genes in different vertebrates for revealing the origins of brain complexity and diversity.

ACKNOWLEDGMENTS

This work supported by grants from Spanish MICINN and the UCM (Grant numbers: BFU2009-12315 and BSCH-UCM GR58/08).

REFERENCES

Abellán, A., and Medina, L. (2009). Subdivisions and derivatives of the chicken subpallium based on expression of LIM and other regulatory genes and markers of neuron subpopulations during development. *J. Comp. Neurol.* 515, 465–501.

Acampora, D., Postiglione, M. P., Avantaggiato, V., Di Bonito, M., Vaccarino, F. M., Michaud, J., and Simeone, A. (1999). Progressive impairment of developing neuroendocrine cell lineages in the hypothalamus of mice lacking the orthopedia gene. *Genes Dev.* 13, 2787–2800.

Bachy, I., Failli, V., and Rétaux, S. (2002). A LIM-homeodomain code for development and evolution of forebrain connectivity. *Neuroreport* 13, A23–A27.

Bachy, I., Vernier, P., and Retáux, S. (2001). The LIM-homeodomain gene family in the developing *Xenopus* brain: conservation and divergences with the mouse related to the evolution of the forebrain. *J. Neurosci.* 21, 7620–7629.

Bardet, S. M., Cobos, I., Puelles, E., Martínez-De-La-Torre, M., and Puelles, L. (2006). Chicken lateral septal organ and other circumventricular organs form in a striatal subdomain abutting the molecular striatopallidal border. *J. Comp. Neurol.* 499, 745–767.

Bardet, S. M., Ferran, J. L., Sánchez-Arrones, L., and Puelles, L. (2010). Ontogenetic expression of sonic hedgehog in the chicken subpallium. *Front. Neuroanat.* 4:28. doi: 10.3389/fnana.2010.00028

Bardet, S. M., Martínez-de-la-Torre, M., Northcutt, R. G., Rubenstein, J. L., and Puelles, L. (2008). Conserved pattern of OTP-positive cells in the paraventricular nucleus and other hypothalamic sites of tetrapods. *Brain Res. Bull.* 75, 231–235.

Blechman, J., Borodovsky, N., Eisenberg, M., Nabel-Rosen, H., Grimm, J., and Levkowitz, G. (2007). Specification of hypothalamic neurons by dual regulation of the homeodomain protein orthopedia. *Development* 134, 4417–4426.

Brinkmann, H., Venkatesh, B., Brenner, S., and Meyer, A. (2004a). Nuclear protein-coding genes support lungfish and not the coelacanth as the closest living relatives of land vertebrates. *Proc. Natl. Acad. Sci. U.S.A.* 101, 4900–4905.

Brinkmann, H., Denk, A., Zitzler, J., Joss, J. J., and Meyer, A. (2004b). Complete mitochondrial genome sequences of the South American and the Australian lungfish: testing of the phylogenetic performance of mitochondrial data sets for phylogenetic problems in tetrapod relationships. *J. Mol. Evol.* 59, 834–848.

Brox, A., Puelles, L., Ferreiro, B., and Medina, L. (2003). Expression of the genes GAD67 and distal-less-4 in the forebrain of *Xenopus laevis* confirms a common pattern in tetrapods. *J. Comp. Neurol.* 461, 370–393.

Bruce, L. L. (2008). "Evolution of the hypothalamus in amniotes," in *Encyclopedic Reference of Neuroscience*, eds M. D. Binder and N. Hirokawa (Springer-Verlag), 1363–1367.

Butler, A., and Hodos, W. (2005). *Comparative Vertebrate Neuroanatomy*. Hoboken, NJ: Wiley.

Chiang, C., Litingtung, Y., Lee, E., Young, K. E., Corden, J. L., Westphal, H., and Beachy, P. A. (1996). Cyclopia and defective axial patterning in mice lacking sonic hedgehog gene function. *Nature* 383, 407–413.

Clack, J. A. (2002). Patterns and processes in the early evolution of the tetrapod ear. *J. Neurobiol.* 53, 251–264.

Couly, G. F., and Le Douarin, N. M. (1987). Mapping of the early neural primordium in quail-chick chimeras. II. The prosencephalic neural plate and neural folds: implications for the genesis of cephalic human congenital abnormalities. *Dev. Biol.* 120, 198–214.

Davis, A. M., Seney, M. L., Stallings, N. R., Zhao, L., Parker, K. L., and Tobet, S. A. (2004). Loss of steroidogenic factor 1 alters cellular topography in the mouse ventromedial nucleus of the hypothalamus. *J. Neurobiol.* 60, 424–436.

Del Giacco, L., Pistocchi, A., Cotelli, F., Fortunato, A. E., and Sordino, P. (2008). A peek inside the neurosecretory brain through Orthopedia lenses. *Dev. Dyn.* 237, 2295–2303.

Del Giacco, L., Sordino, P., Pistocchi, A., Andreakis, N., Tarallo, R., Di Benedetto, B., and Cotelli, F. (2006). Differential regulation of the zebrafish orthopedia 1 gene during fate determination of diencephalic neurons. *BMC Dev. Biol.* 6, 50. doi: 10.1186/1471-213X-6-50

Domínguez, L., González, A., and Moreno, N. (2010). Sonic hedgehog expression during *Xenopus laevis* forebrain development. *Brain Res.* 1347, 19–32.

Eagleson, G. W., and Harris, W. A. (1990). Mapping of the presumptive brain regions in the neural plate of *Xenopus laevis. J. Neurobiol.* 21, 427–440.

Eaton, J. L., and Glasgow, E. (2007). Zebrafish orthopedia (otp) is required for isotocin cell development. *Dev. Genes Evol.* 217, 149–158.

Eaton, J. L., Holmqvist, B., and Glasgow, E. (2008). Ontogeny of vasotocin-expressing cells in zebrafish: selective requirement for the transcriptional regulators orthopedia and single-minded 1 in the preoptic area. *Dev. Dyn.* 237, 995–1005.

Flames, N., Pla, R., Gelman, D. M., Rubenstein, J. L., Puelles, L., and Marín, O. (2007). Delineation of multiple subpallial progenitor domains by the combinatorial expression of transcriptional codes. *J. Neurosci.* 27, 9682–9695.

García-López, M., Abellán, A., Legaz, I., Rubenstein, J. L., Puelles, L., and Medina, L. (2008). Histogenetic compartments of the mouse centromedial and extended amygdala based on gene expression patterns during development. *J. Comp. Neurol.* 506, 46–74.

García-López, R., Pombero, A., and Martínez, S. (2009). Fate map of the chick embryo neural tube. *Dev. Growth Differ.* 51, 145–165.

González, A., López, J. M., and Marín, O. (2002a). Expression pattern of the homeobox protein NKX2-1 in the developing *Xenopus* forebrain. *Brain Res. Gene Expr. Patterns* 1, 181–185.

González, A., López, J. M., Sánchez-Camacho, C., and Marín, O. (2002b). Regional expression of the homeobox gene NKX2-1 defines pallidal and interneuronal populations in the basal ganglia of amphibians. *Neuroscience* 114, 567–575.

González, A., and Northcutt, R. G. (2009). An immunohistochemical approach to lungfish telencephalic organization. *Brain Behav. Evol.* 74, 43–55.

Goshu, E., Jin, H., Lovejoy, J., Marion, J. F., Michaud, J. L., and Fan, C. M. (2004). Sim2 contributes to neuroendocrine hormone gene expression in the anterior hypothalamus. *Mol. Endocrinol.* 18, 1251–1262.

Hallstrom, B. M., and Janke, A. (2009). Gnathostome phylogenomics utilizing lungfish EST sequences. *Mol. Biol. Evol.* 26, 463–471.

Hedges, S. B., Hass, C. A., and Maxson, L. R. (1993). Relations of fish and tetrapods. *Nature* 363, 501–502.

Hodos, W. (2008). "Evolution of the hypothalamus in anamniotes," in *Encyclopedic Reference of Neuroscience*, eds M. D. Binder and N. Hirokawa (Springer-Verlag), 1361–1363.

Inoue, T., Nakamura, S., and Osumi, N. (2000). Fate mapping of the mouse prosencephalic neural plate. *Dev. Biol.* 219, 373–383.

Joly, J. S., Osorio, J., Alunni, A., Auger, H., Kano, S., and Rétaux, S. (2007). Windows of the brain: towards a developmental biology of circumventricular and other neurohemal organs. *Semin. Cell Dev. Biol.* 18, 512–524.

Kimura, S., Hara, Y., Pineau, T., Fernández-Salguero, P., Fox, C. H., Ward, J. M., and González, F. J. (1996). The T/ebp null mouse: thyroid-specific enhancer-binding protein is essential for the organogenesis of the thyroid, lung, ventral forebrain, and pituitary. *Genes Dev.* 10, 60–69.

Kuratani, S., Kuraku, S., and Murakami, Y. (2002). Lamprey as an evo-devo model: lessons from comparative embryology and molecular phylogenetics. *Genesis* 34, 175–183.

Labosky, P. A., Winnier, G. E., Jetton, T. L., Hargett, L., Ryan, A. K., Rosenfeld, M. G., Parlow, A. F., and Hogan, B. L. (1997). The winged helix gene, Mf3, is required for normal development of the diencephalon and midbrain, postnatal growth and the milk-ejection reflex. *Development* 124, 1263–1274.

Manning, L., Ohyama, K., Saeger, B., Hatano, O., Wilson S. A., Logan, M., and Placzek, M. (2006). Regional morphogenesis in the hypothalamus: a BMP-Tbx2 pathway coordinates fate and proliferation through Shh downregulation. *Dev. Cell* 11, 873–885.

Marín, O., Baker, J., Puelles, L., and Rubenstein, J. L. (2002). Patterning of the basal telencephalon and hypothalamus is essential for guidance of cortical projections. *Development* 129, 761–773.

Marín, O., Smeets, W. J., and González, A. (1998). Evolution of the basal ganglia in tetrapods: a new perspective based on recent studies in amphibians. *Trends Neurosci.* 21, 487–494.

Medina, L. (2008). "Evolution and embryological development of forebrain," in *Encyclopedic Reference of Neuroscience*, eds M. D. Binder and N. Hirokawa (Springer-Verlag), 1172–1192.

Menuet, A., Alunni, A., Joly, J. S., Jeffery, W. R., and Rétaux, S. (2007). Expanded expression of sonic hedgehog in astyanax cavefish: multiple consequences on forebrain development and evolution. *Development* 134, 845–855.

Meyer, A., and Dolven, S. I. (1992). Molecules, fossils, and the origin of tetrapods. *J. Mol. Evol.* 35, 102–113.

Meyer, A., and Wilson, A. C. (1990). Origin of tetrapods inferred from their mitochondrial DNA affiliation to lungfish. *J. Mol. Evol.* 31, 359–364.

Michaud, J. L. (2001). The developmental program of the hypothalamus and its disorders. *Clin. Genet.* 60, 255–263.

Michaud, J. L., Rosenquist, T., May, N. R., and Fan, C. M. (1998). Development of neuroendocrine lineages requires the bHLH-PAS transcription factor SIM1. *Genes Dev.* 12, 3264–3275.

Moreno, N., Bachy, I., Rétaux, S., and González, A. (2004). LIM-homeodomain genes as developmental and adult genetic markers of *Xenopus* forebrain functional subdivisions. *J. Comp. Neurol.* 472, 52–72.

Moreno, N., Bachy, I., Rétaux, S., and González, A. (2005). LIM-homeodomain genes as territory markers in the brainstem of adult and developing *Xenopus laevis*. *J. Comp. Neurol.* 485, 240–254.

Moreno, N., Domínguez, L., Rétaux, S., and González, A. (2008a). Islet1 as a marker of subdivisions and cell types in the developing forebrain of *Xenopus*. *Neuroscience* 154, 1423–1439.

Moreno, N., Rétaux, S., and González, A. (2008b). Spatio-temporal expression of Pax6 in *Xenopus* forebrain. *Brain Res.* 1239, 92–99.

Moreno, N., González, A., and Rétaux, S. (2009). Development and evolution of the subpallium. *Semin. Cell Dev. Biol.* 20, 735–743.

Moreno, N., Morona, R., López, J. M., and González, A. (2010). Subdivisions of the turtle *Pseudemys scripta* subpallium based on the expression of regulatory genes and neuronal markers. *J. Comp. Neurol.* 518, 4877–4902.

Mueller, T., Vernier, P., and Wullimann, M. F. (2004). The adult central nervous cholinergic system of a neurogenetic model animal, the zebrafish *Danio rerio*. *Brain Res.* 1011, 156–169.

Murakami, Y., Ogasawara, M., Sugahara, F., Hirano, S., Satoh, N., and Kuratani, S. (2001). Identification and expression of the lamprey Pax6 gene: evolutionary origin of the segmented brain of vertebrates. *Development* 128, 3521–3531.

Murakami, Y., Uchida, K., Rijli, F. M., and Kuratani, S. (2005). Evolution of the brain developmental plan: insights from agnathans. *Dev. Biol.* 280, 249–259.

Northcutt, R. G. (1970). *The Telencephalon of the Western Painted Turtle (Chrysemys picta bellis)*. Chicago: University of Illinois Press.

Ogasawara, M., Shigetani, Y., Suzuki, S., Kuratani, S., and Satoh, N. (2001). Expression of thyroid transcription factor-1 (TTF-1) gene in the ventral forebrain and endostyle of the agnathan vertebrate, *Lampetra japonica*. *Genesis* 30, 51–58.

Osorio, J., Mazan, S., and Rétaux, S. (2005). Organisation of the lamprey (*Lampetra fluviatilis*) embryonic brain: insights from LIM-homeodomain, pax and hedgehog genes. *Dev. Biol.* 288, 100–112.

Osorio, J., Megias, M., Pombal, M. A., and Rétaux, S. (2006). Dynamic expression of the LIM-homeodomain gene Lhx15 through larval brain development of the sea lamprey (*Petromyzon marinus*). *Gene Expr. Patterns* 6, 873–878.

Osorio, J., and Rétaux, S. (2008). The lamprey in evolutionary studies. *Dev. Genes Evol.* 218, 221–235.

Pérez, S. E., Yañez, J., Marín, O., Anadón, R., González, A., and Rodríguez-Moldes, I. (2000). Distribution of choline acetyltransferase (ChAT) immunoreactivity in the brain of the adult trout and tract-tracing observations on the connections of the nuclei of the isthmus. *J. Comp. Neurol.* 428, 450–474.

Pombal, M. A., El Manira, A., and Grillner, S. (1997a). Afferents of the lamprey striatum with special reference to the dopaminergic system: a combined tracing and immunohistochemical study. *J. Comp. Neurol.* 386, 71–91.

Pombal, M. A., El Manira, A., and Grillner, S. (1997b). Organization of the lamprey striatum – transmitters and projections. *Brain Res.* 766, 249–254.

Pombal, M. A., Marín, O., and González, A. (2001). Distribution of choline acetyltransferase-immunoreactive structures in the lamprey brain. *J. Comp. Neurol.* 431, 105–126.

Price, M., Lazzaro, D., Pohl, T., Mattei, M. G., Ruther, U., Olivo, J. C., Duboule, D., and Di Lauro, R. (1992). Regional expression of the homeobox gene Nkx-2.2 in the developing mammalian forebrain. *Neuron* 8, 241–255.

Puelles, L., Kuwana, E., Puelles, E., Bulfone, A., Shimamura, K., Keleher, J., Smiga, S., and Rubenstein, J. L. (2000). Pallial and subpallial derivatives in the embryonic chick and mouse telencephalon, traced by the expression of the genes Dlx-2, Emx-1, Nkx-2.1, Pax-6, and Tbr-1. *J. Comp. Neurol.* 424, 409–438.

Puelles, L., and Rubenstein, J. L. (1993). Expression patterns of homeobox and other putative regulatory genes in the embryonic mouse forebrain suggest a neuromeric organization. *Trends Neurosci.* 16, 472–479.

Puelles, L., and Rubenstein, J. L. (2003). Forebrain gene expression domains and the evolving prosomeric model. *Trends Neurosci.* 26, 469–476.

Reiner, A., Medina, L., and Veenman, C. L. (1998). Structural and functional evolution of the basal ganglia in vertebrates. *Brain Res. Brain Res. Rev.* 28, 235–285.

Rétaux, S., Rogard, M., Bach, I., Failli, V., and Besson, M. J. (1999). Lhx9: a novel LIM-homeodomain gene expressed in the developing forebrain. *J. Neurosci.* 19, 783–793.

Rohr, K. B., Barth, K. A., Varga, Z. M., and Wilson, S. W. (2001). The nodal pathway acts upstream of hedgehog signaling to specify ventral telencephalic identity. *Neuron* 29, 341–351.

Roth, M., Bonev, B., Lindsay, J., Lea, R., Panagiotaki, N., Houart, C., and Papalopulu, N. (2010). FoxG1 and TLE2 act cooperatively to regulate ventral telencephalon formation. *Development* 137, 1553–1562.

Rubenstein, J. L., Shimamura, K., Martínez, S., and Puelles, L. (1998). Regionalization of the prosencephalic neural plate. *Annu. Rev. Neurosci.* 21, 445–477.

Ryu, S., Mahler, J., Acampora, D., Holzschuh, J., Erhardt, S., Omodei, D., Simeone, A., and Driever, W. (2007). Orthopedia homeodomain protein is essential for diencephalic dopaminergic neuron development. *Curr. Biol.* 17, 873–880.

Sánchez-Arrones, L., Ferran, J. L., Rodríguez-Gallardo, L., and Puelles, L. (2009). Incipient forebrain boundaries traced by differential gene expression and fate mapping in the chick neural plate. *Dev. Biol.* 335, 43–65.

Scholpp, S., Wolf, O., Brand, M., and Lumsden, A. (2006). Hedgehog signalling from the zona limitans intrathalamica orchestrates patterning of the zebrafish diencephalon. *Development* 133, 855–864.

Schonemann, M. D., Ryan, A. K., McEvilly, R. J., O'Connell, S. M., Arias, C. A., Kalla, K. A., Li, P., Sawchenko, P. E., and Rosenfeld, M. G. (1995). Development and survival of the endocrine hypothalamus and posterior pituitary gland requires the neuronal POU domain factor Brn-2. *Genes Dev.* 9, 3122–3135.

Shimada, M., and Nakamura, T. (1973). Time of neuron origin in mouse hypothalamic nuclei. *Exp. Neurol.* 41, 163–173.

Shimamura, K., Hartigan, D. J., Martínez, S., Puelles, L., and Rubenstein, J. L. (1995). Longitudinal organization of the anterior neural plate and neural tube. *Development* 121, 3923–3933.

Shimogori, T., Lee, D. A., Miranda-Angulo, A., Yang, Y., Wang, H., Jiang, L., Yoshida, A. C., Kataoka, A., Mashiko, H., Avetisyan, M., Qi, L., Qian, J., and Blackshaw, S. (2010). A genomic atlas of mouse hypothalamic development. *Nat. Neurosci.* 13, 767–775.

Simeone, A., D'Apice, M. R., Nigro, V., Casanova, J., Graziani, F., Acampora, D., and Avantaggiato, V. (1994). Orthopedia, a novel homeobox-containing gene expressed in the developing CNS of both mouse and *Drosophila*. *Neuron* 13, 83–101.

Soma, M., Aizawa, H., Ito, Y., Maekawa, M., Osumi, N., Nakahira, E., Okamoto, H., Tanaka, K., and Yuasa, S. (2009). Development of the mouse amygdala as revealed by enhanced green fluorescent protein gene transfer by means of in utero electroporation. *J. Comp. Neurol.* 513, 113–128.

Stoykova, A., Treichel, D., Hallonet, M., and Gruss, P. (2000). Pax6 modulates the dorsoventral patterning of the mammalian telencephalon. *J. Neurosci.* 20, 8042–8050.

Sussel, L., Marín, O., Kimura, S., and Rubenstein, J. L. (1999). Loss of Nkx2.1 homeobox gene function results in a ventral to dorsal molecular respecification within the basal telencephalon: evidence for a transformation of the pallidum into the striatum. *Development* 126, 3359–3370.

Szábo, N. E., Zhao, T., Cankaya, M., Theil, T., Zhou, X., and Alvarez-Bolado, G. (2009). Role of neuroepithelial Sonic hedgehog in hypothalamic patterning. *J. Neurosci.* 29, 6989–7002.

Takezaki, N., Figueroa, F., Zaleska-Rutczynska, Z., Takahata, N., and Klein, J. (2004). The phylogenetic relationship of tetrapod, coelacanth, and lungfish revealed by the sequences of forty-four nuclear genes. *Mol. Biol. Evol.* 21, 1512–1524.

ten Donkelaar, H. J. (1998). "Anurans," in *The Central Nervous System of Vertebrates. Urodela, Anura and Reptiles*, eds R. Nieuwenhuys, H. J. ten Donkelaar, and C. Nicholson (London: Springer), 1145–1524.

Tohyama, Y., Ichimiya, T., Kasama-Yoshida, H., Cao, Y., Hasegawa, M., Kojima, H., Tamai, Y., and Kurihara, T. (2000). Phylogenetic relation of lungfish indicated by the amino acid sequence of myelin DM20. *Brain Res. Mol. Brain Res.* 80, 256–259.

van den Akker, W. M., Brox, A., Puelles, L., Durston, A. J., and Medina, L. (2008). Comparative functional analysis provides evidence for a crucial role for the homeobox gene Nkx2.1/Titf-1 in forebrain evolution. *J. Comp. Neurol.* 506, 211–223.

Vieira, C., Pombero, A., García-López, R., Gimeno, L., Echevarria, D., and Martínez, S. (2010). Molecular mechanisms controlling brain development: an overview of neuroepithelial secondary organizers. *Int. J. Dev. Biol.* 54, 7–20.

Wang, W., and Lufkin, T. (2000). The murine Otp homeobox gene plays an essential role in the specification of neuronal cell lineages in the developing hypothalamus. *Dev. Biol.* 227, 432–449.

Wehr, R., Mansouri, A., de Maeyer, T., and Gruss, P. (1997). Fkh5-deficient mice show dysgenesis in the caudal midbrain and hypothalamic mammillary body. *Development* 124, 4447–4456.

Wullimann, M. F., and Mueller, T. (2004). Teleostean and mammalian forebrains contrasted: evidence from genes to behavior. *J. Comp. Neurol.* 475, 143–162.

Yun, K., Potter, S., and Rubenstein, J. L. (2001). Gsh2 and Pax6 play complementary roles in dorsoventral patterning of the mammalian telencephalon. *Development* 128, 193–205.

Zardoya, R., Cao, Y., Hasegawa, M., and Meyer, A. (1998). Searching for the closest living relative(s) of tetrapods through evolutionary analyses of mitochondrial and nuclear data. *Mol. Biol. Evol.* 15, 506–517.

Zardoya, R., and Meyer, A. (2001a). On the origin of and phylogenetic relationships among living amphibians. *Proc. Natl. Acad. Sci. U.S.A.* 98, 7380–7383.

Zardoya, R., and Meyer, A. (2001b). The evolutionary position of turtles revised. *Naturwissenschaften* 88, 193–200.

Zhao, T., Szabo, N., Ma, J., Luo, L., Zhou, X., and Alvarez-Bolado, G. (2008). Genetic mapping of Foxb1-cell lineage shows migration from caudal diencephalon to telencephalon and lateral hypothalamus. *Eur. J. Neurosci.* 28, 1941–1955.

Conflict of Interest Statement: The authors declare that the research was conducted in the absence of any commercial or financial relationships that could be construed as a potential conflict of interest.

3

Nonapeptides and the evolution of social group sizes in birds

James L. Goodson* and Marcy A. Kingsbury

Department of Biology, Indiana University, Bloomington, IN, USA

Edited by:
Fernando Martinez-Garcia, Universidad de Valencia, Spain

Reviewed by:
Enrique Lanuza, Universidad de Valencia, Spain
Jacques Balthazart, University of Liege, Belgium

****Correspondence:***
James L. Goodson, Department of Biology, Indiana University, 1001 East 3rd Street, Bloomington, IN 47405, USA.
e-mail: jlgoodso@indiana.edu

Species-typical patterns of grouping have profound impacts on many aspects of physiology and behavior. However, prior to our recent studies in estrildid finches, neural mechanisms that titrate species-typical group-size preferences, independent of other aspects of social organization (e.g., mating system and parental care), have been wholly unexplored, likely because species-typical group size is typically confounded with other aspects of behavior and biology. An additional complication is that components of social organization are evolutionarily labile and prone to repeated divergence and convergence. Hence, we cannot assume that convergence in social structure has been produced by convergent modifications to the same neural characters, and thus any comparative approach to grouping must include not only species that differ in their species-typical group sizes, but also species that exhibit convergent evolution in this aspect of social organization. Using five estrildid finch species that differ selectively in grouping (all biparental and monogamous) we have demonstrated that neural motivational systems evolve in predictable ways in relation to species-typical group sizes, including convergence in two highly gregarious species and convergence in two relatively asocial, territorial species. These systems include nonapeptide (vasotocin and mesotocin) circuits that encode the valence of social stimuli (positive–negative), titrate group-size preferences, and modulate anxiety-like behaviors. Nonapeptide systems exhibit functional and anatomical properties that are biased toward gregarious species, and experimental reductions of nonapeptide signaling by receptor antagonism and antisense oligonucleotides significantly decrease preferred group sizes in the gregarious zebra finch. Combined, these findings suggest that selection on species-typical group size may reliably target the same neural motivation systems when a given social structure evolves independently.

Keywords: aggression, bird, evolution, mesotocin, oxytocin, sociality, vasopressin, vasotocin

INTRODUCTION: EVOLUTION AND DIVERSITY IN SOCIAL PHENOTYPES

Vertebrate animals affiliate in multiple contexts, but sexual behavior is likely the only context of affiliation that is nearly ubiquitous across vertebrate species. Thus, the various forms of social contact that we observe across species are subject to independent evolution in different taxa, although some forms are conserved across very large clades. The provision of maternal care to offspring post-hatching or post-parturition is a good example. This kind of behavior typifies most mammals and most birds, but mammals and birds have evolved extended maternal care independently (Alcock, 2009; Goodenough et al., 2010). Studies of many vertebrate taxa demonstrate that the neural mechanisms of sexual behavior are strongly conserved (Goodson, 2005; Martinez-Garcia et al., 2008), and limited evidence suggests that mechanisms of parental care are at least grossly similar in mammals and birds, as well (Buntin et al., 2006). However, almost no generalizations can be made regarding the mechanisms of evolutionarily labile aspects of social behavior, such as cooperative breeding, mating systems, and grouping. These variables represent major defining features of species-specific social structures and have therefore garnered an extraordinary amount of attention from evolutionary biologists and behavioral ecologists. However, evolutionarily labile behaviors pose fairly extreme challenges for comparative neurobiology, largely for reasons of feasibility. For instance, after two decades of intensive research, the neural mechanisms of selective partner preference (a hallmark of monogamy), paternal care, and alloparental care are reasonably well understood for only a single species, the monogamous prairie vole (*Microtus ochrogaster*), and we know a limited amount about the critical variables that differentiate prairie voles from other non-monogamous vole species (Carter et al., 2008; Donaldson and Young, 2008; Aragona and Wang, 2009; Ross and Young, 2009; McGraw and Young, 2010). What we do not yet know is whether neural mechanisms have evolved convergently in other monogamous or alloparental species, although this is a matter of substantial current interest (Fink et al., 2006; Goodson and Thompson, 2010; Turner et al., 2010).

This example points out a fundamental difference in the approaches to social organization that are employed by evolutionary biologists and neuroethologists. Evolutionary biologists can often bring extensive information to bear on a given question, perhaps using data from dozens or hundreds of species, and analyze it in a phylogenetically corrected way that allows the extrapolation of general patterns. To some extent, neurobiologists can employ similar techniques if they are based on anatomical characteristics or genes (Northcutt, 2008; Pollen and Hofmann, 2008). Nonetheless, we cannot make any strong claims about evolutionary patterns of regulation if the experimental approaches of behavioral neuroscience are not employed, and it simply not feasible to replicate experiments in dozens or hundreds of species. For this reason, neuroethological approaches to questions about evolutionarily labile behaviors will likely continue to be somewhat different from evolutionary biological approaches, even when both are employed by the same investigators. However, if neuroethologists want to establish predictive validity for other species, comparative experimentation focused on divergent and convergent evolution is essential. In the sections that follow, we describe a quasi-experimental approach that we have taken to study convergent and divergent evolution in grouping behavior within the estrildid finch family. Although only five species have been used (**Table 1**), they have been carefully selected and our findings should therefore have good predictive validity for other estrildid finches. Whether our findings can be extrapolated to other vertebrate taxa is a matter of greater speculation, and a topic that we will return to in the Section "Conclusion."

A COMPARATIVE APPROACH TO GROUPING

Sociality *sensu stricto*, as defined by grouping behavior (Alexander, 1974), has broad influences on other important variables such as reproductive behavior, disease transmission, resource exploitation, and defense (Moller and Birkhead, 1993; Krause and Ruxton, 2002; Silk, 2007), but has not previously been examined in neurobiological studies, likely because grouping is difficult to isolate from other aspects of ecology and behavior, such as mating system and patterns of parental care. For instance, rodent species that differ in their grouping behavior also differ in whether they are monogamous or polygamous, and whether the father contributes to parental care (King, 1968; Tamarin, 1985). However, if we want to examine the neural mechanisms that titrate species-typical group-size preferences, control for such variables is very important, given that shared mechanisms (particularly neuroendocrine mechanisms) often regulate numerous aspects of social behavior (e.g., pair bonding, parental care, and affiliation) and related aspects of physiology (e.g., hormone levels and stress physiology; Carter et al., 2008; Neumann, 2009; Goodson and Thompson, 2010).

Birds offer excellent opportunities to study grouping, since we can identify closely related species that are virtually identical in most aspects of behavior and ecology, but that nonetheless exhibit extreme variation in sociality, ranging from territorial pairs to massive flocks. The finch family Estrildidae is a standout in this regard. The majority of estrildid species (approximately 141 total; Clements, 2007) form small groups of about 6–12 birds when they are not breeding, and then loosely distribute themselves for nesting without strong territoriality. Defense of a breeding territory has evolved in five to six species across three genera. Colonial breeding has also evolved in several genera, although most colonies are small (perhaps 5–10 breeding pairs). Available evidence suggests that all estrildids exhibit biparental care and long-term (typically life-long), socially monogamous pair bonds (Immelmann, 1965; Goodwin, 1982).

Table 1 | Behavioral and ecological characteristics of estrildid finch species that have been used for studies of grouping behavior. For relevant references, see footnote 1.

Species	Grouping behavior	Mating system	Parental care	Distribution	Breeding cycle
Melba finch (*Pytilia melba*)	Territorial pairs	Long-term socially monogamous	Biparental	Wide distribution in sub-Saharan Africa; desert and dry savannah	Opportunistic; in years with late rains, may delay breeding by several months relative to modal timing, which coincides with peaks in seeding grasses and insect abundance
Violet-eared waxbill (*Uraeginthus granatina*)	Territorial pairs	Long-term socially monogamous	Biparental	Southern Africa; desert and dry savannah	Comparable to Melba finch (above)
"Angolan" blue waxbill[1] (*Uraeginthus angolensis*)	Modestly gregarious (groups of 8–40); loosely distribute for breeding, but small foraging parties are still observed	Long-term socially monogamous	Biparental	Southern Africa; desert and dry savannah	Comparable to Melba finch (above)
Spice finch[2] (*Lonchura punctulata*)	Highly gregarious and colonial; flocks may contain >1000 birds, but typically fewer	Long-term socially monogamous	Biparental	Wide distribution in Indo-Asia; both arid and mesic grasslands, rice paddies	Opportunistic; may breed during any month dependent upon rainfall and seeding grasses, but with strong post-monsoonal peaks that are fairly seasonal
Zebra finch (*Taeniopygia guttata*)	Highly gregarious and colonial; average group size of ~100 with occasional groups up to 300	Long-term socially monogamous; low promiscuity	Biparental	Wide distribution in arid regions of Australia, including central Outback	Highly opportunistic; may breed during any month dependent upon rainfall and seeding grasses

[1]*The genus Uraeginthus contains three species of blue waxbill that are each known by multiple common names. Thus, although U. angolensis is most typically referred to as simply "blue waxbill," we have referred to this species as "Angolan blue waxbill" in our publications in order to clearly differentiate them from other species.*
[2]*This species is commonly encountered in the scientific literature, but under a variety of common names, including spotted munia, nutmeg mannikin, and spice finch.*

We have collected five estrildid finch species that exhibit large and seasonally stable differences in grouping, but are otherwise closely matched in behavior and ecology (**Table 1**). In addition to being socially monogamous and biparental, as already noted, all of these species live in arid or semi-arid grassland scrub and breed opportunistically or semi-opportunistically in relation to rainfall (Skead, 1975; Goodwin, 1982; Zann, 1996; Goodson et al., 2006). These include two territorial African species that live as male–female pairs year-round (violet-eared waxbill, *Uraeginthus granatina*, and melba finch, *Pytilia melba*); two highly gregarious, colonially breeding species that exhibit modal group sizes of approximately 100 (zebra finch, *Taeniopygia guttata*, and spice finch, *Lonchura punctulata*); and a moderately gregarious species, the Angolan blue waxbill (*Uraeginthus angolensis*), which exhibits a modal group size of approximately 20. The two territorial species have evolved their territorial behavior independently and the two colonial species have also evolved their extreme sociality independently[1] (Goodson et al., 2006). The gregarious Angolan blue waxbill is sympatric with both the Melba finch and violet-eared waxbill, and our laboratory population of these three species has been established through the breeding of birds that were caught from a single location in the Kalahari thornscrub of South Africa in 2001. We have obtained zebra finches and wild-caught spice finches (likely of an Indian subspecies) from commercial suppliers.

The inclusion of the zebra finch is an important asset to our research program because domestic zebra finches are both behaviorally robust and readily available, which makes them an ideal species for extensive laboratory studies. Domestic zebra finches are behaviorally indistinguishable from wild-caught zebra finches (Morris, 1958) and virtually their full range of social behavior can be observed in the lab. For instance, we are able to quantify over 20 behaviors while zebra finches are interacting in a colony environment, and can readily track the natural formation of monogamous pair bonds (Goodson et al., 1999; Kabelik et al., 2009).

NEURAL CIRCUITS OF TERRITORIAL AGGRESSION, AVERSION, AND SOCIALITY IN SONGBIRDS

Vertebrates possess a core social behavior network within the basal ("limbic") forebrain and midbrain (**Figure 1**) that is evolutionarily conserved across all taxa, but is particularly stable across the amniote clades giving rise to birds and mammals, as demonstrated by a wide range of functional and anatomical studies. This network includes the medial extended amygdala (including the medial bed nucleus of the stria terminalis, BSTm), lateral septum (LS), anterior hypothalamus (AH), ventromedial hypothalamus (VMH), midbrain central gray (CG; or periaqueductal gray), and the ventral tegmental area, although these structures are not strictly social in function and contribute to other core networks for the regulation of behavior and physiology. All of these areas express high densities of sex steroid receptors, and in contrast to most other areas of the brain that influence social behavior, they are absolutely essential for basic functions such as the expression of sexual, aggressive, and parental behaviors, and also for the regulation of anxiety, social recognition, and approach–avoidance processes (Newman, 1999; Goodson, 2005).

Birds exhibit mammal-like patterns of immediate early gene (IEG) induction in this network across a variety of social contexts, including territorial aggression, a context that is strongly relevant to

[1]We have compiled information on estrildid sociality from available sources, but most particularly Goodwin (1982), who provides an extensive review of estrildid biology and good summaries of much non-English literature (including a number of relevant works in German by K. Immelmann, G. Immelmann, P. Kunkel and J. Nicolai). We additionally consulted English-language publications by Immelmann (1965), Payne (1998), Skead (1975), Harrison (1962), Zann (1996), and Ziegler (1971). *Estrildid systematics:* Estrildid systematics have been argued for many decades (Delacour, 1943; Mayr, 1968; Christidis, 1987a,b), but fortunately, the various arrangements are largely irrelevant to our conclusions regarding convergent evolution in territoriality and extreme coloniality. A species-level molecular phylogeny is not yet available for the Estrildidae, but a genus-level molecular phylogeny has been published by Sorenson et al. (2004). Note that Sorenson has place the violet-eared waxbills into a new genus *Granatina* (two species), a closely related sister genus of *Uraeginthus*. However, pending a species-level phylogeny, we still assign the violet-eared waxbill to *Uraeginthus*, largely for purposes of consistency with our previous publications and the synthetic work of Goodwin (1982). *Independent evolution of territoriality*: The majority of estrildid species form small parties outside of the breeding season and loosely distribute for breeding, without aggressive defense of a territory. Territoriality is exhibited in three genera (*Euschistospiza, Pytilia, and Uraeginthus*), and the closest outgroups for each of these three genera are typical, non-territorial estrildids. Of the five species in the *Uraeginthus* genus, only the violet-eared waxbill (*U. granatina)* and the closely related purple grenadier (*U. ianthinogaster*) aggressively maintain exclusive breeding territories (these species are assigned to *Granatina* by Sorenson et al., 2004). Immelmann (cited in Goodwin, 1982) reports that the territories of *U. granatina* are several hundred meters square and that intruders are promptly driven out. Although *U. ianthinogaster* appears to be much the same, this species is occasionally encountered in small parties during the non-breeding season (Goodwin, 1982), whereas adult pairs of *U. granatina* do not associate with other pairs (B. M. Mines and J. L. Goodson, unpublished observations; includes 3 years of field observations by B. M. Mines). Other *Uraeginthus* species are much more social; e.g., the Angolan blue waxbill (or blue-breasted cordon bleu, *U. angolensis*) tends to breed in a semi-colonial manner, with each pair occupying a clump of bushes (Skead, 1975; Goodwin, 1982). The closest outgroups to *Uraeginthus*, the bluebills (*Spermophaga*; three species) and seedcrackers (*Pyrenestes*; three species) are also typical of the estrildids, in that they may be encountered in small parties when not breeding, and loosely distribute for breeding without defending territories. Hence, the evolution of territoriality in the violet-eared waxbill and closely related purple grenadier appears to be a shared derived character of these two species alone. Similarly, the Melba finch is the only territorial species within *Pytilia* (five species), and the closest outgroup to the *Pytilia* genus, *Lagonosticta*, is comprised of 10 firefinch species that are all typical, social estrildids. *Independent evolution of extreme coloniality:* Zebra finches and spice finches belong to a large group of predominantly Australasian finches, although this group is largely divisible into two distinct clades, one containing the zebra finch (approximately 11 species) and the other containing the spice finch (approximately 30 species). Most species in the zebra finch clade are modestly gregarious, at least during the non-breeding season, and many form small, loose colonies. However, there are also a few species that are markedly less social, particularly the *Stagonopleura* (firetail) and *Oreostruthus* (mountain firetail) species, and despite the fact that numerous species in the zebra finch clade are social during breeding, a high level of coloniality has evolved only in the zebra finch and chestnut-eared finch (*T. castanotis*; historically considered a subspecies of the zebra finch; Goodwin, 1982; Zann, 1996). Based on a large number of counts by Zann and colleagues (reviewed in Zann, 1996), the average zebra finch breeding colony includes 66 adults (an unknown number of dependent young would also be present), and the average non-breeding flock contains 107 birds. The owl finch (*T. bichenovii*), which is arguably the next most social species in the zebra finch clade, displays a level of sociality well below that of the zebra finch, with typical flocks numbering only 4–20 individuals (Immelmann, 1965). Thus, parsimony strongly suggests that the zebra finch's uniquely high level of colonial behavior is not ancestral for its clade. Similarly, only three of the species in the other Australasian clade exhibit a level of coloniality that is comparable to the zebra finch, including the spice finch (see Immelmann, 1965). Several species form only small non-breeding parties and distribute for breeding, while the majority of species form non-breeding flocks and breed with a few pairs close together. These observations, combined with the considerations of the zebra finch clade, firmly support the view that extremely gregarious behavior, characterized by large colonies and non-breeding flocks of hundreds to thousands of individuals, has evolved independently in the spice finch and zebra finch.

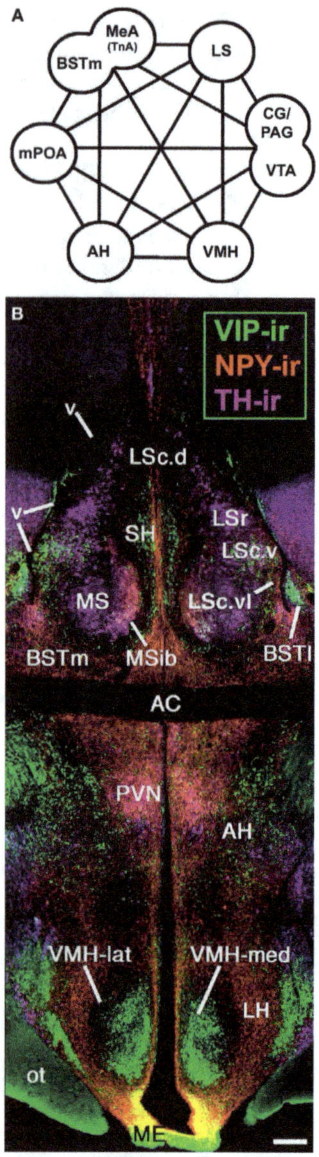

FIGURE 1 | An evolutionarily conserved suite of brain regions that regulate vertebrate social behavior. (A) The core components of the social behavior network include numerous areas of the basal forebrain – the medial extended amygdala (medial amygdala, MeA, or taenial amygdala, TnA, plus the medial bed nucleus of the stria terminalis, BSTm), medial preoptic area (mPOA), anterior hypothalamus (AH), ventromedial hypothalamus (VMH), and lateral septum (LS), as well as areas of the midbrain, most notably the central gray (CG; or periaqueductal gray, PAG) and the ventral tegmental area (VTA). Modified from Newman (1999) and Maney et al. (2008). **(B)** A photomontage of a female zebra finch brain at the level of the anterior commissure (AC). Immunocytochemical triple-labeling for vasoactive intestinal polypeptide (VIP), neuropeptide Y (NPY), and tyrosine hydroxylase (TH) shows the location of the AH and multiple zones of the LS, BST, and VMH. The topography shown here is very similar across vertebrate groups, particularly among amniotes. Scale bar = 200 μm. Modified from Goodson, 2005. Other abbreviations: BSTl, lateral bed nucleus of the stria terminalis; Hp, hippocampus; LH, lateral hypothalamus; LSc, caudal division of the lateral septum (dorsal, ventrolateral, and ventral zones denoted as LSc.d, LSc.vl, and LSc.v, respectively); LSr, rostral division of the lateral septum; ME, median eminence; MS, medial septum; MSib, internal band of the medial septum; ot, optic tract; OM, occipitomesencephalic tract; PVN, paraventricular nucleus of the hypothalamus; SH, septohippocampal septum; v, lateral ventricle.

species differences in sociality. IEG proteins such as Fos and egr-1 are rapidly inducible transcription factors that are proxy markers of neuronal activity. Following resident–intruder encounters in territorial rodents (Kollack-Walker et al., 1997; Motta et al., 2009) and simulated territorial intrusion (STI; playback of song and presentation of a caged decoy male) in male song sparrows, significant activation is observed in forebrain areas such as the BSTm, LS, paraventricular nucleus of the hypothalamus (PVN), AH, and the lateral portion of the VMH (Goodson and Evans, 2004; Goodson et al., 2005b), as well as midbrain areas such as the CG (Maney and Ball, 2003). IEG results are extensively comparable in winter and summer sparrows (Goodson and Evans, 2004; Goodson et al., 2005b). Notably, IEG responses of the AH, PVN, and multiple zones of the LS correlate *negatively* with aggression (Goodson et al., 2005b), and the case is much the same in hamsters and mice, such that fighting-induced Fos expression is higher in subordinate versus dominant animals (Kollack-Walker et al., 1997; Motta et al., 2009). This applies to most aggression-related areas in the brain, and we have obtained very similar results in the territorial violet-eared waxbill (J. L. Goodson, S. E. Schrock, and M. A. Kingsbury, unpublished observations).

Neural circuitry that regulates grouping is substantially less well known. As an initial approach to this issue, we examined the neural responses of territorial and gregarious estrildids to same-sex conspecifics (Goodson et al., 2005a). Subjects were isolated in a quiet room and then exposed to a same-sex conspecific through a wire barrier. Importantly, this manipulation elicits very little overt behavior and thus species differences in neural response should primarily reflect species differences in perceptual or motivational processes. Despite the simplicity of this paradigm, Fos and egr-1 responses clearly distinguish the territorial from gregarious (flocking) species, including differences between the two sympatric *Uraeginthus* species described in the previous section. Overall, territorial birds exhibit significantly greater IEG responses in the medial extended amygdala (especially the BSTm), ventrolateral LS, AH, lateral VMH, and CG (and adjacent "intercollicular" territory that is now known to be homologous to the dorsal and dorsolateral CG of mammals; Goodson et al., 2005a; Kingsbury et al., 2011). This pattern is virtually identical to a pattern associated with aversive social stimulation in rodents (Sheehan et al., 2001; providing a good example of deep functional conservation in the social behavior circuits of vertebrate brains), but possible mechanisms of gregariousness were not evident at this level of analysis. This may partially reflect the fact that functionally distinct neurons are intercalated with one another in the various brain areas that influence social behavior (e.g., Choi et al., 2005). For instance, as described in the next section, Fos induction within arginine vasotocin (VT) neurons of the BSTm is strictly associated with affiliation-related stimuli, and following same-sex exposure, the gregarious species show greater Fos induction in the VT neurons than do territorial species (Goodson and Wang, 2006). However, as just noted, the *overall* Fos response of the BSTm is greater in the territorial birds (Goodson et al., 2005a), suggesting that the VT neurons are intermingled with other neurons that exhibit opposing profiles of response. These hypothetical "aversion" neurons have not yet been identified, although aromatase-expressing neurons, which are numerous in the BSTm and mostly negative for VT (Kabelik et al., 2010), are possible candidates. Consistent with this idea, recent findings in mice suggest that estrogen signaling within the BSTm is important for the regulation of resident–intruder aggression (Trainor et al., 2006, 2007) and inhibits affiliative behavior in male prairie voles (Lei et al., 2010).

NONAPEPTIDE SYSTEMS: PHENOTYPIC DIVERSITY AND THE SPECIES-SPECIFIC ASSIGNMENT OF SOCIAL VALENCE

The nine amino acid neuropeptides, or "nonapeptides," are among the most interesting modulators of social behavior identified to date. Although many anatomical and functional properties of nonapeptide systems are strongly conserved across all vertebrate taxa (and in the case of neurosecretory magnocellular neurons, perhaps across all bilaterians; Tessmar-Raible et al., 2007), there is substantial diversity in receptor distributions and nonapeptides have been extensively linked to behavioral variation across individuals, sexes, and species (Goodson and Bass, 2001; De Vries and Panzica, 2006; Donaldson and Young, 2008; Goodson, 2008).

Duplication of the VT gene in early jawed vertebrates gave rise to two nonapeptide lineages, which include the mammalian peptides arginine vasopressin (VP; homolog of VT) and oxytocin (OT). Most non-mammalian vertebrates express VT and an OT-like peptide, such as isotocin, found in ray-finned fishes, or mesotocin (MT), which is ubiquitously expressed in non-mammalian tetrapods (Acher, 1972; Hoyle, 1999). All jawed vertebrates express their two nonapeptide forms in both magnocellular and parvocellular neurons of the preoptic area and hypothalamus, which in amniotes are located primarily within the supraoptic nucleus of the hypothalamus and the PVN (Moore and Lowry, 1998; Goodson, 2008). In rats, the parvocellular neurons of the PVN give rise to widespread projections in the brain (De Vries and Buijs, 1983), and this is almost certainly the same in other vertebrates. Lesions of the PVN in rats virtually eliminate VP projections to the caudal brainstem, but not other areas, and eliminate OT projections throughout the brain (De Vries and Buijs, 1983). Thus, given the strong similarities of MT and OT systems, it is likely the case that extrahypothalamic MT projections in birds are exclusively or almost exclusively derived from the PVN.

In addition to these hypothalamic cell groups, most tetrapods exhibit a very unique VT/VP cell group of the BSTm, which in some mammals extends into medial amygdala proper. With only a few exceptions, these neurons and their projections to the LS and other basal forebrain areas have been found to be seasonally variable, exquisitely dependent on sex steroids, and sexually dimorphic (males > females). In each of these respects, the extrahypothalamic VT/VP circuitry arising in the BSTm is among the most extremely plastic systems in the brain. Indeed, as demonstrated for many species of mammals, amphibians, birds, and reptiles, this circuitry typically disappears in animals that are in non-reproductive condition or otherwise deprived of sex steroids (Goodson and Bass, 2001; De Vries and Panzica, 2006). However, in estrildids that exhibit opportunistic breeding and have no apparent endogenous reproductive cycles, no such collapse is observed, although basal transcriptional activity [as measured by constitutive expression of Fos protein in VT-immunoreactive (-ir) neurons] is nonetheless regulated by androgens (Kabelik et al., 2010). Thus, of the finches that we have examined, large seasonal fluctuations in VT immunoreactivity are found only for the spice finch, a species that exhibits photorefractoriness and endogenous rhythms of reproductive physiology that correlate with monsoon cyclicity (Goodwin, 1982; Chaturvedi and Prasad, 1991; Sikdar et al., 1992; Hahn and MacDougall-Shackleton, 2008).

The VT/VP neurons of the BSTm project to numerous other areas of the basal forebrain where VT/VP modulates aggression, parental behavior, social recognition, and various affiliative and anxiety-like behaviors; and at least in male prairie voles, VP release in the ventral pallidum promotes partner preference (Donaldson and Young, 2008; Veenema and Neumann, 2008; Goodson and Thompson, 2010; Insel, 2010). Although these basal forebrain sites likely receive VT/VP from multiple hypothalamic cell groups in addition to the BSTm population, the relative contributions of the different cell groups are difficult to ascertain, given the extensive evidence for paracrine signaling and volumetric release from dendrites and soma (Ludwig and Leng, 2006; Goodson and Kabelik, 2009).

In order to determine the kinds of stimuli that different VT/VP cell groups respond to (particularly those of the BSTm), we have conducted several experiments in which we have exposed animals to social stimuli or control conditions, and then sacrificed the animals 90 min later for immunohistochemical colocalization of VT and Fos (see **Table 2** for a summary of studies). Experimental induction of Fos is still robust at 90 min, but the half-life of Fos protein is only 45 min (Herdegen and Leah, 1998), and thus if cellular activity is depressed by our social manipulations, we can detect this as a *reduction* in Fos expression. These experiments did not include analyses of MT–Fos colocalization, since MT behavioral functions were unknown at the time, but we are now conducting these analyses with alternate tissue series from the same animals.

Using this approach, our experiments have demonstrated a remarkable sensitivity of the BSTm VT/VP cells to social valence (**Figure 2**). Relative to handled controls, VT-ir neurons in the territorial estrildid species decrease their Fos expression in response to same-sex stimuli (exposed through a wire barrier as described above), but increase Fos expression in response to their pairbond partner. In contrast, in colonial birds that form mixed-sex flocks, VT-ir cells in the BSTm *increase* their activity in response to both same-sex stimuli and competitive courtship interactions, but not following intense subjugation (Goodson and Wang, 2006). No sex differences were observed in any of these results and similar effects were not observed for VT–Fos colocalization in the PVN (J. L. Goodson and Y. Wang, unpublished observations). Notably, although the modestly gregarious Angolan blue waxbill shows only a small (and not significant) increase in VT–Fos colocalization following exposure to a same-sex conspecific, the response profile of this species is still significantly different from its territorial congener, the violet-eared waxbill. Species differences in VT signaling may be further magnified based on VT-ir cell numbers, which are approximately 10 times more abundant in the colonial species relative to other species (Goodson and Wang, 2006). Finally, adding onto the remarkable response profile of this cell group, recent experiments in male zebra finches demonstrate that the BSTm VT

Table 2 | A summary of main findings from studies of nonapeptide systems in territorial (T), moderately gregarious (MG), and highly gregarious (HG) species of estrildid finches.

Variable or manipulation	Result
Fos response of VT-ir neurons in the BSTm[1]	To same-sex conspecifics: T < MG < HG
	Socially negative stimuli decrease VT–Fos colocalization or have no effect
	Socially positive stimuli increase VT–Fos colocalization
Constitutive VT–Fos colocalization in the BSTm (early AM baseline)[1]	T < MG = HG
VT-ir cell number in the BSTm[1]	T = MG < HG
Fos response of VT-ir neurons in the PVN to same-sex conspecific stimuli[2]	T = MG = HG
^{125}I–V_{1a} antagonist binding in the LS[3]	T < MG = HG
VT infusions into the LS for tests of aggression[4]	Inhibit territorial (resident–intruder) aggression in male violet-eared waxbills
	Facilitate aggression in the context of mate competition in male zebra finches
V_{1a} antagonist infusions into the LS (male zebra finches)[5]	Potently decrease gregariousness (% of total contact time spent with the larger of two groups) with no effects on total contact time
	Potently increase anxiety-like behavior
	Reduce mate competition aggression
Knockdown of VT production in the BSTm by antisense oligonucleotides (male zebra finches)[6]	Potently decreases gregariousness
	Increases anxiety-like behavior
	Modestly increases social contact time
^{125}I–OT antagonist binding in the LS[7]	Dorsal (pallial): T < MG = HG
	Ventral (subpallial): T = MG < HG ($P = 0.06$)
	Dorsal–ventral ratio: T < MG = HG
OT antagonist administrations (peripheral, intraventricular, and intraseptal; zebra finches)[7]	Decrease preferences for the larger of two groups with no effect on total contact time
	Decrease preferences for familiar versus novel groups
	Some effects are female-specific

[1] *Goodson and Wang (2006), also see Goodson et al. (2009b).*
[2] *J. L. Goodson and Y. Wang (unpublished observation).*
[3] *Goodson et al. (2006).*
[4] *Goodson (1998), Goodson and Adkins-Regan (1999), Goodson et al. (2004).*
[5] *Goodson et al. (2004), Kelly et al. (2011).*
[6] *Kelly et al. (2011).*
[7] *Goodson et al. (2009c).*

neurons increase their Fos expression selectively in response to a positive social stimulus, but show no response to a positive non-social stimulus (Goodson et al., 2009b).

Our results in birds are consistent with other recent findings in mice, and may therefore represent a common feature of BSTm VT/VP neurons across all tetrapods. In male C57BL/6J mice, BSTm VP neurons exhibit robust Fos responses to copulation (which is clearly a positive, affiliation-related stimulus) and very modest responses to non-aggressive same-sex chemoinvestigation, but show no greater Fos response to aggressive interactions than simple chemoinvestigation (Ho et al., 2010). Notably, the sensitivity of amygdala neurons to valence has been extensively characterized through neurophysiological and neuroimaging studies in mammals (Nishijo et al., 1988; Paton et al., 2006; also see Goodson and Thompson, 2010), but specific cell types that process valence have not previously been identified. Neurophysiological studies in monkeys demonstrate that neurons which exhibit stable preferences for positive or negative stimuli are intercalated (Paton et al., 2006), and thus the neurochemical identification of valence-sensitive populations represents an important step toward understanding how social value is encoded and used by the brain to regulate behavior.

EVOLUTIONARY CONVERGENCE AND DIVERGENCE IN NEUROPEPTIDE RECEPTOR DISTRIBUTIONS: A SPECIAL STATUS FOR THE LATERAL SEPTUM?

Species differences in the response profiles of various brain areas and specific cell group are likely coordinated, at least to an extent, by the differential expression of receptors for neuromodulators. In fact, using the five finch species already introduced, we have obtained good evidence that the distributions of binding sites for vasoactive intestinal polypeptide (VIP), VT, and MT all exhibit convergent and divergent evolution in relation to sociality (based on quantitative autoradiography using ^{125}I–VIP and iodinated antagonists of OT and V_{1a} receptors; Goodson et al., 2006, 2009c). Remarkably, binding sites for all three peptides exhibit sociality-related evolution within the LS, indicating that the LS plays a special role in grouping. In order

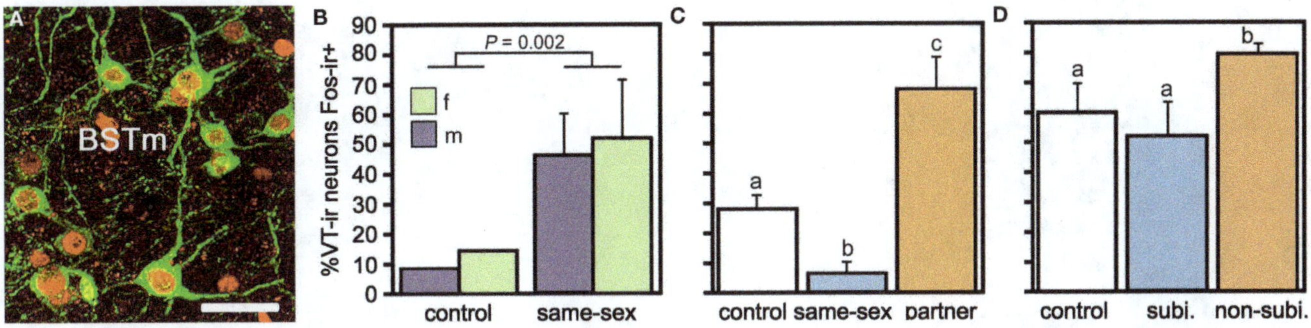

FIGURE 2 | Valence sensitivity of vasotocin (VT) neurons in the medial bed nucleus of the stria terminalis (BSTm), as demonstrated by socially induced changes in the immunocytochemical colocalization of VT and the proxy activity marker Fos. (A) Representative colocalization of VT (green) and Fos (red) in the BSTm of a male zebra finch following a courtship interaction. Note that most VT neurons express Fos. Scale bar = 20 μm. **(B)** In the zebra finch, which is a highly gregarious species, isolation in a quiet room followed by exposure to a same-sex conspecific through a wire barrier produces a robust increase in VT neuronal activity in both males and females. Total n = 10. **(C)** This same manipulation produces a significant decrease in VT–Fos colocalization in the territorial violet-eared waxbill, a species that does not naturally exhibit same-sex affiliation, but exposure to the subject's pairbond partner (a presumably positive stimulus), produces a robust increase in neuronal activity. Sexes are shown pooled. Total n = 16. **(D)** VT–Fos colocalization increases in zebra finches following competition with a same-sex individual for courtship access to an opposite-sex bird, but not if the subject is paired with a highly aggressive partner and intensely subjugated. Subjugated animals were aggressively displaced or attacked 71–210 times during a 10-min interaction, demonstrating that social arousal alone does not increase VT–Fos colocalization in the BSTm. Sexes are shown pooled. Total n = 15. **(A)** is modified from Goodson et al. (2009b); **(B–D)** are modified from Goodson and Wang (2006).

to be interpreted as "sociality-related," we require that binding densities differ significantly between the two territorial and three flocking species (defined as contrast A) and differ significantly between the two territorial and two colonial species (contrast B), with the modestly gregarious species being intermediate or falling in line with the two colonial species. The most convincing comparisons are those that meet these criteria, with additional significant differences between the territorial and gregarious *Uraeginthus* species, which are sympatric (contrast C). Sociality-related differences that meet this highest criterion are described as fitting an "ABC" pattern (Goodson et al., 2006). **Figure 3** shows one such pattern for the density of V_{1a}-like receptor density in the dorsal LS, and similar ABC species differences are observed in several other LS zones for both V_{1a}-like, OT-like and VIP binding sites (Goodson et al., 2006, 2009c). Binding densities are mostly biased toward the gregarious species, although sociality-related differences in OT-like binding densities reverse along a dorso-ventral gradient, and the *relative density* between the pallial and subpallial LS provides the clearest differentiation of territorial and flocking species (Goodson et al., 2009c; **Figure 4**), suggesting that sociality is reflected in a complex neuromodulatory balance across the LS subnuclei. Outside of the LS, sociality-related differences in the finches are observed for VIP binding in the BSTm, which are biased toward the gregarious species (Goodson et al., 2006).

Densities of nonapeptide receptors in the LS are also highly variable in mammals, although the relevance of these species differences to behavior has largely been a matter of speculation (Insel et al., 1991, 1994; Campbell et al., 2009; Turner et al., 2010). However, recent findings suggest that OT receptor densities may reflect species differences in the provision of alloparental care by juvenile females, and alloparental care in female prairie voles is negatively correlated with OT receptor densities in the LS (Olazábal and Young, 2006). In male prairie voles, social investigation behavior is positively correlated with V_{1a} receptor densities and negatively with OT receptor densities in the LS (Ophir et al., 2009).

NONAPEPTIDES PROMOTE FLOCKING

The relevance of nonapeptide receptors to grouping behavior has been directly confirmed by a series of recent experiments using central antagonist and antisense manipulations in zebra finches. Based on the well known effects of OT and OT receptors on affiliation in mammals (Carter et al., 2008; Goodson and Thompson, 2010), we began by blocking OT-like receptors (as in mammals, a single OT-like receptor has been identified in birds, VT3; Baeyens and Cornett, 2006). Using the choice apparatus shown in **Figure 5A**, in which subjects can choose between groups of 10 or 2 same-sex conspecifics (or not spend time near either), we first showed that subcutaneous and lateral ventricle infusions of an OT antagonist reduce preferences for the larger group (**Figures 5B–E**) without influencing the amount of time that subjects spent in close proximity to other birds (hereafter "contact time"). The peripheral effect was female-specific and ventricular infusions of MT produced a female-specific increase in the amount of time that subjects spent with large group, again with no effect on contact time. Infusions of the OT antagonist directly into the LS replicated the peripheral and ventricular antagonist effects in females, whereas control infusions into the medial striatum (adjacent to the ventricle) did not (Goodson et al., 2009c).

As described in the previous sections, gregarious species show a relatively greater social induction of Fos within VT neurons, more VT-ir neurons in the BSTm, and a higher density of VT V_{1a}-like receptors in the LS than do territorial species (Goodson and Wang, 2006; Goodson et al., 2006), suggesting the hypothesis that VT projections from the BSTm to the LS promote sociality. Indeed, recent experiments in male zebra finches

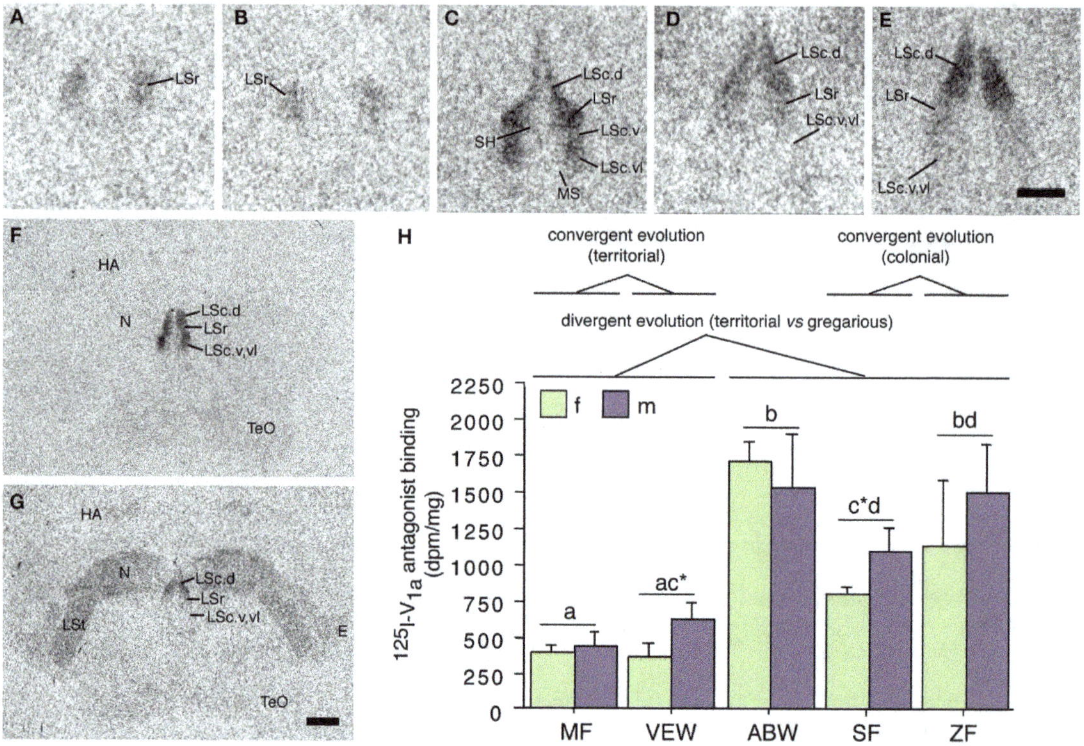

FIGURE 3 | Species differences in linear ^{125}I–V$_{1a}$ antagonist binding in the lateral septum (LS) reflect evolutionary convergence and divergence in flocking and territoriality. (A–E) Representative ^{125}I–V$_{1a}$ antagonist binding in the LS of the territorial Melba finch [MF; **(A)**], territorial violet-eared waxbill [VEW; **(B)**], moderately gregarious Angolan blue waxbill [ABW; **(C)**], colonial spice finch [SF; **(D)**], and colonial zebra finch [ZF; **(E)**]. The scale bar in **(E)** corresponds to 500 µm in **(A–E)**. **(F,G)** Representative sections for a male Angolan blue waxbill and male spice finch (colonial), respectively, showing species differences in binding for the nidopallium (N) and other areas of the forebrain. The scale bar in **(G)** corresponds to 1 mm in **(F,G)**. **(H)** Linear ^{125}I–V$_{1a}$ antagonist binding in the dorsal (pallial) portion of the LS, shown as decompositions per min/mg (dpm/mg; means ± SEM). Different letters above the error bars denote significant species differences (Fisher's PLSD following significant ANOVA; $P < 0.0001$). Asterisks denote near-significant species differences ($P = 0.06$). Modified from Goodson et al. (2006). Abbreviations: E, entopallium; HA, apical part of the hyperpallium; LSc, caudal division of the lateral septum (dorsal, ventrolateral, and ventral zones denoted as LSc.d, LSc.vl, and LSc.v, respectively); LSr, rostral division of the lateral septum; LSt, lateral striatum; MS, medial septum; N, nidopallium; SH, septohippocampal septum; TeO, optic tectum.

demonstrate that knockdown of VT production in the BSTm by antisense oligonucleotides potently reduces gregariousness relative to subjects infused with scrambled oligonucleotides, with a median reduction of 80%. "Gregariousness" in this experiment was defined as the percent of contact time that was spent next to a group of 10 conspecifics versus a group of 2 (Kelly et al., 2011). Surprisingly, this same manipulation increased contact time modestly relative to scrambled oligonucleotide controls (median difference of 25%), although intraseptal infusions of a V$_{1a}$ antagonist produce no effects on contact time (and convincingly so). As with the VT antisense, intraseptal V$_{1a}$ antagonist infusions virtually eliminated subjects' preferences for the large group while concomitantly increasing the amount of time that subjects spent with the small group. The median reduction in gregariousness was again 80%. We have further replicated this effect in both males and females using a novel V$_{1a}$ antagonist that crosses the blood–brain barrier (JNJ-17308616; J. L. Goodson and S. E. Schrock, unpublished observations). In conjunction with both the antisense and central antagonist studies, we also conducted tests of anxiety-like behavior (novelty-suppressed feeding and exploration of a novel environment), which produced particularly intriguing results: whereas septal VP is usually found to be anxiogenic in rodents, it appears to be strongly anxiolytic in zebra finches (Kelly et al., 2011). Whether this difference is the result of unique receptor distributions and/or is an important factor in the social evolution of zebra finches remains to be determined. However, it is interesting in this light to note that septal VP may promote active stress coping in rats (Ebner et al., 1999), which are more social than laboratory mice and hamsters.

CONCLUSION

Using five finch species that are all socially monogamous and biparental, we have shown that (1) receptor distributions for multiple neuropeptide systems (VT/MT, VIP, and CRF) exhibit divergent and convergent evolution in relation to species-typical group size, particularly within the LS, (2) VT cells in the BSTm exhibit an exquisite sensitivity to the valence of social stimuli, thereby

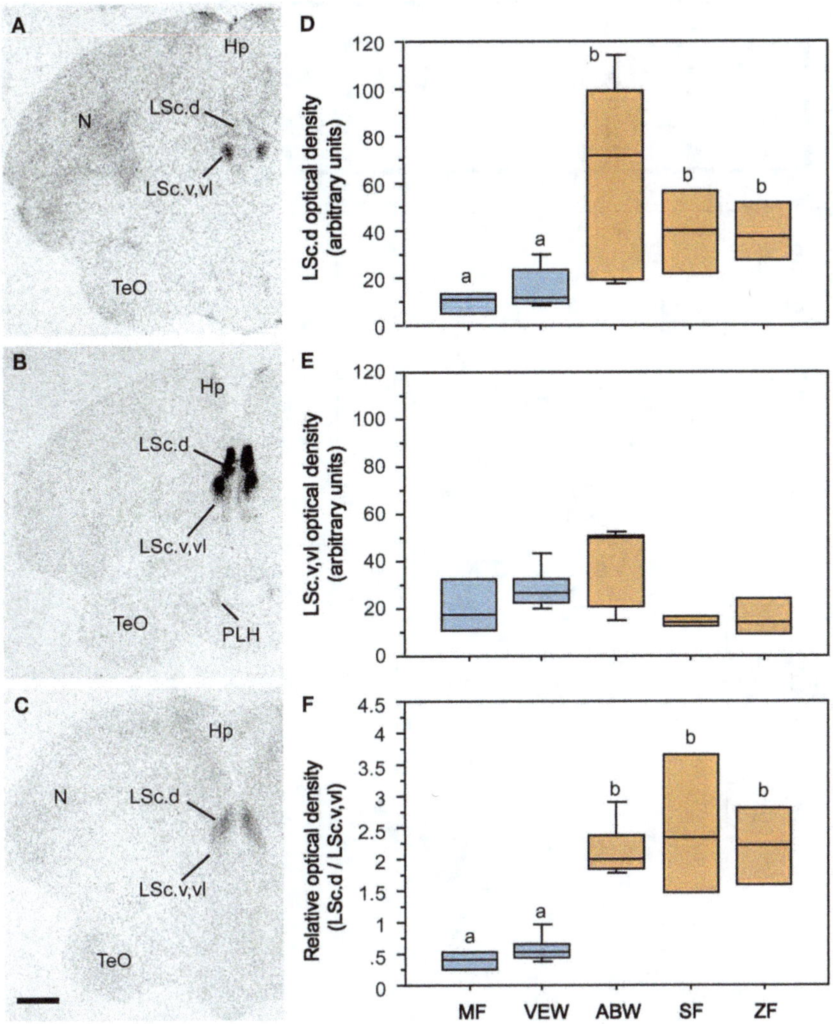

FIGURE 4 | Species-specific distributions of oxytocin-like binding sites reflect evolutionary convergence and divergence in flocking and territoriality. (A–C) Representative autoradiograms of ^{125}I–OT antagonist binding sites in the caudal LS (LSc) in two sympatric, congeneric finches – the territorial violet-eared waxbill **(A)** and the gregarious Angolan blue waxbill **(B)**, plus the highly gregarious zebra finch **(C)**. **(D)** Densities of binding sites in the dorsal (pallial) LSc of two territorial species (Melba finch, MF, and violet-eared waxbill, VEW), a moderately gregarious species (Angolan blue waxbill, ABW), and two highly gregarious species (spice finch, SF, and zebra finch, ZF). No sex differences are observed and sexes were pooled. Total $n = 23$. Different letters above the boxes denote significant species differences (Mann–Whitney $P < 0.05$) following significant Kruskal–Wallis. **(E)** Binding densities tend to reverse in the subpallial LSc ($P = 0.06$), suggesting that species differences in sociality are most closely associated with the relative densities of binding sites along a dorso-ventral gradient, as confirmed in the bottom **(F)** using a dorsal:ventral ratio. Abbreviations: Hp, hippocampus; LSc.d, dorsal zone of the LSc; LSc.v,vl, ventral, and ventrolateral zones of the LSc; N, nidopallium; PLH, posterolateral hypothalamus; TeO, optic tectum. Modified from Goodson et al. (2009c).

creating differences between gregarious and territorial species in the response of their BSTm VT neurons to same-sex conspecifics, (3) endogenous nonapeptide signaling via V_{1a}- and OT-like receptors in the LS promotes preferences for larger groups in zebra finches without effects on social contact time, and (4) in male zebra finches, antisense knockdown of VT production in the BSTm profoundly reduces gregariousness. Although not discussed above, we have also found that the three flocking finch species exhibit relatively more dopamine neurons than do territorial species in a caudal subpopulation of cells in the ventral tegmental area that has also been implicated in appetitive courtship behavior (Goodson et al., 2009a).

A major remaining question is whether our results are predictive for other taxa. All of the neurochemical systems just mentioned influence myriad behavioral and physiological functions, thus we might expect that those systems may not evolve in relation to grouping, and in an estrildid-like manner, if other species-specific behavioral and physiological functions constrain the evolutionary process. This may occur if a given neural mechanism is under strong selection in relation to something other than grouping. At the same time, nonapeptides influence basic social behaviors across a wide range of vertebrates, suggesting that they may be common or even ubiquitous targets of selection during social evolution.

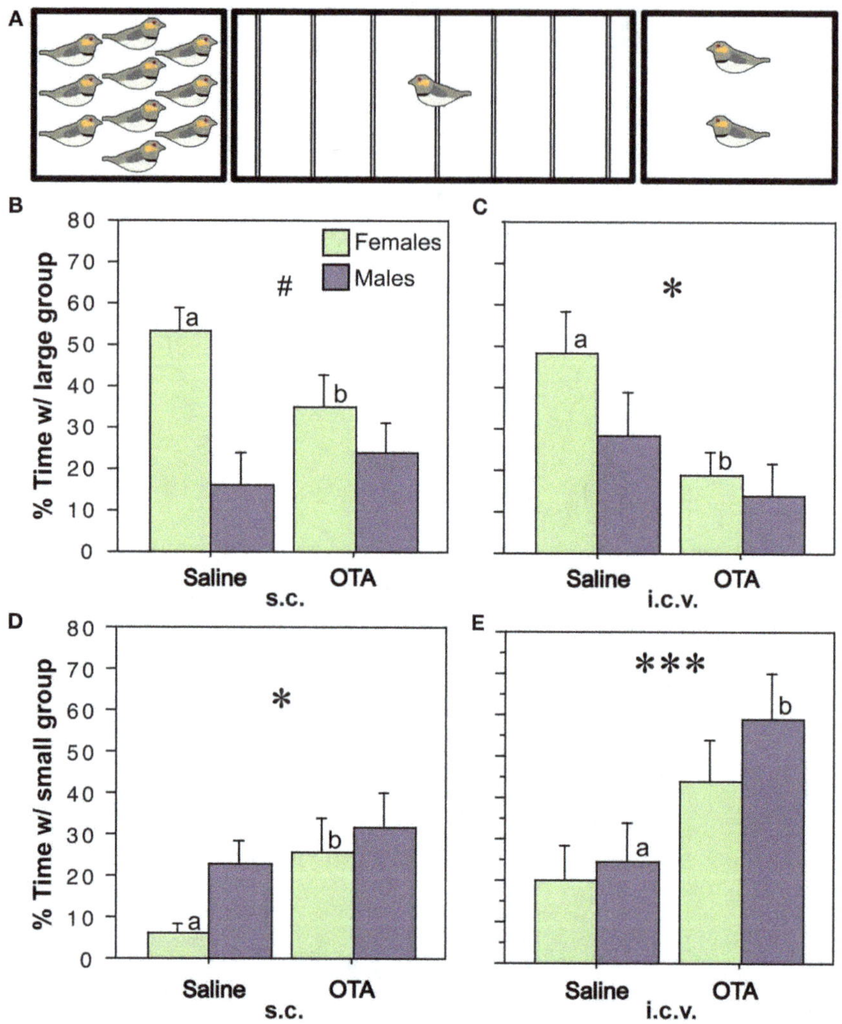

FIGURE 5 | Endogenous activation of oxytocin-like receptors promotes preferences for larger groups. (A) Choice apparatus design. A 1-m wide testing cage was subdivided into zones by seven perches (thin lines). Subjects were considered to be within close proximity when they were within 6 cm of a stimulus cage (i.e., on the perches closest to the sides of the testing cage). The stimulus cages contained either 2 or 10 same-sex conspecifics. **(B–E)** Relative to vehicle treatments, subcutaneous (s.c.) or intracerebroventricular (i.c.v.) administrations of the oxytocin antagonist desGly–NH_2, $d(CH_2)_5$[Tyr(Me)^2, Thr^4]OVT (OTA; 250 ng), reduce the amount of time that zebra finches spend in close proximity to the large group **(B,C)** and increase time in close proximity to the small group **(D,E)**. *$P < 0.05$, ***$P < 0.001$, main effect of Treatment; #$P < 0.5$ Sex*Treatment; n = 12 m, 12 f. Letters above the error bars denote significant within-sex effects. Modified from Goodson et al. (2009c).

ACKNOWLEDGMENTS

Our thanks to Aubrey M. Kelly, Richmond R. Thompson, Kristin Hoffbuhr, Sara E. Schrock, Brandon Waxman, David Kabelik, Yiwei Wang, James D. Klatt, Andrew K. Evans, and Jacob Rinaldi for significant contributions to the work described here. Support for this work was provided by the National Institute of Mental Health grant MH062656 to James L. Goodson.

REFERENCES

Acher, R. (1972). *Chemistry of the Neurohypophysial Hormones: An Example of Molecular Evolution*, Endocrinology, 119–130. Washington, DC: American Physiological Society.

Alcock, J. (2009). *Animal Behavior: An Evolutionary Approach*, 9th Edn. Sunderland, MA: Sinauer Associates.

Alexander, R. D. (1974). The evolution of social behavior. *Annu. Rev. Ecol. Syst.* 5, 325–383.

Aragona, B. J., and Wang, Z. (2009). Dopamine regulation of social choice in a monogamous rodent species. *Front. Behav. Neurosci.* 3:15. doi: 10.3389/neuro.08.015.2009

Baeyens, D. A., and Cornett, L. E. (2006). The cloned avian neurohypophysial hormone receptors. *Comp. Biochem. Physiol. B* 143, 12–19.

Buntin, L., Berghman, L. R., and Buntin, J. D. (2006). Patterns of Fos-like immunoreactivity in the brains of parent ring doves (*Streptopelia risoria*) given tactile and nontactile exposure to their young. *Behav. Neurosci.* 120, 651–664.

Campbell, P., Ophir, A. G., and Phelps, S. M. (2009). Central vasopressin and oxytocin receptor distributions in two species of singing mice. *J. Comp. Neurol.* 516, 321–333.

Carter, C. S., Grippo, A. J., Pournajafi-Nazarloo, H., Ruscio, M. G., and Porges, S. W. (2008). Oxytocin, vasopressin and sociality. *Prog. Brain Res.* 170, 331–336.

Chaturvedi, C. M., and Prasad, S. K. (1991). Timed daily injections of neurotransmitter precursors alter the gonad and body weights of spotted munia, *Lonchura punctulata*, maintained under short daily photoperiods. *J. Exp. Zool.* 260, 194–201.

Choi, G. B., Dong, H. W., Murphy, A. J., Valenzuela, D. M., Yancopoulos, G. D., Swanson, L. W., and Anderson, D. J. (2005). Lhx6 delineates a pathway mediating innate reproductive behaviors from the amygdala to the hypothalamus. *Neuron* 46, 647–660.

Christidis, L. (1987a). Biochemical systematics within paleotropic finches (Aves: Estrildidae). *Auk* 104, 380–392.

Christidis, L. (1987b). Phylogeny and systematics of estrildine finches and their relationships to other seed-eating passerines. *Emu* 87, 119–123.

Clements, J. F. (2007). *Birds of the World: A Checklist*, 6th Edn. Sussex: Pica Press.

De Vries, G. J., and Buijs, R. M. (1983). The origin of the vasopressinergic and oxytocinergic innervation of the rat brain with special reference to the lateral septum. *Brain Res.* 273, 307–317.

De Vries, G. J., and Panzica, G. C. (2006). Sexual differentiation of central vasopressin and vasotocin systems in vertebrates: different mechanisms, similar endpoints. *Neuroscience* 138, 947–955.

Delacour, J. (1943). A revision of the subfamily Estrildinae of the family Ploceidae. *Zoologica* 28, 69–86.

Donaldson, Z. R., and Young, L. J. (2008). Oxytocin, vasopressin, and the neurogenetics of sociality. *Science* 322, 900–904.

Ebner, K., Wotjak, C. T., Holsboer, F., Landgraf, R., and Engelmann, M. (1999). Vasopressin released within the septal brain area during swim stress modulates the behavioural stress response in rats. *Eur. J. Neurosci.* 11, 997–1002.

Fink, S., Excoffier, L., and Heckel, G. (2006). Mammalian monogamy is not controlled by a single gene. *Proc. Natl. Acad. Sci. U.S.A.* 103, 10956–10960.

Goodenough, J., McGuire, B., and Jakob, E. (2010). *Perspectives on Animal Behavior*, 3rd Edn. Hoboken, NJ: John Wiley and Sons, Inc.

Goodson, J. L. (1998). Vasotocin and vasoactive intestinal polypeptide modulate aggression in a territorial songbird, the violet-eared waxbill (Estrildidae: *Uraeginthus granatina*). *Gen. Comp. Endocrinol.* 111, 233–244.

Goodson, J. L. (2005). The vertebrate social behavior network: evolutionary themes and variations. *Horm. Behav.* 48, 11–22.

Goodson, J. L. (2008). Nonapeptides and the evolutionary patterning of sociality. *Prog. Brain Res.* 170, 3–15.

Goodson, J. L., and Adkins-Regan, E. (1999). Effect of intraseptal vasotocin and vasoactive intestinal polypeptide infusions on courtship song and aggression in the male zebra finch (*Taeniopygia guttata*). *J. Neuroendocrinol.* 11, 19–25.

Goodson, J. L., and Bass, A. H. (2001). Social behavior functions and related anatomical characteristics of vasotocin/vasopressin systems in vertebrates. *Brain Res. Rev.* 35, 246–265.

Goodson, J. L., Eibach, R., Sakata, J., and Adkins-Regan, E. (1999). Effect of septal lesions on male song and aggression in the colonial zebra finch (*Taeniopygia guttata*) and the territorial field sparrow (*Spizella pusilla*). *Behav. Brain Res.* 98, 167–180.

Goodson, J. L., and Evans, A. K. (2004). Neural responses to territorial challenge and nonsocial stress in male song sparrows: segregation, integration, and modulation by a vasopressin V1 antagonist. *Horm. Behav.* 46, 371–381.

Goodson, J. L., Evans, A. K., Lindberg, L., and Allen, C. D. (2005a). Neuro-evolutionary patterning of sociality. *Proc. R. Soc. Lond., B, Biol. Sci.* 272, 227–235.

Goodson, J. L., Evans, A. K., and Soma, K. K. (2005b). Neural responses to aggressive challenge correlate with behavior in nonbreeding sparrows. *Neuroreport* 16, 1719–1723.

Goodson, J. L., Evans, A. K., and Wang, Y. (2006). Neuropeptide binding reflects convergent and divergent evolution in species-typical group sizes. *Horm. Behav.* 50, 223–236.

Goodson, J. L., and Kabelik, D. (2009). Dynamic limbic networks and social diversity in vertebrates: from neural context to neuromodulatory patterning. *Front. Neuroendocrinol.* 30:4. doi: 10.1016/j.yfrne.2009.05.007

Goodson, J. L., Kabelik, D., Kelly, A. M., Rinaldi, J., and Klatt, J. D. (2009a). Midbrain dopamine neurons reflect affiliation phenotypes in finches and are tightly coupled to courtship. *Proc. Natl. Acad. Sci. U.S.A.* 106, 8737–8742.

Goodson, J. L., Rinaldi, J., and Kelly, A. M. (2009b). Vasotocin neurons in the bed nucleus of the stria terminalis preferentially process social information and exhibit properties that dichotomize courting and non-courting phenotypes. *Horm. Behav.* 55, 197–202.

Goodson, J. L., Schrock, S. E., Klatt, J. D., Kabelik, D., and Kingsbury, M. A. (2009c). Mesotocin and nonapeptide receptors promote estrildid flocking behavior. *Science* 325, 862–866.

Goodson, J. L., Lindberg, L., and Johnson, P. (2004). Effects of central vasotocin and mesotocin manipulations on social behavior in male and female zebra finches. *Horm. Behav.* 45, 136–143.

Goodson, J. L., and Thompson, R. R. (2010). Nonapeptide mechanisms of social cognition, behavior and species-specific social systems. *Curr. Opin. Neurobiol.* 20, 784–794.

Goodson, J. L., and Wang, Y. (2006). Valence-sensitive neurons exhibit divergent functional profiles in gregarious and asocial species. *Proc. Natl. Acad. Sci. U.S.A.* 103, 17013–17017.

Goodwin, D. (1982). *Estrildid Finches of the World.* Ithaca, NY: Cornell University Press.

Hahn, T. P., and MacDougall-Shackleton, S. A. (2008). Adaptive specialization, conditional plasticity and phylogenetic history in the reproductive cue response systems of birds. *Philos. Trans. R. Soc. Lond., B, Biol. Sci.* 363, 267–286.

Harrison, C. J. O. (1962). An ethological comparison of some waxbills (Estrildini) and its relevance to their taxonomy. *Proc. Zool. Soc. Lond.* 139, 261–282.

Herdegen, T., and Leah, J. D. (1998). Inducible and constitutive transcription factors in the mammalian nervous system: control of gene expression by Jun, Fos and Krox, and CREB/ATF proteins. *Brain Res. Rev.* 28, 370–490.

Ho, J. M., Murray, J. H., Demas, G. E., and Goodson, J. L. (2010). Vasopressin cell groups exhibit strongly divergent responses to copulation and male-male interactions in mice. *Horm. Behav.* 58, 368–377.

Hoyle, C. H. V. (1999). Neuropeptide families and their receptors: evolutionary perspectives. *Brain Res.* 848, 1–25.

Immelmann, K. (1965). *Australian Finches in Bush and Aviary.* Sydney: Angus and Robertson.

Insel, T. R. (2010). The challenge of translation in social neuroscience: a review of oxytocin, vasopressin, and affiliative behavior. *Neuron* 65, 768–779.

Insel, T. R., Gelhard, R., and Shapiro, L. E. (1991). The comparative distribution of forebrain receptors for neurohypophyseal peptides in monogamous and polygamous mice. *Neuroscience* 43, 623–630.

Insel, T. R., Wang, Z. X., and Ferris, C. F. (1994). Patterns of brain vasopressin receptor distribution associated with social organization in microtine rodents. *J. Neurosci.* 14, 5381–5392.

Kabelik, D., Klatt, J. D., Kingsbury, M. A., and Goodson, J. L. (2009). Endogenous vasotocin exerts context-dependent behavioral effects in a semi-naturalistic colony environment. *Horm. Behav.* 56, 101–107.

Kabelik, D., Morrison, J. A., and Goodson, J. L. (2010). Cryptic regulation of vasotocin neuronal activity but not anatomy by sex steroids and social stimuli in opportunistic desert finches. *Brain Behav. Evol.* 75, 71–84.

Kelly, A. M., Kingsbury, M. A., Hoffbuhr, K., Schrock, S. E., Waxman, B., Kabelik, D., Thompson, R. R., and Goodson, J. L. (2011). Vasotocin neurons and septal V1a-like receptors potently modulate finch flocking and responses to novelty. *Horm. Behav.* doi: 10.1016/j.yhbeh.2011.01.012. [Epub ahead of print].

King, J. A. (ed.). (1968). *Biology of Peromyscus (Rodentia).* Stillwater, MN: American Society of Mammalogists.

Kingsbury, M. A., Kelly, A. K., Schrock, S. E., and Goodson, J. L. (2011). Mammal-like organization of the avian midbrain central gray and a reappraisal of the intercollicular nucleus. *PLoS ONE* (in press).

Kollack-Walker, S., Watson, S. J., and Akil, H. (1997). Social stress in hamsters: defeat activates specific neurocircuits within the brain. *J. Neurosci.* 17, 8842–8855.

Krause, J., and Ruxton, G. D. (2002). *Living in Groups.* Oxford: Oxford University Press.

Lei, K., Cushing, B. S., Musatov, S., Ogawa, S., and Kramer, K. M. (2010). Estrogen receptor-alpha in the bed nucleus of the stria terminalis regulates social affiliation in male prairie voles (*Microtus ochrogaster*). *PLoS ONE* 5, e8931. doi: 10.1371/journal.pone.0008931

Ludwig, M., and Leng, G. (2006). Dendritic peptide release and peptide-dependent behaviours. *Nat. Rev. Neurosci.* 7, 126–136.

Maney, D. L., and Ball, G. F. (2003). Fos-like immunoreactivity in catecholaminergic brain nuclei after territorial behavior in free-living song sparrows. *J. Neurobiol.* 56, 163–170.

Maney, D. L., Goode, C. T., Lange, H. S., Sanford, S. E., and Solomon, B. L. (2008). Estradiol modulates neural responses to song in a seasonal songbird. *J. Comp. Neurol.* 511, 173–186.

Martinez-Garcia, F., Novejarque, A., and Lanuza, E. (2008). Two interconnected functional systems in the amygdala of amniote vertebrates. *Brain Res. Bull.* 75, 206–213.

Mayr, E. (1968). The sequence of genera in the Estrildidae (Aves). *Breviora* 287, 1–14.

McGraw, L. A., and Young, L. J. (2010). The prairie vole: an emerging model organism for understanding the social brain. *Trends Neurosci.* 33, 103–109.

Moller, A. P., and Birkhead, T. R. (1993). Cuckoldry and sociality: a comparative study in birds. *Am. Nat.* 142, 118–140.

Moore, F. L., and Lowry, C. A. (1998). Comparative neuroanatomy of vasotocin and vasopressin in amphibians and other vertebrates. *Comp. Biochem. Physiol. C Pharmacol. Toxicol. Endocrinol.* 119, 251–260.

Morris, D. (1958). The comparative ethology of grassfinches (Erythrurae) and mannikins (Amadinae). *Proc. Zool. Sci. Lond.* 131, 389–439.

Motta, S. C., Goto, M., Gouveia, F. V., Baldo, M. V. C., Canteras, N. S., and Swanson, L. W. (2009). Dissecting the brain's fear system reveals the hypothalamus is critical for responding in subordinate conspecific intruders. *Proc. Natl. Acad. Sci. U.S.A.* 106, 4870–4875.

Neumann, I. D. (2009). The advantage of social living: brain neuropeptides mediate the beneficial consequences of sex and motherhood. *Front. Neuroendocrinol.* 30:4. doi: 10.1016/j.yfrne.2009.04.012

Newman, S. W. (1999). The medial extended amygdala in male reproductive behavior: a node in the mammalian social behavior network. *Ann. N. Y. Acad. Sci.* 877, 242–257.

Nishijo, H., Ono, T., and Nishino, H. (1988). Single neuron responses in amygdala of alert monkey during complex sensory stimulation with affective significance. *J. Neurosci.* 8, 3570–3583.

Northcutt, R. G. (2008). Forebrain evolution in bony fishes. *Brain Res. Bull.* 75, 191–205.

Olazábal, D. E., and Young, L. J. (2006). Species and individual differences in juvenile female alloparental care are associated with oxytocin receptor density in the striatum and the lateral septum. *Horm. Behav.* 49, 681–687.

Ophir, A. G., Zheng, D.-J., Eans, S., and Phelps, S. M. (2009). Social investigation in a memory task relates to natural variation in septal expression of oxytocin receptor and vasopressin receptor 1a in prairie voles (*Microtus ochrogaster*). *Behav. Neurosci.* 123, 979–991.

Paton, J. J., Belova, M. A., Morrison, S. E., and Salzman, C. D. (2006). The primate amygdala represents the positive and negative value of visual stimuli during learning. *Nature* 439, 865–870.

Payne, R. B. (1998). A new species of firefinch *Lagonosticta* from northern Nigeria and its association with the Jos Plateau indigobird *Vidua maryae. Ibis* 140, 368–381.

Pollen, A. A., and Hofmann, H. A. (2008). Beyond neuroanatomy: novel approaches to studying brain evolution. *Brain Behav. Evol.* 72, 145–158.

Ross, H. E., and Young, L. J. (2009). Oxytocin and the neural mechanisms regulating social cognition and affiliative behavior. *Front. Neuroendocrinol.* 30:4. doi: 10.1016/j.yfrne.2009.05.004

Sheehan, T. P., Paul, M., Amaral, E., Numan, M. J., and Numan, M. (2001). Evidence that the medial amygdala projects to the anterior/ventromedial hypothalamic nuclei to inhibit maternal behavior in rats. *Neuroscience* 106, 341–356.

Sikdar, M., Kar, A., and Prakash, P. (1992). Role of humidity in the seasonal reproduction of male spotted munia, *Lonchura punctulata. J. Exp. Zool.* 264, 82–84.

Silk, J. B. (2007). The adaptive value of sociality in mammalian groups. *Philos. Trans. R. Soc. Lond., B, Biol. Sci.* 362, 539–559.

Skead, D. M. (1975). Ecological studies of four estrildines in the central Transvaal. *Ostrich* 11 (Suppl.), 1–55.

Sorenson, M. D., Balakrishnan, C. N., and Payne, R. B. (2004). Clade-limited colonization in brood parasitic finches (*Vidua* spp.). *Syst. Biol.* 53, 140–153.

Tamarin, R. H. (ed.). (1985). *Biology of New World Microtus.* Stillwater, OK: American Society of Mammalogists.

Tessmar-Raible, K., Raible, F., Christodoulou, F., Guy, K., Rembold, M., Hausen, H., and Arendt, D. (2007). Conserved sensory-neurosecretory cell types in annelid and fish forebrain: insights into hypothalamus evolution. *Cell* 129, 1389–1400.

Trainor, B. C., Greiwe, K. M., and Nelson, R. J. (2006). Individual differences in estrogen receptor α in select brain nuclei are associated with individual differences in aggression. *Horm. Behav.* 50, 338–345.

Trainor, B. C., Lin, S., Finy, M. S., Rowland, M. R., and Nelson, R. J. (2007). Photoperiod reverses the effects of estrogens on male aggression via genomic and nongenomic pathways. *Proc. Natl. Acad. Sci. U.S.A.* 104, 9840–9845.

Turner, L. M., Young, A. R., Rompler, H., Schoneberg, T., Phelps, S. M., and Hoekstra, H. E. (2010). Monogamy evolves through multiple mechanisms: evidence from V1aR in deer mice. *Mol. Biol. Evol.* 27, 1269–1278.

Veenema, A. H., and Neumann, I. D. (2008). Central vasopressin and oxytocin release: regulation of complex social behaviours. *Prog. Brain Res.* 170, 261–276.

Zann, R. A. (1996). *The Zebra Finch: A Synthesis of Field and Laboratory Studies.* Oxford: Oxford University Press.

Ziegler, A. P. (1971). Habitat and breeding of the grey-headed olive-back *Nesocharis capistrata* in northern Uganda. *Ibis* 113, 238–240.

Conflict of Interest Statement: The authors declare that the research was conducted in the absence of any commercial or financial relationships that could be construed as a potential conflict of interest.

4

Ontogenetic distribution of the transcription factor Nkx2.2 in the developing forebrain of *Xenopus laevis*

Laura Domínguez, Agustín González and Nerea Moreno*

Faculty of Biology, Department of Cell Biology, University Complutense of Madrid, Madrid, Spain

Edited by:
Fernando Martinez-Garcia, Universidad de Valencia, Spain

Reviewed by:
Loreta Medina, Universidad de Lleida, Spain
Isabel Rodríguez-Moldes, University of Santiago de Compostela, Spain

***Correspondence:**
Nerea Moreno, Faculty of Biology, Department of Cell Biology, University Complutense of Madrid, C/José Antonio Novais 2, Madrid E-28040, Spain.
e-mail: nerea@bio.ucm.es

The expression of the Nkx2.2 gene is involved in the organization of the alar-basal boundary in the forebrain of vertebrates. Its expression in different diencephalic and telencephalic regions, helped to define distinct progenitor domains in mouse and chick. Here we investigated the pattern of Nkx2.2 protein distribution throughout the development of the forebrain of the anuran amphibian, *Xenopus laevis*. We used immunohistochemical and *in situ* hybridization techniques for its detection in combination with other essential territorial markers in the forebrain. No expression was observed in the telencephalon. In the alar hypothalamus, Nkx2.2 positive cells were scattered in the suprachiasmatic territory, but also in the supraopto-paraventricular area, as defined by the expression of the transcription factor Orthopedia (Otp) and the lack of xDll4. In the basal hypothalamus Nkx2.2 expressing cells were localized in the tuberal region, with the exception of the arcuate nucleus, rich in Otp expressing cells. In the diencephalon it was expressed in all three prosomeres (P1–P3) and not in the *zona limitans intrathalamica*. The presence of Nkx2.2 expressing cells in P3 was restricted to the alar portion, as well as in prosomere P2, whereas in P1 the Nkx2.2 expressing cells were located in the basal plate and identified the alar/basal boundary. These results showed that Nkx2.2 and Sonic hedgehog are expressed in parallel adjacent stripes along the anterior–posterior axis. The results of this study showed a conserved distribution pattern of Nkx2.2 among vertebrates, crucial to recognize subdivisions that are otherwise indistinct, and supported the relevance of this transcription factor in the organization of the forebrain, particularly in the delineation of the alar/basal boundary of the forebrain.

Keywords: prosencephalon, hypothalamus, *in situ* hybridization, evolution, forebrain patterning, thalamus

INTRODUCTION

During the last 10 years our understanding of the organization of the developing forebrain has dramatically changed, in part as a consequence of the impressive number of morphological, chemoarchitectonic, embryological, and, primarily, genoarchitectonic data. In most of the recent studies, the columnar conception of the brain organization (Herrick, 1910) has been frequently challenged by the interpretation of the data in a current prosomeric model (Puelles and Rubenstein, 1993, 2003), which is emerging as the most useful tool in the evolutionary genoarchitectonic analysis. In this scheme, a prosomere, as all neural segments, is composed of four longitudinal zones: roof, alar plate, basal plate, and floor. Their boundaries are defined by molecular patterns and cellular fates commonly established by dorso-ventral patterning of the forebrain wall (Puelles and Rubenstein, 1993, 2003) that show an impressive grade of conservation across vertebrates in morphological and gene expression terms (Puelles et al., 2000; Bachy et al., 2001, 2002; Brox et al., 2003, 2004; Moreno et al., 2003, 2004, 2005, 2008a,b, 2010; Osorio et al., 2005, 2006; Flames et al., 2007; Bardet et al. 2008, 2010; García-Lopez et al., 2008; Abellán and Medina, 2009; Ferran et al., 2009; Domínguez et al., 2010; Morona et al., 2011).

In this scenario, the expressions of key patterning genes involved both in regional and cellular specification processes are currently being analyzed in detail in the main vertebrate models, in order to establish precise traits of the forebrain evolution. Among these developmental regulators is Nkx2.2, a member of the vertebrate homeodomain transcription factor gene family homologous to the Drosophila NK2/ventral nervous system defective (vnd) gene (Kim and Nirenberg, 1989; Price et al., 1992; Jiménez et al., 1995). It was originally identified as a gene that is expressed in ventral regions of the developing vertebrate central nervous system (Price et al., 1992), and is closely related to Sonic hedgehog (Shh), a powerful morphogen that controls progenitor proliferation, regional patterning, and cell fate in the developing brain (for review see Fuccillo et al., 2006). It is involved in a wide range of regionalization mechanisms including the early specification of progenitor cell identity and cell fate processes in the ventral neural tube, in response to graded Shh signaling (Briscoe and Ericson, 1999; Briscoe et al., 2000). It is also implicated in the establishment of the alar-basal boundary (Puelles and Rubenstein, 1993; Vieira et al., 2005) and in the specification of the diencephalic patterning, helping to define distinct progenitor domains (Ericson et al., 1997; Vue et al., 2007; Kataoka and Shimogori, 2008; Ferran et al., 2009).

Most of the data about Nkx2.2 expression in the forebrain were obtained in amniotes, primarily mouse, and chick, and only fragmentary data on Nkx2.2 expression have been reported in anamniotes, especially fishes and amphioxus (Holland et al., 1998; Schäfer et al., 2005). Surprisingly, the expression of Nkx2.2 has not been analyzed in the forebrain of amphibians, which constitute the only anamniote group of tetrapods. Of interest, in numerous recent studies it is shown that the forebrain organization in amphibians shares many key features with amniotes, mainly in terms of genetic specification, as revealed when the prosomeric paradigm is used in the interpretation of many territorial gene expression patterns (Bachy et al., 2001, 2002; Brox et al., 2003, 2004; Moreno et al., 2004, 2008a,b; van den Akker et al., 2008; Domínguez et al., 2010; Morona et al., 2011). In particular, we have recently reported the distribution of xShh in the forebrain of the anuran amphibian *Xenopus laevis* during development (Domínguez et al., 2010) and, following this line of research, herein we have analyzed the pattern of distribution of Nkx2.2, a functionally and anatomically related transcription factor in vertebrates. The comparative analysis, following the prosomeric model, serves to assess evolutionary trends. We have characterized phenotypically the developing Nkx2.2 expressing forebrain subdivisions and neurons by means of the combination of Nkx2.2 expression with forebrain essential regulators and markers, such as Nkx2.1, Tbr1, Pax6, GABA, Pax7, Orthopedia (Otp), xDll4, xShh, tyrosine hydroxylase (TH), mesotocin (MST), and somatostatin (SOM). The results of this study showed an extremely conserved distribution pattern of Nkx2.2 among vertebrates, crucial to delineate subdivisions that were otherwise indistinct, and supported the relevance of this transcription factor in the establishment and organization of the forebrain.

MATERIALS AND METHODS

ANIMALS AND TISSUE PROCESSING

For the present study, adults, juveniles, and tadpoles of *X. laevis* were used. Embryos and larvae were classified according to Nieuwkoop and Faber (1967). Embryonic (42–45), premetamorphic (46–52), prometamorphic (53–58), and metamorphic (59–65) stages were used, minimizing as much as possible the number of animals used. All animals were treated according to the regulations and laws of the European Union (86/609/EEC) and Spain (Royal Decrees 1201/2005) for care and handling of animals in research, after approval from the University to conduct the experiments described.

Adult *Xenopus* were purchased from commercial suppliers (Xenopus Express; France), and the different developing specimens were obtained by *in vitro* fertilization and maintained in tap water at 20°C throughout their development. At appropriate times, embryos and larvae were deeply anesthetized in a 0.4-mg/ml solution of tricaine methanesulfonate (MS222, Sigma-Aldrich, Steinheim, Germany). The adults, juveniles, and late larvae were perfused transcardially with 0.9% sodium chloride, followed by cold 4% paraformaldehyde in a 0.1-M phosphate buffer (PB, pH 7.4). The brains were removed and kept in the same fixative for 2–3 h. Subsequently, they were immersed in a solution of 30% sucrose in PB for 4–6 h at 4°C until they sank, embedded in a solution of 20% gelatin with 30% sucrose in PB, and stored for 6 h in a 3.7% formaldehyde solution at 4°C. The brains were cut on a freezing microtome at 40 μm (adults) or 20–30 μm (juveniles and late larvae) in the transverse or sagittal plane and sections were collected and rinsed in cold PB. The embryos and premetamorphic larvae were fixed by immersion overnight at 4°C in MEMFA [0.1 M MOPS (4-morpholinopropanesulfonic acid) 2 mM ethyleneglycoltetraacetic acid, 1 mM $MgSO_4$, 3.7% formaldehyde], then they were processed *in toto* and finally sectioned at 14–16 μm thickness in the transverse, horizontal, or sagittal plane on a freezing microtome.

IMMUNOCHEMISTRY

Single immunohistochemistry for Nkx2.2

A immunohistofluorescence procedure was conducted with the primary antibody on the free-floating sections that, in all cases, was diluted in 5–10% normal serum of the species in which the secondary antibody was raised in PB with 0.1% Triton X-100 (Sigma) and 2% bovine serum albumin (BSA, Sigma). The protocol included two steps, as follows: (1) Incubation for 72 h at 4°C in the dilution of the primary antibody mouse anti-Nkx2.2 (1:500; Developmental Studies Hybridoma Bank, DSHB, Iowa City, USA. Clone: 74.5A5) and (2) the second incubation was conducted for 90 min at room temperature with the labeled secondary antibody Alexa 488-conjugated goat anti-mouse (1:500; Molecular Probes; catalog reference: A21042). After being rinsed, the sections were mounted on glass slides and coverslipped with Vectashield mounting medium (Vector Laboratories, Burlingame, CA, USA; catalog number: H1000).

Double immunohistochemistry for Nkx2.2/Otp, Nkx2.2/MST, Nkx2.2/SOM, Nkx2.2/Nkx2.1, Nkx2.2/Tbr1, Nkx2.2/TH, Nkx2.2/Pax6, and Nkx2.2/GABA

The cocktails of primary antibodies were diluted in PB with 0.1% Triton X-100 and used for 60 h at 4°C. They always included mouse anti-Nkx2.2 (1:500; DSHB) in combination with: rabbit anti-Otp (1:1000; produced by "PickCell laboratories" Amsterdam, The Netherlands; according to the protocol described in Lin et al., 1999), rabbit anti-MST (diluted 1:2000; donated by Dr. J. M. Guerné Université de Strasbourg, France), rabbit anti-SOM (1:1000; Incstar, Wisconsin, USA, Code number: 20067), rabbit anti-Nkx2.1 (1:500; Biopat Immunotechnologies, Italy, Code number: PA0100), rabbit anti-Tbr1 (1:250; Santa Cruz Biotechnology, Inc., USA, Code number: sc-48816), rabbit anti-TH (diluted 1:1000; Chemicon International, Inc., USA, Code number: P22941), rabbit anti-Pax6 (1:200; Covance, California, USA, Code number: PBR-278P), and rabbit anti-GABA (1:3000; Sigma-Aldrich, Steinheim, Germany, Code number: A2052). The secondary antibodies were used in appropriated combinations and were: Alexa 488-conjugated goat anti-mouse (1:500, Molecular Probes) and Alexa 594-conjugated goat anti-rabbit (1:500, Molecular Probes; catalog number: A11012). In all cases, secondary antibodies were diluted in PB with 0.1% Triton X-100 for 90 min at room temperature. After rinsing, the sections were mounted on glass slides and coverslipped with Vectashield.

IN SITU HYBRIDIZATION

Double labeling with in situ hybridization and immunohistochemistry: Nkx2.2/xShh and Nkx2.2/xDll4

For double histofluorescence labeling experiments, we combined the immunohistochemistry for Nkx2.2 with *in situ* hybridization for the following markers: xShh (provided by Dr. Randal Moon. University of Washington; Ekker et al., 1995) and xDll4 (provided by Dr. Nancy Papalopulu. University of Manchester; Papalopulu and Kintner, 1993).

For *in situ* hybridization, which was performed first, antisense digoxigenin (DIG)-labeled riboprobes for these markers were synthesized according to the protocol described in Bachy et al. (2001), linearizing the clones in Bluescript KS with Bam H1 (Promega, Madison, USA) and transcribing with T3 (Promega) for xShh, with Not1 (Promega, Madison, USA) and T3 (Promega) for xDll4. The embryos and premetamorphic larvae were processed *in toto* after progressive rehydration and pretreatments (see Bachy et al., 2001), and the late larvae were processed in floating sections (see Moreno et al., 2004).

Hybridization step was done with 3 μl/ml of a DIG-labeled RNA probe, in a 50% formamide containing medium overnight at 55°C. The solution used for prehybridization (at 60°C for 1 h) and hybridization contained 50% deionized formamide (Fluka, Steinheim, Germany), 5× standard saline citrate (Sigma-Aldrich, Steinheim, Germany), 2% blocking reagent (Roche Diagnostics, Mannheim, Germany), 0.1% Tween-20, 0.5% 3-[(3-cholamidopropyl)-dimethylammonio]-1-propanesulfonate (CHAPS; Sigma-Aldrich), 1 mg/ml of yeast tRNA (Sigma-Aldrich), 5 mM of ethylenediaminetetraacetic acid (Sigma-Aldrich), and 50 g/ml of heparin (Sigma-Aldrich) in water.

Hybridization was detected using an alkaline phosphatase coupled anti-DIG antibody (Roche Diagnostics, dilution 1:1500). Alkaline phosphatase staining was developed with Fast red tablets (Roche Diagnostics). The *in situ* hybridization was followed by the immunohistochemistry for mouse anti-Nkx2.2 (1:500; DSHB) revealed with Alexa 488-conjugated goat anti-mouse (diluted 1:500, Molecular Probes). Subsequently, embryos and early larvae were immersed in a solution of 30% sucrose in PB until they sank, embedded in a solution of 20% gelatin and 30% sucrose in PB, and stored overnight at 4°C in a solution of 4% formaldehyde and 30% sucrose in PB. Sections were cut at 14–25 μm thickness in the frontal, sagittal, and horizontal plane on a freezing microtome.

IMAGING

The sections were analyzed with an Olympus BX51 microscope that was equipped for fluorescence with appropriate filter combinations. Selected sections were photographed by using a digital camera (Olympus DP72). Contrast and brightness of the photomicrographs were adjusted in Adobe PhotoShop CS3 (Adobe Systems, San Jose, CA) and figures were mounted in Canvas 11 (ACD Systems, Canada).

RESULTS

The distribution of the Nkx2.2 protein has been analyzed in the prosencephalon of *X. laevis* from embryonic stages through the adult. In the following sections we analyze, using both immunohistochemistry and *in situ* hybridization procedures, the spatio-temporal sequence of Nkx2.2 expression during forebrain development in single (**Figure 1**) and double (**Figures 2–5**) stained material. All of the markers used in combination with Nkx2.2 have been previously used in the analysis of the *Xenopus* forebrain development, and the nomenclature used in the present study largely follows that used in our preceding mapping studies of the anuran forebrain (Moreno et al., 2004, 2008a,b; Morona and González, 2008; Domínguez et al., 2010; Morona et al., 2011). A schematic representation of the Nkx2.2 distribution in the case of the early (premetamorphic) forebrain is shown in **Figure 6**.

Nkx2.2 DISTRIBUTION IN THE DEVELOPING PROSENCEPHALON

In *Xenopus*, Nkx2.2 immunoreactive (Nkx2.2-ir) cells were not observed in telencephalic areas, neither evaginated nor non-evaginated territories, from early developmental stages through the juvenile, when the brain morphology is close to that observed in adults (**Figure 1**).

The most anterior expression detected was observed in the hypothalamic territory, helping to the identification of the alar and basal domains (**Figures 1A–D**). Form early (**Figures 1A,B**) to late (**Figures 1C,D**) developmental stages, Nkx2.2-ir cells were observed in the supraopto-paraventricular (SPV) region of the alar hypothalamus (**Figures 1E–H**). At embryonic developmental stages (**Figure 1E**), virtually all the cells observed in the ventricular (vz) and subventricular layers (svz) of this zone were Nkx2.2-ir, whereas from early larval (**Figures 1F,G**) through juvenile stages the cells decreased notably occupying a band in the svz (**Figure 1H**). In addition, in the alar hypothalamus scattered Nkx2.2 cells were observed in the suprachiasmatic (SC) territory that became more numerous from late developmental stages and through the adulthood (**Figures 1A–D,G,H,P**). These cells formed a continuous band above the optic chiasm (oc) that was especially evident in sagittal sections (**Figures 1C,D**). In the basal hypothalamus (BH), scarce Nkx2.2-ir cells were found in the svz of the medial part of the tuberal region, whereas the most posterior portion of this basal region was devoid of Nkx2.2 positive cells (**Figures 1I–L**). Caudally, Nkx2.2 expressing cells were detected in the diencephalon, defining the midbrain-diencephalic boundary (MDB; **Figures 1A–D**) with the exception of the *zona limitans intrathalamica* (Zli), which was devoid of Nkx2.2 expression (**Figures 1A–D,M–P**). In prosomeres 2 (P2) and 3 (P3) Nkx2.2 positive cells were restricted to the alar portion (**Figures 1M–P**). At early stages of development, these cells were observed in the vz and svz of P2 and P3, respectively (**Figures 1M,N**), whereas from prometamorphic stages Nkx2.2-ir cells were only detected in the svz and mz (**Figures 1O,P**). In P1, the Nkx2.2-ir cells were located in the alar/basal boundary, representing the ventral limit of the pretectum (**Figures 1I–L**).

Nkx2.2 DISTRIBUTION IN RELATION TO PROSENCEPHALIC MARKERS

In order to further characterize the localization of Nkx2.2-ir cells within the forebrain, we carried out double labeling experiments throughout development, using different prosencephalic markers (**Figures 2–5**).

To analyze the distribution of the Nkx2.2-ir cells in the alar hypothalamus we combined Nkx2.2 with the transcription factor Orthopedia (Otp; **Figures 2A,B,E**), the neuropeptides mesotocin (MST; **Figures 2C,F**) and somatostatin (SOM; **Figure 2D**), the dopaminergic marker tyrosine hydroxylase (TH; **Figures 2G,H**), and the transcription factor xDll4 (**Figure 2I**). From early premetamorphic stages, the double staining for Nkx2.2/Otp (**Figure 2A**) defined the position of a restricted population of Nkx2.2 expressing cells in the svz of the SPV. Whereas almost all the SPV cells expressed Otp (**Figure 2B**), only a subpopulation of the SPV cells coexpressed Nkx2.2 and Otp (see arrowhead in **Figure 2B**), just in the most posterior portion of the SPV, defining the limit between the SPV and the SC (**Figures 2E,E′**). This was also confirmed by the double labeling Nkx2.2/MST (**Figure 2C**) and Nkx2.2/SOM (**Figure 2D**).

At SC levels, the double staining for Nkx2.2/MST (**Figure 2F**), Nkx2.2/TH (**Figures 2G,H**), and Nkx2.2/xDll4 (**Figure 2I**) confirmed the position of Nkx2.2-ir cells in this territory, anterior to the oc and posterior to the SPV (**Figure 2F′**). In this area, the Nkx2.2-ir cells were found in the catecholaminergic (**Figures 2G,H**) and xDll4-expressing region (**Figure 2I**). During the development the Nkx2.2 expressing cells were numerous and from the early larvae

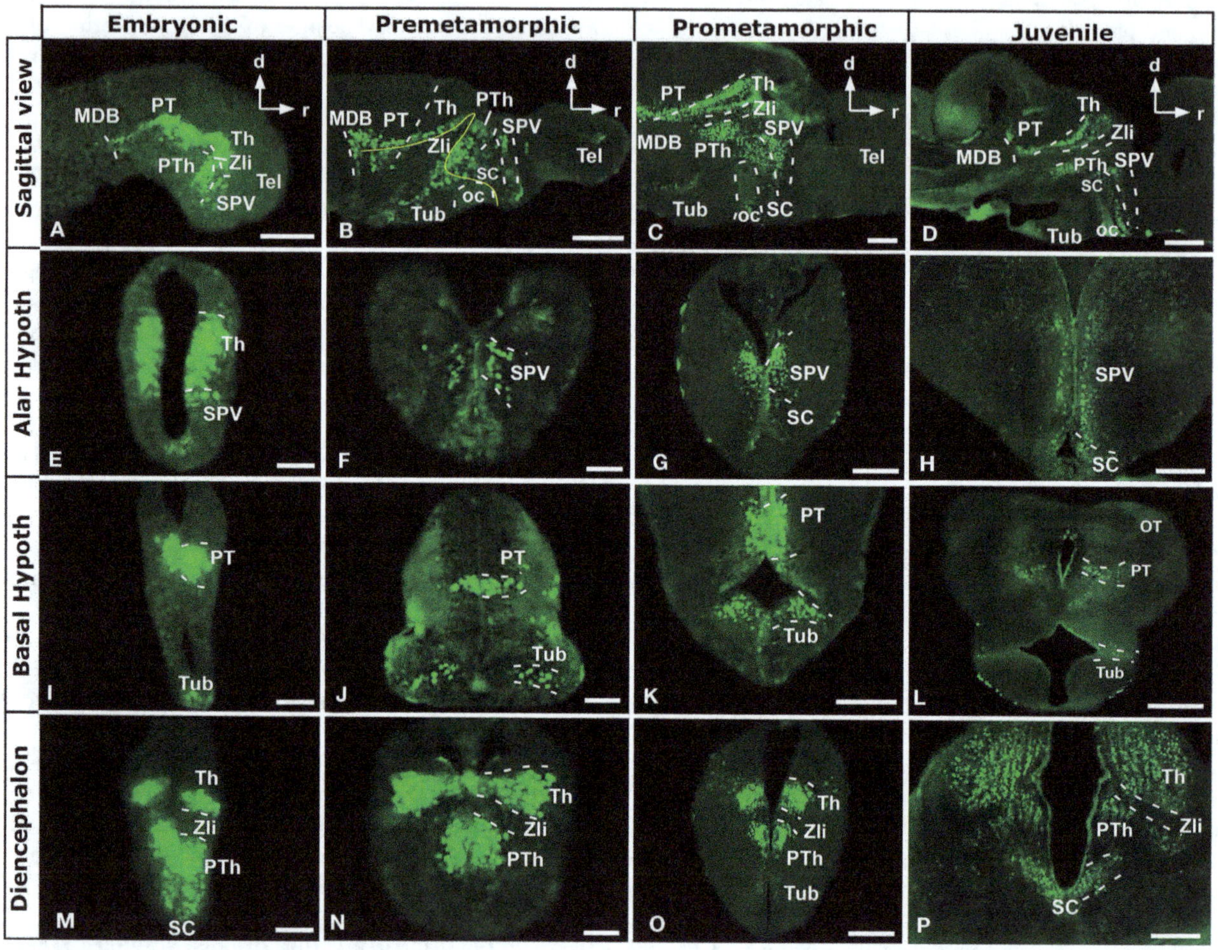

FIGURE 1 | Photomicrographs of sagittal (A–D) and transverse (E–P) sections through the *Xenopus* forebrain subdivisions along the different representative developmental stages. The sagittal sections show the almost continuous Nkx2.2 expression from anterior hypothalamic areas to the most caudal regions of the forebrain **(A–D)**. Nkx2.2 is not expressed in telencephalic areas, from embryonic stages through the adult. Nkx2.2 expression starts in the SPV territory of the alar hypothalamus **(E–H)**. In the basal hypothalamus Nkx2.2 expression is restricted to the tuberal hypothalamus **(I–L)**. In the diencephalon, Nkx2.2 is observed in the three prosomeres (P1–P3) and the Zli lacks Nkx2.2 expressing cells **(I–P)**. Abbreviations: Arc, nucleus arcuatus; BH, basal hypothalamus; MB, mammillary band; MDB, midbrain-diencephalic boundary; OB, olfactory bulb; oc, optic chiasm; OT, optic tectum; P1-P3, diencephalic prosomeres 1–3; Pa, pallium; POC, preoptic commissural area/commissural septo-preoptic area; PO, preoptic area; PT, pretectum; PTh, prethalamus; PThE, prethalamic eminence; PV, paraventricular nucleus; SC, suprachiasmatic nucleus; SPa, subpallium; SPV, supraopto-paraventricular area; Tel, telencephalon; Th, thalamus; TP, posterior tubercle; Tub, tuberal area; ZI, zona incerta; Zli, zona limitans intrathalamica. Scale bars: 500 µm **(D,L)**, 200 µm **(C,G,H,K,O,P)**, 100 µm **(A,B)**, and 50 µm **(E,F,I,J,M,N)**.

stages these cells showed a clear patterning, however it is from late developmental stages when these cells clearly formed an independent and exclusive subpopulation in the SC, situated in the ventral portion avoiding the anterior region (see asterisk in **Figure 2F′**).

From early premetamorphic stages, the double staining for Nkx2.2/Nkx2.1 (**Figure 3A**) confirmed the Nkx2.2 expression in the svz of the BH. The double staining Nkx2.2/Otp confirmed the position of Nkx2.2 positive cells in the tuberal area of the BH, but avoiding the nucleus arcuatus (Arc), and the mammillary band (MB), both rich in Otp expressing cells (**Figures 3B,C**). In addition, the lack of Nkx2.2 expression in the mammillary region was confirmed by the Nkx2.2/TH (**Figure 3D**) and Nkx2.2/xDll4 double staining (**Figure 3E**).

Caudally in the diencephalon, the banded staining pattern obtained for the pair Nkx2.2/Tbr1 confirmed the lack of Nkx2.2 expressing cells in the prethalamic eminence (PThE), rich in Tbr1 expression (**Figure 4A**), but allowed the identification of Nkx2.2-ir cells in the thalamus and prethalamus. The expression observed in the alar portion of P3 and P2 was confirmed by the double staining Nkx2.2/Pax6 (**Figure 4B**), Nkx2.2/xDll4 (**Figure 4C**), and Nkx2.2/GABA (**Figure 4D**). In addition, specifically the Nkx2.2-ir cells in P3 were noted in the zona incerta (ZI; **Figures 4E,F**), where Nkx2.1 expression is present (Moreno et al., 2008a) and a conserved catecholaminergic group is located (Smeets and González, 2000). The combination of Nkx2.2/xShh confirmed the lack of Nkx2.2 expressing cells in the *zona limitans intrathalamica* (Zli; **Figure 4G**) defined by the xShh-expression (Domínguez et al., 2010).

Finally, Nkx2.2 has been functionally related to the morphogen Shh implied in the alar-basal boundary establishment (for review see Fuccillo et al., 2006). We have recently reported the

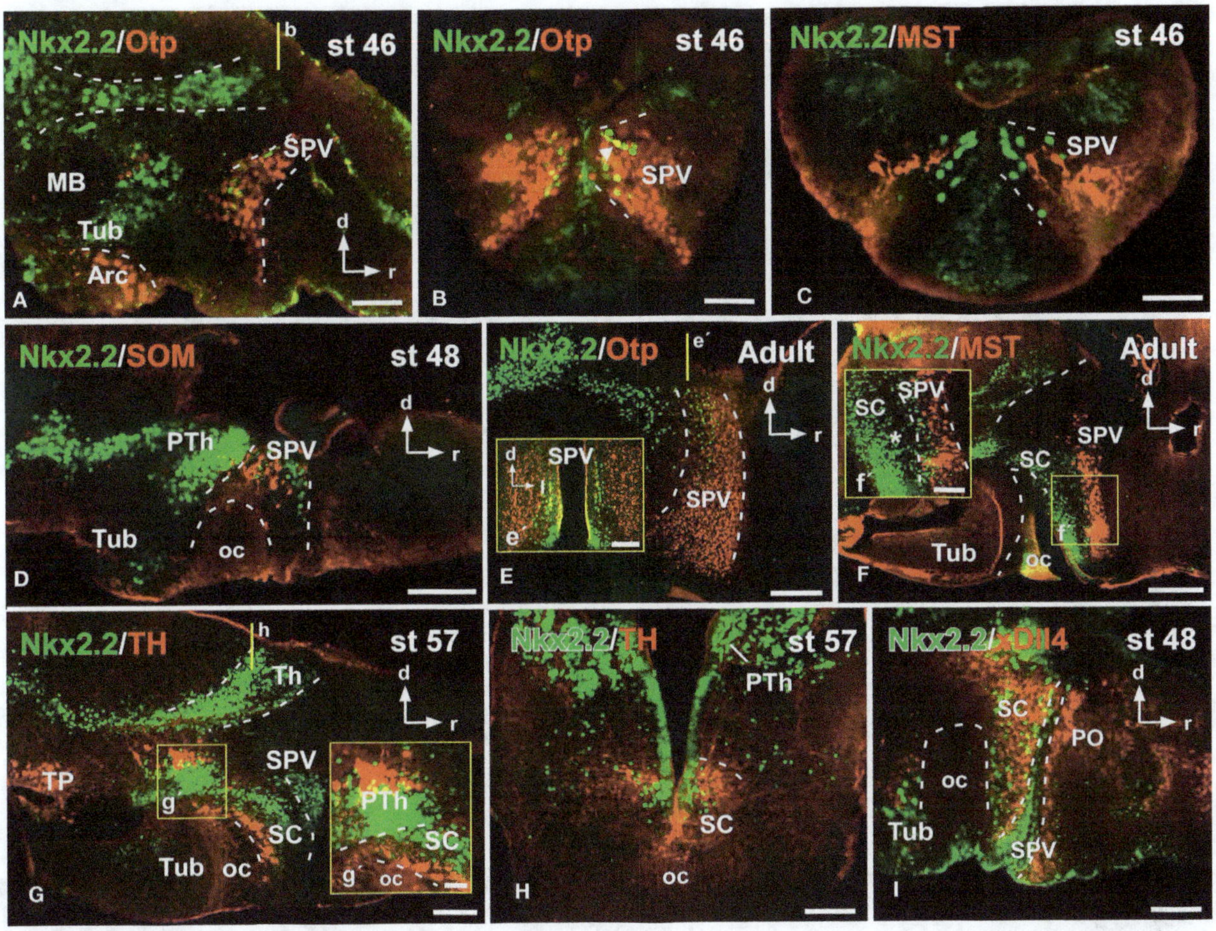

FIGURE 2 | Photomicrographs of sagittal (A,D–G,I) and transverse (B,C,E′,H) sections through the alar hypothalamus illustrating the Nkx2.2 expression in combination with several hypothalamic markers. The most anterior Nkx2.2 expressing cells are observed in the SPV (the Otp expressing territory) during development **(A,B,E,E′)**, in the region where it colocalizes with mesotocin **(C,F,F′)** and somatostatin **(D)**, but only a subpopulation of the SPV cells coexpress Nkx2.2 and Otp [see arrow in **(B,E,E′)**]. At suprachiasmatic levels, the Nkx2.2 positive cells are located in the catecholaminergic **(G,G′,H)** and xDll4 **(I)** expressing region, constituting an independent territory within this domain **(G–I)**. The yellow lines in **(A,E,G)** indicate the level of the sections of **(B,E′,H)**, respectively. Yellow boxes in **(F,G)** indicate the higher magnifications shown in **(F′,G′)**, respectively. Abbreviations as in **Figure 1**. Scale bars: 500 μm **(F)**, 200 μm **(E,E′,G)**, 100 μm **(D,H)** and 50 μm **(A,B,C,F′,G′,I)**.

precise distribution of xShh in the *Xenopus* developing forebrain (Domínguez et al., 2010) and in the present study we have analyzed the extent of the Nkx2.2 expressing cells along the entire forebrain in combination with xShh, in transverse (**Figures 5A,B**) and horizontal sections (**Figure 5C**) to analyze their relation with the *Xenopus* forebrain axis. Of note, this double labeling shows that the pattern of distribution of Nkx2.2-ir cells formed a series of bands that extended along the anterior–posterior axis in parallel to adjacent stripes labeled for xShh (**Figure 5**).

All the results obtained from the double labeling analysis confirmed the localization of the Nkx2.2-ir cells in the regions described above and summarized in **Figure 6**.

DISCUSSION

Nkx2.2 was the first gene of the NK2 homeobox class to be demonstrated in all the deuterostomes, showing homology in all the models analyzed. Even possible homologies were suggested in the nervous system between invertebrates and vertebrates given the high conservations in the expression and function of this gene (Holland et al., 1998). The presence of two paralogs, Nkx2.2a and Nkx2.2b, was demonstrated in zebrafish and phylogenetic and expression analysis suggests that these genes arose by a fish-specific gene duplication and acquired differential transcriptional control. Subsequently one paralog was lost and only the Nkx2.2a is considered ortholog of the mammal gene (Schäfer et al., 2005) and, in addition, its expression domain is very conserved. However, both paralogs are regulated by Shh (Barth and Wilson, 1995; Schäfer et al., 2005).

In general terms, in the vertebrate central nervous system Nkx2.2 has been implicated in the ventral neuronal patterning, at early developmental stages (Briscoe and Ericson, 1999), defining the alar/basal boundary along to Shh-expression (Puelles and Rubenstein, 1993; Vieira et al., 2005). This is found even in amphioxus, in which there is not obvious anatomical boundary separating alar and basal regions along the dorso-ventral axis of the cerebral vesicle (Holland et al., 1998).

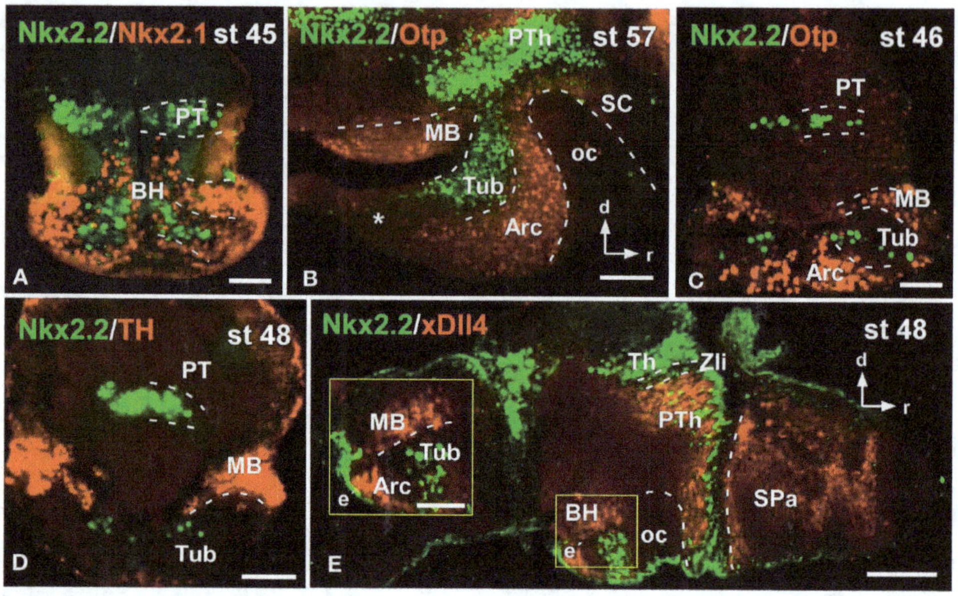

FIGURE 3 | Photomicrographs of transverse (A,C,D) and sagittal (B,E) sections through the basal hypothalamus illustrating the Nkx2.2 expression in combination with several hypothalamic markers. The Nkx2.1 expression confirms that the limited Nkx2.2 expression found in the basal hypothalamic territory is situated in the tuberal region **(A)**, restricted to the anterior part [asterisk in **(B)**] and avoiding the nucleus arcuatus, labeled for Otp **(B,C)**, and the mammillary band, defined by TH **(D)** and xDll4 **(E,E′)**. Yellow box in e indicates the area shown in higher magnification in e´. Abbreviations as in **Figure 1**. Scale bars: 100 μm **(B,E)**, 50 μm **(A,C,D,E′)**.

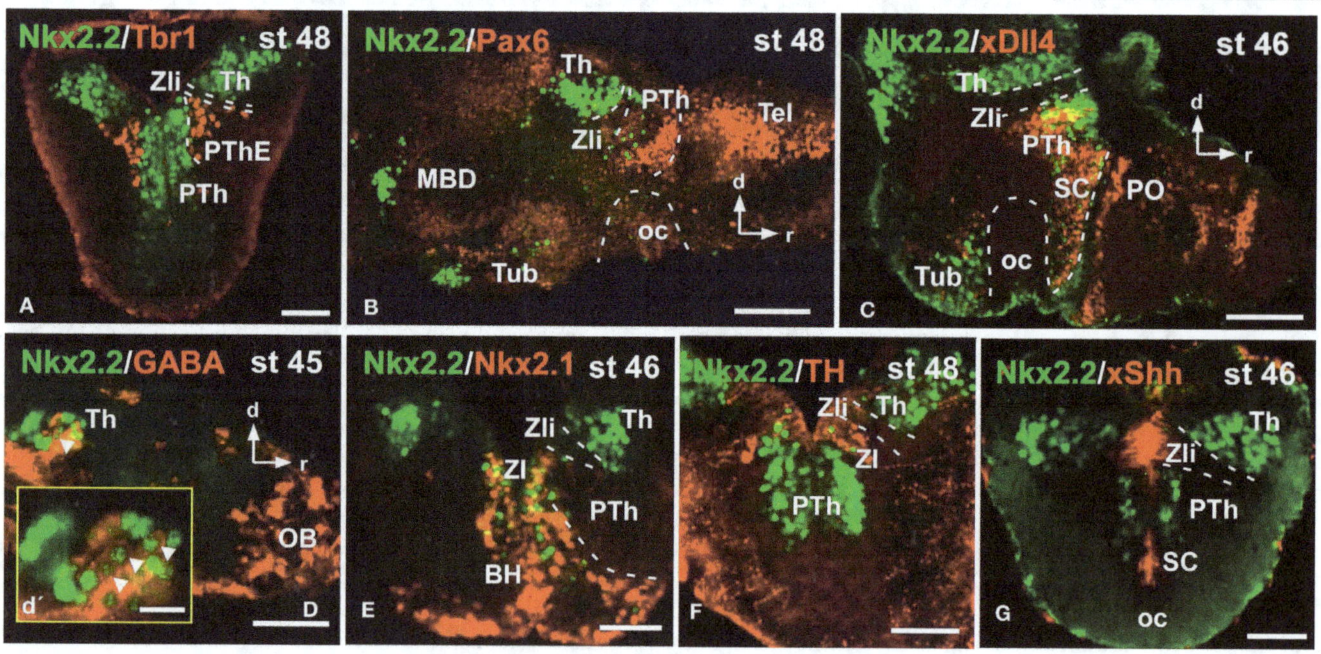

FIGURE 4 | Photomicrographs of transverse (A,E,F,G) and sagittal (B,C,D) sections through the diencephalon illustrating the Nkx2.2 expression in combination with diverse diencephalic markers. The prethalamic eminence, rich in Tbr1 **(A)**, was devoid of Nkx2.2 expression, in contrast to the prethalamus, defined by the Pax6 **(B)** and xDll4 expressions **(C)**. The yellow box in d shows a higher magnification of the Nkx2.2/GABA double labeled cells found in the thalamus [see arrowheads in **(D,D′)**]. The double labeling Nkx2.2/Nkx2.1 **(E)** and Nkx2.2/TH **(F)** define the position of the Nkx2.2 cells in the zona incerta of the prethalamus. The xShh diencephalic expression defines the lack of Nkx2.2 expression in the Zli (*zona limitans intrathalamica*) **(G)**. Abbreviations as in **Figure 1**. Scale bars: 100 μm **(B,C,D)**, 50 μm **(A,E,F,G)**, 25 μm **(D′)**.

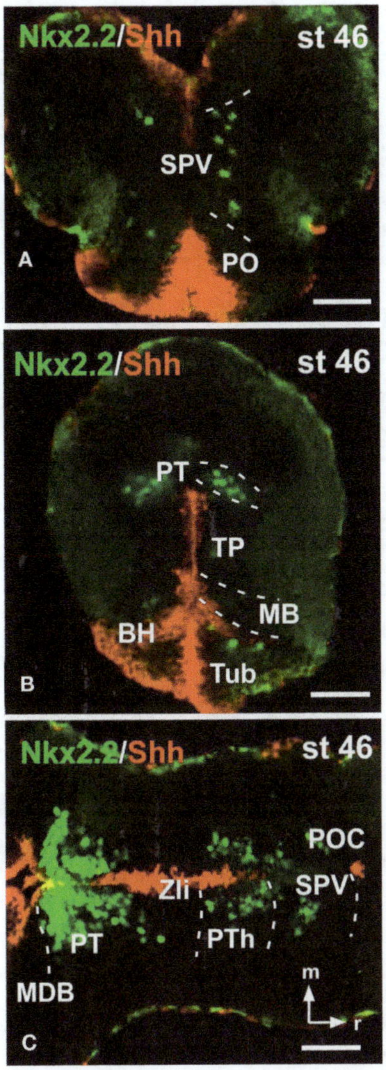

FIGURE 5 | Photomicrographs of transverse (A,B) and horizontal (C) sections through the forebrain illustrating Nkx2.2 expression in combination with xShh. The expressions of Nkx2.2 and xShh extend along the anterior–posterior axis in parallel adjacent stripes, forming longitudinal columns along the forebrain. Abbreviations as in **Figure 1**. Scale bars: 50 µm.

Nkx2.2 EXPRESSION IN THE FOREBRAIN AND COMPARISON WITH OTHER VERTEBRATES: CONSERVATIVE TRAITS AND EVOLUTIONARY IMPORTANCE

In all vertebrates analyzed Nkx2.2 is expressed in the prosencephalon where it is known to be involved in the specification of progenitor domains and in establishing regionalization patterns. Moreover, it contributes to the differentiation of distinct areas and their compartmentalization, as well as to the acquisition of cellular identity and the regulation of the distribution of the earliest neurons in the brain (Wilson et al., 1993; Barth and Wilson, 1994; Vieira and Martínez, 2006; Vue et al., 2007). Thus, the analysis in anamniote and amniote vertebrates of the spatio-temporal distribution of this transcription factor is considered of relevance in the understanding of the establishment of the different subdivisions within the forebrain and in evaluating the degree of conservation across vertebrates (Price et al., 1992; Barth and Wilson, 1995; Holland et al., 1998; Schäfer et al., 2005; Vieira and Martínez, 2006; Vue et al., 2007; Ferran et al., 2009). In the present study we have provided for the first time in amphibians a detailed analysis of its distribution in *X. laevis*, a tetrapod anamniote with a forebrain organization that in genoarchitectonic terms shares many features with its counterpart in amniotes (Bachy et al., 2001, 2002; Brox et al., 2003, 2004; Moreno et al., 2004, 2008a,b; van den Akker et al., 2008; Domínguez et al., 2010; Morona et al., 2011). To fully understand the precise topological distribution of Nkx2.2 expression, its combination with the respective expression of different forebrain markers has been shown to be extremely useful. Thus, we have analyzed the distribution of Nkx2.2 in combination with the localization of Nkx2.1, Otp, Pax6, GABA, Tbr1, TH, MST, and SOM, and *in situ* hybridization for the detection of xShh and xDll4.

The expression of Nkx2.1 has been deeply analyzed in the prosencephalon of many vertebrates and it has served to identify the preoptic (PO), SC, and tuberal territories (Tub) during development (Rohr et al., 2001; González et al., 2002a,b; Moreno et al., 2008a; van den Akker et al., 2008), like the developmental regulatory gene xDll4 (Papalopulu and Kintner, 1993; Puelles and Rubenstein, 1993; Shimamura and Rubenstein, 1997; Puelles et al., 2000; Bachy et al., 2002; Marín et al., 2002; Brox et al., 2003). In addition, the localization of TH highlighted the regionalization of the SC and the ZI in P3 (González et al., 1993, 1994; Milán and Puelles, 2000; Smeets and González, 2000). Specifically in the hypothalamus, Otp expression served in the identification of the SPV region and it also defines the Arc and the MB within the BH (Bardet et al., 2008; Domínguez et al., 2010). The presence of MST (or its homolog oxytocin) and SOM in the magnocellular neurons of the SPV is also a shared feature between amniotes and anamniotes (Bläsher and Heinrichs, 1982; González et al., 1995, 2003; Petkó and Orosz, 1996; López et al., 2007). In the diencephalon, the morphogen xShh was crucial to delimit the Zli, as well as to define the alar-basal boundary and the longitudinal columns that establish the dorso-ventral patterning (Puelles and Rubenstein, 2003; Domínguez et al., 2010). The homeobox gene Tbr1 was extremely useful in the recognition of the PThE (Puelles et al., 2000; Brox et al., 2004) and the relative expression of xDll4, Pax6, and GABA served to identify the boundaries of the three diencephalic prosomeres (Bachy et al., 2002; Brox et al., 2003; Moreno et al., 2008b; Morona et al., 2011).

Telencephalon

In mammals, the most anterior Nkx2.2 expression was observed in the medial ganglionic eminence (MGE), also called pallidal domain, which consists of, at least, five progenitor domains globally defined by the strong expression of Nkx2.1, weak expression of Nkx2.2, and lack of Pax6 and Shh-expressions (Flames et al., 2007). In the case of the chicken, three subdivisions were recently identified in the pallidal domain, comparable to those described for mammals (Abellán and Medina, 2009). In chicken, the Nkx2.2 expression was not described in detail but it seems to be weakly expressed in the subpallium (see Figures 4F,G in Vieira et al., 2005 and see Figures 1K,Q in Bardet et al., 2010) in contrast to the strong expression found in mammals (Flames et al., 2007). Differently, in

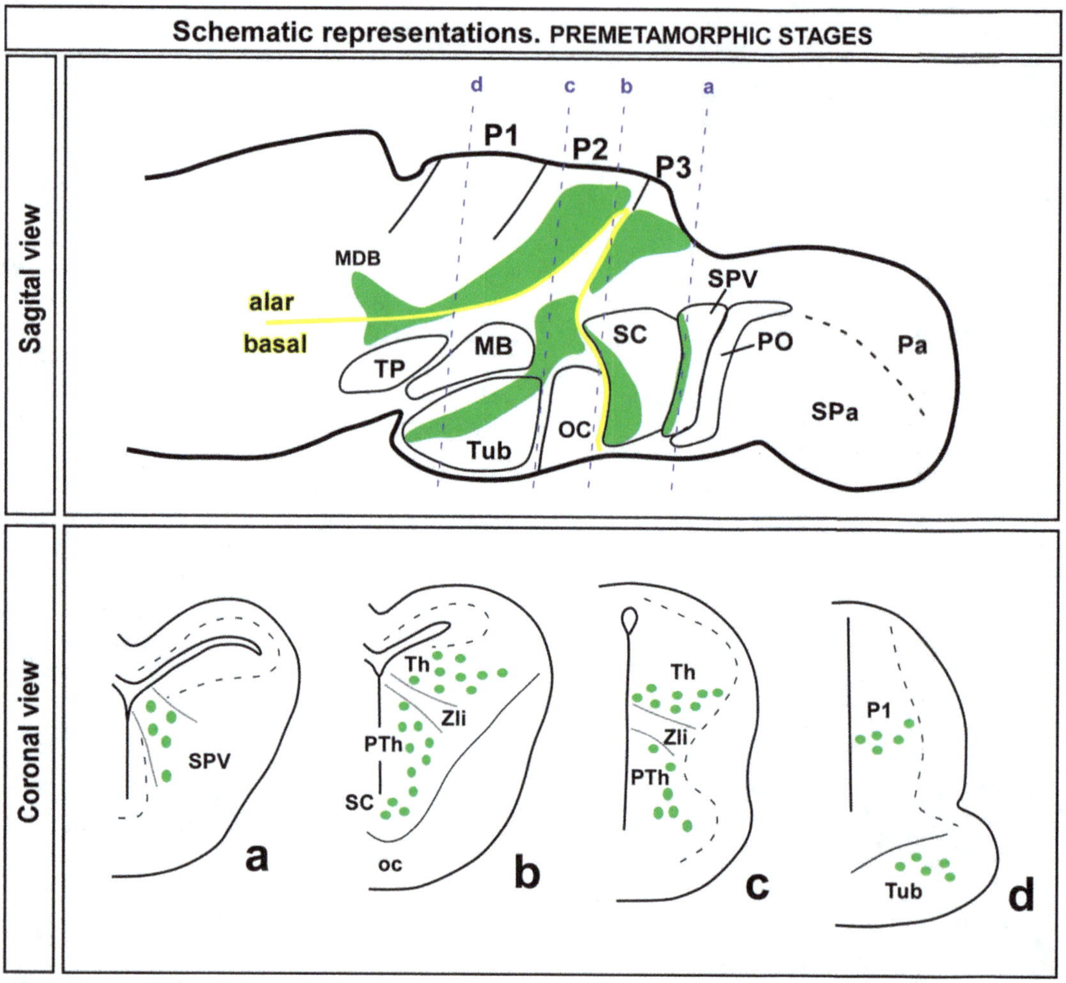

FIGURE 6 | Schematic drawings of sagittal and coronal sections through a premetamorphic brain of *Xenopus laevis* illustrating the distribution of Nkx2.2 expressing zones (green regions in the sagittal view) and cells (green dots in the coronal view) along the forebrain. The appropriated levels of the coronal sections are indicated in the sagittal view. Abbreviations as in **Figure 1**.

Xenopus (present results) and in the turtle (Moreno et al., 2010) Nkx2.2 expression has not been observed in the svz of the MGE. This interesting result might be in correlation with the presence of Shh-expression in the subventricular zone of the mouse MGE (García-Lopez et al., 2008) and chicken (Abellán and Medina, 2009) and its absence in the pallidal region of amphibians (Domínguez et al., 2010). However, Shh and Nkx2.2 are not always expressed in the same regions.

Also in the telencephalon, the PO region in mammals contains at least two distinct progenitor domains (Flames et al., 2007). The ventricular zone of the PO is uniquely defined by the simultaneous expression of Nkx2.1, Nkx2.2, and Shh, and most prominently by the lack of detectable levels of Gsh2, Lhx6, Lhx7, or Olig2 expression (Flames et al., 2007). Like in the case of the MGE, in *Xenopus* (present results) but also in turtle (Moreno et al., 2010), there is not Nkx2.2 expression in the POA. However, in this case it is not correlated with the lack of the Shh-expression, because Shh-expression is observed in the preoptocommissural area (Domínguez et al., 2010).

The boundary between the telencephalon and the hypothalamus has been recently defined, first in chicken (Bardet et al., 2006) and later in mouse (Flames et al., 2007), as the preoptohypothalamic zone (POH). It constitutes the border of the subpallium and was described by its characteristic and specific expression of Nkx2.2 as a narrow territory separating longitudinally the PO from the magnocellular hypothalamus (Bardet et al., 2006). This region contains progenitor cells that express Dlx2, Dlx5, Pax6, Olig2, and Gsh2, lacks expression of Nkx2.1, Shh, Nkx6.2, and Dbx1 and can be further subdivided into two areas because the POH1, but not the POH2, expresses high levels of Nkx2.2 in mammals (Flames et al., 2007; Bardet et al., 2010). In *Xenopus*, Nkx2.2 expression is not detected in a comparable region, given that the most anterior expression found coincides with the Otp SPV expressing zone within the hypothalamus (see below).

Hypothalamus

The hypothalamus constitutes a very complex structure, as regards its functionality, cell complexity, hodology, development, and morphology. Therefore, it is not surprising that the elucidation of its genoarchitecture is particularly important to understand how is generated and maintained the diversity in the hypothalamus. That is one of the reasons that makes fascinating the hypothalamus and, thereby, the focus of analysis in many comparative studies. This has as its counterparts the numerous studies in which the nomenclature and interpretation of the nuclei and boundaries are constantly under debate (Szabó et al., 2009b; Bardet et al., 2010; Domínguez et al., 2010; Shimogori et al., 2010).

On the basis of combined expression analysis, at least two different longitudinal alar domains have been proposed in the chick hypothalamus: the Dlx- and Shh-negative SPV area, which lies under the border of the FoxG1-positive telencephalic field, and the subparaventricular area, which lies under it and is adjacent to the Shh-positive basal plate, and expresses Dlx5 and Nkx2.2 (Bardet et al., 2010). In *Xenopus*, the most anterior Nkx2.2 positive cells were localized in a Shh−/Nkx2.1−/xDll4−/Otp+ territory forming a thin strip of cells that delimit the region just anterior to the SC (present results) and their localization within this distinct region is highlighted because some of these cells contain both Otp and Nkx2.2.

The SC region is complex in terms of nuclei organization that most likely reflects a complex genetic specification. In general, the SC is defined as a Dlx-expressing zone in all vertebrates analyzed (Bachy et al., 2002; Brox et al., 2003; Puelles and Rubenstein, 2003; Flames et al., 2007; present results). In mammals, this region does not express Nkx2.1 and Shh, in contrast to the situation in other amniotes (Medina, 2008) and anamniotes (Medina, 2008; Moreno et al., 2008a; Domínguez et al., 2010). In particular, although these two markers were not specifically described in the SC region of the chick, their presence can be inferred from the published mapping studies (compare Figures 6I,J from Puelles et al., 2000 and Figures 1D,P,F,J from Bardet et al., 2010) suggesting possible evolutionary differences between birds and mammals in this area and/or the existence of different progenitor domains.

The SC of *X. laevis* has been carefully studied in the last years, mapping the distribution of numerous markers that identified different regions within this territory. In general terms, mainly on the basis of calcium binding proteins expression, rostral, and caudal SC zones were defined (Milán and Puelles, 2000; Morona and González, 2008). In addition, based on the expression of neuropeptide Y and TH (Kramer et al., 2001) three different nuclei were identified, the ventrolateral, dorsomedial, and caudal nuclei. All of them differ from each other in location, shape, number of cells, and function (Kramer et al., 2001) and, therefore, it is logic to think that also in genetic specification. In terms of genoarchitecture, the expression of several genes of the LIM-homeodomain family appears to define distinct territories within this SC area (Moreno et al., 2004, 2008a). Among others, Islet1 is expressed in a cell population that forms a curved band surrounding externally the Nkx2.1/Shh vz expression, i.e., the only area where Nkx2.2, TH, and xGAD67/xDll4 populations seem to be intermingled (present results; Brox et al., 2003; Moreno et al., 2008a; Domínguez et al., 2010). Noteworthy, it is known that Nkx2.2 and Shh are involved in the control of the development of midbrain dopaminergic neurons (Prakash and Wurst, 2006) and, given the close spatial relationship between Shh, Nkx2.2, and TH expressing neurons in the SC of *Xenopus*, a possible implication of Shh/Nkx2.2 may exist for the acquisition of the dopaminergic phenotype in this region.

Finally in the BH, like in the rest of the forebrain regions, the elucidation of genetic combinatorial expression patterns has served to characterize and define regions, and their comparative analysis in different vertebrates has been used as a useful tool to establish their grade of conservation. Thus, it was defined that Nkx2.1 expression in the BH is required to maintain molecular characteristics of the developing hypothalamus (Kimura et al., 1996; Takuma et al., 1998; Sussel et al., 1999; Marín et al., 2002; van den Akker et al., 2008), but other members of this gene family also seem to have roles in hypothalamic formation because, for example, Nkx2.2 or Nkx6.1 mutant mice have ventral to dorsal transformations (Briscoe and Ericson, 1999; Sander et al., 2000). In addition, in all vertebrates studied the transcription factor Otp is expressed in the arcuate nucleus and the oblique perimammillary band of the BH (Simeone et al., 1994; Puelles and Rubenstein, 2003; Del Giacco et al., 2006; Bardet et al., 2008), where contributes to progenitor cell proliferation, survival, and migration (Goshu et al., 2004), and operates in the proper differentiation of several neurohormone-secreting nuclei (Acampora et al., 1999, 2000; Wang and Lufkin, 2000; Michaud, 2001; Blechman et al., 2007; Eaton and Glasgow, 2007; Ryu et al., 2007; Del Giacco et al., 2008; Eaton et al., 2008). Additionally, the activity of Otp is essential for the induction of the dopaminergic phenotype in the hypothalamus of vertebrates (Del Giacco et al., 2008). In *Xenopus*, the mammillary area has been defined by TH and dopamine or histamine immunohistochemistry (Airaksinen and Panula, 1990; González et al., 1993, 1994; Milán and Puelles, 2000) and further identified by the expression of Otp (Domínguez et al., 2010) and the lack of Nkx2.2 (present results). In contrast, the Nkx2.2 combinatorial expression patterns identified different zones within the Nkx2.1 expressing tuberal hypothalamus in *Xenopus*: an intermediate Nkx2.2+/Otp− zone and the Nkx2.2−/Otp+ zone that constitutes the arcuate nucleus (Bardet et al., 2008; Domínguez et al., 2010; present results). Of note, the lack of Nkx2.2 expressing cells in the most posterior region of the tuberal area, coincides with a total absence of xShh-expression in the same territory (Domínguez et al., 2010).

Diencephalon

In the last 10 years an impressive number of morphological, chemo- and genoarchitectural data has helped to the interpretation in the diencephalon of the boundaries, extent of the areas and identification of distinct nuclei and subnuclei. These data have often been gathered not only for mammals but also in a number of non-mammalian species and the evolutionary perspective shows the impressive degree of conservation of this forebrain region, not only regarding the expression of different genes but also their functions. In all vertebrates analyzed, the alar diencephalon early develops into three major neuroepithelial domains along the anterior–posterior (A/P) axis, known as the prethalamus (P3), the thalamus (P2), and the pretectum (P1), and it is limited by two boundaries, the most anterior one that lies along the supraopto-mammillary region and the posterior one that lies between the pretectum and the mesencephalon (Puelles and Rubenstein, 2003;

Moreno et al., 2004, 2008b; Vieira et al., 2005; Ferran et al., 2009; Morona et al., 2011). Also in all the vertebrates exists the Zli as a secondary morphogenetic organizer in diencephalic histogenesis that appears as a transverse ventricular ridge between the prethalamus and the thalamus from neural tube stages (Echevarría et al., 2003; Puelles and Rubenstein, 2003). The final position, boundaries, organizations, and functions are in the end defined by signaling molecules such as Shh or Fgf8 (Echevarría et al., 2003; Vieira et al., 2005, 2010; Kataoka and Shimogori, 2008), which act regulating the expression of developmental genes that will specify compartmentalization and cell fate in the diencephalon (Echevarría et al., 2003; Hashimoto-Torii et al., 2003; Kiecker and Lumsden, 2004).

In mammals, from early embryonic stages Nkx2.2 is expressed in a distinct pattern in all three diencephalic prosomeres (Price et al., 1992; Puelles and Rubenstein, 2003; Vue et al., 2007; Kataoka and Shimogori, 2008) and is induced by Shh, which diffuses from the ventral territory and from the Zli, and is directly or indirectly repressed by Pax6 (Pratt et al., 2000; Kiecker and Lumsden, 2004). However, the interaction Pax6–Nkx2.2 it is not simple and reciprocal given that the downregulation of Pax6 in the posterior thalamus is not followed by the upregulation of Nkx2.2 (Pratt et al., 2000). In many studies, the influence of Shh over Nkx2.2 has been demonstrated (Barth and Wilson, 1995; Kiecker and Lumsden, 2004; Vieira and Martínez, 2006), however there are also evidences about their independence in different models. This is the case of the mammalian Nkx2.2 expression in the posterior region of the Zli, which is under the control of Fgf8 and not Shh (Kataoka and Shimogori, 2008), but also in the cave-living form of the teleost fish *Astyanax mexicanus*, which shows a clear expansion of Shh-expression at the ventral midline but is not correlated with a larger Nkx2.2 expression domain; in contrast to other transcription factors expressed in the forebrain such us Nkx2.1 (Menuet et al., 2007).

In the diencephalon of mouse and chicken, the gene Nkx2.2 is expressed during development in a rostroventral band of the thalamus (Puelles and Rubenstein, 1993; Martínez-de-la-Torre et al., 2002). On the basis of the Nkx2.2 expression, a distinct progenitor domain has been characterized in the developing thalamus (also marked by Mash1; Vue et al., 2007; Kataoka and Shimogori, 2008), which is controlled by FGF signaling, with independence of the Shh activity (Kataoka and Shimogori, 2008). Later in the thalamic development, the expressions of Nkx2.2 and Gad67 were detected in different nuclei (Vue et al., 2007; Kataoka and Shimogori, 2008), specifically in the posterior ventral lateral geniculate nucleus (vLGN), concluding that at least a portion of the vLGN, classically a considered a prethalamic nuclei (Kitamura et al., 1997), belongs to the set of retinorecipient thalamic nuclei that do not project to the cortex (Paxinos, 1994) and arises from the thalamic domain (Vue et al., 2007; Kataoka and Shimogori, 2008).

In the chick, the combined expression of Gbx2, Nkx2.2, and Pax6 (Martínez-de-la-Torre et al., 2002), the cadherin expression (Redies, 2000), and fate maps analysis (García-Lopez et al., 2004) allowed the identification in the thalamus of four subdivisions, the anteroventral, dorsal, intermediate, and ventral regions. Interestingly, Nkx2.2 expression was only detected into the anteroventral region (adjacent to the Zli) and its derivatives, among which are the set retinorecipient thalamic nuclei (Martínez-de-la-Torre et al., 2002) that express Nkx2.2 and are proposed as thalamic derivates (Vue et al., 2007).

In *Xenopus*, we have found an extended Nkx2.2 positive region along the developing thalamus that might define a distinct progenitor domain whose cells would contribute to the formation of other diencephalic nuclei. The Nkx2.2 thalamic expression is observed in different nuclei expressing diverse transcription factors such as x-Lhx2/9 (Moreno et al., 2004) and scattered GAD67 (Brox et al., 2003). In addition, it is suggested that in *Xenopus* the Nkx2.2 gene is a good candidate involved in the acquisition of the GABAergic phenotype in the thalamus, the pretectum, and the basal plate of the caudal diencephalon, where there is not Dll expression (Brox et al., 2003; present results). In mammals and chick it has been proposed that the area adjacent to the Shh-expression of the Zli is induced by Shh to express Nkx2.2, and this area has been proposed to be the source of the subpopulation of GABAergic interneurons observed in the thalamus (Fode et al., 2000; Martínez-de-la-Torre et al., 2002; Puelles et al., 2004). In this context, we have observed Nkx2.2/GABA double labeled cells in the thalamus (present results), a region devoid of Dll4 expression (Brox et al., 2003; present results), suggesting that Nkx2.2 could be implicated in the acquisition of the GABAergic phenotype, like in amniotes.

Interestingly, also in *Xenopus*, Nkx2.2 expression is observed in the prethalamus, and its precise localization is corroborated by the colocalization of the Nkx2.2 expressing cells in the territory of P3 that is xDll4+/Nkx2.1+/Pax6+/TH+/xShh+ (present results; Bachy et al., 2002; Brox et al., 2003; Moreno et al., 2008a,b; Domínguez et al., 2010).

As regards the Zli, it expresses Shh in all vertebrates analyzed and is involved in the correct acquisition of the P2 and P3 gene expression and regionalization pattern (Braun et al., 2003; Hashimoto-Torii et al., 2003; Kiecker and Lumsden, 2004; Scholpp et al., 2006; Szabó et al., 2009a). In this context, Nkx2.2 expression in the thalamus and prethalamus is induced by Shh secreted by Zli cells (Kiecker and Lumsden, 2004; Vieira et al., 2005; Vieira and Martínez, 2006). Thus, the xShh-expression in the Zli found in *Xenopus* suggests that also in amphibians Shh is likely involved in the specification of the diencephalic territory (Domínguez et al., 2010), and that xShh-expression in the Zli could lead to establish the Nkx2.2 expression pattern in the P2/P3 territory of amphibians, like in amniotes.

Finally, the Nkx2.2 expression observed in the thalamus of the mouse and chicken continues into P1 (Puelles and Rubenstein, 1993; Martínez-de-la-Torre et al., 2002). Studies about the pretectal molecular regionalization in chick and *Xenopus* have described that the precise Nkx2.2 expression within P1 marks the alar/basal boundary, representing a tentative ventral limit of the pretectum (Ferran et al., 2009; Morona et al., 2011; present results).

ACKNOWLEDGMENTS

This work supported by grants from Spanish MICINN and the UCM (Grant numbers: BFU2009-12315 and BSCH-UCM GR58/08). We are grateful to Dr. Ruth Morona for the fruitful discussions about the diencephalic regionalization and to Dr. Jesús M. López for the critical reading of the manuscript.

REFERENCES

Abellán, A., and Medina, L. (2009). Subdivisions and derivatives of the chicken subpallium based on expression of LIM and other regulatory genes and markers of neuron subpopulations during development. *J. Comp. Neurol.* 515, 465–501.

Acampora, D., Postiglione, M. P., Avantaggiato, V., Di Bonito, M., and Simeone, A. (2000). The role of Otx and Otp genes in brain development. *Int. J. Dev. Biol.* 44, 669–677.

Acampora, D., Postiglione, M. P., Avantaggiato, V., Di Bonito, M., Vaccarino, F. M., Michaud, J., and Simeone, A. (1999). Progressive impairment of developing neuroendocrine cell lineages in the hypothalamus of mice lacking the orthopedia gene. *Genes Dev.* 13, 2787–2800.

Airaksinen, M. S., and Panula, P. (1990). Comparative neuroanatomy of the histaminergic system in the brain of the frog *Xenopus laevis*. *J. Comp. Neurol.* 292, 412–423.

Bachy, I., Berthon, J., and Rétaux, S. (2002). Defining pallial and subpallial divisions in the developing *Xenopus* forebrain. *Mech. Dev.* 117, 163–172.

Bachy, I., Vernier, P., and Rétaux, S. (2001). The LIM-homeodomain gene family in the developing *Xenopus* brain: conservation and divergences with the mouse related to the evolution of the forebrain. *J. Neurosci.* 21, 7620–7629.

Bardet, S. M., Cobos, I., Puelles, E., Martínez-De-La-Torre, M., and Puelles, L. (2006). Chicken lateral septal organ and other circumventricular organs form in a striatal subdomain abutting the molecular striatopallidal border. *J. Comp. Neurol.* 499, 745–767.

Bardet, S. M., Ferran, J. L., Sánchez-Arrones, L., and Puelles, L. (2010). Ontogenetic expression of sonic hedgehog in the chicken subpallium. *Front. Neuroanat.* 4:28. doi: 10.3389/fnana.2010.00028

Bardet, S. M., Martínez-de-la-Torre, M., Northcutt, R. G., Rubenstein, J. L., and Puelles, L. (2008). Conserved pattern of OTP-positive cells in the paraventricular nucleus and other hypothalamic sites of tetrapods. *Brain Res. Bull.* 75, 231–235.

Barth, K. A., and Wilson, S. W. (1994). Specification of neuronal identity in the embryonic CNS. *Semin. Dev. Biol.* 5, 349–358.

Barth, K. A., and Wilson, S. W. (1995). Expression of zebrafish nk2.2 is influenced by sonic hedgehog/vertebrate hedgehog-1 and demarcates a zone of neuronal differentiation in the embryonic forebrain. *Development* 121, 1755–1768.

Bläsher, S., and Heinrichs, M. (1982). Immunoreactive neuropeptide systems in avian embryos (domestic mallard, domestic fowl, Japanese quail). *Cell Tissue Res.* 223, 287–303.

Blechman, J., Borodovsky, N., Eisenberg, M., Nabel-Rosen, H., Grimm, J., and Levkowitz, G. (2007). Specification of hypothalamic neurons by dual regulation of the homeodomain protein orthopedia. *Development* 134, 4417–4426.

Braun, M. M., Etheridge, A., Bernard, A., Robertson, C. P., and Roelink, H. (2003). Wnt signaling is required at distinct stages of development for the induction of the posterior forebrain. *Development* 130, 5579–5587.

Briscoe, J., and Ericson, J. (1999). The specification of neuronal identity by graded sonic hedgehog signalling. *Semin. Cell Dev. Biol.* 10, 353–362.

Briscoe, J., Pierani, A., Jessell, T. M., and Ericson, J. (2000). A homeodomain protein code specifies progenitor cell identity and neuronal fate in the ventral neural tube. *Cell* 101, 435–445.

Brox, A., Puelles, L., Ferreiro, B., and Medina, L. (2003). Expression of the genes GAD67 and distal-less-4 in the forebrain of *Xenopus laevis* confirms a common pattern in tetrapods. *J. Comp. Neurol.* 461, 370–393.

Brox, A., Puelles, L., Ferreiro, B., and Medina, L. (2004). Expression of the genes Emx1, Tbr1, and Eomes (Tbr2) in the telencephalon of *Xenopus laevis* confirms the existence of a ventral pallial division in all tetrapods. *J. Comp. Neurol.* 474, 562–577.

Del Giacco, L., Pistocchi, A., Cotelli, F., Fortunato, A. E., and Sordino, P. (2008). A peek inside the neurosecretory brain through orthopedia lenses. *Dev. Dyn.* 237, 2295–2303.

Del Giacco, L., Sordino, P., Pistocchi, A., Andreakis, N., Tarallo, R., Di Benedetto, B., and Cotelli, F. (2006). Differential regulation of the zebrafish orthopedia 1 gene during fate determination of diencephalic neurons. *BMC Dev. Biol.* 6, 50. doi: 10.1186/1471-213X-6-50

Domínguez, L., González, A., and Moreno, N. (2010). Sonic hedgehog expression during *Xenopus laevis* forebrain development. *Brain Res.* 1347, 19–32.

Eaton, J. L., and Glasgow, E. (2007). Zebrafish orthopedia (otp) is required for isotocin cell development. *Dev. Genes Evol.* 217, 149–158.

Eaton, J. L., Holmqvist, B., and Glasgow, E. (2008). Ontogeny of vasotocin-expressing cells in zebrafish: selective requirement for the transcriptional regulators orthopedia and single-minded 1 in the preoptic area. *Dev. Dyn.* 237, 995–1005.

Echevarría, D., Vieira, C., Gimeno, L., and Martínez, S. (2003). Neuroepithelial secondary organizers and cell fate specification in the developing brain. *Brain Res. Brain Res. Rev.* 43, 179–191.

Ekker, S. C., McGrew, L. L., Lai, C. J., Lee, J. J., von Kessler, D. P., Moon, R. T., and Beachy, P. A. (1995). Distinct expression and shared activities of members of the hedgehog gene family of *Xenopus laevis*. *Development* 121, 2337–2347.

Ericson, J., Rashbass, P., Schedl, A., Brenner-Morton, S., Kawakami, A., van Heyningen, V., Jessell, T. M., and Briscoe, J. (1997). Pax6 controls progenitor cell identity and neuronal fate in response to graded Shh signaling. *Cell* 90, 169–180.

Ferran, J. L., de Oliveira, E. D., Merchán, P., Sandoval, J. E., Sánchez-Arrones, L., Martínez-De-La-Torre, M., and Puelles, L. (2009). Genoarchitectonic profile of developing nuclear groups in the chicken pretectum. *J. Comp. Neurol.* 517, 405–451.

Flames, N., Pla, R., Gelman, D. M., Rubenstein, J. L., Puelles, L., and Marín, O. (2007). Delineation of multiple subpallial progenitor domains by the combinatorial expression of transcriptional codes. *J. Neurosci.* 27, 9682–9695.

Fode, C., Ma, Q., Casarosa, S., Ang, S. L., Anderson, D. J., and Guillemot, F. (2000). A role for neural determination genes in specifying the dorsoventral identity of telencephalic neurons. *Genes Dev.* 14, 67–80.

Fuccillo, M., Rutlin, M., and Fishell, G. (2006). Removal of Pax6 partially rescues the loss of ventral structures in Shh null mice. *Cereb. Cortex* 16(Suppl. 1), 96–102.

García-Lopez, M., Abellán, A., Legaz, I., Rubenstein, J. L., Puelles, L., and Medina, L. (2008). Histogenetic compartments of the mouse centromedial and extended amygdala based on gene expression patterns during development. *J. Comp. Neurol.* 506, 46–74.

García-Lopez, R., Vieira, C., Echevarría, D., and Martínez, S. (2004). Fate map of the diencephalon and the zona limitans at the 10-somites stage in chick embryos. *Dev. Biol.* 268, 514–530.

González, A., López, J. M., and Marín, O. (2002a). Expression pattern of the homeobox protein NKX2-1 in the developing *Xenopus* forebrain. *Brain Res. Gene Expr. Patterns* 1, 181–185.

González, A., López, J. M., Sánchez-Camacho, C., and Marín, O. (2002b). Regional expression of the homeobox gene NKX2-1 defines pallidal and interneuronal populations in the basal ganglia of amphibians. *Neuroscience* 114, 567–575.

González, A., Marín, O., Tuinhof, R., and Smeets, W. J. (1994). Ontogeny of catecholamine systems in the central nervous system of anuran amphibians: an immunohistochemical study with antibodies against tyrosine hydroxylase and dopamine. *J. Comp. Neurol.* 346, 63–79.

González, A., Moreno, N., Morona, R., and López, J. M. (2003). Somatostatin-like immunoreactivity in the brain of the urodele amphibian *Pleurodeles waltl*. Colocalization with catecholamines and nitric oxide. *Brain Res.* 965, 246–258.

González, A., Muñóz, A., Muñóz, M., Marín, O., and Smeets, W. J. (1995). Ontogeny of vasotocinergic and mesotocinergic systems in the brain of the South African clawed frog *Xenopus laevis*. *J. Chem. Neuroanat.* 9, 27–40.

González, A., Tuinhof, R., and Smeets, W. J. (1993). Distribution of tyrosine hydroxylase and dopamine immunoreactivities in the brain of the South African clawed frog *Xenopus laevis*. *Anat. Embryol. (Berl.)* 187, 193–201.

Goshu, E., Jin, H., Lovejoy, J., Marion, J. F., Michaud, J. L., and Fan, C. M. (2004). Sim2 contributes to neuroendocrine hormone gene expression in the anterior hypothalamus. *Mol. Endocrinol.* 18, 1251–1262.

Hashimoto-Torii, K., Motoyama, J., Hui, C. C., Kuroiwa, A., Nakafuku, M., and Shimamura, K. (2003). Differential activities of sonic hedgehog mediated by Gli transcription factors define distinct neuronal subtypes in the dorsal thalamus. *Mech. Dev.* 120, 1097–1111.

Herrick, C. J. (1910). The Morphology of the forebrain in amphibia and reptilia. *J. Comp. Neurol.* 20, 413–547.

Holland, L. Z., Venkatesh, T. V., Gorlin, A., Bodmer, R., and Holland, N. D. (1998). Characterization and developmental expression of AmphiNk2-2, an NK2 class homeobox gene from *Amphioxus*. (phylum chordata; subphylum cephalochordata). *Dev. Genes Evol.* 208, 100–105.

Jiménez, F., Martin-Morris, L. E., Velasco, L., Chu, H., Sierra, J., Rosen, D. R., and White, K. (1995). vnd, a gene required for early neurogenesis of *Drosophila*, encodes a homeodomain protein. *EMBO J.* 14, 3487–3495.

Kataoka, A., and Shimogori, T. (2008). Fgf8 controls regional identity in the developing thalamus. *Development* 135, 2873–2881.

Kiecker, C., and Lumsden, A. (2004). Hedgehog signaling from the ZLI regulates diencephalic regional identity. *Nat. Neurosci.* 7, 1242–1249.

Kim, Y., and Nirenberg, M. (1989). Drosophila NK-homeobox genes.

Proc. Natl. Acad. Sci. U.S.A. 86, 7716–7720.

Kimura, S., Hara, Y., Pineau, T., Fernández-Salguero, P., Fox, C. H., Ward, J. M., and González, F. J. (1996). The T/ebp null mouse: thyroid-specific enhancer-binding protein is essential for the organogenesis of the thyroid, lung, ventral forebrain, and pituitary. *Genes Dev.* 10, 60–69.

Kitamura, K., Miura, H., Yanazawa, M., Miyashita, T., and Kato, K. (1997). Expression patterns of Brx1 (Rieg gene), sonic hedgehog, Nkx2.2, Dlx1 and Arx during zona limitans intrathalamica and embryonic ventral lateral geniculate nuclear formation. *Mech. Dev.* 67, 83–96.

Kramer, B. M., Welting, J., Berghs, C. A., Jenks, B. G., and Roubos, E. W. (2001). Functional organization of the suprachiasmatic nucleus of *Xenopus laevis* in relation to background adaptation. *J. Comp. Neurol.* 432, 346–355.

Lin, X., State, M. W., Vaccarino, F. M., Greally, J., Hass, M., and Leckman, J. F. (1999). Identification, chromosomal assignment, and expression analysis of the human homeodomain containing gene Orthopedia (OTP). *Genomics* 60, 96–104.

López, J. M., Moreno, N., Morona, R., Muñóz, M., Domínguez, L., and González, A. (2007). Distribution of somatostatin-like immunoreactivity in the brain of the caecilian *Dermophis mexicanus* (amphibia: gymnophiona): comparative aspects in amphibians. *J. Comp. Neurol.* 501, 413–340.

Marín, O., Baker, J., Puelles, L., and Rubenstein, J. L. (2002). Patterning of the basal telencephalon and hypothalamus is essential for guidance of cortical projections. *Development* 129, 761–773.

Martínez-de-la-Torre, M., Garda, A. L., Puelles, E., and Puelles, L. (2002). Gbx2 expression in the late embryonic chick dorsal thalamus. *Brain Res. Bull.* 57, 435–438.

Medina, L. (2008). "Evolution and embryological development of forebrain," in *Enciclopedic Reference of Neuroscience*, eds M. D. Binder and N. Hirokawa (Springer-Verlag), 1172–1192.

Menuet, A., Alunni, A., Joly, J. S., Jeffery, W. R., and Rétaux, S. (2007). Expanded expression of sonic hedgehog in *Astyanax* cavefish: multiple consequences on forebrain development and evolution. *Development* 134, 845–855.

Michaud, J. L. (2001). The developmental program of the hypothalamus and its disorders. *Clin. Genet.* 60, 255–263.

Milán, F. J., and Puelles, L. (2000). Patterns of calretinin, calbindin, and tyrosine-hydroxylase expression are consistent with the prosomeric map of the frog diencephalon. *J. Comp. Neurol.* 419, 96–121.

Moreno, N., Bachy, I., Rétaux, S., and González, A. (2003). Pallial origin of mitral cells in the olfactory bulbs of *Xenopus. Neuroreport* 14, 2355–2358.

Moreno, N., Bachy, I., Rétaux, S., and González, A. (2004). LIM-homeodomain genes as developmental and adult genetic markers of *Xenopus* forebrain functional subdivisions. *J. Comp. Neurol.* 472, 52–72.

Moreno, N., Bachy, I., Rétaux, S., and González, A. (2005). LIM-homeodomain genes as territory markers in the brainstem of adult and developing *Xenopus laevis. J. Comp. Neurol.* 485, 240–254.

Moreno, N., Domínguez, L., Rétaux, S., and González, A. (2008a). Islet1 as a marker of subdivisions and cell types in the developing forebrain of *Xenopus. Neuroscience* 154, 1423–1439.

Moreno, N., Rétaux, S., and González, A. (2008b). Spatio-temporal expression of Pax6 in *Xenopus* forebrain. *Brain Res.* 1239, 92–99.

Moreno, N., Morona, R., López, J. M., and González, A. (2010). Subdivisions of the turtle *Pseudemys scripta subpallium* based on the expression of regulatory genes and neuronal markers. *J. Comp. Neurol.* 518, 4877–4902.

Morona, R., Ferran, J. L., Puelles, L., and González, A. (2011). Embryonic genoarchitecture of pretectum in *Xenopus laevis*: a conserved pattern in tetrapods. *J. Comp. Neurol.* 519, 1024–1050.

Morona, R., and González, A. (2008). Calbindin-D28k and calretinin expression in the forebrain of anuran and urodele amphibians: further support for newly identified subdivisions. *J. Comp. Neurol.* 511, 187–220.

Nieuwkoop, P. D., and Farber, J. (1967). *Normal Table of Xenopus laevis (Daudin)*. Amsterdam: North-Holland.

Osorio, J., Mazan, S., and Rétaux, S. (2005). Organization of the lamprey (*Lampetra fluviatilis*) embryonic brain: insights from LIM-homeodomain, Pax and hedgehog genes. *Dev. Biol.* 288, 100–112.

Osorio, J., Megías, M., Pombal, M. A., and Rétaux, S. (2006). Dynamic expression of the LIM-homeodomain gene Lhx15 through larval brain development of the sea lamprey (*Petromyzon marinus*). *Gene Expr. Patterns* 6, 873–878.

Papalopulu, N., and Kintner, C. (1993). *Xenopus* distal-less related homeobox genes are expressed in the developing forebrain and are induced by planar signals. *Development* 117, 961–975.

Paxinos, G. (1994). *Atlas of the Developing Rat Nervous System*. New York: Academy press.

Petkó, M., and Orosz, V. (1996). Distribution of somatostatin-immunoreactive structures in the central nervous system of the frog, *Rana esculenta. J. Hirnforsch.* 37, 109–120.

Prakash, N., and Wurst, W. (2006). Genetic networks controlling the development of midbrain dopaminergic neurons. *J. Physiol.* 575, 403–410.

Pratt, T., Vitalis, T., Warren, N., Edgar, J. M., Mason, J. O., and Price, D. J. (2000). A role for Pax6 in the normal development of dorsal thalamus and its cortical connections. *Development* 127, 5167–5178.

Price, M., Lazzaro, D., Pohl, T., Mattei, M. G., Rüther, U., Olivo, J. C., Duboule, D., and Di Lauro, R. (1992). Regional expression of the homeobox gene Nkx-2.2 in the developing mammalian forebrain. *Neuron* 8, 241–255.

Puelles, L., Kuwana, E., Puelles, E., Bulfone, A., Shimamura, K., Keleher, J., Smiga, S., and Rubenstein, J. L. (2000). Pallial and subpallial derivatives in the embryonic chick and mouse telencephalon, traced by the expression of the genes Dlx-2, Emx-1, Nkx-2.1, Pax-6, and Tbr-1. *J. Comp. Neurol.* 424, 409–438.

Puelles, L., Martínez, S., Martínez-de-la-Torre, M., and Rubenstein, J. L. (2004). "Gene maps and related histogenetic domains in the forebrain and midbrain," in *The Rat Nervous System*, 3rd Edn, ed. G. Paxinos (San Diego: Elsevier), 3–25.

Puelles, L., and Rubenstein, J. L. (1993). Expression patterns of homeobox and other putative regulatory genes in the embryonic mouse forebrain suggest a neuromeric organization. *Trends Neurosci.* 16, 472–479.

Puelles, L., and Rubenstein, J. L. (2003). Forebrain gene expression domains and the evolving prosomeric model. *Trends Neurosci.* 26, 469–476.

Redies, C. (2000). Cadherins in the central nervous system. *Prog. Neurobiol.* 61, 611–648.

Rohr, K. B., Barth, K. A., Varga, Z. M., and Wilson, S. W. (2001). The nodal pathway acts upstream of hedgehog signaling to specify ventral telencephalic identity. *Neuron* 29, 341–351.

Ryu, S., Mahler, J., Acampora, D., Holzschuh, J., Erhardt, S., Omodei, D., Simeone, A., and Driever, W. (2007). Orthopedia homeodomain protein is essential for diencephalic dopaminergic neuron development. *Curr. Biol.* 17, 873–880.

Sander, M., Paydar, S., Ericson, J., Briscoe, J., Berber, E., German, M., Jessell, T. M., and Rubenstein, J. L. (2000). Ventral neural patterning by Nkx homeobox genes: Nkx6.1 controls somatic motor neuron and ventral interneuron fates. *Genes Dev.* 14, 2134–2139.

Schäfer, M., Kinzel, D., Neuner, C., Schartl, M., Volff, J. N., and Winkler, C. (2005). Hedgehog and retinoid signalling confines nkx2.2b expression to the lateral floor plate of the zebrafish trunk. *Mech. Dev.* 122, 43–56.

Scholpp, S., Wolf, O., Brand, M., and Lumsden, A. (2006). Hedgehog signalling from the zona limitans intrathalamica orchestrates patterning of the zebrafish diencephalon. *Development* 133, 855–864.

Shimamura, K., and Rubenstein, J. L. (1997). Inductive interactions direct early regionalization of the mouse forebrain. *Development* 124, 2709–2718.

Shimogori, T., Lee, D. A., Miranda-Angulo, A., Yang, Y., Wang, H., Jiang, L., Yoshida, A. C., Kataoka, A., Mashiko, H., Avetisyan, M., Qi, L., Qian, J., and Blackshaw, S. (2010). A genomic atlas of mouse hypothalamic development. *Nat. Neurosci.* 13, 767–775.

Simeone, A., D'Apice, M. R., Nigro, V., Casanova, J., Graziani, F., Acampora, D., and Avantaggiato, V. (1994). Orthopedia, a novel homeobox-containing gene expressed in the developing CNS of both mouse and *Drosophila. Neuron* 13, 83–101.

Smeets, W. J., and González, A. (2000). Catecholamine systems in the brain of vertebrates: new perspectives through a comparative approach. *Brain Res. Brain Res. Rev.* 33, 308–379.

Sussel, L., Marín, O., Kimura, S., and Rubenstein, J. L. (1999). Loss of Nkx2.1 homeobox gene function results in a ventral to dorsal molecular respecification within the basal telencephalon: evidence for a transformation of the pallidum into the striatum. *Development* 126, 3359–3370.

Szabó, N. E., Zhao, T., Zhou, X., and Alvarez-Bolado, G. (2009a). The role of sonic hedgehog of neural origin in thalamic differentiation in the mouse. *J. Neurosci.* 29, 2453–2466.

Szabó, N. E., Zhao, T., Cankaya, M., Theil, T., Zhou, X., and Alvarez-Bolado, G. (2009b). Role of neuroepithelial sonic hedgehog in hypothalamic patterning. *J. Neurosci.* 29, 6989–7002.

Takuma, N., Sheng, H. Z., Furuta, Y., Ward, J. M., Sharma, K., Hogan, B. L., Pfaff, S. L., Westphal, H., Kimura, S., and Mahon, K. A. (1998). Formation of Rathke's pouch requires dual induction from the diencephalon. *Development* 125, 4835–4840.

van den Akker, W. M., Brox, A., Puelles, L., Durston, A. J., and Medina, L. (2008). Comparative functional analysis provides evidence for a crucial role for the homeobox gene Nkx2.1/Titf-1 in forebrain evolution. *J. Comp. Neurol.* 506, 211–223.

Vieira, C., Garda, A. L., Shimamura, K., and Martínez, S. (2005). Thalamic development induced by Shh in the chick embryo. *Dev. Biol.* 284, 351–363.

Vieira, C., and Martínez, S. (2006). Sonic hedgehog from the basal plate and the zona limitans intrathalamica exhibits differential activity on diencephalic molecular regionalization and nuclear structure. *Neuroscience* 143, 129–140.

Vieira, C., Pombero, A., García-Lopez, R., Gimeno, L., Echevarría, D., and Martínez, S. (2010). Molecular mechanisms controlling brain development: an overview of neuroepithelial secondary organizers. *Int. J. Dev. Biol.* 54, 7–20.

Vue, T. Y., Aaker, J., Taniguchi, A., Kazemzadeh, C., Skidmore, J. M., Martin, D. M., Martin, J. F., Treier, M., and Nakagawa, Y. (2007). Characterization of progenitor domains in the developing mouse thalamus. *J. Comp. Neurol.* 505, 73–91.

Wang, W., and Lufkin, T. (2000). The murine Otp homeobox gene plays an essential role in the specification of neuronal cell lineages in the developing hypothalamus. *Dev. Biol.* 227, 432–449.

Wilson, S. W., Placzek, M., and Furley, A. (1993). Border disputes: do boundaries play a role in growth-cone guidance? *Trends Neurosci.* 16, 316–322.

Conflict of Interest Statement: The authors declare that the research was conducted in the absence of any commercial or financial relationships that could be construed as a potential conflict of interest.

5

Developmental modes and developmental mechanisms can channel brain evolution

Christine J. Charvet[1]* and Georg F. Striedter[1,2]

[1] Department of Neurobiology and Behavior, Center for the Neurobiology of Learning and Memory, University of California, Irvine, CA, USA
[2] Department of Ecology and Evolutionary Biology, University of California, Irvine, CA, USA

Edited by:
Fernando Martinez-Garcia, Universidad de Valencia, Spain

Reviewed by:
Ann B. Butler, George Mason University, USA
John Kirn, Wesleyan University, USA

***Correspondence:**
Christine J. Charvet, Department of Psychology, Cornell University, 229 Uris Hall, Ithaca, NY 14853-7601, USA.
e-mail: charvetcj@gmail.com

Anseriform birds (ducks and geese) as well as parrots and songbirds have evolved a disproportionately enlarged telencephalon compared with many other birds. However, parrots and songbirds differ from anseriform birds in their mode of development. Whereas ducks and geese are precocial (e.g., hatchlings feed on their own), parrots and songbirds are altricial (e.g., hatchlings are fed by their parents). We here consider how developmental modes may limit and facilitate specific changes in the mechanisms of brain development. We suggest that altriciality facilitates the evolution of telencephalic expansion by delaying telencephalic neurogenesis. We further hypothesize that delays in telencephalic neurogenesis generate delays in telencephalic maturation, which in turn foster neural adaptations that facilitate learning. Specifically, we propose that delaying telencephalic neurogenesis was a prerequisite for the evolution of neural circuits that allow parrots and songbirds to produce learned vocalizations. Overall, we argue that developmental modes have influenced how some lineages of birds increased the size of their telencephalon and that this, in turn, has influenced subsequent changes in brain circuits and behavior.

Keywords: bird, mode, development, proliferation, evolution

INTRODUCTION

Parrots, songbirds, and anseriform birds (ducks and geese) have evolved a disproportionately large telencephalon compared with many other birds (**Figure 1**; Portmann, 1947a; Boire and Baron, 1994; Iwaniuk and Hurd, 2005). Although the proportional size of the telencephalon in ducks and geese rivals that in parrots and songbirds, the latter taxa differ from ducks and geese in numerous respects. First, parrots and songbirds are altricial (their hatchlings are fed by their parents), whereas ducks and geese are precocial (their hatchlings feed on their own; Starck and Ricklefs, 1998). Second, parrots and songbirds enlarge their telencephalon by delaying telencephalic neurogenesis (Striedter and Charvet, 2008; Charvet and Striedter, 2009a), whereas ducks and geese enlarge their telencephalon before telencephalic neurogenesis begins (Charvet and Striedter, 2009b). Finally, parrots and songbirds have evolved a set of telencephalic nuclei responsible for vocal learning (Nottebohm, 1972; Nottebohm et al., 1976; Doupe and Kuhl, 1999), whereas anseriform birds have evolved an expanded trigeminal system that is related to feeding (Dubbeldam and Visser, 1987; Gutiérrez-Ibáñez et al., 2009). Thus, anseriform birds differ form parrots and songbirds in their developmental modes, in brain development, in brain anatomy, and in behavior.

Recent analyses of avian phylogenetic relationships indicate that parrots are the sister group of passerines, which include songbirds and suboscines (manakins, antbirds, tyrant-flycatchers; Ericson et al., 2006; Hackett et al., 2008). Anseriform birds are the sister group of galliform birds (e.g., chickens), which are distantly related to songbirds and parrots (Ericson et al., 2006; Hackett et al., 2008). Therefore, it is most parsimonious to conclude that the expansion of the telencephalon evolved at least twice independently among birds: once in the lineage leading to anseriform birds and at least once in the group that gave rise to parrots and songbirds. In this review we show that distinct developmental mechanisms underlie these two independent evolutionary changes in telencephalon size. We next examine how ancestral developmental modes may have influenced changes in developmental mechanisms, which in turn influenced evolutionary changes in behavioral flexibility and learning capacity.

ALTRICIALITY IS A PRE-ADAPTATION FOR DELAYED BRAIN MATURATION

Most land birds (e.g., parrots, songbirds, suboscines, owls, kingfishers, falcons) are altricial (**Figure 2**; Starck and Ricklefs, 1998). That is, their hatchlings are relatively immobile and receive extensive post-hatching parental care. However, the degree of helplessness at hatching varies among land birds (Starck and Ricklefs, 1998). For instance, falcons and owls are considered semi-altricial in that their hatchlings are covered with down. Parrots, songbirds, and suboscines are among the most altricial avian species (Starck and Ricklefs, 1998; Londoño, 2003; Greeny et al., 2004, 2005). Their hatchlings are naked, have their eyes closed, and are fed for several weeks after hatching. In general, the most salient difference between altricial and precocial species is that parents feed altricial hatchlings whereas precocial hatchlings feed on their own.

Altricial and precocial species also differ in the timing of brain maturation. Specifically, altricial species delay some aspects of brain maturation into the post-hatching period relative to precocial species. This is most evident from the observation that altricial (including semi-altricial) species such as parrots, songbirds,

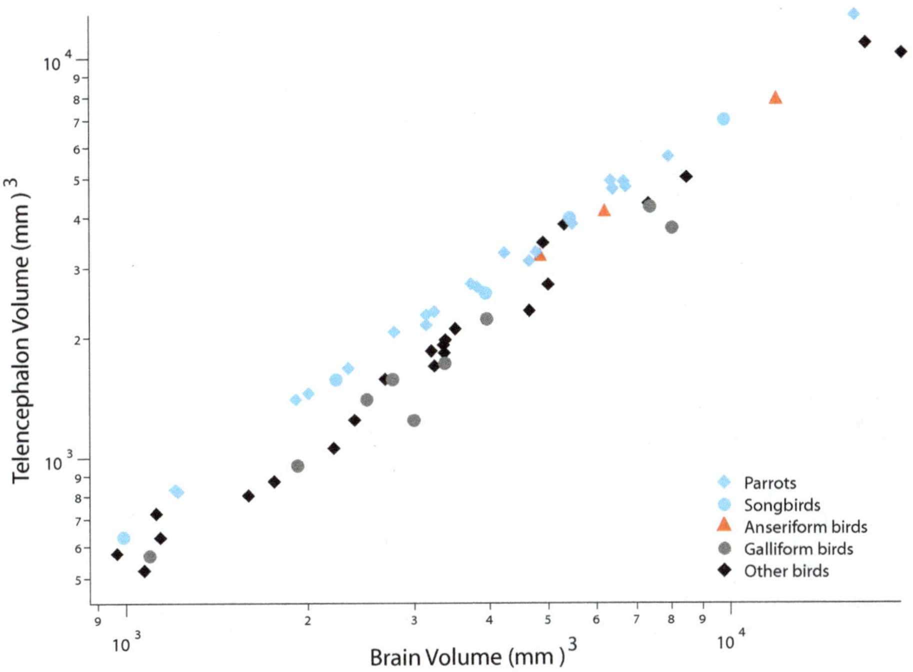

FIGURE 1 | A plot of telencephalon volume versus overall brain volume shows that the telencephalon is disproportionately large in parrots, songbirds (i.e., oscine passerines), and anseriform birds (ducks and geese) compared with galliform birds and diverse other avian species. The other avian species in this graph include mainly pigeons, shorebirds and falcons. Data are from Iwaniuk and Hurd (2005).

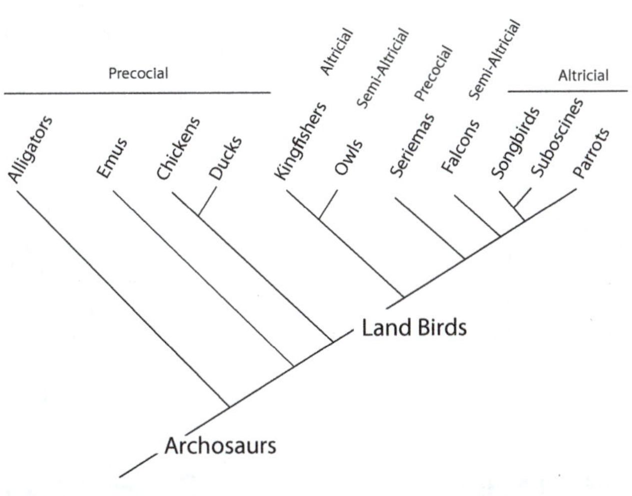

FIGURE 2 | Phylogeny of archosaurs (alligators and birds) shows their modes of development. Parrots, songbirds, suboscines (manakins, antbirds, tyrant-flycatchers), and kingfishers are altricial, whereas falcons and owls are semi-altricial. Because most land birds (e.g., suboscines and falcons) are either altricial or semi-altricial, the ancestors of parrots and songbirds were probably either altricial or semi-altricial. This, in turn, implies that the expansion of the telencephalon in parrots and songbirds evolved in a lineage that was at least semi-altricial. In contrast, many reptiles (e.g., alligators), paleognaths (e.g., emus), and basal lineages of Neoaves (e.g., galliform and anseriform birds) are precocial. Thus, ducks and geese were probably precocial when they expanded their telencephalon. The phylogeny is based on Hackett et al. (2008).

owls, and pigeons generally exhibit more post-hatching brain growth than precocial species (**Figure 3**). Given this delayed brain growth, we can infer that late-born brain regions, such as the telencephalon, are functionally immature at hatching in altricial species (Portmann, 1947b; Finlay and Darlington, 1995; Ling et al., 1997; Finlay et al., 1998; Striedter and Charvet, 2008). This delayed brain maturation presumably renders altricial hatchlings relatively helpless and dependent on their parents.

Parrots and songbirds exhibit even more post-hatching brain growth than other altricial species (e.g., pigeons, owls; **Figure 3**; Portmann, 1947b; Starck and Ricklefs, 1998). Most of the post-hatching brain growth in parrots and songbirds is due to a late expansion of the telencephalon, which is associated with a general delay and extension of telencephalic neurogenesis (Striedter and Charvet, 2008; Charvet and Striedter, 2009a). Post-hatching neurogenesis has only been examined in a few parrots (parakeets) and songbirds (canaries, chickadees, zebra finches; Paton and Nottebohm, 1984; Kirn and DeVoogd, 1989; Barnea and Nottebohm, 1994). Previous work shows that the telencephalon in parakeets (*Melopsittacus undulatus*) and zebra finches (*Taeniopygia guttata*) harbors an expanded pool of precursor cells, which persists well into the post-hatching period (Charvet and Striedter, 2008; Striedter and Charvet, 2009). In zebra finches, the major period of telencephalic neurogenesis ends approximately 1 week after hatching, although a limited amount of telencephalic neurogenesis persists into adulthood (DeWulf and Bottjer, 2005; Charvet and Striedter, 2009a; Kirn, 2010). In parakeets, the major period of telencephalic neurogenesis wanes approximately 2 weeks after hatching (Striedter and Charvet,

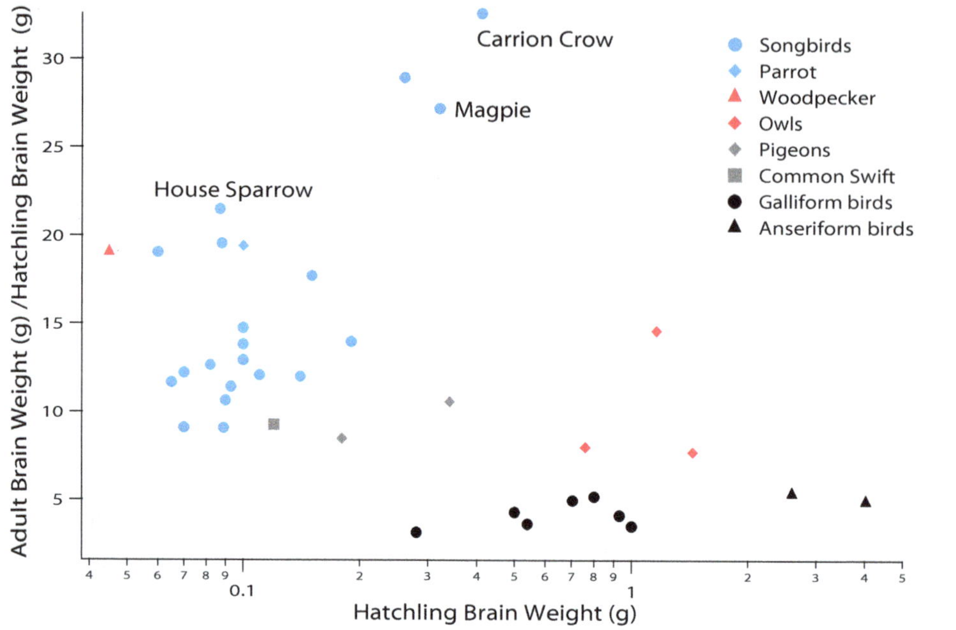

FIGURE 3 | Comparative analysis of avian post-hatching brain growth is measured by the ratio of adult to hatchling brain weight. Altricial species with proportionally small telencephalons (e.g., swifts and pigeons) exhibit more post-hatching brain growth than precocial species (e.g., anseriform and galliform birds). Parrots and songbirds (i.e., oscine passerines) exhibit even more post-hatching brain growth than many other altricial species. Among songbirds, corvids (carrion crows, magpies) exhibit some of the largest post-hatching brain growth. Because the telencephalon is born late in development, post-hatching brain growth is due primarily to the expansion of the telencephalon (see Striedter and Charvet, 2008; Charvet and Striedter, 2009a). Data are from Portmann (1947b).

2008), but the extent to which telencephalic neurogenesis persists in adult parrots is unclear. Because of the extension of telencephalic neurogenesis into the post-hatching period, the brains of parrots and songbirds are relatively immature at hatching. This immaturity presents no major problem, however, because parrot and songbird hatchlings receive extensive parental care.

Because most land birds are either altricial or semi-altricial, it is likely that altriciality evolved before the origin of parrots and passerines (songbirds and suboscines; **Figure 2**). This suggests that telencephalic expansion in the ancestors of modern songbirds and parrots, relative to suboscines, falcons and kingfishers (Day et al., 2005; Iwaniuk and Hurd, 2005; Charvet, 2010), occurred after the evolution of altriciality. Based on these observations, we hypothesize that altriciality may have been a pre-adaptation for telencephalic expansion and its associated delays of telencephalic neurogenesis and maturation in parrots and songbirds.

PRECOCIALITY REQUIRES AN ALTERNATE MECHANISM FOR TELENCEPHALIC EXPANSION

Although a disproportionately expanded telencephalon appears to be more common among altricial species than among precocial species (Iwaniuk and Nelson, 2003), ducks and geese are precocial and have evolved an enlarged telencephalon (Iwaniuk and Hurd, 2005). However, unlike parrots and songbirds, ducks and geese do not enlarge their telencephalon by delaying telencephalic neurogenesis. This is evident from the observation that post-hatching brain growth and neurogenesis timing are conserved in precocial anseriform and galliform birds (Portmann, 1947b; Charvet and Striedter, 2009b, 2010). Furthermore, the major period of neurogenesis is thought to be largely complete by hatching in precocial species (quail, chicken) although a limited amount of neurogenesis persists after hatching (Tsai et al., 1981; Nikolakopoulou et al., 2006; Striedter and Charvet, 2008). Instead of delaying neurogenesis, ducks (*Anas platyrhynchos*) and geese (*Anser anser*) enlarge their presumptive telencephalon early in development, before telencephalic cells exit the cell cycle (Charvet and Striedter, 2009b). Thus, the enlarged telencephalon of adult ducks and geese can be traced back to an expansion of the telencephalon precursor pool before neurogenesis begins.

Ducks and geese belong to a basal clade of neognathous birds (Hackett et al., 2008) and are closely related to paleognathous birds (e.g., emus; **Figure 2**). Because these lineages are all precocial (Starck and Ricklefs, 1998; see Burley and Johnson, 2002; Zhou and Zhang, 2004), the expansion of the telencephalon in anseriform birds probably evolved in precocial ancestors. We suggest that this ancestral precociality did not allow ducks and geese to enlarge their telencephalon by delaying telencephalic growth and maturation. Instead, anseriform birds enlarged their telencephalon by an alternate mechanism that probably involved a shift in the expression boundaries of genes or shortening cell cycle duration in the presumptive telencephalon prior to neurogenesis (Menuet et al., 2007; Charvet and Striedter, 2010; see McGowan et al., 2010; Sylvester et al., 2010). However, more work is needed to determine the developmental mechanisms underlying the early expansion of the telencephalon in ducks and geese.

DELAYED BRAIN MATURATION FACILITATES LEARNING

Delays in brain maturation probably foster behavioral flexibility and innovation. Although some innovative behaviors (e.g., bait-fishing, rock-throwing) have been reported in a variety of avian species such as vultures and wading birds (e.g., herons; van Lawick-Goodall and van Lawick, 1966; Higuchi, 1985; Post et al., 2009), many innovative behaviors have been reported in songbirds and parrots (Jones and Kamil, 1973; Tebbich et al., 2001; Lefebvre et al., 2002; Huber and Gajdon, 2006; Lefebvre and Sol, 2008; Prior et al., 2008; Pepperberg, 2010). Delays in brain maturation may promote the evolution of flexible and innovative behaviors, such as tool use and manufacture by some crows (Hunt, 1996; Emery and Clayton, 2004, 2009). Most spectacularly, parrots and songbirds have evolved specialized telencephalic circuits that allow them to produce learned vocalizations (Nottebohm, 1972; Nottebohm et al., 1976; Striedter, 1994; Mooney, 2009; Pepperberg, 2010). The telencephalic cell groups involved in vocal learning generally mature long after hatching, at least in songbirds (Bottjer et al., 1985; Alvarez-Buylla et al., 1992; Bottjer and Arnold, 1997; Kirn, 2010; Roberts et al., 2010). For instance, neurogenesis in the higher vocal control center (HVC) is high when zebra finches learn their vocalization, though it decreases substantially after zebra finches crystallize their song (Wilbrecht and Kirn, 2004). In contrast, neurogenesis in precocial birds is largely complete by hatching (Tsai et al., 1981; Striedter and Charvet, 2008). Therefore, we propose that the delayed maturation in songbirds and parrots is causally linked to delayed maturation of the entire telencephalon in parrots and songbirds. In other words, we suggest that the developmental mechanism used to expand the telencephalon in parrots and songbirds facilitated the emergence of vocal learning.

Primates resemble parrots and songbirds in that they are also capable of vocal learning and delay brain maturation into the post-hatching or post-natal period (Coqueugniot et al., 2004; Locke and Bogin, 2006). However, not all species that delay neurogenesis and brain maturation are capable of vocal learning. For instance, marsupials delay brain maturation well into the post-natal period (Darlington et al., 1999) but they are not known to learn complex vocalizations. Furthermore, several species of primates delay isocortical neurogenesis (Clancy et al., 2001), but humans are the only primates that learn complex vocalizations. Thus, all studied vocal learners delay telencephalic maturation into the juvenile period, but not all species that delay telencephalic maturation are vocal learners. These findings are consistent with our proposal that delaying telencephalic neurogenesis and maturation fosters the evolution of learned vocalizations.

CONCLUSION

Recent work has shown that nature has produced diverse developmental mechanisms for expanding specific brain regions, such as the telencephalon. These mechanisms include evolutionary changes in gene expression patterns, neurogenesis timing, and cell cycle rates (Finlay and Darlington, 1995; Bachy et al., 2001; Clancy et al., 2001; Menuet et al., 2007; Dyer et al., 2009; Abellan et al., 2010; Charvet and Striedter, 2010; Finlay et al., 2010; Sylvester et al., 2010). We here explain some of this diversity in developmental mechanisms by examining evolutionary changes in developmental modes. Specifically, we suggest that ducks and geese could not expand their telencephalon by delaying telencephalic neurogenesis because their ancestors were precocial. In contrast, songbirds and parrots were able to expand their telencephalon by delaying neurogenesis because their ancestors were already altricial and, therefore, prepared to care for helpless hatchlings. Post-hatching neurogenesis and brain maturation, in turn, may have facilitated the emergence of specialized circuits that mediate vocal learning. Whether delays in brain maturation also made songbirds and parrots more flexible and innovative in other aspects of behavior remains an interesting question.

ACKNOWLEDGMENTS

We thank Dr. Andrew Iwaniuk for kindly providing his data on brain size in birds. We thank Dr. Nancy Burley for very helpful comments on the manuscript. This work was supported by an NSF grant # IOS-0744332.

REFERENCES

Abellan, A., Menuet, A., Dehay, C., Medina, L., and Rétaux, S. (2010). Differential expression of LIM-homeodomain factors in Cajal–Retzius cells of primates, rodents, and birds. *Cereb. Cortex* 20, 1788–1798.

Alvarez-Buylla, A., Ling, C. Y., and Nottebohm, F. (1992). High vocal center growth and its relation to neurogenesis, neuronal replacement and song acquisition in juvenile canaries. *J. Neurobiol.* 23, 396–406.

Bachy, I., Vernier, P., and Retaux, S. (2001). The LIM-homeodomain gene family in the developing *Xenopus* brain: conservation and divergences with the mouse related to the evolution of the forebrain. *J. Neurosci.* 21, 7620–7629.

Barnea, A., and Nottebohm, F. (1994). Seasonal recruitment of hippocampal neurons in adult free-ranging black-capped chickadees. *Proc. Natl. Acad. Sci. U.S.A.* 91, 11217–11221.

Boire, D., and Baron, G. (1994). Allometric comparison of brain and main brain subdivisions in birds. *J. Hirnforsch.* 35, 49–66.

Bottjer, S. W., and Arnold, A. P. (1997). Developmental plasticity in neural circuits for a learned behavior. *Annu. Rev. Neurosci.* 20, 459–481.

Bottjer, S. W., Glaessner, S. L., and Arnold, A. P. (1985). Ontogeny of brain nuclei controlling song learning and behavior in zebra finches. *J. Neurosci.* 5, 1556–1562.

Burley, N. T., and Johnson, K. (2002). The evolution of avian parental care. *Philos. Trans. R. Soc. Lond., B, Biol. Sci.* 357, 241–250.

Charvet, C. (2010). *Developmental Origins of Brain Diversity in Birds and Reptiles.* Ph.D. thesis, University of California, Irvine.

Charvet, C. J., and Striedter, G. F. (2008). Developmental species differences in brain cell cycle rates between bobwhite quail (*Colinus virginianus*) and parakeets (*Melopsittacus undulatus*): implications for mosaic brain evolution. *Brain Behav. Evol.* 72, 295–306.

Charvet, C. J., and Striedter, G. F. (2009a). Developmental origins of mosaic brain evolution: morphometric analysis of the developing zebra finch brain. *J. Comp. Neurol.* 514, 203–213.

Charvet, C. J., and Striedter, G. F. (2009b). Developmental basis for telencephalon expansion in waterfowls: enlargement prior to neurogenesis. *Proc. Biol. Sci.* 276, 3421–3427.

Charvet, C. J., and Striedter, G. F. (2010). Bigger brains cycle faster before neurogenesis begins: a comparison in brain development between chickens and bobwhite quail. *Proc. Biol. Sci.* 277, 3469–3475.

Clancy, B., Darlington, R. B., and Finlay, B. L. (2001). Translating developmental time across mammalian species. *Neuroscience* 105, 7–17.

Coqueugniot, H., Hublin, J. J., Veillon, F., Houët, F., and Jacob, T. (2004). Early brain growth in *Homo erectus* and implications for cognitive ability. *Nature* 431, 299–302.

Darlington, R. B., Dunlop, S. A., and Finlay, B. L. (1999). Neural development in metatherian and eutherian mammals: variation and constraint. *J. Comp. Neurol.* 411, 359–368.

Day, L. B., Fusani, L., and Schlinger, B. A. (2005). Sex differences in brain areas related to courtship display in manakins. *Soc. Neurosci. Abstr.* 762, 9.

DeWulf, V., and Bottjer, S. W. (2005). Neurogenesis within the juvenile zebra finch telencephalic ventricular zone: a map of proliferative activity. *J. Comp. Neurol.* 481, 70–83.

Doupe, A. J., and Kuhl, P. K. (1999). Birdsong and human speech: common themes and mechanisms. *Annu. Rev. Neurosci.* 22, 567–631.

Dubbeldam, J. L., and Visser, A. M. (1987). The organization of the nucleus basalis-neostriatum complex of the mallard (*Anas platyrhynchos* L.) and its connections with the archistriatum and the paleostriatum complex. *Neuroscience* 21, 487–517.

Dyer, M. A., Martins, R., da Silva Filho, M., Muniz, J. A., Silveira, L. C., Cepko C. L., and Finlay, B. L. (2009). Developmental sources of conservation and variation in the evolution of the primate eye. *Proc. Natl. Acad. Sci. U.S.A.* 106, 8963–8968.

Emery, N. J., and Clayton, N. S. (2004). The mentality of crows: convergent evolution of intelligence in corvids and apes. *Science* 306, 1903–1907.

Emery, N. J., and Clayton, N. S. (2009). Tool use and physical cognition in birds and mammals. *Curr. Opin. Neurobiol.* 19, 27–33.

Ericson, P. G., Anderson, C. L., Britton, T., Elzanowski, A., Johansson, U. S., Källersjö, M., Ohlson, J. I., Parsons, T. J., Zuccon, D., and Mayr, G. (2006). Diversification of Neoaves: integration of molecular sequence data and fossils. *Biol. Lett.* 2, 543–547.

Finlay, B. L., Clancy, B., and Darlington, R. B. (2010). Late stills equals large. *Brain Behav. Evol.* 75, 4–6.

Finlay, B. L., and Darlington, R. B. (1995). Linked regularities in the development and evolution of mammalian brains. *Science* 268, 1578–1584.

Finlay, B. L., Hersman, M. N., and Darlington, R. B. (1998). Patterns of vertebrate neurogenesis and the paths of vertebrate evolution. *Brain Behav. Evol.* 52, 232–242.

Greeny, H. F., Dobbs, R. C., and Gelis, R. A. (2005). The nest, eggs, nestlings, and parental care of the Bronze-olive Pygmy-Tyrant (*Pseudotriccus pelzelni*). *Ornitol. Neotrop.* 16, 511–518.

Greeny, H. F., Krabbe, N., Lysinger, M., and Funk, W. C. (2004). Observations on the breeding and vocalizations of the Fulvous-breasted Flatbill (*Rhynchocyclus fulvipectus*) in eastern Ecuador. *Ornitol. Neotrop.* 15, 365–370.

Gutiérrez-Ibáñez, C., Iwaniuk, A. N., and Wylie, D. R. (2009). The independent evolution of the enlargement of the principal sensory nucleus of the trigeminal nerve in three different groups of birds. *Brain Behav. Evol.* 74, 280–294.

Hackett, S. J., Kimball, R. T., Reddy, S., Bowie, R. C., Braun, E. L., Braun, M. J., Chojnowski, J. L., Cox, W. A., Han, K. L., Harshman, J., Huddleston, C. J., Marks, B. D., Miglia, K. J., Moore, W. S., Sheldon, F. H., Steadman, D. W., Witt, C. C., and Yuri, T. (2008). A phylogenomic study of birds reveals their evolutionary history. *Science* 320, 1763–1768.

Higuchi, H. (1985). Bait-fishing by the Green-backed Heron *Ardeola striata* in Japan. *Ibis* 128, 285–290.

Huber, L., and Gajdon, G. K. (2006). Technical intelligence in animals: the kea model. *Anim. Cogn.* 9, 295–305.

Hunt, G. R. (1996). Manufacture and use of hook-tools by New Caledonian Crows. *Nature* 379, 249–251.

Iwaniuk, A. N., and Hurd, P. L. (2005). The evolution of cerebrotypes in birds. *Brain Behav. Evol.* 65, 215–230.

Iwaniuk, A. N., and Nelson, J. E. (2003). Developmental differences are correlated with relative brain size in birds: a comparative analysis. *Can. J. Zool.* 81, 1913–1928.

Jones, T. B., and Kamil, A. C. (1973). Tool-making and tool-using in the Northern Blue Jay. *Science* 180, 1076–1078.

Kirn, J. R. (2010). The relationship of neurogenesis and growth of brain regions to song learning. *Brain Lang.* 115, 29–44.

Kirn, J. R., and DeVoogd, T. J. (1989). Genesis and death of vocal control neurons during sexual differentiation in the zebra finch. *J. Neurosci.* 9, 3176–3187.

Lefebvre, L., Nicolakakis, N., and Boire, D. (2002). Tools and brains in birds. *Behaviour* 139, 939–973.

Lefebvre, L., and Sol, D. (2008). Brains, lifestyles and cognition: are there general trends? *Brain Behav. Evol.* 72, 135–144.

Ling, C., Zuo, M., Alvarez-Buylla, A., and Cheng, M. F. (1997). Neurogenesis in juvenile and adult ring doves. *J. Comp. Neurol.* 379, 300–312.

Locke, J. L., and Bogin, B. (2006). Language and life history: a new perspective on the development and evolution of human language. *Behav. Brain Sci.* 29, 259–280.

Londoño, G. A. (2003). First description of the nest and eggs of the Plumbeous (*Myrmeciza hyperythra*) and the Blackfaced (*Myrmoborus myototerinus*) antbirds. *Ornitol. Neotrop.* 14, 405–410.

McGowan, L., Kuo, E., Martin, A., Monuki, E. S., and Striedter, G. (in press). Species differences in early patterning of the avian brain. *Evolution* doi: 10.1111/j.1558-5646.2010.01126.x

Menuet, A., Alunni, A., Joly, J. S., Jeffrey, W. R., and Rétaux S. (2007). Expanded expression of Sonic Hedgehog in *Astyanax* cavefish: multiple consequences on forebrain development and evolution. *Development* 134, 845–855.

Mooney, R. (2009). Neural mechanisms for learned birdsong. *Learn. Mem.* 16, 655–669.

Nikolakopoulou, A. M., Parpas, A., Panagis, L., Zikopoulos, B., and Dermon, C. R. (2006). Early post-hatching sex differences in cell proliferation and survival in the quail telencephalic ventricular zone and intermediate medial mesopallium. *Brain Res. Bull.* 70, 107–116.

Nottebohm, F. (1972). The origins of vocal learning. *Am. Nat.* 106, 116–140.

Nottebohm, F., Stokes, T. M., and Leonard, C. M. (1976). Central control of song in the canary, *Serinus canarius*. *J. Comp. Neurol.* 165, 457–486.

Paton, J. A., and Nottebohm, F. N. (1984). Neurons generated in the adult brain are recruited into functional circuits. *Science* 225, 1046–1048.

Pepperberg, I. M. (2010). Vocal learning in Grey parrots: a brief review of perception, production, and cross-species comparisons. *Brain Lang.* 115, 81–91.

Portmann, A. (1947a). Étude sur la cérébralisation chez les oiseaux. II. Les indices intracérébraux. *Alauda* 15, 1–15.

Portmann, A. (1947b). Étude sur la cérébralisation chez les oiseaux. III. Cérébralisation et mode ontogénétique. *Alauda* 15, 161–171.

Post, R. J., Post C. P. K., and Walsh, J. F. (2009). Little Egret (*Egretta garzetta*) and Grey Heron (*Ardea cinerea*) using bait for fishing in Kenya. *Waterbirds* 32, 450–452.

Prior, H., Schwarz, A., and Güntürkün, O. (2008). Mirror-induced behavior in the magpie (*Pica pica*): evidence of self-recognition. *PLoS Biol.* 6, e202. doi: 10.1371/journal.pbio.0060202

Roberts, T. F., Tschida, K. A., Klein, M. E., and Mooney, R. (2010). Rapid spine stabilization and synaptic enhancement at the onset of behavioural learning. *Nature* 463, 948–952.

Starck, J. M., and Ricklefs, R. E. (1998). *Avian Growth and Development: Evolution Within the Altricial-Precocial Spectrum*. New York: Oxford University Press.

Striedter, G. F. (1994). The vocal control pathways in budgerigars differ from those in songbirds. *J. Comp. Neurol.* 343, 35–56.

Striedter, G. F., and Charvet, C. J. (2008). Developmental origins of species differences in telencephalon and tectum size: morphometric comparisons between a parakeet (*Melopsittacus undulatus*) and a quail (*Colinus virgianus*). *J. Comp. Neurol.* 507, 1663–1675.

Striedter, G. F., and Charvet, C. J. (2009). Telencephalon enlargement by the convergent evolution of expanded subventricular zones. *Biol. Lett.* 5, 134–137.

Sylvester, J. B., Rich, C. A., Loh, Y. H., van Staaden, M. J., Fraser, G. J., and Streelman, J. T. (2010). Brain diversity evolves via differences in patterning. *Proc. Natl. Acad. Sci. U.S.A.* 107, 9718–9723.

Tebbich, S., Taborsky, M., Fessl, B., and Blomqvist, D. (2001). Do woodpecker finches acquire tool-use by social learning? *Proc. Biol. Sci.* 268, 2189–2193.

Tsai, H. M., Garber, B. B., and Larramendi, L. M. (1981). 3H-thymidine autoradiographic analysis of telencephalic histogenesis in the chick embryo: I. Neuronal birthdates of telencephalic compartments in situ. *J. Comp. Neurol.* 198, 275–292.

van Lawick-Goodall, J., and van Lawick, H. (1966). Use of tools by the Egyptian vulture, *Neophron percnopterus*. *Nature* 212, 1468–1469.

Wilbrecht, L., and Kirn, J. R. (2004). Neuron addition and loss in the song system: regulation and function. *Ann. N. Y. Acad. Sci.* 1016, 659–683.

Zhou Z., and Zhang F. (2004). A precocial avian embryo from the Lower Cretaceous of China. *Science* 306, 653.

Conflict of Interest Statement: The authors declare that the research was conducted in the absence of any commercial or financial relationships that could be construed as a potential conflict of interest.

6

The evolution of dopamine systems in chordates

Kei Yamamoto and Philippe Vernier*

Neurobiology and Development (UPR3294), Institute of Neurobiology Alfred Fessard, CNRS, Gif-sur-Yvette, France

Edited by:
Agustín González, Universidad Complutense de Madrid, Spain

Reviewed by:
Mario F. Wullimann, Ludwig Maximilians University, Germany
Nilima Prakash, Helmholtz Center Munich, Germany

***Correspondence:**
Philippe Vernier, Neurobiology and Development (UPR3294), Institute of Neurobiology Alfred Fessard, CNRS, Gif-sur-Yvette 91198, France.
e-mail: vernier@inaf.cnrs-gif.fr

Dopamine (DA) neurotransmission in the central nervous system (CNS) is found throughout chordates, and its emergence predates the divergence of chordates. Many of the molecular components of DA systems, such as biosynthetic enzymes, transporters, and receptors, are shared with those of other monoamine systems, suggesting the common origin of these systems. In the mammalian CNS, the DA neurotransmitter systems are diversified and serve for visual and olfactory perception, sensory–motor programming, motivation, memory, emotion, and endocrine regulations. Some of the functions are conserved among different vertebrate groups, while others are not, and this is reflected in the anatomical aspects of DA systems in the forebrain and midbrain. Recent findings concerning a second tyrosine hydroxylase gene (*TH2*) revealed new populations of DA-synthesizing cells, as evidenced in the periventricular hypothalamic zones of teleost fish. It is likely that the ancestor of vertebrates possessed *TH2* DA-synthesizing cells, and the *TH2* gene has been lost secondarily in placental mammals. All the vertebrates possess DA cells in the olfactory bulb, retina, and in the diencephalon. Midbrain DA cells are abundant in amniotes while absent in some groups, e.g., teleosts. Studies of protochordate DA cells suggest that the diencephalic DA cells were present before the divergence of the chordate lineage. In contrast, the midbrain cell populations have probably emerged in the vertebrate lineage following the development of the midbrain–hindbrain boundary. The functional flexibility of the DA systems, and the evolvability provided by duplication of the corresponding genes permitted a large diversification of these systems. These features were instrumental in the adaptation of brain functions to the very variable way of life of vertebrates.

Keywords: tyrosine hydroxylase, monoamine transporters, monoamine receptors, vertebrates, protochordates, gene duplication, forebrain, hypothalamus

INTRODUCTION

Since the seminal discovery that it could be a neurotransmitter in the central nervous system (CNS) of vertebrates (Carlsson et al., 1958), dopamine (DA) has received a lot of attention due to its role in many cerebral functions and its implication in a number of major human diseases. Indeed, DA acts to modulate early steps of sensory perception in the olfactory bulb and the retina, motor programming, learning, and memory, affective and motivational processes in the forebrain, control of body temperature, food intake, and several other hypothalamic functions as well as chemosensitivity in the area postrema and solitary tract, to cite only the main of the DA-controlled functions. Dysfunction of DA neurotransmission was initially shown in Parkinson's disease (Hornykiewicz, 1962), fostering an enormous interest for this neurotransmitter. In addition, DA has now been shown to significantly contribute to the pathophysiology of several psychiatric disorders such as schizophrenia, addiction to drugs, or attention deficit with hyperactivity.

Implication of DA in such a large range of otherwise unrelated functions, its wide distribution in a number of brain nuclei, and fast-growing knowledge about the differentiation of these DA neuronal groups strongly suggest that there is not a unique DA system, but several, independent anatomo-physiological systems, with DA as the only common denominator. It is thus of importance to trace back the origin of these different DA systems in the course of the evolution of chordate animals, the group to which vertebrates belong, in order to gain clues of the adaptive constraints which led to select each of the DA systems, and to understand better the nature of functions that DA exerts in the brain and how it can become maladaptive in neuropsychiatric diseases. In this review, we integrate recent data with established features of DA systems, to shed a new light on their origin and evolution in chordates.

MOLECULAR COMPONENTS DEFINING THE PHENOTYPE OF DA NEURONS AND THEIR PHYLOGENY

Dopamine is a catecholamine that is an amine derivative of catechol (2-hydroxyphenol). DA is certainly one of the oldest neurotransmitters, since it is being used as such in a very wide range of metazoans including diblastic species (Carlberg and Anctil, 1993). DA can also be a precursor of melanin pigments in many animals. For example, it plays a role in immunity and cuticle hardening in insects (Tang, 2009), and produces neuromelanin of the substantia nigra in humans (Fedorow et al., 2005).

Dopamine is derived from the aromatic amino acid tyrosine through two enzymatic stages. The first and limiting step is catalyzed by tyrosine hydroxylase [TH; an aromatic amino acid hydroxylase (AAAH)] and the second step is catalyzed by an aromatic amino acid decarboxylase (AADC; **Figure 1A**). Since the supply of tyrosine in food is short, most of the tyrosine used for dopamine synthesis is derived from another aromatic amino acid, phenylalanine, which is present *ad libitum* in food. Phenylalanine is transformed into tyrosine by the enzyme phenylalanine hydroxylase (PAH), which is also a member of the AAAH family.

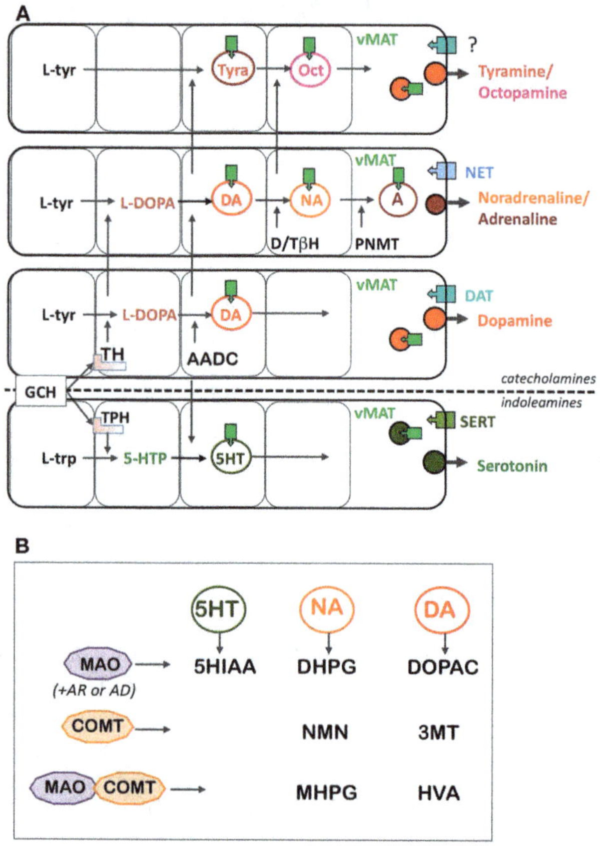

FIGURE 1 | Schematic representation of the metabolic (A) and catabolic (B) pathways of DA and other monoamines. (A) The biosynthesis of DA is highly modular and shares several molecular components with biosynthetic pathways of other monoamines. Catecholamines are synthesized from the aromatic amino acid l-tyrosine, and indoleamines synthesized from the aromatic amino acid l-tryptophan, but TH and TPH display many common characteristics, including the same co-factor (tetrahydrobiopterin, pinkish square under TH and TPH). Tyramine and octopamine come from the same pathways than the other catecholamines, without the primary action of TH. Then, AADC and vMAT are components shared by all the pathways, including indoleamines. Finally, the membrane transporters, DAT, NET, and SERT, responsible for the re-uptake of the monoamines are more specific of the different monoamine pathways based on their cell-expression pattern, although their functional specificity is weak, especially for the DAT and NET (see text). **(B)** The catabolic enzymes are also essentially shared by all the monoamines. MAO is an intracellular enzyme, whose direct metabolites are rapidly transformed by aldehyde reductases (AR) and aldehyde dehydrogenase (AD) in compounds (5HIAA for serotonin, DHPG for noradrenaline, and DOPAC for dopamine) easy to assay and which reflect the utilization of the transmitters. The effect of COMT, combined to that of MAO, provides metabolites assayable in body fluid such as CSF, blood, or urine, reflecting preferentially the utilization of monoamines at the periphery of the body. Abbreviations: 3MT, 3-methoxytyramine; 5HIAA, 5-hydroxy-acetic acid; 5-HTP, 5-hydroxytryptophan; AADC, aromatic amino acid decarboxylase; AD, aldehyde dehydrogenase; AR, aldehyde reductase; COMT, catechol-*O*-methyl transferase; DAT, dopamine transporter; DHPG, 3,4-dihydroxyphenyl-ethylene-glycol; DOPAC, 3,4-dihydroxyphenylacetate; D/TβH, dopamine/tyramine β-hydroxylase; GCH, GTP cyclohydrolase; HVA, homovanillic acid; l-trp, l-tryptophan; l-tyr, l-tyrosine; MAO, monoamine oxidase; MHPG, 3-methoxy-4-hydroxyphenyl-ethylene-glycol; NET, noradrenaline transporter; NMN, normetanephrine; Oct, octopamine; PNMT, phenylethanolamine-*N*-methyl transferase; SERT, serotonine transporter; TH, tyrosine hydroxylase; Tyra, tyramine; vMAT, vesicular monoamine transporter.

Dopamine is also a precursor of two other catecholamines, noradrenaline, and adrenaline. Noradrenaline is produced through the action of the enzyme dopamine/tyramine β-hydroxylase (DBH). Adrenaline requires an additional step catalyzed by phenylethanolamine-*N*-methyl transferase (PNMT; **Figure 1A**). Catecholamines are included in a larger category of intercellular transmitters, the monoamines, which was initially defined by their property to be degraded by monoamine oxidases (MAO). Monoamines also comprise indolamines (e.g., serotonin, melatonin) and trace amines (tyramine, octopamine), the latter present in low amount in vertebrates. Histamine is also often included into the monoamines, although it is a diamine degraded by diamine oxidase.

The synthesized DA is then stored in synaptic vesicles by vesicular monoamine transporter 2 (vMAT2). DA is released at nerve terminal or dendrites upon neuronal depolarization. Neurotransmitter release is controlled by the synaptic machinery and triggered upon depolarization of the terminals and calcium entry (Pucak and Grace, 1994). The release of the different monoamines seems to depend on the differential contribution of synaptic molecules such as synapsins. This may be relevant to specific mode of release regulation depending on the monoamine neurotransmitters. Dendritic release also occurs by a vesicular mechanism controlled by local calcium concentration. Its role in regulating the presynaptic activity of dopamine neurons in areas such as the substantia nigra is critical to the overall regulation of mesostriatal, mesocortico-limbic systems, and related functions (Pucak and Grace, 1994). The released, extracellular DA is taken up by the dopamine transporter (DAT) located into the plasma membrane of nerve terminals, to terminate the neurotransmission. DA is then degraded inside the cells by monoamine oxidase (MAO) and catechol-*O*-methyl transferase (COMT).

Many of the molecular components used in dopamine neurotransmission are shared with the other monoamine neurons (**Figure 1**). This is the case for AADC, vMAT2, and MAO, for example. Other components of dopamine, noradrenaline, or serotonin neurons are members of the same gene/protein family. This is the case of dopamine, noradrenaline, and serotonin membrane transporters (DAT, NET, and SERT), or of the synthesizing enzymes TH, TPH, and PAH. It is thus important to discuss the evolution of these molecules together. We here present the various molecular components such as synthesizing and catabolic enzymes, transporters, and receptors, which define the phenotype of the dopamine systems. We also present and discuss the phylogenies of the molecular components of monoamine systems.

TYROSINE HYDROXYLASE (TH)

The active form of TH, as for the other AAAH, is a tetramer coordinated by one iron atom and binding a co-factor, tetrahydrobiopterin (BH4), synthesized by the enzyme GTP cyclohydrolase. TH sequence can be broadly divided into two domains, a catalytic C-terminal domain (two-third of the protein sequence), the structure of which has been resolved (Goodwill et al., 1997; Teigen et al., 2004) and which is highly conserved in all metazoans, and a N-terminal regulatory domain which bears several phosphorylation sites, and which is much more variable, both in length and sequence (Kumer and Vrana, 1996). In vertebrates phosphorylation sites for the MAP kinase ERK, for the protein kinase A, and protein kinase C are highly conserved, and in every species where it has been tested, TH phosphorylation is required for the enzyme to be active (Dunkley et al., 2004). In addition, in several vertebrate species – mostly mammals but also other amniotes – alternative splicing of the *TH* mRNA generates several isoforms of TH, which allow a tissues-specific, differential regulation of TH activity by phosphorylation (Kumer and Vrana, 1996; Nakashima et al., 2009).

The structural requirements for enzyme activity impose heavy constraints on TH sequence, highlighted by its strong conservation in both protostomes and deuterostomes. Only one *TH* gene has been found in the protostomes. The protostome *TH* is clearly homologous to deuterostome *TH* (including vertebrates), suggesting that the two animal groups share a common ancestral gene. In basal deuterostomes, only one *TH* gene has been found (in sea urchin, ascidia, and amphioxus for example), which is also a clear homolog of protostome and vertebrate *TH* genes. Inside vertebrates, the situation is more complex. Two *TH* genes (*TH1* and *TH2*) have been recently shown to exist in most gnathostomes (jawed vertebrates) except in eutherian mammals (Candy and Collet, 2005; Yamamoto et al., 2010; **Figure 2A**). A *TH2*-related gene is indeed present in prototherians (platypus) and metatherians (opossum). Phylogenetic analyses and gene synteny strongly suggest that the two *TH* genes were duplicated before or close to the divergence of the jawed vertebrates, and secondarily lost in the eutherian lineage (Yamamoto et al., 2010). The exact timing of the duplication cannot be ascertained until completion of the genome sequence in agnathostomes (jawless vertebrate; e.g., lamprey). A recent study showed that the lamprey *Petromyzon marinus* possess at least one TH gene (Barreiro-Iglesias et al., 2010). The phylogenetic analysis shows that the lamprey TH gene belongs to the clade of *TH1* of jawed vertebrates rather than being an outgroup of TH1 and TH2. This favors that the TH duplication occurred before the separation of the gnathostomes and agnathostomes. However, more genomic information is required to know if lamprey has second *TH* gene (**Figure 2A**).

Incidentally, the evolutionary history of TH genes is shared by the other members of AAAH family, PAH, and tryptophan hydroxylase (TPH), the key-enzyme of indoleamine biosynthesis. Only one copy of each AAAH gene (*TH, TPH, PAH*) is found in the non-vertebrate bilaterians. In contrast, in most groups of jawed vertebrates, at least two *TH* and *TPH* genes are found, while *PAH* gene exhibits only one copy. Interestingly, the *TPH1* gene is located on the same chromosome as *TH1* (e.g., in human, chicken, and zebrafish), while *TPH2* and *PAH* tend to be on the same chromosome as *TH2*. In case of non-mammals, *PAH* and *TH2* are next to each other on the same chromosome. It is thus likely that an ancestral chromosome was bearing the three genes (*TH, TPH,* and *PAH*), and they have been duplicated early in the vertebrate evolution, probably corresponding to one of the whole genome duplications proposed to have occurred close to vertebrate emergence (Panopoulou and Poustka, 2005). Considering the presence of only one *PAH* gene throughout the vertebrates, one copy of *PAH* (close the *TH1* locus) should have been lost early during vertebrate evolution, while the two *TH* and *TPH* genes were kept (*TPH* went through an additional duplication in the teleostean lineage). The evolution of the paralogous regions of the human chromosome 11 and 12 have been already described in relation to the evolution of AAAHs and insulin-related genes (Patton et al., 1998), and our observations are consistent with this hypothesis.

AROMATIC AMINO ACID DECARBOXYLASE (AADC)

The aromatic amino acid decarboxylase (AADC) catalyzes the transformation of L-DOPA into dopamine, and as such it is often called "DOPA decarboxylase" (encoded by the *ddc* gene). However, it does not use only L-DOPA as a substrate, but also 5-HTP, the precursor of indoleamines such as serotonin (5HT). As for the catecholamines, AADC catalyzes the second step of 5HT synthesis, that is the transformation of 5-HTP into 5HT. It is a member of decarboxylase genes, which form a large protein family involved in the catabolism of amino acids, the products of which are also used as neurotransmitters (e.g., histidine decarboxylase for the synthesis of histamine, glutamate decarboxylase for GABA). The evolutionary history of orthologous and paralogous decarboxylase genes is rather complex (Saenz-de-Miera and Ayala, 2004). However, a *bona fide* AADC is present in both protostomes and deuterostomes, indicating that this enzyme was probably ancestral to all the bilaterians. It has been duplicated in insects (providing the paralogous *amd* gene) but not in deuterostomes including vertebrates. Although a single *ddc* gene exists in all the vertebrates species analyzed so far, alternative transcription provides at least two forms of transcripts in mammals, one of them being specifically expressed in the nervous system.

VESICULAR MONOAMINE TRANSPORTER

Dopamine is actively transported into vesicles by exchange of protons across the vesicular membrane (two protons for one monoamine molecule) promoted by the vMAT2 (or slc18a2; reviewed in Parsons, 2000; Eiden et al., 2004). Two *vMAT* genes are present in jawed vertebrates, *vMAT1* (*slc18a1*) localized exclusively in peripheral neuroendocrine cells, and *vMAT2*, present both in some neuroendocrine cells and in the neurons of the peripheral and CNS (Weihe and Eiden, 2000). vMAT2 is not specific to DA, but allows the accumulation of all sort of monoamines, with similar affinity and efficacy, leading to a 10,000 higher concentration of DA inside the vesicle than in the cytoplasm. In addition, the uptake of DA or other monoamines into vesicles protects the cells against the toxic effect of auto-oxidized monoamines, in particular quinones, which are important factors of oxidative stress and may predispose brain areas synthesizing high amounts of monoamines to neurodegenerative disorders, such as Parkinson's disease and supranuclear palsy for example (Vernier et al., 2004; Guillot and Miller, 2009). The existence of the two *vMAT* genes (*vMAT1* and *vMAT2*) is certainly the result of a craniate/vertebrate duplication, as it was also the case for *TH* and other genes encoding monoaminergic markers (**Figure 2A**). But, again the duplication time cannot be inferred due to absence of data in jawless vertebrates. Orthologs of *vMAT* are present in other chordates such as ascidians, and also in protostomes such as drosophila and *Caenorhabditis elegans* (Guillot and Miller, 2009) revealing that they are major components of the monoamine neurons throughout the evolution of bilaterian animals.

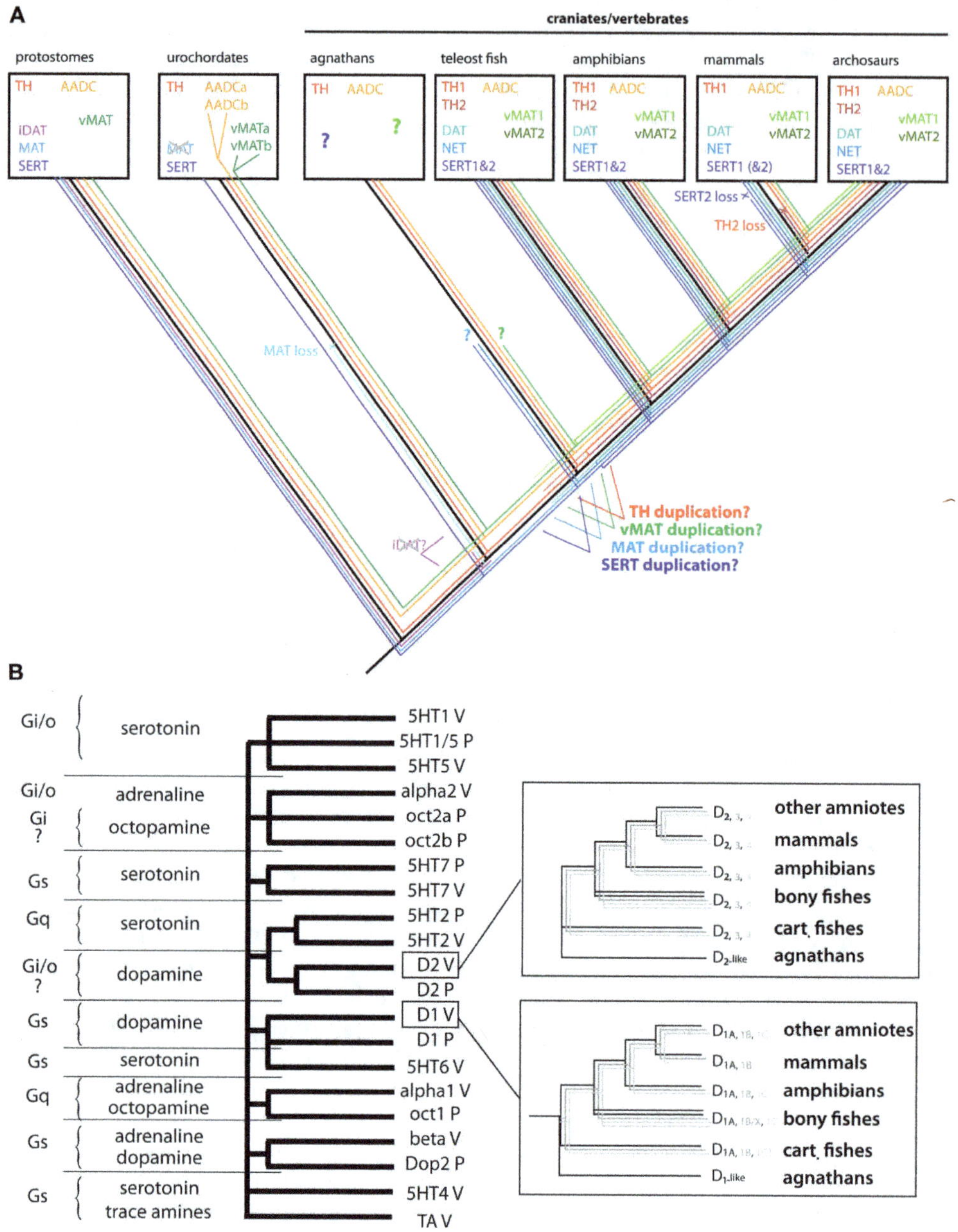

FIGURE 2 | Evolution of the molecular components of the monoaminergic systems in chordates. (A) Protochordates have all the basic molecular components of the monoamine pathways found in vertebrates. In urochordates, both MAT and iDAT do not exist but since MAT is present in amphioxus, it may have been lost specifically in urochordates. The loss of iDAT may have occurred earlier since it is not present in amphioxus. In vertebrates, MAT has been duplicated to provide DAT and NET, which are not thus orthologous to invertebrate iDAT but to invertebrate MAT. Similarly, SERT has been duplicated in jawed vertebrates. vMAT and AADC have been specifically duplicated in the urochordate lineage. Close to the emergence of vertebrates, TH, AADC, and vMAT have been duplicated. But since no genomic data are available yet in agnathans, it is currently impossible to known if this duplication took place before or after the emergence of jawed vertebrates. TH2 and SERT2 have been lost in placental mammals. Abbreviations and colors: AADC, aromatic amino acid decarboxylase (orange); iDAT and DAT, invertebrate form (i), and vertebrate form of dopamine transporter (light blue); MAT, monoamine transporter (blue); NET, noradrenaline transporter (blue); SERT, serotonine transporter (marine blue); TH, tyrosine hydroxylase (red); vMAT, vesicular monoamine transporter (green). **(B)** The molecular phylogeny of monoamine receptor in bilaterian animals reveals that most classes of monoamine receptors predated the origin of chordates and vertebrates. Classes of orthologous receptors in vertebrates and protostomes (most sequences come from ecdysozoan insects and nematodes) are transducing signals in cells via the same G protein (question marks correspond to the cases when the nature of G protein in not known), highlighting one of the major constraint on the conservation of the receptor sequences throughout bilaterian evolution. For example, α_1 adrenergic receptors are orthologous to octopamine 1 receptors (Oct1) and α_2 adrenergic receptors are orthologous to octopamine 2 receptors (Oct2), but both D_1-like and D_2-like receptors are also dopaminergic in protostomes. The topology of the tree also shows that receptor classes that bind the same natural ligand (e.g., DA) are not grouped together, suggesting that each class of receptor acquired independently and convergently the ability to bind a given neurotransmitter. Inside the rectangle, a simplified version of the phylogenetical relationships of the D_1 and D_2 receptor is presented. Three subtypes of receptor exist in each class, with the notable exception of mammals.

DOPAMINE TRANSPORTER

After DA release into the extracellular space, the DAT (or slc6a3) located at the plasma membrane of nerve terminals is the main controller of the duration of the signal transmission, by taking up the extracellular neurotransmitter. In addition to DAT, two other monoamine transporters (MAT) exist in vertebrates, one for noradrenalin (NET or slca2) and one for serotonin (SERT or slc6a4), all belonging to the same protein family of solute carriers (slc6; Torres et al., 2003). The DAT has the capacity to transport both DA and noradrenaline, and the NET has an even better affinity for DA than noradrenaline (Apparsundaram et al., 1997; Roubert et al., 2001). However, both have several hundred orders of magnitude less affinity for serotonin.

In the mammalian prefrontal cortex (PFC), where DAT is found to be expressed at only a very low level, NET plays a major role for DA re-uptake (Moron et al., 2002; Carboni and Silvagni, 2004; Valentini et al., 2004). Also, when a given membrane MAT has been blocked or inactivated, the other remaining transporters are able to compensate, at least partially for the transporter loss-of-function (Sulzer and Edwards, 2005). Re-uptake of DA and NA by SERT (Vizi et al., 2004; Kannari et al., 2006), and re-uptake of 5HT by DAT and NET (Daws et al., 1998; Zhou et al., 2005; Mossner et al., 2006) have been described. Also, in the protochordate ascidia, SERT is expressed in DA-synthesizing cells of the sensory vesicle (Razy-Krajka et al., unpublished). When the evolution of these gene families is taken into account, these heterologous interactions may not be so surprising, given the close relationships between many of these monoaminergic markers, several of which are used simultaneously by several biosynthetic pathways.

The evolution of membrane MAT has been well documented (Caveney et al., 2006), although some refinements can be made owing to recent genome data. Molecular phylogenies of MAT-related sequences show the existence of three classes of molecules inside the slc6 clade; a DAT restricted to invertebrates (iDAT), and two other groups of transporters, a catecholamine/phenolamine MAT, and an SERT. Vertebrate DAT and NET belong to the MAT branch, and there is no ortholog of the iDAT branch in vertebrates. Thus gene encoding DAT in vertebrates and in protostomes (iDAT) are not orthologous, but paralogous. It is suggested that the three genes iDAT, MAT, and SERT were present in basal bilaterians. In the chordate lineage, iDAT was lost while MAT was kept. MAT was then duplicated early in vertebrate evolution to give rise to DAT and NET found in contemporary vertebrates. The duplication occurred probably after separation of the cephalochordate lineage, because only one MAT gene is present in the amphioxus genome. In urochordates (e.g., ascidians), only SERT has been found but no other MAT-related sequences, and these species thus seem to have secondarily lost MAT at their ancestral stage. Finally SERT is likely to be duplicated in the stem vertebrate since two copies of SERT (SERT1 and SERT2) are found in each taxon except eutherian mammals (Caveney et al., 2006; our unpublished data). Gene synteny supports the lost of SERT2 in eutherian mammals, in a way reminiscent of the evolutionary history of TH in mammals (see above; Caveney et al., 2006).

DEGRADATION ENZYMES: MONOAMINE OXIDASE (MAO)

Dopamine, when freed into the cytoplasm, can be degraded into 3,4-dihydroxyphenylacetaldehyde (DOPAL), by monoamine oxidase (MAO), an homodimeric enzyme using FAD as co-factor and located on the external membrane of mitochondria. DOPAL is further oxidized by aldehyde dehydrogenase to 3,4-dihydroxyphenylacetate (DOPAC), often used as an index of DA catabolism and turn-over (reviewed in Nagatsu, 2004). Two MAO exist in most vertebrate species, MAO-A and MAO-B, with different relative affinities for catecholamines and indoleamines. MAO-A preferentially oxidizes phenylethylamine and DA, and it is located mostly in catecholamine-containing cell groups, such as the substantia nigra, the locus coeruleus, or the periventricular region of the hypothalamus. MAO-B uses 5HT as a degradation substrate and is localized mostly in serotoninergic neurons of the raphe nuclei, for example (Westlund et al., 1985; Willoughby et al., 1988; Anichtchik et al., 2006). The gene duplication that gave rise to the two *MAO* paralogs is a tandem duplication, as evidenced in the sequenced genomes of amniotes and amphibians (on the X chromosome in human). Interestingly, only one MAO exists in several teleost fish, with functional characteristics clearly closer to those of MAO-A than to those of MAO-B (Anichtchik et al., 2006; Sallinen et al., 2009). Whether the duplication of the *MAO* gene in vertebrates occurred before of after the emergence of teleosts cannot be established presently. However, it has to be stressed that MAO present in teleosts is mostly used in the 5HT system to regulate its metabolism, and its precise role in the regulation of the metabolism of other monoamines, including DA, needs to be investigated further.

The presence of MAO-A and -B is of importance for human pathophysiology since the neurotoxic MPTP is metabolized by MAO-A into MMP$^+$ in non-dopaminergic neurons, but it becomes toxic when taken up by DAT (and not NET or SERT) into DA neurons, where it promotes mitochondria-dependent apoptosis and a syndrome close to idiopathic Parkinson's disease. Accordingly, different species have differential susceptibility to MPTP, zebrafish, mouse, and primates being rather sensitive to the toxic, but rats are much more resistant, for example.

Since MAO sequence has not been described yet in cartilaginous fish or in jawless vertebrates, it is not clear when the duplication of two MAO genes occurred. Since there is only one MAO gene in teleosts, it is possible that the duplication happened in the tetrapod lineage. In addition, the evolutionary origin of the vertebrate MAO is unclear since no ortholog of vertebrate MAO exists in protostomes (MacHeroux et al., 2001). However, a vertebrate-like MAO exists in protochordate genomes (amphioxus and ascidian, unpublished). Thus, it may be possible that an ancestral L-amino acid oxidase (another member of flavin-containing amine oxidoreductases) has been co-opted in the deuterostome lineage leading to protochordates and vertebrates. Then this MAO has been conserved in chordates, with the occurrence of MAO duplication in jawed vertebrates.

DEGRADATION ENZYMES: CATECHOL-*O*-METHYL TRANSFERASE (COMT)

Dopamine can also be degraded into 3-methoxytyramine (3-MT) by catechol-*O*-methyl transferase (COMT) located essentially at extraneuronal sites. COMT is an intracellular enzyme that catalyzes the transfer of a methyl group from *S*-adenosylmethionine to catecholamines, either the neurotransmitters or xenobiotic catechols. COMT has a very widespread distribution in the vertebrate body, and its distribution, even in the CNS is mostly non-neuronal. The combined action of MAO and COMT on dopamine yield one of its most commonly measured extracellular metabolites, homovanillic acid (HVA). The balance of neurotransmitter production, recycling, and degradation is reflected in the ratio of the DOPAC or HVA metabolites to neurotransmitter, and these metabolites can be assayed in the cerebrospinal fluid (CSF) or the blood as a reflection of DA metabolism and dysfunction (Eisenhofer et al., 1985).

In mammals, COMT is found in two forms in cells, a soluble form and a membrane-bound form, generated by different gene promoters and alternative translation initiation sites. As far as we know, there is only one gene in the available genome sequences of jawed vertebrates. Orthologous COMT sequences are present in protochordates, but they are not found in sea urchin genome sequences or in the protostome genomes sequenced so far. Thus, as for MAO, it is possible that a COMT was acquired only in the chordate lineage, transformed from one of the numerous methyl transferase genes found in most living species.

To summarize our view of the evolution of the molecular components of the DA metabolic pathways, it could be stressed that several of the corresponding genes have been duplicated in jawed vertebrates (TH, TPH, vMAT, membrane transporters, MAO, but not AADC and COMT). These duplicated genes exhibit a clear differential expression in the vertebrate brain, reflecting both subfunctionalization and neofunctionalization. These derived characters drove the conservation of the duplicated genes, and were probably used for adaptation of the DA systems to the large anatomical and functional changes that can be evidenced in the different groups of vertebrates. In this respect, it is quite remarkable that placental mammals have lost most of these duplicated genes. It is very likely that placental mammals have found different ways of using highly adaptive DA systems than the other jawed vertebrates do.

DOPAMINE RECEPTORS

Most of the cellular receptors for monoamines are membrane proteins with seven transmembrane segments coupled to heterotrimeric G protein (G protein coupled receptors or GPCR). GPCRs act as exchange factors for G proteins that regulate many different cellular processes or signaling pathways (Neves et al., 2002). The dopamine receptors are divided into two classes of GPCR, D_1- and D_2-class receptors (reviewed in Missale et al., 1998; Callier et al., 2003). Members of the D_1 receptor class are structurally characterized by a short third cytoplasmic loop and a very long C-terminal tail. They are coupled to the G_s/G_{olf} class of G proteins and accordingly they activate adenylyl cyclase. In contrast, receptors of the D_2 class are coupled to G_i/G_o proteins and they display a long third cytoplasmic loop and a short cytoplasmic C-terminal end. D_2 receptors have been initially described as mediating adenylyl cyclase inhibition, but their major cellular effects in adult vertebrates are the modulation of neuronal excitability through inhibition of voltage-sensitive Ca^{++} and activation of K^+ channels. D_2-like receptors are able to regulate other signaling pathways related to changes of cell shape or mitosis (Missale et al., 1998; O'Keeffe et al., 2009).

The nomenclature of DA receptors is quite confusing. Originally one excitatory and one inhibitory DA subtype were found, and they are named to be D_1 and D_2. Molecular cloning techniques led finding of additional subtypes, and they were named D_3, D_4, and D_5, however, later characterization of the subtypes defined that D_5 is rather close to D_1 (D_1-class) and D_3 and D_4 are close to D_2 (D_2-class). D_1 and D_5 are often called D_{1A} and D_{1B} respectively in non-human, and especially in non-mammalian vertebrate species, according findings of additional D_1-class receptors; D_{1C} (*Xenopus*; Sugamori et al., 1994), D_{1D} (chicken; Demchyshyn et al., 1995), and D_{1X} (carp; Hirano et al., 1998).

Molecular phylogenies are the best way to classify the DA receptors, especially when analyzed together with other classes of monoamine receptors; the adrenergic (α_1, α_2, β), serotoninergic ($5HT_1$, $5HT_2$, $5HT_4$, $5HT_5$, $5HT_6$, and $5HT_7$), or trace amine receptors. A first important observation made by such a molecular analysis is that the different receptor classes binding the same neurotransmitter (D_1 and D_2 receptors for example) are not more related to each other than to other classes of monoamine receptors (**Figure 2B**). This observation implicates that DA receptors have acquired independently (by convergence) the ability to bind DA, as it was also the case for the other classes of monoamine GPCR.

Inside each class of monoamine receptors, several subtypes exist in jawed vertebrates (D_{1A}, D_{1B}, D_{1C}, D_{1D}, and D_{1X} in the D_1 receptor class for example), which resulted from gene duplications that had occurred rather early in the vertebrate lineage. Amphioxus possesses only one D_1-like gene (AmphiAmR1; Burman et al., 2009) which is an outgroup of all the D_1 receptor subtypes of vertebrates. Since the genome sequence data currently available for jawless vertebrates such as lamprey or hagfish are too scarce, it is impossible to draw a reliable assumption about the timing of the duplication of the ancestral receptor genes. Several molecular phylogenies and hypotheses on their evolution have been published (Callier et al., 2003; Le Crom et al., 2003). However, recent findings changed our view of the D_1 receptor relationships.

It was previously thought that D_{1C} and D_{1D} were different subtypes, based on their distinct pharmacological and cellular functional characteristics as well as on molecular phylogenies using a limited number of species. However, recent phylogenic analyses including more sequences from a larger range of species, as well better knowledge of gene synteny, strongly suggest that D_{1C} (mostly found in anamniotes) and D_{1D} receptor subtypes (described in sauropsids) are in fact encoded by orthologous genes (Yamamoto et al., unpublished). The $D_{1C/D}$ receptor subtype is found in all the jawed vertebrate groups except mammals, and thus likely to have been secondarily lost in the mammalian lineage. Teleost fishes possess additional copies of D_1 receptor genes. This fact is most likely to be a consequence of the teleost-specific genome duplication (Postlethwait et al., 2000; Vandepoele et al., 2004; Volff, 2005). In addition, a phylogenic analysis suggests that the D_{IX} receptor gene, which is found only in teleost genomes, may be a paralog of the vertebrate D_{IB} receptor gene (Yamamoto et al., in preparation). Thus, the molecular phylogeny of the D_1 receptors class may now be simplified to three subtypes; the D_{1A}, $D1_{B/X}$, and $D_{1C/D}$ receptor subtypes. As for the molecular components of the DA metabolism, it should be mentioned that mammals have reduced the genetic diversity of the dopamine receptors as compared to the other groups of jawed vertebrates, at odd with the common view that mammals, especially human, could be more "complex" than the other vertebrates groups.

Similar overall statements could be made for the D_2-class receptors. The D_2-class receptors comprise three subtypes in jawed vertebrates, the D_2, D_3, and D_4 receptor subtypes (more logically to be named D_{2A}, D_{2B}, D_{2C}, which were envisaged at one time, but not retained by usage). These D_2 receptor subtypes are found in most of the sequenced vertebrate species, thus it is likely that the ancestral jawed vertebrates already possessed all of them. Additional duplication within the subtypes occurred specifically in the teleost lineage, with many species-specific differences. While many fishes possess two to three paralogs of D_2 and D_4 receptor genes, there is only one D_3 receptor gene in all teleosts analyzed so far. The timing of the duplication giving rise to the three D_2-like receptor subtypes is unclear, as only one D_2-like receptor has been found in lamprey. In addition, there is no D_2-like receptor gene found in protochordates so far (in ascidians and amphioxus published genomes). It is, however, very likely to be a secondary loss in the protochordate lineage, since protostomes have D_2 receptor orthologs.

Finally, as described above for the transporters, some heterologous interactions with other monoamine systems also exist for the receptors. In several vertebrates, it has been shown that DA can interact with adrenergic receptors, either α_1 (Ruffolo and Morgan, 1984; Aguayo and Grossie, 1994; Rey et al., 2001), α_2 (Ruffolo and Morgan, 1984; Aguayo and Grossie, 1994; Zhang et al., 1999; Rey et al., 2001; Cornil et al., 2005; Cornil and Ball, 2008), or β (Ruffolo and Morgan, 1984; Lee et al., 1998) adrenergic receptors. Conversely, noradrenaline and adrenaline can interact with D_1 or D_2 receptors (Lanau et al., 1997; Newman-Tancredi et al., 1997). Indeed the chemical differences between the natural catecholaminergic ligands are not huge, and the binding site of one class of receptors has some degree of flexibility and adaptability to accommodate related ligands (Xhaard et al., 2006). The heterologous ligand–receptor interactions are probably less efficient compared to the homologous interaction (for example, affinity of dopamine to adrenergic α_2 receptor is 3–30 times less than that of noradrenaline), nonetheless, they can play a physiologically significant role in the brain. It has been demonstrated that DA modulates quail male sexual behaviors via α_2 adrenergic receptors in the preoptic area (Cornil et al., 2005).

COMPARATIVE ANATOMY OF DOPAMINE SYSTEMS IN VERTEBRATES

The localization of monoamine neurotransmitters including DA was first demonstrated by histochemical detection of MAO. According to the improved formaldehyde-induced fluorescence (FIF) method, catecholaminergic cell populations were described in the rat brain and designated as A1–A12 from the medulla oblongata to the hypothalamus (Dahlstrom and Fuxe, 1964). Later development of specific antibodies recognizing individual catecholamine enzymes revealed additional A13–A17 cell groups (Björklund and Lindvall, 1984; Hökfelt et al., 1984). This nomenclature is still often used, because DAergic cells are not always located in a single distinct nucleus, and also because the distribution of the cell groups remarkably varies even among mammalian species. Indeed a one to one homology is difficult to determine among distant vertebrate groups, and some caution should be kept, since similar hodological/functional aspects of DA systems in different vertebrate groups may be the result of conservation, but alternatively of convergence (see **Figure 3**).

Extensive reviews have been given of the distribution and organization of DA cell groups in the vertebrate brain (Smeets and Reiner, 1994; Smeets and González, 2000). In this paper, we are restricting our overview to the DAergic neurons of the forebrain and midbrain. As mentioned above, all the TH immunopositive cells in the forebrain and midbrain have been considered to be DAergic, because there is no DBH or PNMT immunoreactivity anterior to the midbrain–hindbrain boundary (MHB). DA cells are generally categorized into the diencephalo-midbrain (A8–A10), diencephalic (A11–A15), olfactory bulb (A16), and retinal (A17) cell groups (Smeets and González, 2000).

Note that the "diencephalon" is defined here in a classical manner (dividing the forebrain into diencephalon and telencephalon) to be consistent with previous works. In this view, the diencephalon includes the pretectal area, thalamus, hypothalamus, and preoptic areas. Then retinal DA cells (A17) can be included in one of the diencephalic DA cell groups, because retina is ontogenetically derived from a territory shared with the hypothalamic anlage. In contrast, the formation of neuromeres during the development of the neural tube allows to describe the forebrain regions as segmented from posterior to anterior into three prosomeres (p1, p2, and p3), and the secondary prosencephalon. Within this frame, the pretectum, thalamus (dorsal thalamus), and prethalamus (ventral thalamus) are the alar part of the p1, p2, and p3 prosomeres respectively, while the hypothalamic and preoptic areas are part of the secondary prosencephalon together with the telencephalon (Puelles and Rubenstein, 2003; Medina, 2008).

DIFFERENTIAL EXPRESSION OF *TH1* AND *TH2* IN THE BRAIN OF VERTEBRATES

It is worth noticing that the DA-synthesizing cell groups described in most publications were expressing the TH1 form of TH, and that TH2-expressing cell populations should be now added to be DA cell groups. Recent accounts demonstrated that the cell populations containing the *TH2* transcripts are not (or very poorly) labeled by commercially available TH antibodies due to their low affinity for the TH2 protein (Yamamoto et al., 2010). Nevertheless, labeling of *TH2* transcripts are co-localized with DA immunoreactivity in the zebrafish brain (Yamamoto et al., 2010, 2011). *TH2* expression is found exclusively in the periventricular zone of diencephalic areas, and its distribution pattern is extremely similar to what has been described as "DA accumulating" CSF-contacting cells found in various non-vertebrate species (Meek, 1994; Smeets and Reiner, 1994; Smeets and González, 2000). Indeed, due to the lack of TH immunolabeling, these DA-immunopositive cells have been considered to accumulate extracellular DA, instead of synthesizing it. Our current knowledge about *TH2* expression strongly suggests that they are in fact DA-synthesizing cells (Yamamoto et al., 2011). Although such data have been obtained in zebrafish only and need to be replicated in other species, the presence of the *TH2* gene in all the non-eutherian classes of jawed vertebrates suggests that the CSF-contacting DA cell populations are common and ancestral to jawed vertebrates. The *TH2* gene has been lost in eutherian mammals (Yamamoto et al., 2010) and one could speculate that adaptation in eutherian mammals, by weakening the physiological role of the TH2-expressing cell populations, was a key-factor of the corresponding gene loss. However, the function of the TH2 cells in

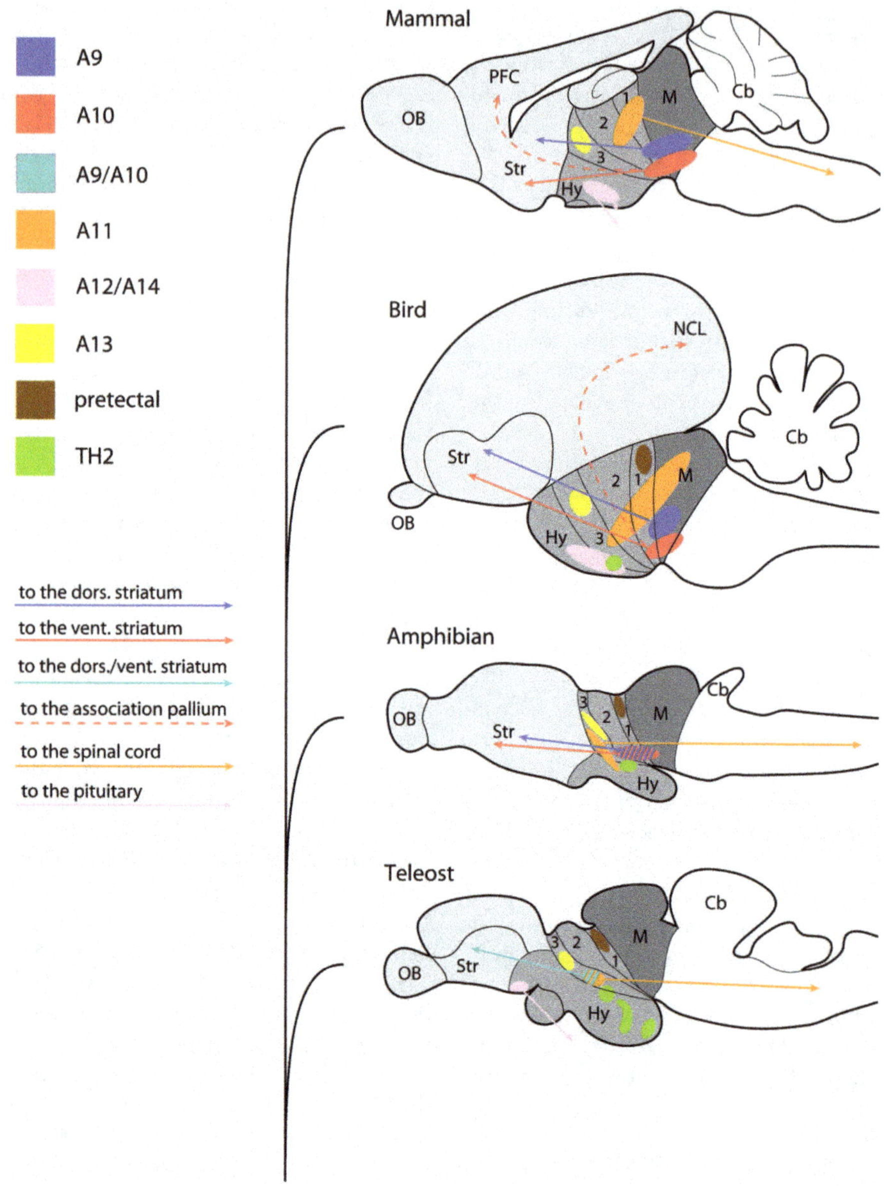

FIGURE 3 | Localization of comparable DA cells among in different groups of vertebrates. A sagittal view of the mammalian (mouse), avian (chicken), amphibian (frog), and teleostean (zebrafish) brains showing comparable DAergic nuclei and their projection patterns. Mammalian A9–A14 DA nuclei are shown in different colors (top), and corresponding colors in other vertebrate groups represent comparative (not necessarily being confirmed to be homologous) DA cell populations. TH2 (green) and pretectal (brown) DA cell groups are commonly found in vertebrates except mammals. Midbrain is shaded with dark gray, diencephalon in gray, and telencephalon in light gray in the brain of each species. The approximate positions of prosomeres p1–p3 are indicated as segmentation within the diencephalon. Abbreviations: Cb, cerebellum; Hy, hypothalamus; M, midbrain; NCL, nidopallium caudolaterale; OB, olfactory bulb; PFC, prefrontal cortex; Str, striatum.

non-eutherian species is unknown, although they may play a role in hypothalamo-hypophyseal regulation as some other hypothalamic CSF-contacting cells do (Vigh-Teichmann and Vigh, 1983).

Except for these restricted TH2 cell populations in the hypothalamic and preoptic areas, the distribution of TH- or DA-immunolabeled cells overlaps with that of *TH1* expression, at least at a regional level. All vertebrate species examined so far possess DA cells in the classical diencephalic areas including the retina, and the olfactory bulb, while teleosts and lampreys are lacking DA cells in the midbrain. Often, DAergic cell populations in the telencephalon (other than the olfactory bulb) are not cited, because there is no detectable TH cell in the adult rat or mouse brains. However, pallial and subpallial DA cells have been found in the lampreys, cartilaginous fishes, and teleosts, and also in primates including humans (Gaspar et al., 1987; Dubach, 1994), although their functions are unknown.

DA CELLS OF THE RETINA

The DA-synthesizing cells in the retina have been found in all the vertebrate species studied so far, including lamprey, with the notable exception of hagfish (Holmberg, 1970; Smeets and González,

2000). Since hagfish are living mostly in the dark and exhibit a highly simplified retina, the absence of DA cells could be a loss in this specific group. Two categories of DA cells have been described in the vertebrate retina, the amacrine cells generally located in the inner nuclear layer or somewhat displaced in the inner plexiform layer, and the interplexiform cells (Masland, 2001). Teleost fish and lampreys have only this latter type of retinal DA cells, whereas typical amacrine cells are found in cartilaginous fishes, amphibians, and amniotes. It now appears that these anatomically distinct cell types have the same ontogenetic origin, and they are all considered as amacrine DA cells (Agathocleous and Harris, 2009). They generally express the whole range of DA markers, although they very often co-express GABA and some of them are able to accumulate 5HT in addition to DA (Huang and Moody, 1998). The amacrine DA cells play a major and conserved role in retinal adaption to light by affecting mechanisms such as retinomotor movements or changes of the size of the receptive fields (Masland, 2001).

DA CELLS OF THE OLFACTORY BULB

Dopamine cells have been found in the olfactory bulb of representatives of all the craniates/vertebrates groups. The DA cells are generally located in a juxtaglomerular position, but they are also found more in the external plexiform layer and in the internal granular layers. There is a considerable diversity in the general location of these DA neurons across species, and very often these cells do not display all DA markers together. In some species, TH immunoreactive cells largely exceed in number the DA positive cells, and in many species, AADC and vMAT2 are poorly expressed (Smeets and González, 2000; Yamamoto et al., 2011). For these reasons, it has been proposed that some TH-expressing neurons of the olfactory bulb could synthesize L-DOPA but not DA (Smeets and Reiner, 1994). In addition, the phenotype of olfactory bulb DA cells is very plastic and changes fast with cellular activities (Cave and Baker, 2009). Neural precursors of the DA cells of the olfactory bulb arise from the subventricular zone of the telencephalon and migrate to the olfactory bulb by the rostral migratory stream. This neurogenesis persists all life long in all vertebrates studied so far, and it is strongly affected by activity (Lazarini and Lledo, 2011). It is thus also possible that some of the discrepancy found for the phenotypes of the DA in the olfactory bulb reflects activity-related changes.

DIENCEPHALIC CELL GROUPS (A11–A15)

Diencephalic DA cell groups consist of five groups in mammals; A11 (caudal diencephalic cell group, giving rise to diencephalo-spinal projections), A12 (tuberal cell group, tubero-infundibular projection), A13 (prethalamic/ventral thalamic cell group; incerto-hypothalamic projection), A14 (rostral periventricular cell group, tubero-hypophysial projection), and A15 (lateral and ventral hypothalamus, local projection in the diencephalon; Björklund and Lindvall, 1984). However, the boundaries of the cell groups are not always clear and, for example, there is no obvious separation between A11 and A13 in some species (Tillet, 1994).

Most of the proposed homologs of A11–A15 in amniotes are based on the topology of TH (TH1) immunoreactive cells (Kiss and Peczely, 1987; Medina et al., 1994; Reiner et al., 1994), although the projections and functional aspects remain to be investigated. One to one comparison with anamniotes is more difficult due to the variation of the brain morphologies. Increasing knowledge of the neuropeptide content, projection patterns, and gene expression profiles allow us, to some extent, to compare the DA nuclei of amniotes and anamniotes.

Dopamine neurons are commonly found in the ventral thalamic area in all the vertebrate groups, which are likely to be homologous to the A13 group (shown in yellow in **Figure 3**). Both mammalian A13 and amphibian ventromedial nucleus (in the alar domain of p3) co-express TH and somatostatin (Inagaki et al., 1981; Meister et al., 1987; Petko and Orosz, 1996). In addition, DA cells of ventral thalamus in zebrafish are located close to Pax6 immunoreactive cells (Wullimann and Rink, 2001), as is the case in the A13 cells in mammals (although half of them co-localize with *Pax6* unlike in the zebrafish ventral thalamus; Vitalis et al., 2000).

Similarly, DA cells located in the periventricular gray matter extending from the mesencephalon to p3 are found in many vertebrates, and they may correspond to the A11 group (reviewed in Smeets and González, 2000). In zebrafish, several diencephalic DA cell groups (located in p3 and hypothalamus), have been proposed to be similar to the mammalian A11 cells (DA groups 2, 4, 5, 6; Ryu et al., 2007; reviewed in Schweitzer and Driever, 2009). These posterior tubercular/hypothalamic DA cells in zebrafish require the transcription factor Orthopedia (Otp) as well as Nkx2.1 for their specification, as it is the case for the mouse A11 (Ryu et al., 2007; Löhr et al., 2009). Furthermore, mammalian A11 is characterized by distal projections to the spinal cord, and cells in the periventricular nucleus of posterior tuberculum (TPp) project to the spinal cord in zebrafish (Becker et al., 1997; Tay et al., 2011). These data indicate that these DA cells of zebrafish posterior tuberculum may be equivalent to the A11 of mammals. A11-like catecholaminergic projections to the spinal cord are found in amphibians as well, and the cell bodies are located in p3 and hypothalamic areas (Sanchez-Camacho et al., 2001), similar to the case in zebrafish. The diencephalo-spinal DA projections are also found in lampreys, but these cells are CSF-contacting neurons, unlike in jawed vertebrates. Thus, although diencephalo-spinal DA systems are commonly found throughout the vertebrates, the homology is currently unclear.

The A12 and A14 DA cells (which are respectively located in the arcuate nucleus and periventricular hypothalamic nucleus in rodents) are well studied and known to regulate prolactin, growth hormone (GH) or gonadotrophins, luteinizing hormone (LH), and follicle stimulating hormone (FSH) in the pituitary (Ben-Jonathan and Hnasko, 2001; Thiery et al., 2002; Dufour et al., 2005; Garcia-Tornadu et al., 2010; Zohar et al., 2010). In amniotes, the A12 cells project to the median eminence where they release DA in the portal blood vessels and regulate some of the anterior pituitary cell populations, whereas A14 send direct projections to the posterior pituitary (intermediate and neural lobes; Zohar et al., 2010). In teleosts, a DAergic regulation similar to that exerted by the A12 cells pituitary is found, with some differences in the projection pattern of the neuronal fibers (review in Busby et al., 2010). In teleosts, the DA cells of the anteroventral part of the preoptic area (PPa) negatively regulate LH release in the anterior pituitary as A12 DA cells, however, unlike mammalian A12, the teleost PPa cells send direct projections to the anterior pituitary (Kah et al., 1984). Many of the DA effects on the pituitary are exerted through the D_2 receptors, and they inhibit the secretion of various pituitary hormones, although there are variations (Busby et al., 2010; Dufour et al., 2010; Zohar et al., 2010). The significance of the DA control on the hypophysis varies depending on the life style of the animals. For example, the DA effects on prolactin is important for regulating lactation in mammals, which is obviously not the case for fish. Instead, DA regulation on prolactin plays an important role for osmoregulation in fish (Liu et al., 2006), and it is probably an ancestral function of hypothalamic DA neurons in vertebrates.

Not much is known about the function A15 cell populations. Their projections are mainly to other diencephalic areas. A15 is the most rostral part of the diencephalic DA cells, and they are located around the optic chiasm including the supraoptic nucleus in mammals. DA cells are consistently found around the supraoptic/suprachiasmatic regions in various vertebrates, and it is possible that they correspond to A15.

In addition to the A11–A15 nuclei, a pretectal DA cell group (alar plate of p1) is consistently found in bony fishes, amphibians, and most amniotes except mammals (reviewed in Smeets and González, 2000). These pretectal neurons are projecting mostly on the optic tectum, in a layer-specific fashion, and they may play a role in the modulation of the retino-tectal visual input (Smeets and Reiner, 1994). In the group of species where no pretectal DA neurons are found (cartilaginous fish and mammals), DA neurons are found in the habenular area, although no role are known for those neurons (Stuesse et al., 1994). However, it is likely that the pretectal DA neuronal population is an ancestral trait of jawed vertebrates (Smeets and Reiner, 1994).

MESENCEPHALO-DIENCEPHALIC CELL GROUPS (A8–A10)

The midbrain populations of DA neurons are the most intensively studied, due to their major contribution to the pathophysiology of Parkinson's disease (Obeso et al., 2010), and also to the mechanisms of drug addition and other psychiatric disorders (schizophrenia, attention deficit with hyperactivity; Wise, 2009). It must be recalled that A8–A10 cells are often called "midbrain" DA cell groups although they are not restricted to the midbrain. Instead, they extend to the ventral diencephalic territories (Medina et al., 1994; Puelles and Medina, 1994; Verney et al., 2001; Vernier and Wullimann, 2009). The DA cell groups of the midbrain/basal diencephalon are characterized in most of vertebrate groups by their projection to the subpallial and pallial areas of the telencephalon.

In mammals, a majority of the DA cells of A9 (substantia nigra pars compacta, SNc) are located in the midbrain, as well as a large part of the A10 neurons (ventral tegmental area, VTA). The A8 group corresponds to the retrorubral component of the DA neurons. Many neurons of the SNc project to the dorsal/somatic striatum in the basal ganglia, controlling mostly sensori-motor programming (nigro-striatal system). In contrast, DA cells in VTA project to areas related to the limbic system such as ventral/visceral basal ganglia (e.g., nucleus accumbens) or amygdala (meso-limbic system), as well as the PFC (meso-cortical system). They play a central role in reward-related behaviors and various cognitive functions such as working memory (Kelley, 2004; Björklund and Dunnett, 2007; Wise, 2009).

Although it may be a too simplified dichotomy (for example some SNc cells also project to the limbic and cortical areas and some VTA cells to the caudate–putamen), the distinct projection pathways to the basal ganglia have been applied to identify the A9 or A10 homologs in the non-mammalian species; DA cell populations projecting to the dorsal striatum were considered to be A9, A10 being those projecting to the ventral striatum (nucleus accumbens). In the avian midbrain, the general configuration is very similar to that of mammals. DA cells providing a massive innervation to the dorsal/somatic striatum are located more dorsolaterally (as is the case in the mammalian SNc), while those projecting to the ventral/visceral striatum are located ventromedially (as the mammalian VTA), and the corresponding regions are now named as SNc and VTA, respectively (Reiner et al., 2004). Similar cell populations are present in reptilian species (Smeets, 1994; Smeets and Reiner, 1994), and as in mammals they extend from the mesencephalon up to the basal part of the two first prosomeres, at least.

In amphibians as well, similar nigro-striatal and meso-limbic pathways are identified, but unlike amniotes, the DAergic cells of amphibians are shifted more rostrally, many of them being located in the diencephalic territories. Then, the neurons giving rise to the two main projection fibers are intermingled rather than segregated (Marin et al., 1997). Midbrain DA cells with extension into the diencephalic posterior tuberculum are also found in cartilaginous fishes with two different populations. One, named the tegmental area is located just anterior to the interpeduncular nucleus, and the other, a putative substantia nigra, is scattered around the red nucleus (Stuesse et al., 1994).

In contrast, there is no midbrain DA cell in teleosts (Meek, 1994; Rink and Wullimann, 2001), or in lampreys (Pierre et al., 1997; Barreiro-Iglesias et al., 2008). In representatives of this very large group of species (more than 24,000 species), DA neurons are found at three main locations, the periventricular nucleus of the posterior tuberculum, the paraventricular organ, and the posterior tuberal nucleus, all located in the basal area of the third prosomere. It was demonstrated that some of the THir cells in the zebrafish posterior tuberculum (periventricular nucleus of posterior tuberculum; TPp) project to the subpallium, and co-express the transcription factor Nurr1/NR4A2, suggesting the presence of teleost counterpart of A9/A10 cells (Rink and Wullimann, 2001; Blin et al., 2008). However, a recent study of zebrafish larval brains demonstrated that the telencephalic projection from DA cells of the posterior tuberculum is scarce, and that the same TH cell of the posterior tuberculum (TPp, group 4) projects to the diencephalon, hindbrain, and spinal cord in addition to the subpallium, (Tay et al., 2011). These cells depend on the transcription factor Otp, suggesting that they resemble the mammalian A11 [see Diencephalic Cell Groups (A11–A15)]. Whether DA cells of the teleostean posterior tuberculum share also molecular determinants and phenotype with the A9/A10-like cells of mammals, and whether older fish may exhibit more prominent ascending projection from the TPp, await more precise characterization. Currently there is no data on the functional role played by the DA neurons of the posterior tuberculum (or other population of DA neurons) in the basal ganglia circuitry in zebrafish, and it is uncertain if a homolog of A8–A10 exists in teleosts. A mesencephalic component of DA neurons has been described in a non-teleost fish, the gar *Lepisosteus osseus*, rendering plausible the hypothesis that the lack of DA cells in the mesencephalon could be specific to teleost (Parent and Northcutt, 1982).

The target area of the A9 DA cells, the dorsal striatum, contains massive THir or DAir terminals, as well as abundant D_{1A} and D_2 receptors in amniotes. In mammals, D_{1A} receptor tends to be co-localize with substance P (SP), while D_2 receptor co-localize with enkephalin (ENK). Functional and pharmacological studies have suggested that DA stimulates SP cells by D_{1A} receptors while D_2 receptors inhibit ENK cells in the striatum, regulating the direct and indirect pathways of the basal ganglia circuitry (Gerfen, 1992). The basal ganglia circuitry for motor output is well studied in birds as well, and known to be essentially similar to that of mammals (Reiner, 2002). Immunohistochemical and hodological studies suggest that amphibians also share the basic basal ganglia organization similar to amniotes (Marin et al., 1998b; Maier et al., 2010). Together with abundant TH terminals (González and Smeets, 1994; Marin et al., 1998a) and D_{1A} receptors (our unpublished data) in the amphibian striatum, it is likely that the role of DA in the basal ganglia motor control is conserved in tetrapods.

The conservation of meso-limbic systems is less clear. DA input to the nucleus accumbens is critical for reward associated behavior, thus intensively studied in the context of the drug addiction. In mammals, D_3 receptor shows particular expression in the island of Calleja and nucleus accumbens (Bouthenet et al., 1991; Landwehrmeyer et al., 1993), while this seems not the case in birds. Based on a study in zebrafinch and chicken (Kubikova et al., 2010), D_3 transcripts are weakly expressed rather in the pallial region, with no remarkable expression in the proposed homologous region of the nucleus accumbens (Reiner et al., 2004; Balint and Csillag, 2007). Midbrain DA input to a proposed nucleus accumbens are found in amphibians, but the receptor distribution is not known.

The meso-cortical system is even more difficult to compare among different vertebrate classes, because there was no homolog of the PFC proposed so far outside of mammals. Nonetheless, behavioral, hodological, neurochemical, and electrophysiological studies suggest that birds also possess a pallial association area functionally equivalent to the PFC (Mogensen and Divac, 1982; Güntürkün, 2005). It is located in the caudal part of the avian pallium named the nidopallium caudolateral (NCL). The avian NCL contains relatively high amount of THir fibers and of D_{1A} receptors as it is also the case in the mammalian PFC. DA depletion or blockade of D_{1A} receptors interferes with working memory and attention task as shown in mammals (Rose et al., 2010). The similar functional properties of NCL and PFC extend from cellular to behavioral levels (Mogensen and Divac, 1982; Güntürkün, 2005). It is likely to be a consequence of convergent evolution, DA being co-opted in each case to support similar function, raising intriguing questions. At the cellular level, DA is known to increase the firing frequency of preactivated neurons via D_1-like receptors in mammals and birds (Güntürkün, 2005). In mammals, D_{1A} receptor subtype is thought to be involved in this property. However, avians possess another subtype of D_1 receptor previously known as D_{1D}, and proposed to be a D_{1C} ortholog (see Dopamine Receptors), which is selectively expressed in the pallial areas including NCL (Kubikova et al., 2010). It is thus possible that the $D_{1C/D}$ subtype, in addition to D_{1A}, plays an important role for cognitive functions in birds. Secondly, the extracellular DA level in the PFC and NCL is higher than in the other dopaminoceptive regions such as the striatum (Sharp et al., 1986; Bast et al., 2002). This may play an important role for a sustained, memory-related activity in these brain areas. In the mammalian PFC, DAT is weakly expressed, and DA is mainly captured by the noradrenaline transporter (NET). Since uptake velocity by NET is not as high as by DAT, it may account for the slow uptake of DA in the PFC. Neither the expression patterns of DAT nor that of NET are known in the avian NCL and this should be interesting to investigate.

DETERMINATION AND DIFFERENTIATION OF THE DOPAMINE NEURON IDENTITY IN THE CENTRAL NERVOUS SYSTEM OF VERTEBRATES

A MASTER GENE OF THE DA PHENOTYPE?

Dopamine neurons of the CNS can be defined as the cells using DA as a neurotransmitter. By this definition, the coincident expression of TH, AADC, vMAT2, and DAT in the same subsets of neurons has been considered to be critical for a functional DA cells, and they are collectively referred to as DA markers. In the model nematode *Caenorhabditis elegans*, it was recently demonstrated that the genes encoding these DA markers were transcribed upon the action of a common transcription factor, *ast-1* (a member of the ETS transcription factor family), which activates a *cis*-regulatory module found in the sequences of each of the genes encoding the DA components (Flames and Hobert, 2009). Since the same authors showed that, in the mouse olfactory bulb, *TH* required Etv1/ER81 (also an ETS factor) to be expressed, it was tempting to propose that the expression of the full dopamine phenotype could depend on a "master gene" of the ETS family, controlling late steps of neuronal differentiation and the determination of neurotransmitter identity of neurons. However, it was subsequently shown that, although Etv1/ER81 was able to transactivate the *TH* gene in the mouse olfactory bulb, it was the case neither for the other components of the DA phenotype (*AADC, vMAT2, DAT*), nor for *TH* in other brain areas. In addition, this action of Etv1/ER81 seems to be rather specific to rodents (Cave et al., 2010). Another ETS transcription factor, Etv5/ERM, which had been suggested to regulate the DA phenotype of the VTA/SNc neurons, was demonstrated to be dispensable. Finally, no other ETS-related factors are expressed at the right place to regulate the expression of the DA markers (Wang and Turner, 2010). Thus, except in *C. elegans*, the notion of a common genetic program governing DA cell differentiation is very unlikely to exist.

GENERAL PRINCIPLES OF DAergic DIFFERENTIATION

As a matter of fact, the DA systems are very heterogeneous in the vertebrate brain. Detailed studies of the relative distribution of the DA markers in the brain of several vertebrate species have shown that they are not always co-localized in the same cells and that their abundance varies significantly from one brain nuclei to another (Lorang et al., 1994; Mel'nikova et al., 2005; Weihe et al., 2006; Björklund and Dunnett, 2007; Yamamoto et al., 2011); reviewed in Björklund and Dunnett (2007). Thus, the DA neuronal groups differ in their molecular phenotypes as well as in the neurological functions they modulate (Cave and Baker, 2009). Accordingly, the molecular mechanisms and gene networks governing the differentiation of the DA systems are also different.

These mechanisms of differentiation vary depending on the location of the DA progenitors in the regionalized neural tube, in line with the concept of a phylotypic period during the embryonic development (Mathis and Nicolas, 2002; Osorio et al., 2010). The regionalization of the neural tube depends on the formation and the positioning of signaling organizing centers, such as the MHB (secreting mostly FGF8), the zona limitans intrathalamica (ZLI, secreting mostly Sonic Hedgehog – Shh), the anterior neural ridge (ANR, secreting mostly FGF8), the notochord and prechordal plate, and the floor plate in the ventral neural tube [secreting mostly BMPs (TGFβ-like factors), Wnts, and Shh], and dorsal midline structures or the roof plate dorsally (secreting mostly BMPs, Wnt, or Wnt inhibitors; Wilson and Houart, 2004; Vieira et al., 2010). These signals are translated into the patterning of antero-posterior, mediolateral, and dorso-ventral morphogenetic units. They are defined as longitudinal columns or plates (floor, basal, alar, and roof plates) and transverse compartments (neuromeres). The neuromeres are named, from posterior to anterior, rhombomeres in the rhombencephalon, then mesencephalon (a neuromere on its own), and prosomeres in the prosencephalon (Puelles, 1995; Vieira et al., 2010). Gene expression is thus controlled in spatially and temporally defined manner, and the combination of genes expressed in each of the neuromere influences the fate and differentiation of neural progenitors and new-born neurons.

The differentiation of all the DA cells takes place anterior to the MHB. This highlights the key role of this structure in the process. Then, DAergic neurogenesis is regulated by distinct genetic networks, depending on the position of the progenitors in the neural tube. Variations around these genetic pathways are certainly at the center of the corresponding disparity of the organization and function of DA cell groups among vertebrate species.

For example, in the olfactory bulb, an anterior telencephalic area, the differentiation of DA neurons depends on the combination of at least three transcription factor encoding-genes, *Etv1/ER81*, *Pax6*, and *Meis2*, as key determinants of the DA phenotypes (Allen et al., 2007). In contrast, the gene networks used for the specification of DA cell groups are very different in the midbrain and diencephalic/hypothalamic cell groups (**Figure 4**).

DIFFERENTIATION OF MESENCEPHALO-DIENCEPHALIC DA CELL POPULATION (A8–A10)

Currently, our knowledge of the differentiation mechanisms of DA neurons mostly comes from mammalian (e.g., mouse) studies on SNc and VTA, and some works have been done in chick embryos as well (reviewed in Ang, 2006; Prakash and Wurst, 2006; Smidt and Burbach, 2007). Seminal work based on loss- and gain-of-function experiments in the mouse suggested that FGF8 secreted at the MHB and Shh secreted by the ventral structures (the notochord and the prechordal plate) were essential for the differentiation of mesencephalic DA cells (reviewed in Hynes and Rosenthal, 1999). Other signals such as Nodal, Wnt-related factors, or BMPs are also crucial for the regulation of different aspects of the DA differentiation, in a spatially and temporally controlled manner (reviewed in Prakash and Wurst, 2006; Smidt and Burbach, 2007).

In addition, the notochord and the prechordal plate may have different signaling properties (Vieira et al., 2010), which may result in differences in the induction and differentiation of ventral DA progenitors in the mesencephalon vs the ventral part of the three first prosomeres (such as the presence of retinaldehyde dehydrogenase in p1–p3 neurons but not in mesencephalic neurons; Smidt and Burbach, 2007). Variations on this theme may exist from one vertebrate species to another. An extreme case is represented by the teleost fishes, in which no DA cells are found in the ventral mesencephalon nor p1–p2 (see Comparative Anatomy of Dopamine Systems in Vertebrates; **Figure 3**). Thus, the role of the signaling pathways involved in the determination and differentiation of DA neurons in front of the MHB in teleost fish may be different from that in amniotes. An illustration of this fact is provided by the FGF8 null zebrafish mutant (*acerebellar – ace –* mutant), which exhibits normal production of DA neuron anterior to the MHB, although the induction of other catecholaminergic neurons posterior to it were strongly affected, as in mammals (locus coeruleus; Holzschuh et al., 2003). The redundancy of FGF signaling is higher in teleost fish (due to an additional gene duplication) than in other species, and the precise role of FGF signaling in the specification of DA progenitors anterior to the MHB remains unclear.

The amniote mesencephalo-diencephalic neurons all derived from the floor plate cells are expressing Shh and *FoxA2* (Ono et al., 2007; Bonilla et al., 2008; Lin et al., 2009). In mouse, the *Otx1/2* genes and LIM-homeodomain genes *Lmx1a/b*, expressed in proliferative ventricular zone, are early determinants of the DA fate (Smidt et al., 2000; Puelles et al., 2004). *Lmx1a*, by activating *Msx1*, promotes the expression of the proneural gene *Ngn2*. This step is important to recruit proliferative progenitors toward a more committed fate also marked by the expression of another proneural gene, *Asc-l1* (*Mash1*; Andersson et al., 2006; Kele et al., 2006). *Lmx1a* continues to be expressed in the same progenitors, but it is also expressed (together with *Lmx1b*) in post-mitotic precursors and differentiating DA neurons. Then, the orphan nuclear receptor *Nurr1/NR4A2* comes into play into post-mitotic progenitors (Zetterström et al., 1997; Saucedo-Cardenas et al., 1998; Smits et al., 2003), and this factor is crucial for the expression of TH, vMAT2, and DAT (but not AADC; Smits et al., 2003). *Ngn2* is transiently expressed in post-mitotic progenitors and involved in the acquisition of generic and subtype specific traits by differentiating DA neurons (Kele et al., 2006). Other parallel pathways such as the Wnt-dependent induction of *Otx2* (required to repress *Nkx2.2*, a determinant of the serotonergic phenotype posterior to the MHB, in the ventral midbrain, Prakash et al., 2006, and for the differentiation of posterior DA progenitors, Omodei et al., 2008), or the FGF8-dependent expression of *En1/2* (Simon et al., 2001), as well as the expression of *Pitx3* (Asbreuk et al., 2002), are critical for the full differentiation and maintenance of midbrain DA neurons throughout life (reviewed in Prakash and Wurst, 2006; Smidt and Burbach, 2007; and references therein). Differences in expression of molecular markers of SNc and VTA DA cells may depend also on specific transcription factors such as Otx2 (Di Salvio et al., 2010).

This pathway is not fully conserved in non-mammalian species, and especially in teleost fishes that lack the mesencephalic and posterior diencephalic components (prosomeres 1 and 2) of DA cells. In the zebrafish, which has no *Ngn2* gene but expresses *Ngn1* instead, the DA progenitors also express *Lmx1b*. However, the sequence of expression of the proneural gene *Asc-l1* (*Zash1a/b*), *Nurr1/NR4A2*, and *TH* is rather different from that in mammals, the population of progenitors labeled by each of these genes being much more temporally segregated from each other (Ryu et al.,

specification of early progenitors	committed progenitors	post-mitotic progenitors	mature neurons
Tgf-β (Nodal) Shh Wnt	Otp Ngn1	Otp	Otp
Tgf-β Shh Fgf-8 Wnt1/5	Otx2 Lmx1a/b Sox2 Ngn2 Asc-l1/2 FoxA2	Lmx1a/b NR4A2/nurr1 Pitx3 En1/2	NR4A2/nurr1 Pitx3 En1/2
Tgf-β (Nodal) Shh Wnt8	Asc-L1 Dbx1 Pax6	Pax6	?

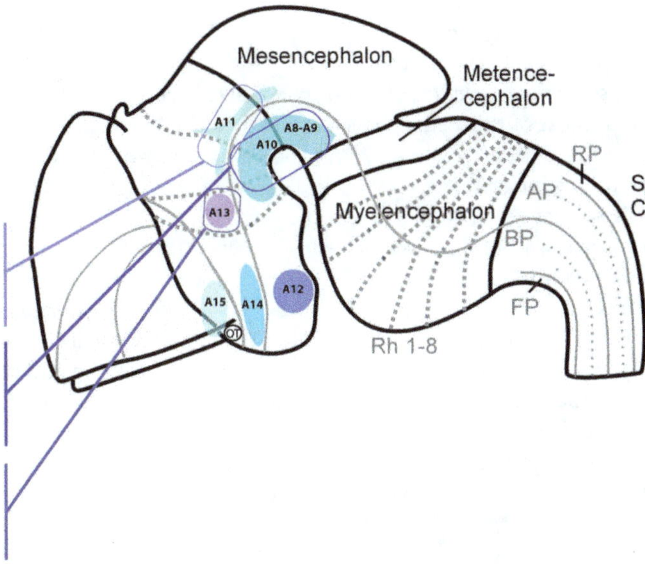

FIGURE 4 | Distinct differentiation pathways for different DA cell groups in mouse. The localization of the main DA-synthesizing nuclei is shown on a neuromeric representation of the mouse embryonic brain. Signaling molecules and genes known to be involved in the differentiation of the A11 (first row) A8–A10 DA nuclei (in the midbrain and first basal diencephalic prosomeres; second row) and A13 DA nuclei (in the ventral thalamus; third row) are indicated as a table. Note that DA cells in the three different areas depend on different signaling and transcription factors expression at each step of the cell differentiation, although little is still known in the case of A11 and A13. This observation supports the hypothesis that different DA neuronal systems have been recruited independently, by different transcriptional mechanisms, probably early in vertebrate evolution.

2006; Filippi et al., 2007; Blin et al., 2008). In addition, although *Lmx1b* is necessary for the commitment of early DA progenitors, *Pitx3* does not seem to play a role in DA terminal differentiation in zebrafish (Ryu et al., 2006; Filippi et al., 2007).

DIFFERENTIATION OF DIENCEPHALO-HYPOTHALAMIC DA CELL POPULATIONS

As compared to the diencephalo-mesencephalic A8–A10 neuronal populations, the differentiation mechanisms of the diencephalo-hypothalamic A11–A15 nuclei are far much less known. The factor Shh secreted from the prechordal plate is crucial to specify hypothalamic and retinal territories in mammals marked by the early expression of key-transcription factors such as Six3 and Rx (reviewed in Wilson and Houart, 2004; Szarek et al., 2010). Later, as shown by experiments made in chick embryos, down-regulation of Shh expression by BMP7 (a TGF-β related factor) is crucial to determine the fate of proliferative progenitors in the tubero-mamillary area, and to specify tuberal hypothalamic DA neurons (corresponding to A12; Manning et al., 2006). This may also be true in mammals, since the sequential effect of Shh and BMP7 can induce the hypothalamic DA cell fate in the mouse embryonic stem cell-derived neural progenitor cells (Ohyama et al., 2005). Mouse A12 DA neurons also depend on the Achaete–scute-like gene *Mash1* at early stages of neurogenesis, but their maintenance requires *Mash1* inhibition at later stages (McNay et al., 2006). In the more dorsally located hypothalamus, the role of *Otp*, *Brn2*, *Sim1/2*, and *Anrt2* on the specification of neuroendocrine neurons is well studied (Acampora et al., 1999; Michaud et al., 2000; Goshu et al., 2004), however, many of them are not specifically focusing on DA neurons.

Genetic experiments in zebrafish showed that, more than Shh, the Nodal pathway (Nodal is a TGFβ signaling factor), and the Wnt pathways are critical for differentiation of the ventral progenitors of the diencephalon and hypothalamus from which DA precursors arise (Mathieu et al., 2002; Kapsimali et al., 2004). These signaling pathways are also likely to play a major role in mammals but Nodal mutants are lethal at early stages and thus the effect of this signal has not been demonstrated on hypothalamus specification (reviewed in Szarek et al., 2010). The role of Nodal in the differentiation of diencephalic DA progenitor could be indirect. Indeed, when *FoxH1*, a Nodal target gene in invalidated (Holzschuh et al., 2003) no DA neurons are found in the ventral diencephalon. However, in a mutant of the Nodal pathway (MZ*oep*, the zebrafish homolog of Cripto a Nodal co-receptor) the rescue of signals emitted by the prechordal mesendoderm (in particular Wnt and Shh signals), permits the specification of DA cell precursors in the diencephalon (Mathieu et al., 2002; reviewed in Schweitzer and Driever, 2009).

Early specification of DA neural progenitors depends at least in part on the Krüppel-like, zinc finger transcription factor Fezf2, which is tightly repressed by the Wnt signals (reviewed in Shimizu and Hibi, 2009). This signaling activity also controls the size of the DA progenitor pool (Russek-Blum et al., 2008). As for the DA precursors of the ventral mesencephalo-diencephalon, proneural genes in the hypothalamus follow a sequence of expression with firstly *Ngn2* (or *Ngn1* in zebrafish) and then *Asc-l1*. *Ngn* expression is controlled by *Fezf2* both in zebrafish and mouse (Jeong et al., 2007; Ryu et al., 2007). *Fezf2* also controls the formation and differentiation of *Dlx1/2–Pax6* expressing neurons of the ventral thalamus (prethalamus; Hirata et al., 2006), which later give rise to the DA neurons of the ventral thalamus (Vitalis et al., 2000; Wullimann and Rink, 2001).

A major target of *Fezf2* is the *Otp* gene, which specifies various hypothalamic cell populations (Bardet et al., 2008; Wang and Lufkin, 2000), as well as DA cells of the mammalian A11 (Ryu et al., 2007). In zebrafish, loss-of-function of *Otp-a/b* severely affects the differentiation of most of the diencephalic/hypothalamic DA cell groups (Blechman et al., 2007; Ryu et al., 2007), including posterior tubercular neurons which project to the subpallium (Tay et al., 2011). These *Otp*-dependent DA cells of zebrafish are also affected by *sim1* or *arnt2* genes, as it is the case for neuroendocrine cells in the mammalian hypothalamus (Löhr et al., 2009; Schweitzer and Driever, 2009).

A lot remains to be done, to understand better the regulatory logic of the expression of the DA phenotypes in the many DA nuclei throughout the forebrain. Nevertheless, based on our current knowledge, the DA nuclei or neurons located in the retina, the olfactory bulb, the hypothalamus, or the mesencephalo-diencephalic areas are each specified and differentiated upon essentially different combination of genes.

DOPAMINE SYSTEMS IN PROTOCHORDATES AND THE ORIGIN OF THE CENTRAL DA SYSTEMS OF VERTEBRATES

Since many DA cell clusters are well conserved in craniates, the roots of the evolution of the vertebrate DA systems have to be searched outside vertebrates. Previous studies in the two sister groups of non-craniate chordates, i.e., urochordates (ascidians and larvaceans) and cephalochordates (amphioxus), have shown that the two groups exhibit DA-containing cells in their CNS (Moret et al., 2004, 2005b). From a phylogenetical point of view, recent molecular data suggest that tunicates are closer to craniates than amphioxus (Delsuc et al., 2006).

Basically, in ascidians and cephalochordates, the organization of the neural tube along antero-posterior axis is to a certain extent similar to that of vertebrates. In the protochordates, the anterior domain (named the sensory vesicle in ascidia, and the cerebral vesicle in amphioxus) expresses *Otx* gene as the vertebrate forebrain/midbrain does. Similarly, a posterior domain and the vertebrate rhombencephalon both express Hox genes (Wada et al., 1998; Holland and Holland, 1999; Ikuta and Saiga, 2007). In vertebrates, the MHB, which is centered on the limit between the *Otx* and *Gbx* territories, expresses *Pax2/5/8* genes, and secretes FGF8. As previously stated [in Differentiation of Mesencephalo-Diencephalic DA Cell Population (A8–A10)], this domain is a major organizing center of the vertebrate brain, and whether there is some equivalent in non-craniate chordates remains debated (Wada et al., 1998; Holland and Holland, 1999; Ikuta and Saiga, 2007; Imai et al., 2009). Although *Otx* and *Gbx* expression domains abut in the amphioxus neural tube, there is no evidence for the existence of a MHB signaling center (Moret et al., 2004; Castro et al., 2006). In contrast, it has been recently shown that FGF8 plays a major role as a signaling component at the boundary between the neck and the visceral ganglion of the ascidian CNS. It allows positioning the expression of *Pax2/5/8* in the neck, just posterior to the *Otx*-expressing domain of the sensory vesicle (Imai et al., 2009).

Comparison of this general organization of the neural tube between vertebrates and protochordates, together with a careful analysis of the localization of their DA cells provides interesting clues on the ancestral chordate situation. In adult amphioxus, three distinct DA cell populations have been identified. Two of them are in the cerebral vesicle (population 1 and 2) and one in the posterior brain (population 3), being close to 5HT-containing neurons, which is reminiscent of the vertebrate situation. This led to a suggestion that, although amphioxus has no true MHB, the topology and competence of the neural tube to express DA neurons have been conserved in amphioxus (Moret et al., 2004). The antero-dorsal population 1 is located close to photoreceptors, and it sends short projections ventrally to the central canal, in a manner reminiscent of some hypothalamic neurons in vertebrates. The population 2 is located more medially and laterally in the cerebral vesicle, and it sends projections to the posterior brain and the spinal cord. It could play a role in modulating the activity of the motor pattern generator in this animal. The third population is located in the posterior cerebral vesicle, and exhibits similarities with the area postrema of the vertebrate hindbrain.

In ascidians, there is only one population of 8–12 DA-synthesizing cells located on the left side of the postero-ventral wall of the sensory vesicle, adjacent to a group of photoreceptors (Moret et al., 2005b). Based on the expression territories of regulatory genes, it was suggested that these ascidian DAergic cells were located in a region of the ventral sensory vesicle somewhat comparable to the vertebrate hypothalamus (Moret et al., 2005a). These DA-immunoreactive cells express *TH* and *AADC*, but *vMAT* gene expression is undetectable (Moret et al., 2005b; Razy-Krajka et al., unpublished). In addition, they express the membrane transporter SERT, enabling these cells to contain both 5HT and DA (no other member of the MAT are present in the ciona genome). Ciona has also lost D_1*-like* or D_2*-like* receptor genes, and instead, DA acts via α_2-like receptors located on DA cells themselves and on some of their probable targets (GABA and glutamate neurons). The very peculiar features of the ascidian DA cells stress the unexpected flexibility or adaptability of the monoamine systems. It may be followed by many gene losses which have taken place in the urochordate lineage, including DA receptor genes and *MAT* genes (*DAT/NET*). This flexible property gives robustness and adaptability to the systems as a whole and this would have been beneficial to many species during evolution.

In another respect, new data on the ascidian DA cells suggest that they share many properties found in DAergic amacrine cells in the vertebrate retina (Razy-Krajka et al., unpublished). For example, ascidian DA cells express transcription factors or other markers found both in hypothalamus and retina such as *six3/6*, *meis*, *pax6*, visual cycle proteins. They also express adrenergic receptors, and contact to glutamatergic and GABAergic neurons, as DA amacrine cells do. In addition, behavioral study demonstrated that they modulate swimming behavior in response to light and one of their roles could be to regulate motor behavior prior to metamorphosis. This important observation led to draw the hypothesis that DA cells in the ancestral chordate were located in a photoreceptive territory of the anterior neural tube, which is homologous to both retina and hypothalamic region (**Figure 5**). These DA cells were probably multifunctional and able to modulate neural functions such as sensory input, motor control, and hormonal regulation.

Together with a better knowledge of the possible evolutionary history of the molecular components of DA neurons, genetic networks controlling DA neuron differentiation, the localization

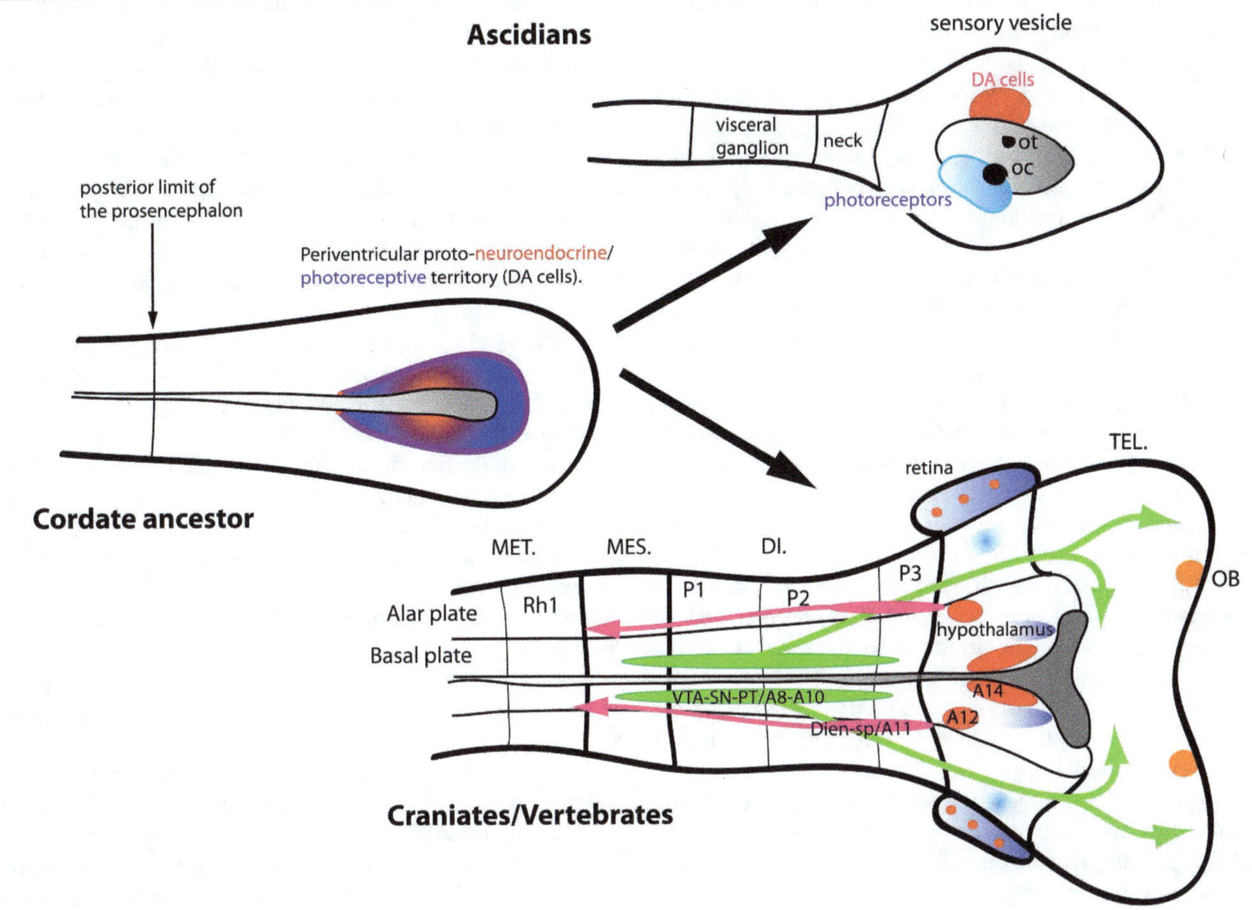

FIGURE 5 | Schematic representation of the hypothetic evolution of DA systems at the protochordate–vertebrate transition. The anterior neural tube of a chordate ancestor contained periventricular photoreceptor cells intermingled with neuroendocrine cells synthesizing dopamine and peptides such as vasopressin or somatostatin. These cells could also be connected to other part of the CNS, in particular a central pattern generator. These cell types are lining the anterior neural ventricle and contact the CSF. A reminiscent but derived situation is found in modern protochordates such as ascidia (superior right part of the schematics) where photoreceptor cells line the ventricle and are adjacent to the DA cells of the sensory vesicle, and which are able to modulate the motor response to light. In craniates/vertebrates, the telencephalon has tremendously increased in size, and the optic vesicle becomes separated from the anterior hypothalamus by bulging out of the neural tube. Several "new" DA systems have been co-opted simultaneously, mostly in the mesencephalon and the basal plate three first prosomeres. These DA cells homologous to those of the SN/VTA project on the dorsal and ventral pallium, representing a major innovation of vertebrates, with strong adaptive properties. The retina comprised several cell types inherited from the protochordate ancestor, including at least photoreceptor cells, pigmented epithelium, and amacrine DA cells.

in the brain, and the new data obtained on the protochordate DA systems, we propose renewed hypothesis of the evolution of DA systems in craniates.

HYPOTHESIS ON THE EVOLUTION OF DA SYSTEMS IN CRANIATES/VERTEBRATES

Dopamine, as a major neuromodulatory transmitter, has certainly played a crucial role in adaptation of animal behavior all along evolution. As described above, the DA phenotype relies on the simultaneous expression of a molecular module consisting of the biosynthetic enzymes TH and AADC, the transporters DAT and vMAT, and the degradation enzymes MAO and COMT. In turn, the action on DA relies on the presence of members of the D_1 and D_2 classes of receptors on target cells. Many of these operational molecules are present in all bilaterian groups (TH, AADC, vMAT, MAT, D_1 and D_2 receptors), while others are in chordates only (MAO, and COMT), as presented in Section "Molecular Components Defining the Phenotype of DA Neurons and their Phylogeny." Thus, all the components of the prototypic DA neurotransmission system found in modern vertebrates were on hand in ancestral chordates. The coordinated cellular expression of these components was mandatory to make a neurotransmission system using DA. It was certainly operant in ancestral chordates also, based on our current knowledge of protochordates. It is however rather difficult to figure out how the ancestral chordate DA system looked like from an anatomical and physiological point of view.

Recent data about the DA systems of ascidia suggest that DA cells of the sensory vesicle on the one hand, and DA cells of the hypothalamus and the retina of vertebrates on the other hand, may have originated from a common neuroendocrine, photoreceptive territory surrounding the ventricle of the neural tube in ancestral chordates (see Section Dopamine Systems in Protochordates and the

Origin of the Central DA Systems of Vertebrates). This hypothesis is reinforced by the situation of amphioxus DA cells, which are located close to photoreceptors in the wall of the cerebral vesicle (Satir, 2000; Vigh et al., 2002); a region proposed to be homologous to the vertebrate prosencephalon (Holland and Holland, 1999; Kozmik et al., 2007). This contention of an ancestral protohypothalamic area, containing both neuroendocrine cells such as DA cells and photoreceptors, resembles the hypothesis of a primordial photoreceptive neuroepithelium folded into the anterior neural tube of ancestral chordates, initially proposed by F. K. Studnicka in 1898 (Walls, 1942; Lamb et al., 2007). It also fits with the observation that the deep brain photoreceptors (CSF-contacting cells of the hypothalamus) and the photoreceptive organs (retina and pineal organ) are all derived from the ventricle-lining prosencephalon (Vigh et al., 2004; **Figure 5**). Thus, based on current data, the ancestral DA neuron population of chordates could have been located in a protohypothalamic periventricular area at the anterior part of the neural tube.

The transition between protochordates and craniates corresponds to the emergence of the "new head," to quote Gans and Northcutt (1983). The encephalization, which accompanied the major development of the neural crest, as well as the emergence of the sensory placodes, were major innovations that transformed the probably small and frail last common ancestor of protochordates and craniates into a much more efficient predator. Obviously, the DA neuronal systems may have followed the tremendous expansion of the forebrain in craniates.

In this respect, the emergence of secondary organizers of the neural tube in the head primordium, such as the prechordal plate, MHB, ANR, ZLI, and also the cephalic neural crest, have certainly been crucial to promote both the spectacular expansion of the prosencephalon and its regionalization (prosomeres). Thus, under the influence of these new signaling networks of the head, regulatory elements of the genes encoding the components of the DA markers should have been co-opted and selected for their expression in permissive, competent territories of the forebrain. The occurrence of duplication of a majority of the molecular components of the DA phenotype, as a part of large genome duplications that took place early in craniate evolution, gave the genes the opportunity to acquire new expression territories. This is particularly the case for TH, vMAT, or DAT/NET transporter (see Molecular Components Defining the Phenotype of DA Neurons and their Phylogeny).

In the framework of this hypothesis, the retinal and hypothalamic DA populations in modern vertebrates are the direct descendants of the putative protohypothalamic DA cells of the ancestral chordate. These cells have undergone segregation and parcelation from ancestral retino-hypothalamic primordium. The role of the Shh signaling pathway in the formation of the retina and hypothalamus is well known, and it is possible that its timely secretion from the prechordal plate, together with the action of Nodal-induced pathways (an other invention of craniates) was a key-event in the dorso-ventral patterning of early craniates, which accompanied the formation of the "new head–new brain." During the early development of the vertebrate neural tube, Nodal and Shh signals are necessary for the future retina to protrude out of the secondary prosencephalon simultaneously with a movement of subduction of the hypothalamus, which pulls apart the two territories (England et al., 2006; Stigloher et al., 2006). In addition, early regionalization of the hypothalamus is still dependent on the Nodal and Shh signals together with the action of Wnts and BMPs. This regionalization probably facilitated the segregation of different DA populations in antero-dorsal (A14, A15 for example) and postero-ventral domains (A12 for example) of the hypothalamus.

Dopamine cell populations have also been recruited in other regions, due to the signaling innovations that pattern the craniate/vertebrate neural tube. The DA population of the olfactory bulb derives from the anterior periventricular area (e.g., the subventricular zone of mammals) and its migratory property was probably secondarily acquired in the earliest craniates. The ventral thalamic population (A13, zona incerta in mammals) and the pretectal DA population are also probably ancestral features of craniates, and represent the most prominent components of the alar domain of the diencephalon.

One of the major innovations among the DA systems of craniates would be the emergence of the DA system of the ventral plate of p1–p2–p3 and ventral mesencephalon (nigro-striato-cortical systems of amniotes, A8–A10). Whether this system was modified from pre-existing hypothalamic DA neurons or it was a true innovation depending on the emergence of the MHB and its signaling properties remains impossible to decipher based on current data. A distinct characteristic of this system is ascending projections to the telencephalon. This allowed DA to act on the newly developed neural area, which took a huge expansion in vertebrates, particularly in amniotes.

As previously stated (Kapsimali et al., 2003), the basic role of DA systems has not significantly changed during vertebrate evolution, as far as the molecular and cellular mechanisms are concerned. None the less, DA modulates sensory information in the retina or the olfactory bulb, regulates many neuroendocrine functions of hypothalamic areas, and controls sensori-motor programming, emotions, motivation, and memory in the telencephalic areas. It is due to the anatomical variations in the craniates/vertebrates accompanied by the quantitative changes of the organization of the CNS. For example, the expansion of the telencephalon and its connectivity with different brain areas determines how sensory perception and motor action are elaborated and how they are used for the adaptation of the life style of animals to their environment. The duplication of genes encoding the molecular components of DA systems, together with the "flexible" use corresponding to the molecular context (see Molecular Components Defining the Phenotype of DA Neurons and their Phylogeny), allowed a large degree of plasticity to the craniate DA systems. The parallel advance of our knowledge on the molecular diversity and on the ontogeny of DA cells in protochordates and vertebrates led to a broader and more precise view of the evolution of DA systems. A better understanding of the physiology and pathology of DA systems is anticipated from such a comparative approach.

ACKNOWLEDGMENTS

Profound thanks to Dr. F. Razy-Krajka, for his advices and discussion on the topic. We also thank Dr. V. V. Gurchenkov for his critical reading of the manuscript and his help with Figure 3. Work in our laboratory is supported by grants from the CNRS and Université Paris-Sud, the Agence Nationale de la Recherche and Fondation de France. Kei Yamamoto was supported by ANR and the Région Île-de-France.

REFERENCES

Acampora, D., Postiglione, M. P., Avantaggiato, V., Di Bonito, M., Vaccarino, F. M., Michaud, J., and Simeone, A. (1999). Progressive impairment of developing neuroendocrine cell lineages in the hypothalamus of mice lacking the Orthopedia gene. *Genes Dev.* 13, 2787–2800.

Agathocleous, M., and Harris, W. A. (2009). From progenitors to differentiated cells in the vertebrate retina. *Annu. Rev. Cell Dev. Biol.* 25, 45–69.

Aguayo, L. G., and Grossie, J. (1994). Dopamine inhibits a sustained calcium current through activation of alpha adrenergic receptors and a GTP-binding protein in adult rat sympathetic neurons. *J. Pharmacol. Exp. Ther.* 269, 503–508.

Allen, Z. J. N., Waclaw, R. R., Colbert, M. C., and Campbell, K. (2007). Molecular identity of olfactory bulb interneurons: transcriptional codes of periglomerular neuron subtypes. *J. Mol. Histol.* 38, 517–525.

Andersson, E., Jensen, J. B., Parmar, M., Guillemot, F., and Bjorklund, A. (2006). Development of the mesencephalic dopaminergic neuron system is compromised in the absence of neurogenin 2. *Development* 133, 507–516.

Ang, S. L. (2006). Transcriptional control of midbrain dopaminergic neuron development. *Development* 133, 3499–3506.

Anichtchik, O., Sallinen, V., Peitsaro, N., and Panula, P. (2006). Distinct structure and activity of monoamine oxidase in the brain of zebrafish (*Danio rerio*). *J. Comp. Neurol.* 498, 593–610.

Apparsundaram, S., Moore, K. R., Malone, M. D., Hartzell, H. C., and Blakely, R. D. (1997). Molecular cloning and characterization of an L-epinephrine transporter from sympathetic ganglia of the bullfrog, *Rana catesbiana*. *J. Neurosci.* 17, 2691–2702.

Asbreuk, C. H. J., Vogelaar, C. F., Hellemons, A., Smidt, M. P., and Burbach, J. P. H. (2002). CNS expression pattern of Lmx1b and coexpression with Ptx genes suggest functional cooperativity in the development of forebrain motor control systems. *Mol. Cell. Neurosci.* 21, 410–420.

Balint, E., and Csillag, A. (2007). Nucleus accumbens subregions: hodological and immunohistochemical study in the domestic chick (*Gallus domesticus*). *Cell Tissue Res.* 327, 221–230.

Bardet, S. M., Martinez-de-la-Torre, M., Northcutt, R. G., Rubenstein, J. L., and Puelles, L. (2008). Conserved pattern of OTP-positive cells in the paraventricular nucleus and other hypothalamic sites of tetrapods. *Brain Res. Bull.* 75, 231–235.

Barreiro-Iglesias, A., Laramore, C., Shifman, M. I., Anadón, R., Selzer, M. E., and Rodicio, M. C. (2010). The sea lamprey tyrosine hydroxylase: cDNA cloning and in situ hybridization study in the brain. *Neuroscience* 168, 659–669.

Barreiro-Iglesias, A., Villar-Cervino, V., Anadon, R., and Rodicio, M. C. (2008). Descending brain-spinal cord projections in a primitive vertebrate, the lamprey: cerebrospinal fluid-contacting and dopaminergic neurons. *J. Comp. Neurol.* 511, 711–723.

Bast, T., Diekamp, B., Thiel, C., Schwarting, R. K., and Gunturkun, O. (2002). Functional aspects of dopamine metabolism in the putative prefrontal cortex analogue and striatum of pigeons (*Columba livia*). *J. Comp. Neurol.* 446, 58–67.

Becker, T., Wullimann, M. F., Becker, C. G., Bernhardt, R. R., and Schachner, M. (1997). Axonal regrowth after spinal cord transection in adult zebrafish. *J. Comp. Neurol.* 377, 577–595.

Ben-Jonathan, N., and Hnasko, R. (2001). Dopamine as a prolactin (PRL) inhibitor. *Endocr. Rev.* 22, 724–763.

Björklund, A., and Dunnett, S. B. (2007). Dopamine neuron systems in the brain: an update. *Trends Neurosci.* 30, 194–202.

Björklund, A., and Lindvall, O. (1984). "Dopamine-containing systems in the CNS," in *Classical Transmitters in the CNS, Part I, Handbook of Chemical Neuroanatomy*, Vol. 2, eds A. Björklund and T. Hökfelt (Amsterdam: Elsevier), 55–122.

Blechman, J., Borodovsky, N., Eisenberg, M., Nabel-Rosen, H., Grimm, J., and Levkowitz, G. (2007). Specification of hypothalamic neurons by dual regulation of the homeodomain protein Orthopedia. *Development* 134, 4417–4426.

Blin, M., Norton, W., Bally-Cuif, L., and Vernier, P. (2008). NR4A2 controls the differentiation of selective dopaminergic nuclei in the zebrafish brain. *Mol. Cell. Neurosci.* 39, 592–604.

Bonilla, S., Hall, A. C., Pinto, L., Attardo, A., Gotz, M., Huttner, W. B., and Arenas, E. (2008). Identification of midbrain floor plate radial glia-like cells as dopaminergic progenitors. *Glia* 56, 809–820.

Bouthenet, M. L., Souil, E., Martres, M. P., Sokoloff, P., Giros, B., and Schwartz, J. C. (1991). Localization of dopamine D3 receptor mRNA in the rat brain using in situ hybridization histochemistry: comparison with dopamine D2 receptor mRNA. *Brain Res.* 564, 203–219.

Burman, C., Reale, V., Srivastava, D. P., and Evans, P. D. (2009). Identification and characterization of a novel amphioxus dopamine D-like receptor. *J. Neurochem.* 111, 26–36.

Busby, E. R., Roch, G. J., and Sherwood, N. M. (2010). "Endocrinology of zebrafish: a small fish with a large gene pool," in *Zebrafish*, eds S. F. Perry, M. Ekker, A. P. Farrell, and C. J. Brauner (London: Academic Press), 173–247.

Callier, S., Snapyan, M., Le Crom, S., Prou, D., Vincent, J. D., and Vernier, P. (2003). Evolution and cell biology of dopamine receptors in vertebrates. *Biol. Cell* 95, 489–502.

Candy, J., and Collet, C. (2005). Two tyrosine hydroxylase genes in teleosts. *Biochim. Biophys. Acta* 1727, 35–44.

Carboni, E., and Silvagni, A. (2004). Dopamine reuptake by norepinephrine neurons: exception or rule? *Crit. Rev. Neurobiol.* 16, 121–128.

Carlberg, M., and Anctil, M. (1993). Biogenic amines in coelenterates. *Comp. Biochem. Physiol. C Comp. Pharmacol. Toxicol.* 106, 1–9.

Carlsson, A., Lindqvist, M., Magnusson, T., and Waldeck, B. (1958). On the presence of 3-hydroxytyramine in brain. *Science* 127, 471.

Castro, L. F., Rasmussen, S. L., Holland, P. W., Holland, N. D., and Holland, L. Z. (2006). A Gbx homeobox gene in amphioxus: insights into ancestry of the ANTP class and evolution of the midbrain/hindbrain boundary. *Dev. Biol.* 295, 40–51.

Cave, J. W., Akiba, Y., Banerjee, K., Bhosle, S., Berlin, R., and Baker, H. (2010). Differential regulation of dopaminergic gene expression by Er81. *J. Neurosci.* 30, 4717–4724.

Cave, J. W., and Baker, H. (2009). Dopamine systems in the forebrain. *Adv. Exp. Med. Biol.* 651, 15–35.

Caveney, S., Cladman, W., Verellen, L., and Donly, C. (2006). Ancestry of neuronal monoamine transporters in the Metazoa. *J. Exp. Biol.* 209, 4858–4868.

Cornil, C. A., and Ball, G. F. (2008). Interplay among catecholamine systems: dopamine binds to alpha2-adrenergic receptors in birds and mammals. *J. Comp. Neurol.* 511, 610–627.

Cornil, C. A., Dejace, C., Ball, G. F., and Balthazart, J. (2005). Dopamine modulates male sexual behavior in Japanese quail in part via actions on noradrenergic receptors. *Behav. Brain Res.* 163, 42–57.

Dahlstrom, A., and Fuxe, K. (1964). Evidence for the existence of monoamine-containing neurons in the central nervous systems. I. Demonstration of monoamines in the cell bodies of brain stem neurons. *Acta Physiol. Scand.* 62, 1–55.

Daws, L. C., Toney, G. M., Gerhardt, G. A., and Frazer, A. (1998). In vivo chronoamperometric measures of extracellular serotonin clearance in rat dorsal hippocampus: contribution of serotonin and norepinephrine transporters. *J. Pharmacol. Exp. Ther.* 286, 967–976.

Delsuc, F., Brinkmann, H., Chourrout, D., and Philippe, H. (2006). Tunicates and not cephalochordates are the closest living relatives of vertebrates. *Nature* 439, 965–968.

Demchyshyn, L. L., Sugamori, K. S., Lee, F. J., Hamadanizadeh, S. A., and Niznik, H. B. (1995). The dopamine D1D receptor. Cloning and characterization of three pharmacologically distinct D1-like receptors from *Gallus domesticus*. *J. Biol. Chem.* 270, 4005–4012.

Di Salvio, M., Di Giovannantonio, L. G., Acampora, D., Prosperi, R., Omodei, D., Prakash, N., Wurst, W., and Simeone, A. (2010). Otx2 controls neuron subtype identity in ventral tegmental area and antagonizes vulnerability to MPTP. *Nat. Neurosci.* 13, 1481–1148.

Dubach, M. (1994). "Telencephalic dopamine cells in monkeys, humans, and rats," in *Phylogeny and Development of Catecholamine Systems in the CNS of Vertebrates*, eds W. J. A. J. Smeets and A. Reiner (Cambridge: Cambridge University Press), 21–47.

Dufour, S., Sebert, M. E., Weltzien, F. A., Rousseau, K., and Pasqualini, C. (2010). Neuroendocrine control by dopamine of teleost reproduction. *J. Fish Biol.* 76, 129–160.

Dufour, S., Weltzien, F. A., Sebert, M. E., Le Belle, N., Vidal, B., Vernier, P., and Pasqualini, C. (2005). Dopaminergic inhibition of reproduction in teleost fishes: ecophysiological and evolutionary implications. *Ann. N. Y. Acad. Sci.* 1040, 9–21.

Dunkley, P. R., Bobrovskaya, L., Graham, M. E., von Nagy-Felsobuki, E. I., and Dickson, P. W. (2004). Tyrosine hydroxylase phosphorylation: regulation and consequences. *J. Neurochem.* 91, 1025–1043.

Eiden, L. E., Schafer, M. K., Weihe, E., and Schutz, B. (2004). The vesicular amine transporter family (SLC18): amine/proton antiporters required for vesicular accumulation and regulated exocytotic secretion of monoamines and acetylcholine. *Pflugers Arch.* 447, 636–640.

Eisenhofer, G., Kopin, I. J., and Goldstein, D. S. (1985). Catecholamine metabolism: a contemporary view with implication for physiology and medicine. *Science* 230, 181–183.

England, S. J., Blanchard, G. B., Mahadevan, L., and Adams, R. J. (2006). A dynamic fate map of the forebrain shows how vertebrate eyes form and explains two causes of cyclopia. *Development* 133, 4613–4617.

Fedorow, H., Tribl, F., Halliday, G., Gerlach, M., Riederer, P., and Double, K. L. (2005). Neuromelanin in human dopamine neurons: comparison with peripheral melanins and relevance to Parkinson's disease. *Prog. Neurobiol.* 75, 109–124.

Filippi, A., Durr, K., Ryu, S., Willaredt, M., Holzschuh, J., and Driever, W. (2007). Expression and function of nr4a2, lmx1b, and pitx3 in zebrafish dopaminergic and noradrenergic neuronal development. *BMC Dev. Biol.* 7, 135. doi: 10.1186/1471-213X-7-135

Flames, N., and Hobert, O. (2009). Gene regulatory logic of dopamine neuron differentiation. *Nature* 458, 885–889.

Gans, C., and Northcutt, R. G. (1983). Neural crest and the origin of vertebrates: a new head. *Science* 220, 268–273.

Garcia-Tornadu, I., Risso, G., Perez-Millan, M. I., Noain, D., Diaz-Torga, G., Low, M. J., Rubinstein, M., and Becu-Villalobos, D. (2010). Neurotransmitter modulation of the GHRH-GH axis. *Front. Horm. Res.* 38, 59–69.

Gaspar, P., Berger, B., Febvret, A., Vigny, A., Krieger-Poulet, M., and Borri-Voltattorni, C. (1987). Tyrosine hydroxylase-immunoreactive neurons in the human cerebral cortex: a novel catecholaminergic group? *Neurosci. Lett.* 80, 257–262.

Gerfen, C. R. (1992). The neostriatal mosaic: multiple levels of compartmental organization in the basal ganglia. *Annu. Rev. Neurosci.* 15, 285–320.

González, A., and Smeets, W. J. A. J. (1994). "Catecholamine systems in the CNS of amphibians," in *Phylogeny and Development of Catecholamine Systems in the CNS of Vertebrates*, eds W. J. A. J. Smeets and A. Reiner (Cambridge: Cambridge University Press), 21–47.

Goodwill, K. E., Sabatier, C., Marks, C., Raag, R., Fitzpatrick, P. F., and Stevens, R. C. (1997). Crystal structure of tyrosine hydroxylase at 2.3 A and its implications for inherited neurodegenerative diseases. *Nat. Struct. Biol.* 4, 578–585.

Goshu, E., Jin, H., Lovejoy, J., Marion, J. F., Michaud, J. L., and Fan, C. M. (2004). Sim2 contributes to neuroendocrine hormone gene expression in the anterior hypothalamus. *Mol. Endocrinol.* 18, 1251–1262.

Guillot, T. S., and Miller, G. W. (2009). Protective actions of the vesicular monoamine transporter 2 (VMAT2) in monoaminergic neurons. *Mol. Neurobiol.* 39, 149–170.

Güntürkün, O. (2005). Avian and mammalian "prefrontal cortices": limited degrees of freedom in the evolution of the neural mechanisms of goal-state maintenance. *Brain Res. Bull.* 66, 311–316.

Hirano, J., Archer, S. N., and Djamgoz, M. B. (1998). Dopamine receptor subtypes expressed in vertebrate (carp and eel) retinae: cloning, sequencing and comparison of five D1-like and three D2-like receptors. *Recept. Channels* 5, 387–404.

Hirata, T., Nakazawa, M., Muraoka, O., Nakayama, R., Suda, Y., and Hibi, M. (2006). Zinc-finger genes Fez and Fez-like function in the establishment of diencephalon subdivisions. *Development* 133, 3993–4004.

Hökfelt, T., Martensson, R., Björklund, A., Kleinau, S., and Goldstein, M. (1984). "Distributional maps of tyrosine-hydroxylase-immunoreactive neurons in the rat brain," in *Classical Transmitters in the CNS, Part I, Handbook of Chemical Neuroanatomy*, Vol. 2, eds A. Björklund and T. Hökfelt (Amsterdam: Elsevier), 277–379.

Holland, L. Z., and Holland, N. D. (1999). Chordate origins of the vertebrate central nervous system. *Curr. Opin. Neurobiol.* 9, 596–602.

Holmberg, K. (1970). The hagfish retina: fine structure of retinal cells in Myxine glutinosa, L., with special reference to receptor and epithelial cells. *Z. Zellforsch. Mikrosk. Anat.* 111, 519–538.

Holzschuh, J., Hauptmann, G., and Driever, W. (2003). Genetic analysis of the roles of Hh, FGF8, and nodal signaling during catecholaminergic system development in the zebrafish brain. *J. Neurosci.* 23, 5507–5519.

Hornykiewicz, O. (1962). Dopamine (3-hydroxytyramine) in the central nervous system and its relation to the Parkinson syndrome in man. *Dtsch. Med. Wochenschr.* 87, 1807–1810.

Huang, S., and Moody, S. A. (1998). Dual expression of GABA or serotonin and dopamine in *Xenopus* amacrine cells is transient and may be regulated by laminar cues. *Vis. Neurosci.* 15, 969–977.

Hynes, M., and Rosenthal, A. (1999). Specification of dopaminergic and serotonergic neurons in the vertebrate CNS. *Curr. Opin. Neurobiol.* 9, 26–36.

Ikuta, T., and Saiga, H. (2007). Dynamic change in the expression of developmental genes in the ascidian central nervous system: revisit to the tripartite model and the origin of the midbrain-hindbrain boundary region. *Dev. Biol.* 312, 631–643.

Imai, K. S., Stolfi, A., Levine, M., and Satou, Y. (2009). Gene regulatory networks underlying the compartmentalization of the *Ciona* central nervous system. *Development* 136, 285–293.

Inagaki, S., Shiosaka, S., Takatsuki, K., Sakanaka, M., Takagi, H., Senba, E., Matsuzaki, T., and Tohyama, M. (1981). Distribution of somatostatin in the frog brain, *Rana catesbeiana*, in relation to location of catecholamine-containing neuron system. *J. Comp. Neurol.* 202, 89–101.

Jeong, J. Y., Einhorn, Z., Mathur, P., Chen, L., Lee, S., Kawakami, K., and Guo, S. (2007). Patterning the zebrafish diencephalon by the conserved zinc-finger protein Fezl. *Development* 134, 127–136.

Kah, O., Chambolle, P., Thibault, J., and Geffard, M. (1984). Existence of dopaminergic neurons in the preoptic region of the goldfish. *Neurosci. Lett.* 48, 293–298.

Kannari, K., Shen, H., Arai, A., Tomiyama, M., and Baba, M. (2006). Reuptake of L-DOPA-derived extracellular dopamine in the striatum with dopaminergic denervation via serotonin transporters. *Neurosci. Lett.* 402, 62–65.

Kapsimali, M., Caneparo, L., Houart, C., and Wilson, S. W. (2004). Inhibition of Wnt/Axin/beta-catenin pathway activity promotes ventral CNS midline tissue to adopt hypothalamic rather than floorplate identity. *Development* 131, 5923–5933.

Kapsimali, M., Le Crom, S., and Vernier, P. (2003). "A natural history of vertebrate dopamine receptors," in *Dopamine Receptors and Transporters*, eds M. Laruelle, A. Sidhu, and P. Vernier (New York: Marcel Dekker Inc.), 1–43.

Kele, J., Simplicio, N., Ferri, A. L., Mira, H., Guillemot, F., Arenas, E., and Ang, S. L. (2006). Neurogenin 2 is required for the development of ventral midbrain dopaminergic neurons. *Development* 133, 495–505.

Kelley, A. E. (2004). Memory and addiction: shared neural circuitry and molecular mechanisms. *Neuron* 44, 161–179.

Kiss, J. Z., and Peczely, P. (1987). Distribution of tyrosine-hydroxylase (TH)-immunoreactive neurons in the diencephalon of the pigeon (*Columba livia domestica*). *J. Comp. Neurol.* 257, 333–346.

Kozmik, Z., Holland, N. D., Kreslova, J., Oliveri, D., Schubert, M., Jonasova, K., Holland, L. Z., Pestarino, M., Benes, V., and Candiani, S. (2007). Pax-Six-Eya-Dach network during amphioxus development: conservation in vitro but context specificity in vivo. *Dev. Biol.* 306, 143–159.

Kubikova, L., Wada, K., and Jarvis, E. D. (2010). Dopamine receptors in a songbird brain. *J. Comp. Neurol.* 518, 741–769.

Kumer, S. C., and Vrana, K. E. (1996). Intricate regulation of tyrosine hydroxylase activity and gene expression. *J. Neurochem.* 67, 443–462.

Lamb, T. D., Collin, S. P., and Pugh, E. N. Jr. (2007). Evolution of the vertebrate eye: opsins, photoreceptors, retina and eye cup. *Nat. Rev. Neurosci.* 8, 960–976.

Lanau, F., Zenner, M. T., Civelli, O., and Hartman, D. S. (1997). Epinephrine and norepinephrine act as potent agonists at the recombinant human dopamine D4 receptor. *J. Neurochem.* 68, 804–812.

Landwehrmeyer, B., Mengod, G., and Palacios, J. M. (1993). Differential visualization of dopamine D2 and D3 receptor sites in rat brain. A comparative study using in situ hybridization histochemistry and ligand binding autoradiography. *Eur. J. Neurosci.* 5, 145–153.

Lazarini, F., and Lledo, P. M. (2011). Is adult neurogenesis essential for olfaction? *Trends Neurosci.* 34, 20–30.

Le Crom, S., Kapsimali, M., Barome, P. O., and Vernier, P. (2003). Dopamine receptors for every species: gene duplications and functional diversification in Craniates. *J. Struct. Funct. Genomics* 3, 161–176.

Lee, T. L., Hsu, C. T., Yen, S. T., Lai, C. W., and Cheng, J. T. (1998). Activation of beta3-adrenoceptors by exogenous dopamine to lower glucose uptake into rat adipocytes. *J. Auton. Nerv. Syst.* 74, 86–90.

Lin, W., Metzakopian, E., Mavromatakis, Y. E., Gao, N., Balaskas, N., Sasaki, H., Briscoe, J., Whitsett, J. A., Goulding, M., Kaestner, K. H., and Ang, S. L. (2009). Foxa1 and Foxa2 function both upstream of and cooperatively with Lmx1a and Lmx1b in a feedforward loop promoting mesodiencephalic dopaminergic neuron development. *Dev. Biol.* 333, 386–396.

Liu, N. A., Liu, Q., Wawrowsky, K., Yang, Z., Lin, S., and Melmed, S. (2006). Prolactin receptor signaling mediates the osmotic response of embryonic zebrafish lactotrophs. *Mol. Endocrinol.* 20, 871–880.

Löhr, H., Ryu, S., and Driever, W. (2009). Zebrafish diencephalic A11-related dopaminergic neurons share a conserved transcriptional network with neuroendocrine cell lineages. *Development* 136, 1007–1017.

Lorang, D., Amara, S. G., and Simerly, R. B. (1994). Cell-type-specific expression of catecholamine transporters in the rat brain. *J. Neurosci.* 14, 4903–4914.

MacHeroux, P., Seth, O., Bollschweiler, C., Schwarz, M., Kurfurst, M., Au, L. C., and Ghisla, S. (2001). L-amino-acid oxidase from the Malayan pit viper *Calloselasma rhodostoma*. Comparative sequence analysis and characterization of active and inactive forms of the enzyme. *Eur. J. Biochem.* 268, 1679–1686.

Maier, S., Walkowiak, W., Luksch, H., and Endepols, H. (2010). An indirect basal ganglia pathway in anuran amphibians? *J. Chem. Neuroanat.* 40, 21–35.

Manning, L., Ohyama, K., Saeger, B., Hatano, O., Wilson, S. A., Logan, M., and Placzek, M. (2006). Regional morphogenesis in the hypothalamus: a BMP-Tbx2 pathway coordinates fate and proliferation through Shh downregulation. *Dev. Cell* 11, 873–885.

Marin, O., Smeets, W. J. A. J., and Gonzalez, A. (1997). Basal ganglia organization in amphibians: catecholaminergic innervation of the striatum and the nucleus accumbens. *J. Comp. Neurol.* 378, 50–69.

Marin, O., Smeets, W. J., and Gonzalez, A. (1998a). Evolution of the basal ganglia in tetrapods: a new perspective based on recent studies in amphibians. *Trends Neurosci.* 21, 487–494.

Marin, O., Smeets, W. J., and Gonzalez, A. (1998b). Basal ganglia organization in amphibians: chemoarchitecture. *J. Comp. Neurol.* 392, 285–312.

Masland, R. H. (2001). The fundamental plan of the retina. *Nat. Neurosci.* 4, 877–886.

Mathieu, J., Barth, A., Rosa, F. M., Wilson, S. W., and Peyrieras, N. (2002). Distinct and cooperative roles for Nodal and Hedgehog signals during hypothalamic development. *Development* 129, 3055–3065.

Mathis, L., and Nicolas, J. F. (2002). Cellular patterning of the vertebrate embryo. *Trends Genet.* 18, 627–635.

McNay, D. E., Pelling, M., Claxton, S., Guillemot, F., and Ang, S. L. (2006). Mash1 is required for generic and subtype differentiation of hypothalamic neuroendocrine cells. *Mol. Endocrinol.* 20, 1623–1632.

Medina, L. (2008). "Evolution and embryological development of forebrain," in *Encyclopedic Reference of Neuroscience*, eds M. D. Binder and N. Hirokawa (Berlin: Springer-Verlag), 1172–1192.

Medina, L., Puelles, L., and Smeets, W. J. (1994). Development of catecholamine systems in the brain of the lizard *Gallotia galloti*. *J. Comp. Neurol.* 350, 41–62.

Meek, J. (1994). "Catecholamines in the brain of Osteichthyes (bony fishes)," in *Phylogeny and Development of Catecholamine Systems in the CNS of Vertebrates*, eds W. J. A. J. Smeets and A. Reiner (Cambridge: Cambridge University Press), 21–47.

Meister, B., Hokfelt, T., Brown, J., Joh, T., and Goldstein, M. (1987). Dopaminergic cells in the caudal A13 cell group express somatostatin-like immunoreactivity. *Exp. Brain Res.* 67, 441–444.

Mel'nikova, V. I., Lavrent'eva, A. V., Kudrin, V. S., Raevskii, K. S., and Ugryumov, M. V. (2005). Dopamine synthesis by non-dopaminergic neurons in the arcuate nucleus of rat fetuses. *Neurosci. Behav. Physiol.* 35, 809–813.

Michaud, J. L., DeRossi, C., May, N. R., Holdener, B. C., and Fan, C. M. (2000). ARNT2 acts as the dimerization partner of SIM1 for the development of the hypothalamus. *Mech. Dev.* 90, 253–261.

Missale, C., Nash, S. R., Robinson, S. W., Jaber, M., and Caron, M. G. (1998). Dopamine receptors: from structure to function. *Physiol. Rev.* 78, 189–225.

Mogensen, J., and Divac, I. (1982). The prefrontal 'cortex' in the pigeon. Behavioral evidence. *Brain Behav. Evol.* 21, 60–66.

Moret, F., Christiaen, L., Deyts, C., Blin, M., Vernier, P., and Joly, J.-S. (2005a). Regulatory gene expressions in the ascidian ventral sensory vesicle: evolutionary relationships with the vertebrate hypothalamus. *Dev. Biol.* 277, 557–566.

Moret, F., Christiaen, L., Deyts, C., Blin, M., Joly, J.-S., and Vernier, P. (2005b). The dopamine-synthesizing cells of the sensory vesicle of the tunicate *Ciona* intestinalis are located only in a hypothalamus-related domain: implications for the origin of vertebrate catecholamine systems. *Eur. J. Neurosci.* 21, 3043–3055.

Moret, F., Guilland, J. C., Coudouel, S., Rochette, L., and Vernier, P. (2004). Distribution of tyrosine hydroxylase, dopamine, and serotonin in the central nervous system of amphioxus (*Branchiostoma lanceolatum*): implications for the evolution of catecholamine systems in vertebrates. *J. Comp. Neurol.* 468, 135–150.

Moron, J. A., Brockington, A., Wise, R. A., Rocha, B. A., and Hope, B. T. (2002). Dopamine uptake through the norepinephrine transporter in brain regions with low levels of the dopamine transporter: evidence from knock-out mouse lines. *J. Neurosci.* 22, 389–395.

Mossner, R., Simantov, R., Marx, A., Lesch, K. P., and Seif, I. (2006). Aberrant accumulation of serotonin in dopaminergic neurons. *Neurosci. Lett.* 401, 49–54.

Nagatsu, T. (2004). Progress in monoamine oxidase (MAO) research in relation to genetic engineering. *Neurotoxicology* 25, 11–20.

Nakashima, A., Hayashi, N., Kaneko, Y. S., Mori, K., Sabban, E. L., Nagatsu, T., and Ota, A. (2009). Role of N-terminus of tyrosine hydroxylase in the biosynthesis of catecholamines. *J. Neural Transm.* 116, 1355–1362.

Neves, S. R., Ram, P. T., and Iyengar, R. (2002). G protein pathways. *Science* 296, 1636–1639.

Newman-Tancredi, A., Audinot-Bouchez, V., Gobert, A., and Millan, M. J. (1997). Noradrenaline and adrenaline are high affinity agonists at dopamine D4 receptors. *Eur. J. Pharmacol.* 319, 379–383.

Obeso, J. A., Rodriguez-Oroz, M. C., Goetz, C. G., Marin, C., Kordower, J. H., Rodriguez, M., Hirsch, E. C., Farrer, M., Schapira, A. H., and Halliday, G. (2010). Missing pieces in the Parkinson's disease puzzle. *Nat. Med.* 16, 653–661.

Ohyama, K., Ellis, P., Kimura, S., and Placzek, M. (2005). Directed differentiation of neural cells to hypothalamic dopaminergic neurons. *Development* 132, 5185–5197.

O'Keeffe, G. C., Barker, R. A., and Caldwell, M. A. (2009). Dopaminergic modulation of neurogenesis in the subventricular zone of the adult brain. *Cell Cycle* 8, 2888–2894.

Omodei, D., Acampora, D., Mancuso, P., Prakash, N., Di Giovannantonio, L. G., Wurst, W., and Simeone, A. (2008). Anterior-posterior graded response to Otx2 controls proliferation and differentiation of dopaminergic progenitors in the ventral mesencephalon. *Development* 135, 3459–3470.

Ono, Y., Nakatani, T., Sakamoto, Y., Mizuhara, E., Minaki, Y., Kumai, M., Hamaguchi, A., Nishimura, M., Inoue, Y., Hayashi, H., Takahashi, J., and Imai, T. (2007). Differences in neurogenic potential in floor plate cells along an anteroposterior location: midbrain dopaminergic neurons originate from mesencephalic floor plate cells. *Development* 134, 3213–3225.

Osorio, J., Mueller, T., Retaux, S., Vernier, P., and Wullimann, M. F. (2010). Phylotypic expression of the bHLH genes Neurogenin2, Neurod, and Mash1 in the mouse embryonic forebrain. *J. Comp. Neurol.* 518, 851–871.

Panopoulou, G., and Poustka, A. J. (2005). Timing and mechanism of ancient vertebrate genome duplications – the adventure of a hypothesis. *Trends Genet.* 21, 559–567.

Parent, A., and Northcutt, R. G. (1982). The monoamine-containing neurons in the brain of the garfish *Lepisosteus osseus*. *Brain Res. Bull.* 9, 189–204.

Parsons, S. M. (2000). Transport mechanisms in acetylcholine and monoamine storage. *FASEB J.* 14, 2423–2434.

Patton, S. J., Luke, G. N., and Holland, P. W. (1998). Complex history of a chromosomal paralogy region: insights from amphioxus aromatic amino acid hydroxylase genes and insulin-related genes. *Mol. Biol. Evol.* 15, 1373–1380.

Petko, M., and Orosz, V. (1996). Distribution of somatostatin-immunoreactive structures in the central nervous system of the frog, *Rana esculenta*. *J. Hirnforsch.* 37, 109–120.

Pierre, J., Mahouche, M., Suderevskaya, E. I., Reperant, J., and Ward, R. (1997). Immunocytochemical localization of dopamine and its synthetic enzymes in the central nervous system of the lamprey *Lampetra fluviatilis*. *J. Comp. Neurol.* 380, 119–135.

Postlethwait, J. H., Woods, I. G., Ngo-Hazelett, P., Yan, Y. L., Kelly, P. D., Chu, F., Huang, H., Hill-Force, A., and Talbot, W. S. (2000). Zebrafish comparative genomics and the origins of vertebrate chromosomes. *Genome Res.* 10, 1890–1902.

Prakash, N., Brodski, C., Naserke, T., Puelles, E., Gogoi, R., Hall, A., Panhuysen, M., Echevarria, D., Sussel, L., Weisenhorn, D. M., Martinez, S., Arenas, E., Simeone, A., and Wurst, W. (2006). A Wnt1-regulated genetic network controls the identity and fate of midbrain dopaminergic progenitors in vivo. *Development* 133, 89–98.

Prakash, N., and Wurst, W. (2006). Genetic networks controlling the development of midbrain dopaminergic neurons. *J. Physiol.* 575, 403–410.

Pucak, M. L., and Grace, A. A. (1994). Regulation of substantia nigra dopamine neurons. *Crit. Rev. Neurobiol.* 9, 67–89.

Puelles, E., Annino, A., Tuorto, F., Usiello, A., Acampora, D., Czerny, T., Brodski, C., Ang, S. L., Wurst, W., and Simeone, A. (2004). Otx2 regulates the extent, identity and fate of neuronal progenitor domains in the ventral midbrain. *Development* 131, 2037–2048.

Puelles, L. (1995). A segmental morphological paradigm for understanding vertebrate forebrains. *Brain Behav. Evol.* 46, 319–337.

Puelles, L., and Medina, L. (1994). "Development of neurons expressing tyrosine hydroxylase and dopamine in the chicken brain: a comparative segmental analysis," in *Phylogeny and Development of Catecholamine Systems in the CNS of Vertebrates*, eds W. J. A. J. Smeets and A. Reiner (Cambridge: Cambridge University Press), 21–47.

Puelles, L., and Rubenstein, J. L. (2003). Forebrain gene expression domains and the evolving prosomeric model. *Trends Neurosci.* 26, 469–476.

Reiner, A. (2002). Functional circuitry of the avian basal ganglia: implications for basal ganglia organization in stem amniotes. *Brain Res. Bull.* 57, 513–528.

Reiner, A., Karle, E. J., Anderson, K. D., Medina, L. (1994). "Catecholaminergic perikarya and fibers in the avian nervous system," in *Phylogeny and Development of Catecholamine Systems in the CNS of Vertebrates*, eds W. J. A. J. Smeets and A. Reiner (Cambridge: Cambridge University Press), 135–181.

Reiner, A., Perkel, D. J., Bruce, L. L., Butler, A. B., Csillag, A., Kuenzel, W., Medina, L., Paxinos, G., Shimizu, T., Striedter, G., Wild, M., Ball, G. F., Durand, S., Gunturkun, O., Lee, D. W., Mello, C. V., Powers, A., White, S. A., Hough, G., Kubikova, L., Smulders, T. V., Wada, K., Dugas-Ford, J., Husband, S., Yamamoto, K., Yu, J., Siang, C., and Jarvis, E. D. (2004). Revised nomenclature for avian telencephalon and some related brainstem nuclei. *J. Comp. Neurol.* 473, 377–414.

Rey, E., Hernandez-Diaz, F. J., Abreu, P., Alonso, R., and Tabares, L. (2001). Dopamine induces intracellular Ca2+ signals mediated by alpha1B-adrenoceptors in rat pineal cells. *Eur. J. Pharmacol.* 430, 9–17.

Rink, E., and Wullimann, M. F. (2001). The teleostean (zebrafish) dopaminergic system ascending to the subpallium (striatum) is located in the basal diencephalon (posterior tuberculum). *Brain Res.* 889, 316–330.

Rose, J., Schiffer, A. M., Dittrich, L., and Güntürkün, O. (2010). The role of dopamine in maintenance and distractability of attention in the "prefrontal cortex" of pigeons. *Neuroscience* 167, 232–237.

Roubert, C., Sagne, C., Kapsimali, M., Vernier, P., Bourrat, F., and Giros, B. (2001). A Na(+)/Cl(−)-dependent transporter for catecholamines, identified as a norepinephrine transporter, is expressed in the brain of the teleost fish medaka (*Oryzias latipes*). *Mol. Pharmacol.* 60, 462–473.

Ruffolo, R. R. Jr., and Morgan, E. L. (1984). Interaction of the novel inotropic agent, ASL-7022, with alpha and beta adrenoceptors in the cardiovascular system of the pithed rat: comparison with dobutamine and dopamine. *J. Pharmacol. Exp. Ther.* 229, 364–371.

Russek-Blum, N., Gutnick, A., Nabel-Rosen, H., Blechman, J., Staudt, N., Dorsky, R. I., Houart, C., and Levkowitz, G. (2008). Dopaminergic neuronal cluster size is determined during early forebrain patterning. *Development* 135, 3401–3413.

Ryu, S., Holzschuh, J., Mahler, J., and Driever, W. (2006). Genetic analysis of dopaminergic system development in zebrafish. *J. Neural Transm. Suppl.* 61–66.

Ryu, S., Mahler, J., Acampora, D., Holzschuh, J., Erhardt, S., Omodei, D., Simeone, A., and Driever, W. (2007). Orthopedia homeodomain protein is essential for diencephalic dopaminergic neuron development. *Curr. Biol.* 17, 873–880.

Saenz-de-Miera, L. E., and Ayala, F. J. (2004). Complex evolution of orthologous and paralogous decarboxylase genes. *J. Evol. Biol.* 17, 55–66.

Sallinen, V., Sundvik, M., Reenila, I., Peitsaro, N., Khrustalyov, D., Anichtchik, O., Toleikyte, G., Kaslin, J., and Panula, P. (2009). Hyperserotonergic phenotype after monoamine oxidase inhibition in larval zebrafish. *J. Neurochem.* 109, 403–415.

Sanchez-Camacho, C., Marin, O., Smeets, W. J., Ten Donkelaar, H. J., and Gonzalez, A. (2001). Descending supraspinal pathways in amphibians. II. Distribution and origin of the catecholaminergic innervation of the spinal cord. *J. Comp. Neurol.* 434, 209–232.

Satir, P. (2000). A comment on the origin of the vertebrate eye. *Anat. Rec.* 261, 224–227.

Saucedo-Cardenas, O., Quintana-Hau, J. D., Le, W. D., Smidt, M. P., Cox, J. J., De Mayo, F., Burbach, J. P., and Conneely, O. M. (1998). Nurr1 is essential for the induction of the dopaminergic phenotype and the survival of ventral mesencephalic late dopaminergic precursor neurons. *Proc. Natl. Acad. Sci. U.S.A.* 95, 4013–4018.

Schweitzer, J., and Driever, W. (2009). "Development of dopamine systems in zebrafish," in *Development and Engineering of Dopamine Neurons*, eds R. J. Pasterkamp, M. P. Smidt, and J. P. H. Burbach (Austin, TX: Landes BioScience), 1–14.

Sharp, T., Zetterstrom, T., and Ungerstedt, U. (1986). An in vivo study of dopamine release and metabolism in rat brain regions using intracerebral dialysis. *J. Neurochem.* 47, 113–122.

Shimizu, T., and Hibi, M. (2009). Formation and patterning of the forebrain and olfactory system by zinc-finger genes Fezf1 and Fezf2. *Dev. Growth Differ.* 51, 221–231.

Simon, H., Saueressig, H., Wurst, W., Goulding, M., and O'Leary, D. (2001). Fate of midbrain dopaminergic neurons controlled by the engrailed genes. *J. Neurosci.* 21, 3126–3134.

Smeets, W. J., and Reiner, A. (1994). "Catecholamines in the CNS of vertebrates: current concepts of evolution and functional significance," in *Phylogeny and Development of Catecholamine Systems in the CNS of Vertebrates*, eds W. J. A. J. Smeets and A. Reiner (Cambridge: Cambridge University Press), 463–481.

Smeets, W. J. A. J. (1994). "Catecholamines in the CNS of reptiles: structure and functional considerations," in *Phylogeny and Development of Catecholamine Systems in the CNS of Vertebrates*, eds W. J. A. J. Smeets and A. Reiner (Cambridge: Cambridge University Press), 21–47.

Smeets, W. J. A. J., and González, A. (2000). Catecholamine systems in the brain of vertebrates: new perspectives through a comparative approach. *Brain Res. Brain Res. Rev.* 33, 308–379.

Smidt, M. P., Asbreuk, C. H., Cox, J. J., Chen, H., Johnson, R. L., and Burbach, J. P. (2000). A second independent pathway for development of mesencephalic dopaminergic neurons requires Lmx1b. *Nat. Neurosci.* 3, 337–341.

Smidt, M. P., and Burbach, J. P. (2007). How to make a mesodiencephalic dopaminergic neuron. *Nat. Rev. Neurosci.* 8, 21–32.

Smits, S. M., Ponnio, T., Conneely, O. M., Burbach, J. P., and Smidt, M. P. (2003). Involvement of Nurr1 in specifying the neurotransmitter identity of ventral midbrain dopaminergic neurons. *Eur. J. Neurosci.* 18, 1731–1738.

Stigloher, C., Ninkovic, J., Laplante, M., Geling, A., Tannhäuser, B., Topp, S., Kikuta, H., Becker, T. S., Houart, C., and Bally-Cuif, L. (2006). Segregation of telencephalic and eye-field identities inside the zebrafish forebrain territory is controlled by Rx3. *Development* 133, 2925–2935.

Stuesse, S. L., Cruce, W. L. R., and Northcutt, R. G. (1994). "Localization of catecholamines in the brains of Chondrichthyes (cartilaginous fishes)," in *Phylogeny and Development of Catecholamine Systems in the CNS of Vertebrates*, eds W. J. A. J. Smeets and A. Reiner (Cambridge: Cambridge University Press), 21–47.

Sugamori, K. S., Demchyshyn, L. L., Chung, M., and Niznik, H. B. (1994). D1A, D1B, and D1C dopamine receptors from *Xenopus laevis*. *Proc. Natl. Acad. Sci. U.S.A.* 91, 10536–10540.

Sulzer, D., and Edwards, R. H. (2005). Antidepressants and the monoamine masquerade. *Neuron* 46, 1–2.

Szarek, E., Cheah, P. S., Schwartz, J., and Thomas, P. (2010). Molecular genetics of the developing neuroendocrine hypothalamus. *Mol. Cell. Endocrinol.* 323, 115–123.

Tang, H. (2009). Regulation and function of the melanization reaction in *Drosophila*. *Fly (Austin)* 3, 105–111.

Tay, T. L., Ronneberger, O., Ryu, S., Nitschke, R., and Driever, W. (2011). Comprehensive catecholaminergic projectome analysis reveals single-neuron integration of zebrafish ascending and descending dopaminergic systems. *Nat. Commun.* 2, 171.

Teigen, K., Dao, K. K., McKinney, J. A., Gorren, A. C., Mayer, B., Froystein, N. A., Haavik, J., and Martinez, A. (2004). Tetrahydrobiopterin binding to aromatic amino acid hydroxylases. Ligand recognition and specificity. *J. Med. Chem.* 47, 5962–5971.

Thiery, J. C., Chemineau, P., Hernandez, X., Migaud, M., and Malpaux, B. (2002). Neuroendocrine interactions and seasonality. *Domest. Anim. Endocrinol.* 23, 87–100.

Tillet, Y. (1994). "Catecholaminergic neuronal systems in the diencephalon of mammals," in *Phylogeny and Development of Catecholamine Systems in the CNS of Vertebrates*, eds W. J. A. J. Smeets and A. Reiner (Cambridge: Cambridge University Press), 207–246.

Torres, G. E., Gainetdinov, R. R., and Caron, M. G. (2003). Plasma membrane monoamine transporters: structure, regulation and function. *Nat. Rev. Neurosci.* 4, 13–25.

Valentini, V., Frau, R., and Di Chiara, G. (2004). Noradrenaline transporter blockers raise extracellular dopamine in medial prefrontal but not parietal and occipital cortex: differences with mianserin and clozapine. *J. Neurochem.* 88, 917–927.

Vandepoele, K., De Vos, W., Taylor, J. S., Meyer, A., and Van de Peer, Y. (2004). Major events in the genome evolution of vertebrates: paranome age and size differ considerably between ray-finned fishes and land vertebrates. *Proc. Natl. Acad. Sci. U.S.A.* 101, 1638–1643.

Verney, C., Zecevic, N., and Puelles, L. (2001). Structure of longitudinal brain zones that provide the origin for the substantia nigra and ventral tegmental area in human embryos, as revealed by cytoarchitecture and tyrosine hydroxylase, calretinin, calbindin, and GABA immunoreactions. *J. Comp. Neurol.* 429, 22–44.

Vernier, P., Moret, F., Callier, S., Snapyan, M., Wersinger, C., and Sidhu, A. (2004). The degeneration of dopamine neurons in Parkinson's disease: insights from embryology and evolution of the mesostriatocortical system. *Ann. N. Y. Acad. Sci.* 1035, 231–249.

Vernier, P., and Wullimann, M. F. (2009). "Evolution of the posterior tuberculum and preglomerular nuclear complex," in *Encyclopedia of Neurosciences*, Part 5, eds M. D. Binder, N. Hirokawa, and U. Windhorst (Berlin: Springer-Verlag), 1404–1413.

Vieira, C., Pombero, A., Garcia-Lopez, R., Gimeno, L., Echevarria, D., and Martinez, S. (2010). Molecular mechanisms controlling brain development: an overview of neuroepithelial secondary organizers. *Int. J. Dev. Biol.* 54, 7–20.

Vigh, B., Manzano e Silva, M. J., Frank, C. L., Vincze, C., Czirok, S. J., Szabó, A., Lukáts, A., and Szél, A. (2004). The system of cerebrospinal fluid-contacting neurons. Its supposed role in the nonsynaptic signal transmission of the brain. *Histol. Histopathol.* 19, 607–628.

Vigh, B., Manzano, M. J., Zádori, A., Frank, C. L., Lukáts, A., Röhlich, P., Szél, A., and Dávid, C. (2002). Nonvisual photoreceptors of the deep brain, pineal organs and retina. *Histol. Histopathol.* 17, 555–590.

Vigh-Teichmann, I., and Vigh, B. (1983). The system of cerebrospinal fluid-contacting neurons. *Arch. Histol. Jpn.* 46, 427–468.

Vitalis, T., Cases, O., Engelkamp, D., Verney, C., and Price, D. J. (2000). Defect of tyrosine hydroxylase-immunoreactive neurons in the brains of mice lacking the transcription factor Pax6. *J. Neurosci.* 20, 6501–6516.

Vizi, E. S., Zsilla, G., Caron, M. G., and Kiss, J. P. (2004). Uptake and release of norepinephrine by serotonergic terminals in norepinephrine transporter knock-out mice: implications for the action of selective serotonin reuptake inhibitors. *J. Neurosci.* 24, 7888–7894.

Volff, J. N. (2005). Genome evolution and biodiversity in teleost fish. *Heredity* 94, 280–294.

Wada, H., Saiga, H., Satoh, N., and Holland, P. W. (1998). Tripartite organization of the ancestral chordate brain and the antiquity of placodes: insights from ascidian Pax-2/5/8, Hox and Otx genes. *Development* 125, 1113–1122.

Walls, G. L. (1942). *The Vertebrate Eye and its Adaptive Radiation.* New York: Hafner, 785.

Wang, S., and Turner, E. E. (2010). Expression of dopamine pathway genes in the midbrain is independent of known ETS transcription factor activity. *J. Neurosci.* 30, 9224–9227.

Wang, W., and Lufkin, T. (2000). The murine Otp homeobox gene plays an essential role in the specification of neuronal cell lineages in the developing hypothalamus. *Dev. Biol.* 227, 432–449.

Weihe, E., Depboylu, C., Schutz, B., Schafer, M. K., and Eiden, L. E. (2006). Three types of tyrosine hydroxylase-positive CNS neurons distinguished by dopa decarboxylase and VMAT2 co-expression. *Cell. Mol. Neurobiol.* 26, 659–678.

Weihe, E., and Eiden, L. E. (2000). Chemical neuroanatomy of the vesicular amine transporters. *FASEB J.* 14, 2435–2449.

Westlund, K. N., Denney, R. M., Kochersperger, L. M., Rose, R. M., and Abell, C. W. (1985). Distinct monoamine oxidase A and B populations in primate brain. *Science* 230, 181–183.

Willoughby, J., Glover, V., and Sandler, M. (1988). Histochemical localisation of monoamine oxidase A and B in rat brain. *J. Neural Transm.* 74, 29–42.

Wilson, S. W., and Houart, C. (2004). Early steps in the development of the forebrain. *Dev. Cell* 6, 167–181.

Wise, R. A. (2009). Roles for nigrostriatal – not just mesocorticolimbic – dopamine in reward and addiction. *Trends Neurosci.* 32, 517–524.

Wullimann, M. F., and Rink, E. (2001). Detailed immunohistology of Pax6 protein and tyrosine hydroxylase in the early zebrafish brain suggests role of Pax6 gene in development of dopaminergic diencephalic neurons. *Brain Res. Dev. Brain Res.* 131, 173–191.

Xhaard, H., Rantanen, V. V., Nyronen, T., and Johnson, M. S. (2006). Molecular evolution of adrenoceptors and dopamine receptors: implications for the binding of catecholamines. *J. Med. Chem.* 49, 1706–1719.

Yamamoto, K., Ruuskanen, J. O., Wullimann, M. F., and Vernier, P. (2010). Two tyrosine hydroxylase genes in vertebrates: comparative distribution with other monoaminergic markers in the zebrafish brain. *Mol. Cell Neurosci.* 43, 394–402.

Yamamoto, K., Ruuskanen, J. O., Wullimann, M. F., and Vernier, P. (2011). Differential expression of dopamine cells markers in the adult zebrafish forebrain. *J. Comp. Neurol.* 519, 576–598.

Zetterström, R. Zetterström, R. H., Solomin, L., Jansson, L., Hoffer, B. J., Olson, L., and Perlmann, T. (1997). Dopamine neuron agenesis in Nurr1-deficient mice. *Science* 276, 248–250.

Zhang, W., Klimek, V., Farley, J. T., Zhu, M. Y., and Ordway, G. A. (1999). Alpha2C adrenoceptors inhibit adenylyl cyclase in mouse striatum: potential activation by dopamine. *J. Pharmacol. Exp. Ther.* 289, 1286–1292.

Zhou, F. M., Liang, Y., Salas, R., Zhang, L., De Biasi, M., and Dani, J. A. (2005). Corelease of dopamine and serotonin from striatal dopamine terminals. *Neuron* 46, 65–74.

Zohar, Y., Munoz-Cueto, J. A., Elizur, A., and Kah, O. (2010). Neuroendocrinology of reproduction in teleost fish. *Gen. Comp. Endocrinol.* 165, 438–455.

Conflict of Interest Statement: The authors declare that the research was conducted in the absence of any commercial or financial relationships that could be construed as a potential conflict of interest.

7

Topography of *somatostatin* gene expression relative to molecular progenitor domains during ontogeny of the mouse hypothalamus

Nicanor Morales-Delgado[1,2†], Paloma Merchan[2†], Sylvia M. Bardet[2,3], José L. Ferrán[2], Luis Puelles[2] and Carmen Díaz[1]*

[1] Department of Medical Sciences, School of Medicine, Regional Centre for Biomedical Research and Institute for Research in Neurological Disabilities, University of Castilla-La Mancha, Albacete, Spain

[2] Department of Human Anatomy and Psychobiology, School of Medicine, University of Murcia, Murcia, Spain

[3] UMR 1061, Unité de Génétique Moléculaire Animale, Institut National de la Recherche Agronomique, University of Limoges, Limoges, France

Edited by:
Fernando Martinez-Garcia, Universidad de Valencia, Spain

Reviewed by:
Nerea Moreno, University Complutense of Madrid, Spain
Hans J. Ten Donkelaar, Radboud University Nijmegen Medical Center, Netherlands

***Correspondence:**
Carmen Díaz, Department of Medical Sciences, School of Medicine, University of Castilla-La Mancha, Almansa Street, 14, Albacete 02006, Spain.
e-mail: carmen.diaz@uclm.es

†Nicanor Morales-Delgado and Paloma Merchan have contributed equally to this work.

The hypothalamus comprises alar, basal, and floor plate developmental compartments. Recent molecular data support a rostrocaudal subdivision into rostral (terminal) and caudal (peduncular) halves. In this context, the distribution of neuronal populations expressing somatostatin (*Sst*) mRNA was analyzed in the developing mouse hypothalamus, comparing with the expression pattern of the genes *Orthopedia* (*Otp*), *Distal-less 5* (*Dlx5*), *Sonic Hedgehog* (*Shh*), and *Nk2 homeobox 1* (*Nkx2.1*). At embryonic day 10.5 (E10.5), *Sst* mRNA was first detectable in the anterobasal nucleus, a *Nkx2.1*-, *Shh*-, and *Otp*-positive basal domain. By E13.5, nascent *Sst* expression was also related to two additional *Otp*-positive domains within the alar plate and one in the basal plate. In the alar plate, *Sst*-positive cells were observed in rostral and caudal ventral subdomains of the *Otp*-positive paraventricular complex. An additional basal *Sst*-expressing cell group was found within a longitudinal *Otp*-positive periretromamillary band that separates the retromamillary area from tuberal areas. Apart of subsequent growth of these initial populations, at E13.5 and E15.5 some *Sst*-positive derivatives migrate tangentially into neighboring regions. A subset of cells produced at the anterobasal nucleus disperses ventralward into the shell of the ventromedial hypothalamic nucleus and the arcuate nucleus. Cells from the rostroventral paraventricular subdomain reach the suboptic nucleus, whereas a caudal contingent migrates radially into lateral paraventricular, perifornical, and entopeduncular nuclei. Our data provide a topologic map of molecularly defined progenitor areas originating a specific neuron type during early hypothalamic development. Identification of four main separate sources helps to understand causally its complex adult organization.

Keywords: forebrain, hypothalamus, *Sst*, *Otp*, *Dlk5*, *Nkx2.1*, *Shh*, *in situ* hybridization

INTRODUCTION

The prosomeric model for the vertebrate forebrain proposes that the hypothalamus is a rostral forebrain entity, lying ventral to the telencephalon and rostral to the diencephalon (Puelles et al., 2004, 2007; Nieuwenhuys et al., 2008; Nieuwenhuys, 2009). Moreover, recent molecular data together with fate map analysis support a definition of the hypothalamus that excludes the preoptic area, considered nowadays a part of subpallial telencephalon (Bulfone et al., 1993; Rubenstein et al., 1998; Puelles et al., 2000; Cobos et al., 2001; Flames et al., 2007; Shimogori et al., 2010). In addition, differential expression of some developmental genes [e.g., *Vax1* in Hallonet et al. (1998), *Distal-less 5* (*Dlx5*), *Six3* in Lagutin et al. (2003) and Puelles and Rubenstein (2003), *Sim1*, *Orthopedia* (*Otp*), *Tbr1* in Puelles et al. (2004) and Bardet (2007), *Sim1*, *Lhx6*, *Lhx8*, *Lhx9*, *Nkx6.2*, *Foxb1* in Shimogori et al. (2010)] support with their presence or absence, or with a dimensional change in their expression domain, a rostrocaudal subdivision of the hypothalamus into two transverse regions recently called *terminal* (rostral) and *peduncular* (caudal) hypothalamus [Allen Developing Mouse Brain Atlas[1] (reference atlas done by Luis Puelles)]. Such a subdivision was already contemplated in earlier sources (Puelles and Rubenstein, 2003; Bardet, 2007; Nieuwenhuys, 2009). The same markers plus additional ones [e.g., *Nk2 homeobox 2* (*Nkx2.2*), *Sonic Hedgehog* (*Shh*), *Nk2 homeobox 1* (*Nkx2.1*)] also support a dorsoventral regionalization of the hypothalamus in alar, basal, and floor longitudinal subdivisions (Puelles and Rubenstein, 2003; Puelles et al., 2004; Bardet, 2007; Shimogori et al., 2010). The peduncular hypothalamus contains the dorsoventrally coursing lateral and medial forebrain bundles and the fornix. Thus, several genes regionalize dorsoventrally and caudo-rostrally the hypothalamus, previously and in parallel to cell differentiation in the mantle. For instance, at early stages of hypothalamic development, expression of *Paired box 6* (*Pax6*) is restricted to the alar plate, whereas *Shh* and *Nkx2.1* expression characterizes the basal plate, and *Nkx2.2*

[1]www.developingmouse.brain-map.org

signal appears in a longitudinal band that overlaps the alar/basal boundary (reviewed in Puelles et al., 2004). Furthermore, the alar hypothalamus is subdivided longitudinally into a ventral domain called subparaventricular area (SPa), characterized by *Dlx* and *Arx* gene expression, and a dorsal domain representing the classic paraventricular area (Pa), which is an *Otp- and Single-minded 1 (Sim1)*-expressing domain (Puelles and Rubenstein, 2003; Bardet et al., 2008; Shimogori et al., 2010).

The differentiation of the hypothalamic hormone-producing neurons implicates a complex hierarchy of genetic interactions among transcription factors that sequentially define each phenotype. Such networks of transcription factors have been partially characterized in cells that populate neurosecretory hypothalamic nuclei such as the anterior periventricular area, the paraventricular nucleus and the supraoptic nucleus, all of them derived from the alar Pa, or the arcuate nucleus (Arc), a separate basal plate derivative. *Otp* and *Sim1/2* are key genes in the proliferation and differentiation of the precursors of cell types producing somatostatin (STT), thyrotropin-releasing hormone, corticotrophin-releasing hormone, arginine vasopressin or oxytocin in the anterior periventricular area, the paraventricular nucleus, and the supraoptic nucleus (Acampora et al., 1999, 2000; Goshu et al., 2004). Moreover, the homeobox-containing transcription factors NKX2.1 and OTP are jointly essential for the specification of SST-producing cells at the Arc (Acampora et al., 1999; Wang and Lufkin, 2000; reviewed by Caqueret et al., 2005).

Somatostatin (also known as somatotropin-release inhibiting factor) is a peptide that was first identified from bovine hypothalamic extracts, which plays an inhibitory role in the secretion of growth hormone (Brazeau et al., 1973) and thyroid-stimulating hormone (Vale et al., 1977) from anterior pituitary cells. In the adult hypothalamus, SST neurons of the anterior periventricular area and the paraventricular nucleus project to the median eminence (ME) and release the peptide into local capillaries; subsequently it reaches the anterior pituitary through the portal vasculature and exerts there its inhibiting neuroendocrine action. Other hypothalamic SST neurons have been located in the Arc, the suprachiasmatic area and the ventromedial hypothalamic nucleus (VMH; Johansson et al., 1984; Cotter and Laemle, 1987). Apart from the hypothalamic locations, STT has a wide distribution in other brain regions such as the amygdala, preoptic area, hippocampus, striatum, cerebral cortex, olfactory regions, and brainstem, where it acts as a neurotransmitter or neuromodulator (Viollet et al., 2008). STT and its receptors have also been implicated in brain development (Yacubova and Komuro, 2002; Le Verche et al., 2009).

In the present work, an attempt was made to analyze in detail the early spatiotemporal developmental distribution of *Sst* across distinct molecular subdivisions (progenitor areas) of the mouse hypothalamus, using *in situ* hybridization. To this end, the location of *Sst*-expressing cell was analyzed in relation to the signal of transcription factor genes such as *Otp*, *Dlx5*, *Shh*, and *Nkx2.1* from embryonic day 9.5 (E9.5) to 15.5 (E15.5). Our data therefore refer exclusively to early differentiating *Sst* neurons, which show a wider distribution than was reported in previous ontogenetic studies (Shiosaka et al., 1982; Bendotti et al., 1990). There are at least four separate early sources of *Sst* cells, and our results suggest the occurrence of early radial and tangential migrations of *Sst* cells within the hypothalamus. It should be noted that we do not address late differentiating hypothalamic *Sst* cell populations, which essentially become observable at late embryonic stages (after E18.5) and postnatally.

MATERIALS AND METHODS

ANIMALS

All protocols involving care and use of laboratory animals were conformed to normative standards of the European Community (86/609/EEC) and the Spanish Government (Royal Decree, 1201/2005; Law 32/2007). *Swiss albino* mice from embryonic days 9.5 (E9.5) to 15.5 were used. For timing pregnancy, the day when vaginal plugs were detected was considered as day 0.5 of gestation (E0.5). For every embryonic age, we examined three to five mouse embryos.

TISSUE PROCESSING

Embryos were quickly removed from pregnant mice and the heads were immediately fixed by immersion in cold 4% paraformaldehyde in 0.1 M phosphate buffered saline (PBS, pH 7.4). Afterward, the dissected brains were post-fixed overnight at 4°C in the same fixative, and then transferred to 30% sucrose in 0.1 M PBS for 24 h at 4°C. Finally, they were embedded in 15% gelatin/20% sucrose and frozen in isopentane at −55°C. Parallel series of sagittal and transversal sections were cut on a cryostat 20 µm-thick and mounted onto Superfrost-plus slides (Menzel-Gläser, Braunschweig, Germany).

RT-PCR

Sst and *Dlx5* cDNA fragments were obtained by RT-PCR. RNA was extracted from fresh dissected brains of *Mus musculus* embryos at stages E10.5, 12.5, and 14.5 using Trizol reagent (10296-028, Invitrogen). The RNA was treated with DNase I (18068-015, Invitrogen) for 15 min at room temperature (RT), and then the enzyme was inactivated at 65°C. The RNA was retro-transcribed into single-stranded cDNA with Superscript II reverse transcriptase and oligo dT anchored primers (11904-018, SuperScript First-Strand Synthesis System for RT-PCR; Invitrogen). The resulting first-strand cDNA (0.5 µl of the reverse transcription reaction) was used as a template for PCR, performed with *Taq* polymerase (M8305, Promega). PCR conditions were as follows: 5 min at 94°C, then 35 cycles (30 s at 94°C, plus 1 min at Tm temperature −58°C, and 1 min at 72°C), followed by 10 min at 72°C. The PCR products were cloned into pGEM-T Easy Vector (Promega) and sequenced (SAI, University of Murcia). Primers: MSstF: 5′-CTGAAGGAGACGCTACCGAAG-3′; MSstR: 5′-TCAATTTCTAATGCAGGGTCAA-3′; MDlx5F: 5′-TAGACCAGAGCAGCTCCACA-3′; MDlx5R: 5′-GGCACCATTG ATAGTGTCCA-3′.

IN SITU HYBRIDIZATION AND IMMUNOHISTOCHEMISTRY

Sense and antisense digoxigenin-labeled riboprobes for mouse *Dlx5*, *Nkx2.1*, *Otp*, *Shh*, and *Sst* were generated by *in vitro* transcription using 1 µg of template, digoxigenin-11-UTP (Roche Diagnostics S.L., Applied Science, Barcelona, Spain), and specific polymerases (Promega). Plasmid information is provided in **Table 1.**

In situ hybridization experiments were performed as described by Hidalgo-Sánchez et al. (2005). Hybridizations were carried out overnight at 72°C (for *Otp* at 68°C). Once hybridization

Table 1 | Characteristics of the gene probes used for ISH.

Gene	NCBI accession no.	Size (bp)	Position	Laboratory
Dlx5	NM_010056.2	1180	106–1285	Present results
Nkx2.1	NM_009385.2	2216	597–2813	Rubenstein J.L.R.
Otp	NM_011021.2	412	179–592	Simeone A.
Shh	NM_009170.2	643	442–1084	McMahon A.
Sst	NM_009215	556	6–561	Present results

was complete, slides were washed under stringent conditions. The probes were detected with an alkaline phosphatase-coupled anti-digoxigenin antibody using nitroblue tetrazolium/5-bromo-4-chloro-3-indolyl phosphate (NBT/BCIP; Roche) for visualization. Exposure times ranged between 1 and 2 days. Sense probes were tested as negative controls and gave no specific signals (data not shown).

The immunohistochemical protocol was described in detail elsewhere (Bardet et al., 2006). The dilution of the polyclonal antiserum against rat NKX2.1 (TTF-1; Biopat Immunotechnologies, Caserta, Italy; no. PA 0100) was 1:1000. After washes, the sections were incubated with biotinylated goat anti-rabbit (Vector Laboratories, CA, USA; 1:200) followed by a streptavidin–peroxidase complex (Vectastain-ABC kit; Vector Laboratories), applied for 1 h at room temperature. Peroxidase activity was developed with 0.03% 3,3′-diaminobenzidine (Sigma; St Louis; MO, USA), plus 0.003% hydrogen peroxidase. We verified the specificity of the antibody by performing parallel control experiments, omitting the primary antibody (data not shown). After hybridization and immunohistochemical labeling, the slides were washed in PBS, air dried and coverslipped with CYTOSEAL™ 60 (Thermo).

IMAGING

Image acquisition of entire slides was carried out with a ScanScope CS digital slide scanner (Aperio Technologies, USA). After scanning, images of adjacent sections were captured by using the software ImageScope. Contrast and focus of singles images were enhanced, artificially pseudocolored (from blue to red) and superimposed using Adobe Photoshop CS3 (Adobe Systems Inc., San José, CA, USA).

RESULTS

PRELIMINARY REMARKS ON HYPOTHALAMIC ORGANIZATION

In order to map *Sst* mRNA expression and to identify different structures in the developing hypothalamus, we have used the updated prosomeric model of the vertebrate forebrain, developed by Luis Puelles for the Allen Developing Mouse Brain Atlas[2]. In this model, the hypothalamus is understood as a portion of the secondary prosencephalon (separated from the classic "diencephalon"). It lies rostral to the diencephalon proper (prethalamus, thalamus, and pretectum) and ventral to the preoptic and innominate/diagonal telencephalic regions (see also Puelles, 1995, 2001; Puelles and Rubenstein, 2003; Puelles et al., 2004; Flames et al., 2007). **Figure 1** summarizes the general position of the hypothalamus, its subdivisions, and major landmark nuclei according to the updated prosomeric model. The hypothalamus is subdivided dorsoventrally into alar, basal, and floor plate developmental components, and a transverse intrahypothalamic limit divides it rostrocaudally into two transverse regions denominated *terminal hypothalamus* and *peduncular hypothalamus* in the model (THy; PHy; **Figures 1A–C**; see also Puelles and Rubenstein, 2003; Puelles et al., 2007; Nieuwenhuys et al., 2008). The model includes a novel subdivision and terminology for the hypothalamic basal plate proposed in preliminary form by Bardet (2007) and further developed in the Allen Developing Mouse Brain Atlas[3]. There is a fundamental dorsoventral division of the basal plate into tuberal/retrotuberal and mamillary/retromamillary regions, each of which has additional subdivisions (Tu/RTu, M/RM; **Figure 1B**). The alar plate is also divided into the Pa (dorsal) and the SPa (ventral; Pa, SPa; **Figure 1B**; Bardet, 2007; Puelles et al., 2007). The Pa forms basically magnocellular and parvocellular neurosecretory populations of the supraopto-paraventricular complex, whereas the SPa forms mainly the suprachiasmatic nucleus, the anterior hypothalamic nucleus, and the subparaventricular zone. The dorsal border of the Pa defines the hypothalamic–telencephalic boundary (**Figure 1A**), which coincides with a plane separating the telencephalic stria terminalis tract from the non-telencephalic stria medullaris tract. All these dorsoventral alar and basal subdivisions are constituted by terminal (THy) and peduncular (PHy) moieties. The areas so delimited are considered independent progenitor areas, within which specific neuronal cell populations are born, forming characteristic nuclei (**Figure 1B**).

As markers of the fundamental hypothalamic subdivisions, helping us to localize the *Sst*-positive cells more precisely, we compared the expression pattern of transcription factors such as *Otp* (Pa and perimamillary/periretromamillary-PM/PRM-areas), *Dlx5* (SPa and Tu/RTu areas), *Shh* and *Nkx2.1* (basal plate in general; **Figures 1C and 2**). Between E10.5 and E15.5, the well-known separate paraventricular and perimamillary domains expressing *Otp* showed practically no overlap with telencephalic and hypothalamic *Dlx5*-positive domains (**Figures 1C and 2A–C**; Bardet et al., 2008). On the other hand, at these stages, *Nkx2.1* was expressed throughout the hypothalamic basal plate, as well as in the telencephalic subpallium (**Figure 2D**), while *Shh* signal was found at the ventricular zone of the hypothalamic basal plate. Early on, *Shh* expression first appears restricted to the floor plate, but its domain soon expands into the adjacent basal plate and is secondarily downregulated in a basal subregion including rostral tuberal and mamillary subareas (**Figure 2E**; Martí et al., 1995). Variations of these patterns will be detailed below.

AT E10.5 AND E11.5, THE EARLIEST *Sst*-POSITIVE CELLS ARE RESTRICTED TO A ROSTRODORSAL BASAL PART OF THE TERMINAL HYPOTHALAMUS

In addition to the marked *Otp* expression mentioned above as characterizing the Pa, less strongly marked *Otp*-positive cells were also found at E10.5 at the immature anterobasal nucleus (ABa), an U-shaped terminal basal derivative distinguished across the midline of the rostrodorsal tuberal region (ABa; **Figures 1B and 3A**).

[2]http://www.developingmouse.brain-map.org/

[3]http://www.developingmouse.brain-map.org/

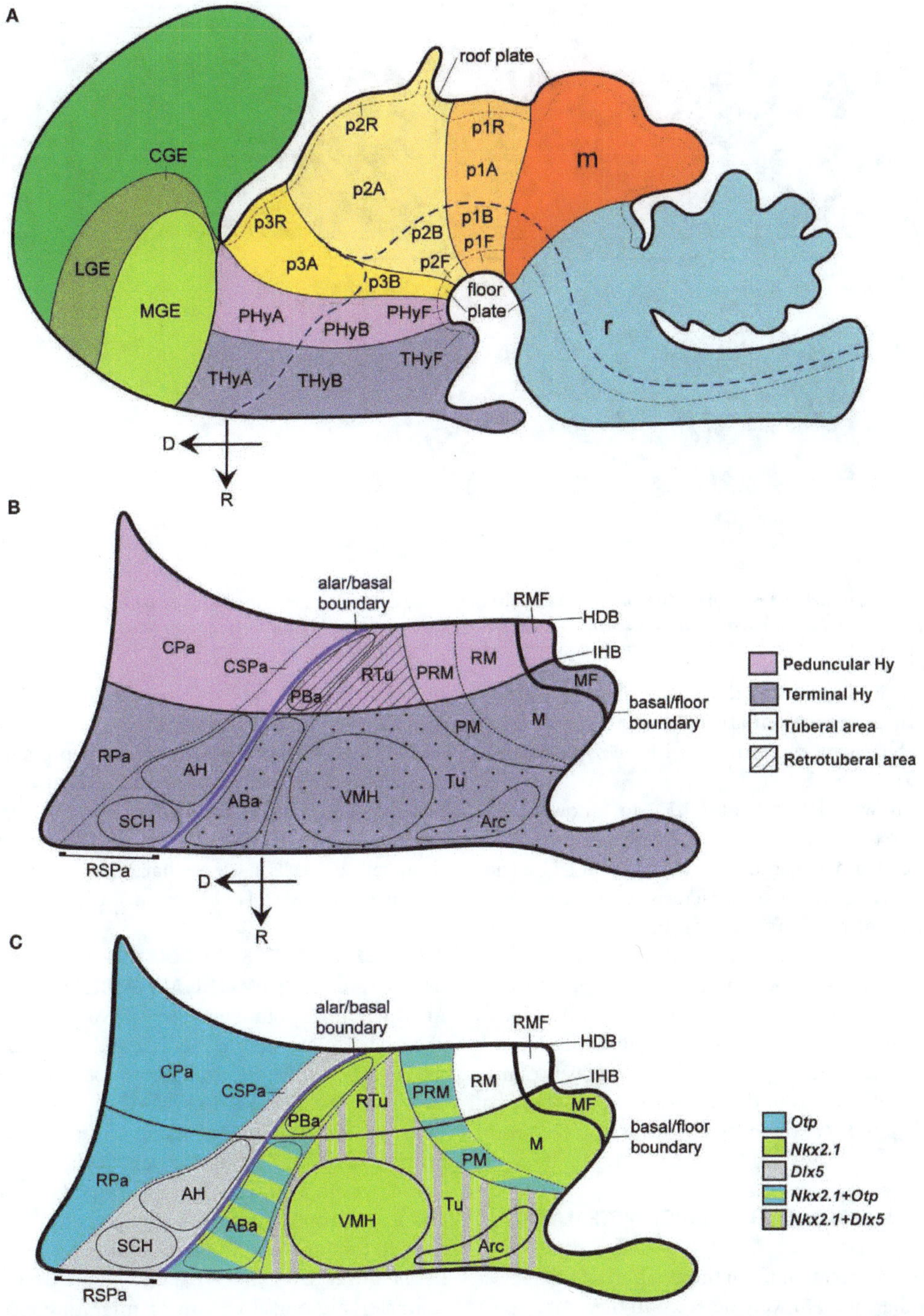

FIGURE 1 | Schematic model of the forebrain, illustrating hypothalamic position and main subdivisions. The rostral (R) and dorsal (D) spatial directions are indicated in **(A,B)**. **(A)** Updated prosomeric model redrawn from the Allen Developing Mouse Brain Atlas (www.developingmouse.brain-map.org), showing the hypothalamo-telencephalic and hypothalamo-diencephalic boundaries, the alar–basal boundary and the main anteroposterior parts, the peduncular and terminal hypothalamic territories (PHy, THy). **(B)** Dorsoventral regional hypothalamic subdivisions across the color-coded PHy and THy (separated by the intrahypothalamic border; IHB). The thick blue line indicates the longitudinal alar–basal boundary. Alar territories are seen on the left [corresponding to PHyA and THyA in **(A)**], and basal territories on the right [PHyB and THyB in **(A)**]. Within the alar plate, a dashed line separates the rostral and caudal paraventricular subdomains (RPa, CPa) from the rostral and caudal subparaventricular subdomains (RSPa, CSPa). The RSPa contains the suprachiasmatic and anterior hypothalamic nuclei (SCH, AH). Within the basal plate, a thin continuous black line separates the tuberal and retrotuberal regions (Tu/RTu; dotted and striped fills, respectively) from the mamillary complex (undotted). A dashed line separates the dorsal Tu/RTu subregion, occupied by the anterobasal and posterobasal nuclei (ABa, PBa) from the main tuberal/retrotuberal region, which contains the VMH, Arc, and DMH nuclei. Another dashed line divides the mamillary body into the dorsal perimamillary/periretromamillary regions (PM, PRM) and the ventral mamillary and retromamillary areas (M, RM). The corresponding parts of the hypothalamic floor lie underneath (MF, RMF). **(C)** Schematic reference gene expression patterns used in our mapping, represented upon the same diagram shown in **(B)**. Striped color patterns imply overlap.

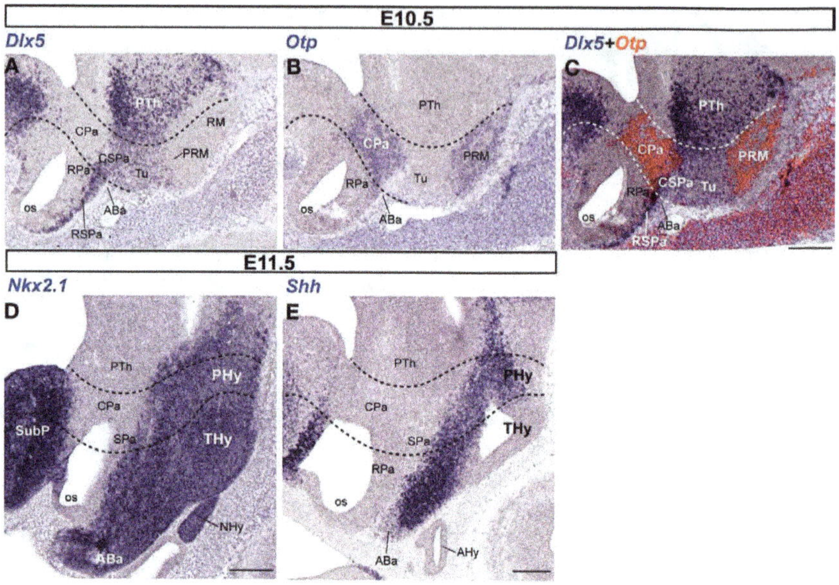

FIGURE 2 | Representative sagittal sections from E10.5 (A–C) and E11.5 (D,E) embryos, showing the expression domains of *Dlx5* (A), *Otp* (B), *Dlx5*+ *Otp* (C; digital overlap with pseudocolor of A,B), *Nkx2.1* (D), and *Shh* (E). The transversal boundaries of the PHy and THy are indicated by dashed lines. Bars = 200 μm.

Altman and Bayer (1986) introduced the ABa term as a preferable alternative to the earlier "retrochiasmatic nucleus/area" name. It is apposite, since it is the rostral-most nucleus of the hypothalamic basal plate (**Figure 3**).

No *Sst* expression was detected at E9.5 (not shown). *Sst*-expressing neurons first appeared in the superficial stratum of the ABa at E10.5 (**Figure 3**) and their number was larger at E11.5 (not shown); this mantle locus shows two characteristic basal markers – *Nkx2.1*, *Shh* – which identify it as a part of the basal hypothalamus, and it always contains *Otp*-expressing cells that are more numerous than the *Sst* ones (**Figures 3A–E,I–K** allow comparison of these four markers); in contrast, the *Dlx5* marker is absent from the ABa at this stage, being restricted to the overlying SPa area (**Figures 3F–H**). *Shh* expression was largely restricted to the ventricular/periventricular zone of the basal hypothalamus and a part of the preoptic area, and was only weakly present at the differentiating ABa cell group (ABa; **Figures 3I,K**).

FIRST APPEARANCE OF *Sst*-POSITIVE CELLS IN THE HYPOTHALAMIC ALAR PLATE AT E12.5

The first *Sst*-positive cells were found in the alar part of the PHy at E12.5. A sparse number of them were detected in the ventral part of the caudal paraventricular nucleus complex (CPa), while the CPa is generally characterized by abundant *Otp*-expressing cells (**Figures 4A–C**). Some *Sst* cells at the borderline with the *Dlx5*-positive SPa may have dispersed into it, also coinciding with scattered *Otp*-positive cells (**Figures 4A–G**). The *Otp*/*Dlx5* (Pa/SPa) boundary is not a clearcut interface (**Figures 4A,D,G**).

However, at E12.5 the majority of *Sst*-positive cells were still concentrated at the rostrodorsal basal plate of the THy, within the superficial and intermediate strata of the ABa mantle zone. This tuberal domain also continued showing extensive *Otp* expression (**Figures 4A–C**), as well as *Nkx2.1* signal and ventricular *Shh* expression (**Figures 4H–N**). Additionally, we observed that some *Sst*- and *Otp*-positive cells were distinguished superficially in the subjacent intermediate tuberal subdivision, also a *Nkx2.1*-positive domain, occupied by the ventromedial hypothalamic and arcuate nuclei (**Figures 1B,C**; arrowheads in **Figures 4B,C,E,F,I,J,L,M**). At this stage, the *Otp*-positive periretromamillary band (PRM) remains free of *Sst* cells, though there appear abundant such cells in the prethalamic tegmentum lying immediately caudal to it (PRM; PTh; **Figures 4A–C**).

PROGRESS OF PRE-EXISTING ALAR AND BASAL *Sst* POPULATIONS AND APPEARANCE OF PERIMAMILLARY *Sst* CELLS AT E13.5

At E13.5, more abundant *Sst*-positive cells were found in the alar plate, particularly at intermediate and superficial strata of the massively *Otp*-positive Pa, and always localized mainly to its ventral part, over the SPa (**Figures 5A–C**). At the CPa domain, populations of *Sst*- and *Otp*-expressing cells are co-localized within the primordia of the lateral paraventricular nucleus (caudally, next to the hypothalamo-prethalamic boundary; LPa; **Figures 5A–D**) and a presumptive perifornical population (rostrally within PHy, close to the intrahypothalamic boundary between PHy and THy; PFx, **Figures 5A–D,L–O**). The *Otp*-positive Pa domain showed a characteristic dorsal stream of migrating cells arching dorsolaterally into the telencephalon under the bottom of the interventricular foramen and connecting with the extended and medial amygdala (Fan et al., 1996; Wang and Lufkin, 2000; Puelles and Rubenstein, 2003; Garcia-Moreno et al., 2010); at E13.5 only a few *Sst* cells appeared mixed with this large *Otp*-positive cell stream (black arrowheads; **Figures 5M,N**). These few elements need to be distinguished from the more numerous suprajacent *Sst* cells apparently associated to the subpallial bed nucleus striae terminalis complex, and, therefore, unrelated to the hypothalamus (white asterisk; BST; **Figures 5M,N**). At the RPa, *Otp* cells start to invade the subpial stratum corresponding to the presumptive supraoptic

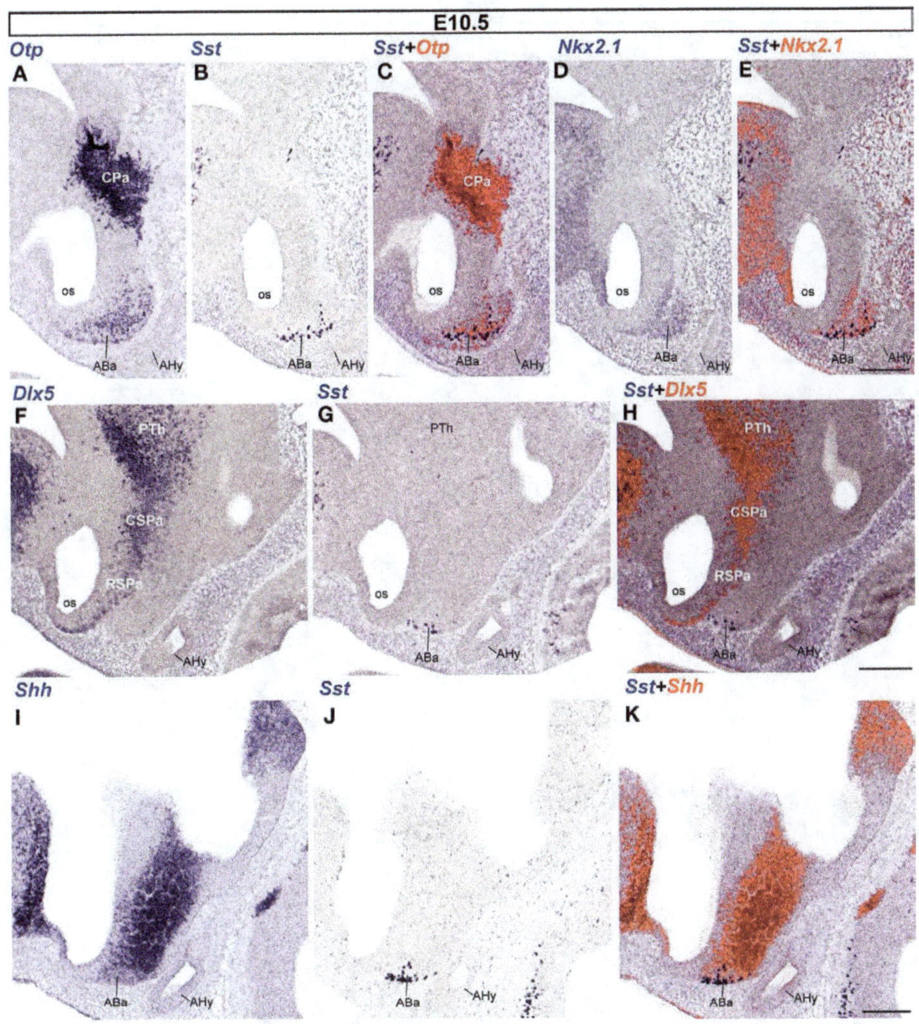

FIGURE 3 | Sagittal sections of E10.5 embryos taken at lateral (A–E), intermediate (F–H), and medial (I–K) levels, correlating the indicated reference markers with the presence of *Sst*-positive cells. Note the topographic coincidence of *Sst* signal with a larger surrounding population of *Otp*-positive cells. Bars = 200 μm.

and suboptic nuclei (SO; **Figure 5A**; we propose here to use "suboptic nucleus" – SbO – as a synonym of the confusing term "retrochiasmatic supraoptic nucleus," given that "retrochiasmatic" is in practice the contrary of "supraoptic" and wrongly refers to the chiasma, whereas the meaning of "suboptic" more clearly suggests the referred topography of this population relative to the optic tract). Suboptic *Sst*-positive cells were observed at this stage at the ventral part of the RPa, in sagittal sections that pass lateral to the suprachiasmatic nucleus primordium (SbO; **Figures 5A–D**). This zone is characterized by relatively dispersed *Otp*-positive cells and is partly intermixed with *Dlx5*-positive RSPa derivatives (**Figures 5A–D**).

The RSPa shows otherwise few dispersed *Sst* cells, whereas the caudal subparaventricular area (CSPa) displays a distinct thin band of such dispersed cells, which overlaps a thin longitudinal alar territory where *Nkx2.1* signal is also found (arrowheads; **Figures 5E–G**; see also Bardet, 2007; Shimogori et al., 2010). It is unclear whether these few cells are newly arisen within CSPa, or correspond to an alignment of cells previously displaced from the CPa.

As regards the basal plate, *Sst*-positive cells at the ABa are more numerous at E13.5, compared to the E12.5 pattern. ABa *Sst* cells were found across the retrochiasmatic median plane, always accompanied by the more numerous *Otp*-positive ABa cells (not shown). We also found scattered *Sst*-positive cells extending toward the intrahypothalamic boundary (THy/PHy) along the entire ABa (**Figures 5B,F,J**). A few *Sst* neurons also seemed to have dispersed caudalward from the ABa into its retrotuberal (peduncular) counterpart, the posterobasal area (PBa; **Figures 5F,G**). Ventrally to the ABa, *Sst*-expressing cells – surrounded by *Otp*-positive cells – were also detected in the intermediate tuberal area, participating in the shell of the ventromedial hypothalamic nucleus (VMHs), stretched around its *Sst*-negative and *Nkx2.1*-positive core, particularly at its rostral aspect (VMHc; **Figures 5A–C,E–G,M–O**). Fewer *Sst*/*Otp* cells were dispersed along the superficial tuberal stratum between the ABa and the superficial part of the arcuate nucleus (Arcs; **Figures 5M–O**). These zones apparently invaded by *Otp* and *Sst* cells produced at the ABa largely correlated topographically with *Shh*/*Nkx2.1*-positive domains (**Figures 5E,G,H,O**).

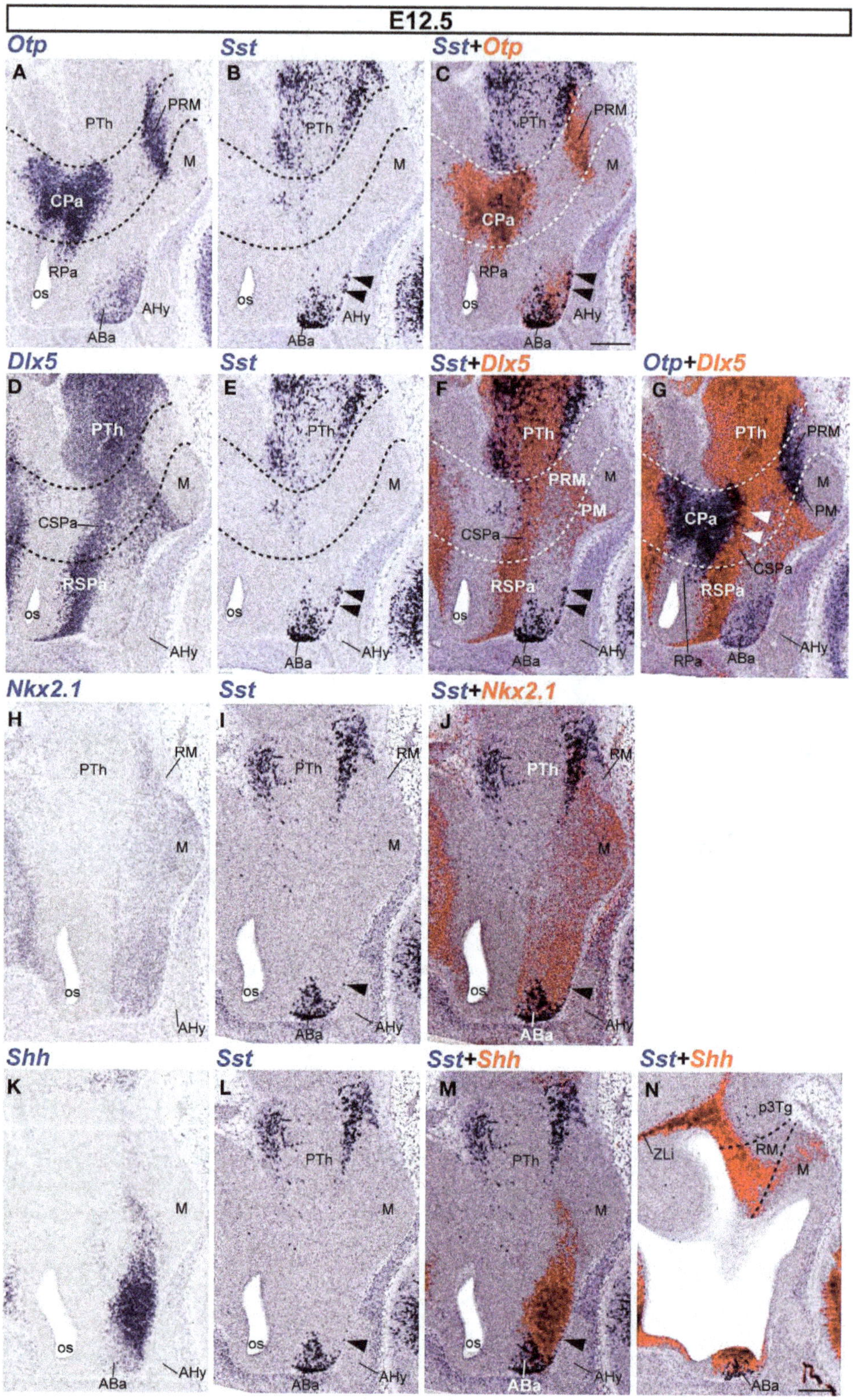

FIGURE 4 | Sagittal sections of E12.5 embryos taken at lateral (A–G) and medial (H–N) levels, correlating the indicated reference markers with the presence of *Sst*-positive cells. The transversal boundaries of the PHy and THy are indicated by dashed lines. Note there are abundant *Sst* cells within basal and alar regions of the prethalamus [PTh; p3Tg in **(N)**], which need to be distinguished from the hypothalamic elements, found rostral to the hypothalamo-diencephalic boundary (caudal dashed line). The black arrowheads mark the incipient ventralward subpial displacement of some ABa-derived *Sst* cells. The white arrowheads in **(G)** indicate the sparse *Otp*-positive cells present within the CSPa subdomain. Bars = 200 μm.

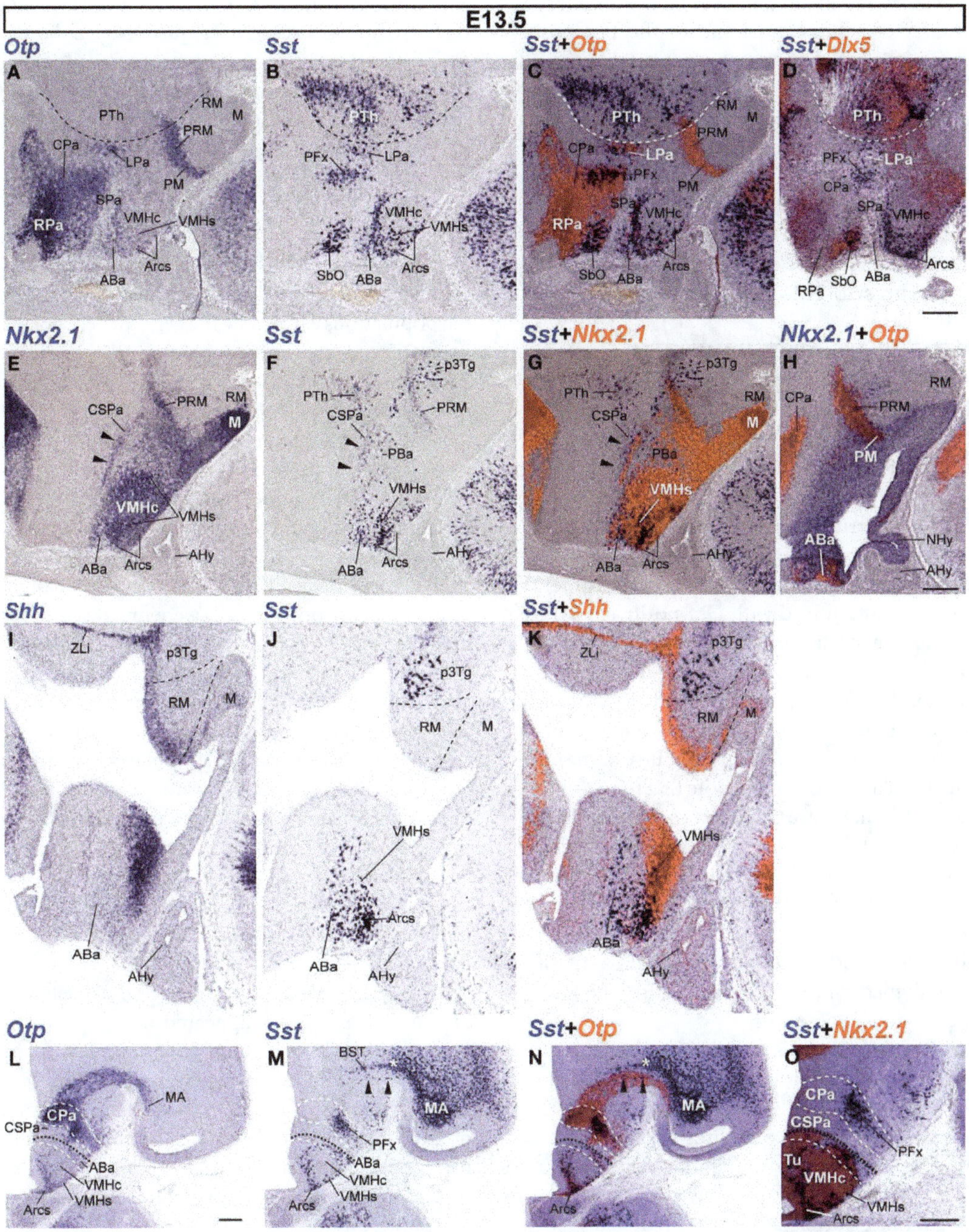

FIGURE 5 | Sagittal (A–K) and transversal (L–O) sections of E13.5 embryos taken at lateral (A–H) and medial (I–K) paramedian levels, correlating the indicated reference markers (*Otp, Nkx2.1, Dlx5*) with the presence of *Sst*-positive cells. (A–G) these images reveal advanced migratory displacement of ABa-derived Sst cells into the underlying VMHs and Arcs formations. **(H)** This nearly median section shows the ventricular domain expressing *Nkx2.1*, as well as its caudal extension along the PM/PRM band. The black arrowheads in **(E–G)** mark the area of overlap between *Nkx2.1*-expressing mantle cells and the sparse *Sst*-positive cell population found within the CSPa. Note also in **(F,G)** a few *Sst*-positive cells lying immediately ventral to the CSPa band, identified by us as the posterobasal nucleus (PBa), where *Nkx2.1* signal is absent. This peculiar retrotuberal basal plate locus (compare **Figure 1B**) corresponds to an area selectively expressing *Lhx9*, recently described by Shimogori et al. (2010). **(I–K)** Dashed lines indicate the HDB and IHB limits demarcating the RM area from the prethalamic tegmentum (p3Tg) and the M area, next to the floor plate. **(L–N)** Correlation of *Otp* and *Sst* signals in adjacent transversal sections (orthogonal to the alar–basal boundary, marked by the black dashed line; white dashed lines indicate the main alar and basal subdivisions). The telencephalic *Otp*-positive migration stream of the CPa area – containing isolated *Sst* cells (black arrowheads in **M,N**) – enters the medial amygdalar area (MA), after passing underneath the *Sst*-positive elements of the subpallial bed nucleus striae terminalis complex (white asterisk; BST). The CPa area itself shows radial stratification of *Otp*-positive derivatives within its mantle layer **(L,N)**. At intermediate levels of this domain, superficially migrated *Sst* cells form an aggregate interpreted as a periforniCal population [PFx **(M,N)**], though it may contain as well elements destined to reach the entopeduncular nucleus, more superficially (not shown). A higher magnification detail of this area is shown in **(O)**. Within the basal plate, both *Otp* and *Sst* cells are observed at the VMHs and Arcs formations, as well as in the overlying ABa. Corresponding overlap between *Nkx2.1* and *Sst* signals is shown in **(O)**. Bars = 200 μm.

Moreover, we also detected at E13.5 a new group of *Sst*-expressing cells centered at the caudal end of the *Otp*-positive periretromamillary area, rostral to a pre-existent magnocellular *Sst*-positive prethalamic tegmental population (**Figures 5C,E–G**; compare **Figures 5H–K**). Interestingly, these *Sst* cells are restricted to the PRM within PHy and do not extend into the similarly *Otp*-positive perimamillary band within THy. This periretromamillary *Otp/Sst*-positive hypothalamic domain overlaps topographically the perimamillary arch of *Nkx2.1* expression that extends into the prethalamic basal plate to end close to the zona limitans intrathalamica (PRM; ZLi; **Figures 5E–H,I–K**).

Sst EXPRESSION PATTERN IN THE HYPOTHALAMUS AT E15.5

The distribution of *Sst* mRNA was on the whole comparable to that obtained at E13.5, although with a larger number of *Sst*-expressing cells.

In the alar plate, the Pa, still identified by dense *Otp* signal and absence of *Dlx5* signal (**Figures 6A,D,G**), contains very few *Sst*-expressing cells at periventricular levels (medial hypothalamus; **Figures 6B–F**). Only sparse small *Sst*-positive cells appear within the CPa (**Figures 6E,F**). In contrast, there are two distinct *Sst*-positive cell aggregates – intermixed with *Otp*-positive cells – that appear displaced radially at caudal and rostral locations within the intermediate CPa level (lateral hypothalamus). These cell groups correspond to the lateral paraventricular nucleus (LPa), found just in front of the hypothalamo-prethalamic boundary, and a perifornical population, detected around the expected course of the fornix, close to the intrahypothalamic boundary; note that the fornix itself was not identified (PFx; LPa; **Figure 6H**). Superficially, the CPa displays as well *Sst*-positive cells at the entopeduncular nucleus, lying interstitial to the cerebral peduncle, dorsal to the level occupied by the subthalamic nucleus and slightly above the level where the optic tract courses longitudinally at the peduncular hypothalamic surface (**Figure 6I**). The underlying *Dlx5*-positive CSPa still shows a sparse number of aligned *Sst* cells (**Figures 6E,F**). The RSPa, in contrast, is practically devoid of them.

Rostrally, close to the optic chiasma and lateral to the suprachiasmatic nucleus primordium, the RSPa appears invaded by a thick bridge of *Otp*-expressing cells that interconnects the overlying RPa – their apparent source, also containing the rounded *Otp*-positive lateral anterior nucleus – with the underlying ABa areas (**Figures 6D,F,H**). Part of these cells possibly converge upon the supraoptic and/or suboptic nuclei. Deeper cells of this bridge may lie at this stage or later within the anterior hypothalamic nucleus (AH; **Figures 6K,L**). The mentioned bridge is however practically devoid of *Sst* cells at this stage (LA; AH; SO; **Figures 6D–H**). In more lateral sections, *Sst*-positive cells unmixed with *Otp*-positive cells appeared quite close to the *Otp*-positive supraoptic nucleus (SO), dorsal the optic tract, and extending into the suboptic nucleus (known as retrochiasmatic or accessory supraoptic nucleus) found under the optic tract (SbO; **Figure 6I**).

Abundant *Sst*-expressing cells were detected in the *Dlx5*-positive and NKX2.1-immunoreactive tuberal region of the hypothalamic basal plate, particularly within its terminal subdivision (ABa, VMHs, Arcs; **Figures 6C,L**). The *Sst* cells always correlated topographically with *Otp*-expressing cell populations (**Figures 6F,H,I**). In contrast, few *Sst* cells were located within the core of the VMH nucleus, which was *Dlx5* and *Otp* negative (VMHc; **Figures 6A–F**), but NKX2.1-immunoreactive (**Figures 6J–L**). We also found at E15.5 an increased number of *Sst*-expressing cells along the peduncular *Otp*-positive periretromamillary area, but not within its terminal continuation, the perimamillary area (PRM; PM; **Figures 6B–H**). Part of the PRM population has migrated radially to intermediate levels of the mantle zone (not shown).

DISCUSSION

This study represents the first to analyze in detail, by means of *in situ* hybridization, the spatiotemporal distribution of the earliest neuronal populations expressing the gene that encodes the SST hormone, in relation to the expression patterns of highly conserved homeobox genes such as *Otp*, *Dlx5*, *Shh*, and *Nkx2.1*, during ontogeny of the mouse hypothalamus. These reference transcription factors have been implicated in the regional patterning of hypothalamus (Shimamura and Rubenstein, 1997; Bertrand and Dahmane, 2006; Yee et al., 2009; Shimogori et al., 2010) and/or the specification of distinct neuroendocrine hypothalamic cells (Acampora et al., 1999; Michaud, 2001; Caqueret et al., 2005; Blechman et al., 2007).

The most relevant results of our study can be summarized as follows: (1) *Sst*-positive cells were first discernible in the basal ABa nucleus at E10.5; (2) as development progressed, *Sst* expression increased particularly within terminal basal hypothalamic areas, apparently extending from the precocious ABa into the subjacent VMHs and Arcs territories; these cells lie within the *Nkx2.1*-positive territory; (3) *Sst*-positive cell populations also developed separately within the alar *Dlx5*-negative and *Otp*-positive CPa and RPa areas, particularly at the ventral part of the paraventricular complex (giving rise caudally mainly to radially migrated lateral paraventricular, perifornical and entopeduncular *Sst*-positive derivatives, and rostrally to the superficially migrated primordium of the suboptic nucleus, also known as retrochiasmatic supraoptic nucleus); an apparent dispersion or migration of alar cells into the subjacent *Dlx5*-positive SPa area was observed as well; (4) a fourth group of *Sst*-expressing cells appeared in the peduncular *Otp*-positive periretromamillary domain; (5) *Sst*-expressing cells generally correlated topographically with more abundant *Otp*-expressing cells, either inside or outside the primarily *Otp*-positive progenitor domains, though there are extensive Pa regions where *Otp* signal is not accompanied by *Sst* signal; and (6) *Sst* cells appearing secondarily at the SPa, VMHs and Arcs domains may represent migratory events.

A remarkable negative observation is that some important *Sst*-expressing cell populations described in the adult mouse brain (e.g., see Allen Developing Mouse Brain Atlas[4]) are not present in our material up to E15.5. The main cell groups missing are those at the anterior periventricular nucleus and the ventral paraventricular nucleus (conventionally identified as "posterior paraventricular nucleus"). Data at the Allen atlas suggest that they differentiate after E18.5, and the full population can be seen at around P28. This heterochronic differentiation pattern does not alter our analysis of early embryonic stages. Our discussion therefore focuses on points 5 and 6 above. First, we examine the progenitor domains where early hypothalamic *Sst*-cells are produced, and, discuss whether

[4]http://www.developingmouse.brain-map.org/

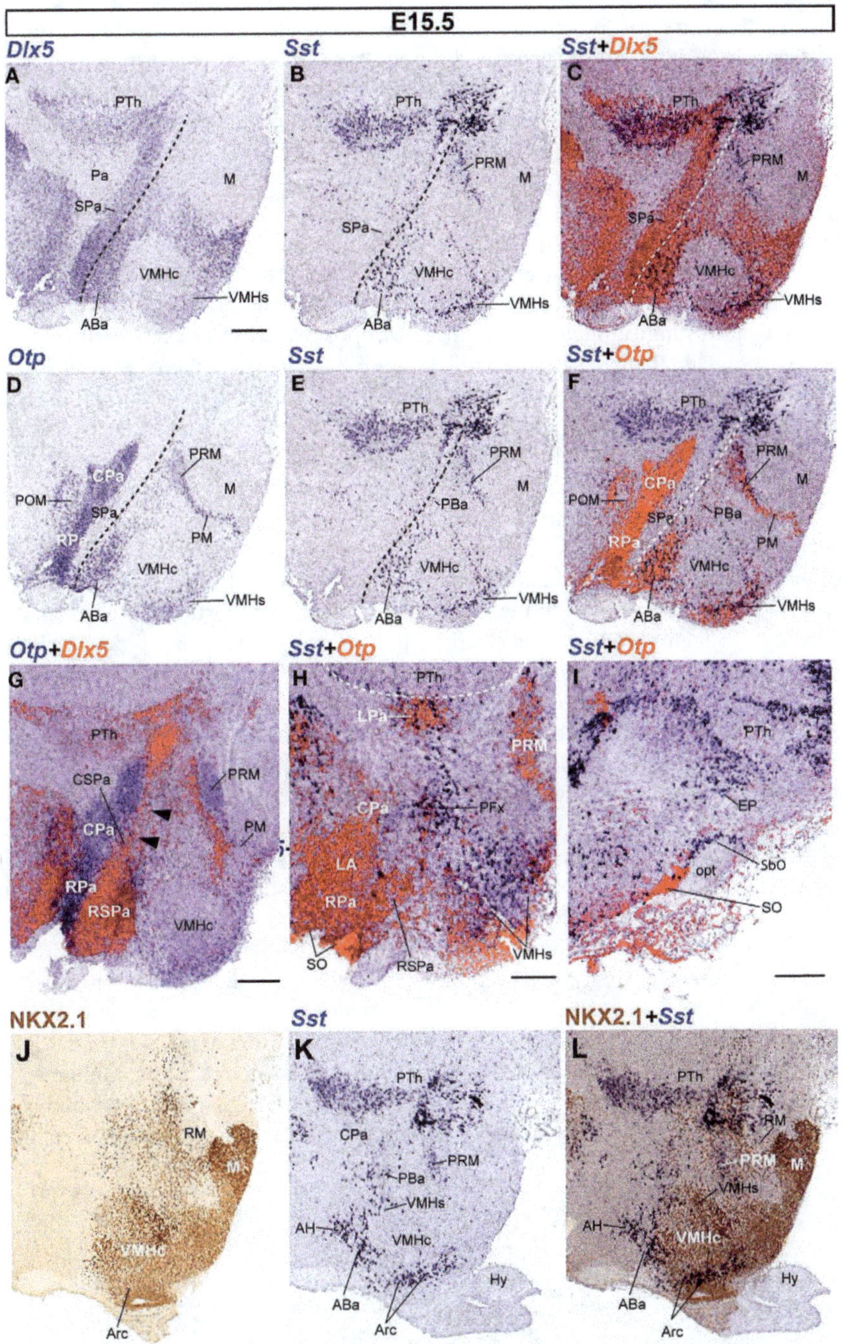

FIGURE 6 | Sagittal sections of E15.5 embryos, correlating the indicated reference markers with the presence of *Sst*-positive cells in adjacent sections. (A–I) This series of sections is a medio-lateral progression, where **(A–F)** represent adjacent sections compared to each other by digital overlap **(C,F)**, and the analogous overlaps shown in **(G–I)** lie progressively more laterally. The dashed lines in **(A–F)** indicate the alar–basal boundary. Note non-hypothalamic *Dlx5* and *Sst* expression in the prethalamus (PTh), but restriction of *Otp* to hypothalamus. The VMHs and Arcs formations express *Dlx5*, whereas the VMHc does not **(C)**. Note as well close neighborhood of *Dlx5* signal to *Otp* signal at the Pa and PRM domains **(G)**. **(J–L)** Sagittal adjacent sections from a different E15.5 embryo, correlating NKX2.1 immunoreaction with the distribution of *Sst* cells. Bars = 200 μm.

there is a shared molecular background that represents a causal common denominator for this neuronal phenotype. This question is relevant because *Sst* cells appear to be distributed widely in the adult hypothalamus. Various recent lines of evidence in other parts of the brain suggest that chemically characterized neuron types usually are produced in specific progenitor domains and may disperse migratorily more or less as they incorporate in the mantle zone and differentiate. This leads to a second issue, whether some *Sst* cell groups migrate from their primary origins into other parts of the hypothalamus.

Sst SOURCE AREAS AND THEIR MOLECULAR BACKGROUND

As regards characterizing the early sources of *Sst* cells, we used comparative mapping in adjacent cryostat sections of gene markers – *Shh, Nkx2.1, Dlx5, Otp* – known to divide the hypothalamic wall into a number of distinct neurogenetic domains. In this way we could distinguish the *alar–basal boundary*, indicated by the interface of the basal markers *Shh* and *Nkx2.1* with the alar marker *Dlx5* (irrespective of the latter also appears later in part of the basal plate). Moreover, *Otp* and *Dlx5* respectively distinguish the *paraventricular* and *subparaventricular areas* within the alar plate, and *Dlx5* becomes secondarily expressed in the *tuberal region* of the basal hypothalamus, stopping at its longitudinal border with the *mamillary body*. The latter shows intercalated between this border and the mamillary and retromamillary nuclear complex the *Otp*-positive *perimamillary/periretromamillary band*. Since we also divide the whole hypothalamus into terminal (THy) and peduncular (PHy) anteroposterior parts (**Figure 1A**; see Allen Developing Mouse Brain Atlas), consistently with gene mappings summarized in the Section "Introduction," the diverse dorsoventral molecular patterns establish a framework of 12 histogenetic areas (**Figure 1C**), where the *Sst* cells can originate and eventually mature. Our data for E10.5–E15.5 embryonic stages clearly pinpointed at least four independent sources for the studied cell type. These correspond to the ABa (a rostrodorsal basal tuberal area), the CPa (a peduncular dorsal alar domain), the RPa (a terminal dorsal alar domain), and the periretromamillary (PRM) domain (a caudal component of the mamillary body; **Figure 7**). A minor cell group observed within the CSPa may represent yet another potential independent contingent, though its non-migratory character is still uncertain. This listing does not pre-empt the possibility that additional progenitor sources may turn out to be relevant in the present context, but show a retarded upregulation of the *Sst* gene in their derivatives, which accordingly only become identifiable perinatally.

The molecular background associated to the four main *Sst* cell sources is variable, as one would expect from the wide anteroposterior and dorsoventral range of the respective topographies across our frame of reference (**Figures 1C and 7**). Nevertheless, this background shows shared aspects that may guide causal analysis of the specification cascade leading to the *Sst* neuronal phenotype. In the first place, there is a clearcut common relationship of emergent *Sst* cells to a surrounding and pre-existent *Otp*-positive cell population. Even migrating *Sst* cells have surrounding, similarly migrating *Otp*-positive cells. Since in several cases the incipient populations observed by us up to E15.5 increase spectacularly perinatally, it is possible to conceive that the *Sst* phenotype differentiates gradually within a pre-existent population labeled by the *Otp* signal.

Secondly, mere expression of *Otp* is not sufficient to condition upregulation of the *Sst* gene, since the large Pa area is full of *Otp*-positive cells from very early stages of development, and only few *Sst* differentiate there between E10.5 and E15.5. Interestingly, these few Pa-derived *Sst* cells are associated to the ventral-most part of both the CPa and RPa, which suggests a relationship with a specific added local causal effect, possibly the expression of *Sim2*, whose deletion causes disappearance of *Sst* and *Trh* cells at the paraventricular nucleus complex (Goshu et al., 2004). Similarly, the *Otp*-positive periretromamillary/perimamillary band develops *Sst* cells between E13.5 and E15.5, but only within its caudal periretromamillary portion (PRM). *Sim1/2* genes are also expressed in this area (Allen Atlas; Shimogori et al., 2010, supplementary data). In both Pa (CPa + RPa) and PRM, the *Otp*-positive area lies adjacent to *Dlx5*-expressing, *Otp/Sst*-negative domains (SPa in the case of the ventral Pa, and tuberal/retrotuberal area in the case of the PRM). The *Arx* gene also appears expressed at the SPa, just under the ventral Pa subdomain, and in a tuberal band adjacent to the PRM, superposed to *Dlx5* (Shimogori et al., 2010).

As regards the terminal ABa domain, *Sst* cells also correlate there with pre-existing numerous *Otp* cells, and there is a neighboring *Dlx5/Arx*-expressing domain, the RSPa. Moreover, its cells express *Nkx2.1*, as happens likewise at the PRM, but not at the Pa domains. The few *Sst* cells that differentiate early on at the ventral CSPa also coincide both with *Otp*-positive cells, a *Dlx5*-positive environment and the expression of *Nkx2.1* (Bardet, 2007; Shimogori et al., 2010). On the other hand, the PBa domain lying caudal to ABa (displaying similar molecular neighborhood relationships as the ABa, but lying at the PHy) produces few *Sst* cells between E10.5 and E15.5, a

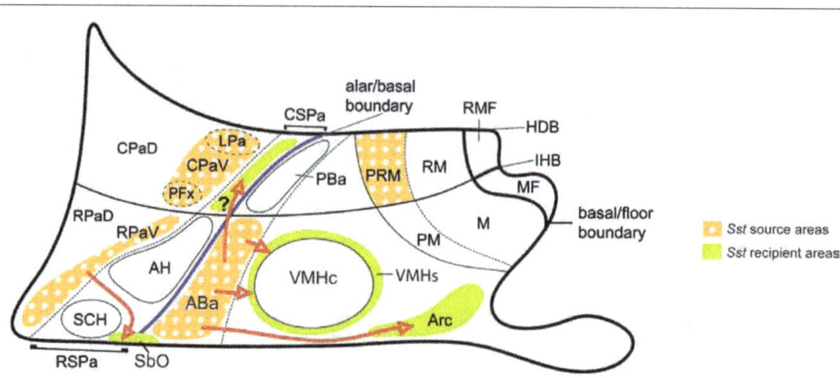

FIGURE 7 | Schematic color-coded mapping (upon our basic schema of Figures 1B,C) of the described *Sst* source areas and the apparent *Sst* recipient areas, involving postulated tangential migrations (red arrows). The migration moving cells potentially from the ABa to the CSPa is marked with an interrogant because the intrinsic versus extrinsic origin of these cells is not clearly distinguishable in our material. Note that we described radial migrations toward intermediate or subpial loci at the ventral subdomains of CPa and RPa (CPaV, RPaV) and PRM areas. Only the radial migration finishing at the suboptic nucleus (SbO; or retrochiasmatic supraoptic nucleus) is represented.

difference in pattern that is not readily understood. Nevertheless the PBa generates many *Sst* cells at later perinatal stages (Allen Atlas). This may be related to the fact that the PBa area coincides with a restricted longitudinal basal domain of the dorsal retrotuberal region where *Nkx2.1* is singularly not expressed (see **Figure 5F**); another peculiar molecular characteristic of this area is its expression of the *Lhx9* gene (Shimogori et al., 2010). It can be conjectured that this distinct molecular code may underlie, at least in part, the observed retarded differentiation pattern.

As is discussed below, we associate the ABa source of *Sst* cells to the subsequent appearance of this sort of neurons at the VMHs and the Arcs domains, presumably due to ventralward tangential migration. We discuss here these populations in the genetic background context. The molecular background conditions discussed above for the primary sources of *Sst* cells do not seem to apply at the VMHs or Arcs. The only connection seems to be the progressive invasion of *Otp/Sst*-positive cells into these differentiating tuberal areas. Interestingly, it has been shown that mice lacking *Otp* function lose the STT-producing or *Sst*-expressing cells both at the Arc and "an adjacent area" (probably the VMHs; Acampora et al., 1999; Wang and Lufkin, 2000). Moreover, N*kx2.1*, a well-known gene expressed early on through most of the basal hypothalamus (Shimamura et al., 1995; Shimamura and Rubenstein, 1997), is likewise required for the development of basal tuberal hypothalamic areas such as the Arc and VMH (Kimura et al., 1996). In addition, *Shh* is expressed even earlier in the notochord and the prechordal plate underlying the forebrain. The peptidic SHH morphogen coded by *Shh* is a diffusible signal that eventually induces its own expression in the hypothalamic floor and basal plate cells, as well as the expression of other genes, such as *Nkx2.1* (Erickson et al., 1995; Dale et al., 1997; Pera and Kessel, 1997; Shimamura and Rubenstein, 1997; Pabst et al., 2000). Considering these data, we postulate that *Shh*, *Nkx2.1*, and *Otp* are part of the genetic network involved in the early specification of the precocious *Sst*-expressing cells at their ABa source. However, basal expression of *Shh*, *Nkx2.1*, and *Dlx5* in the tuberal area may influence the guidance of *Sst* cells into the VMH and Arc territories, as well as their definitive stabilization therein. Restriction of the ABa *Sst* pattern to the peduncular part of the hypothalamus may be related to the general presence of the *Six3* gene at the rostral midline, which is needed to activate *Shh* at this locus (Geng et al., 2008), as well as to the restricted local activity of the *Neurog3* gene (Allen atlas). Curiously, the ABa seemed not be affected in *Nkx2.1* knockout mice, though the Arc and VMH did not develop, or were abnormal, respectively (Kimura et al., 1996). It will be of interest to analyze *Sst* ontogeny in these knockout mice.

CHARACTERIZATION OF *Sst* DIFFERENTIATION AT THE ABa

The ABa progenitor domain had not been related to *Sst* cell production before. *Sst*-positive cells were first identified in our material as early as E10.5 at the ABa, which is known as one of the most precociously differentiating forebrain populations (Shimada and Nakamura, 1973). Other developmental reports on hypothalamic *Sst* cells were apparently less sensitive. In E14 mouse embryos, Bendotti et al. (1990) exclusively reported *Sst* mRNA expression in the entopeduncular nucleus. This observation may correspond to *Sst*-positive cells observed at E13.5 at the intermediate radial level of CPa, some of which subsequently apparently migrate radially into the EP nucleus. SST-immunoreactive cells in the entopeduncular nucleus were detected at E17 in the rat embryo study of Shiosaka et al. (1982). At this stage, these authors also located early SST-positive cells in a region near the root of the mamillothalamic tract; these probably correspond to our *Sst*-expressing cells at the peduncular periretromamillary band, observed from E13.5 onward in the mouse. Surprisingly, the precocious ABa population was not detected in this study. In the mouse, cells at the corresponding location were first distinguished after birth by immunohistochemistry (Forloni et al., 1990) or *in situ* hybridization (Bendotti et al., 1990), while SST-immunoreactive cells were detected at fetal day 19 in the rat (Shiosaka et al., 1982). A secondary perinatal surge of detectable SST is likely related to the functional role of SST in inhibiting the release of growth hormone from the anterior pituitary (Gross and Longer, 1979).

The ABa seems to be a particular area of the basal plate, which forms an U-shaped neuronal formation (there is a median portion and two lateral, caudally oriented wings of the ABa), which is restricted in extent to the terminal part of the basal hypothalamus, just under the alar–basal boundary and dorsal to the VMH nucleus. Data offered at the Allen Developing Mouse Brain Atlas reveal that the proneurogenic *Neurog3* gene is expressed selectively at the terminal ABa locus at E11.5. Moreover, the *Otp* data at the Allen Atlas for this stage corroborate our finding of a precocious *Otp*-positive ABa population, born strictly separately from that appearing at the peduncular and terminal paraventricular subareas. As mentioned above, the ABa was already known as one of the most precociously differentiated forebrain areas (Altman and Bayer, 1978, 1986, 1995) and is comparable to the avian retrochiasmatic nucleus of Puelles et al. (1987). According to our results, the sizeable *Otp*-positive cell population of this primordium also expresses *Nkx2.1* and *Shh* from E10 to E15.5. This strongly supports a basal plate origin. The early *Sst* cells appear as a smaller population intermixed with these *Otp* cells. They accordingly also seem to have a rostral basal origin restricted to the terminal ABa area (rostral–dorsal tuberal area). While numerous *Otp* cells clearly do not express *Sst* (within the sensibility of our ISH protocol), our material does not allow to assess whether all or some *Sst* cells also express *Otp*. Interestingly, *Shh* expression seems to become downregulated at the ABa mantle zone in parallel to the increase in the number of local *Otp*/*Sst*-positive cells. Presence of STT-immunoreactive cells at the retrochiasmatic area (ABa), as well as surrounding the VMH, has been described in adult mammals (Hoffman and Hayes, 1979; Johansson et al., 1984; Scanlan et al., 2003) and in the developing hypothalamus of the rat (Shiosaka et al., 1981).

POSSIBLE MIGRATION OF SOME *Sst* CELL POPULATIONS

The *Sst* cell population formed at the ABa is always paralleled by a *Otp* population, and remarkably involves up to E15.5 a ventralward dispersion of part of both populations. Cells spreading ventrally from the arms of the ABa surround the glutamatergic VMH core nucleus and colonize its shell domain (VMHs; **Figure 7**). Other cells imitate this behavior at the median and paramedian regions of the ABa and penetrate the underlying tuberal region, ingressing centrally into the peripheric shell of the Arc nucleus (Arcs) and more laterally into bilateral wing-shaped subpial domains associated to the Arcs (Arcs; **Figure 7**). The tuberal arcuate nucleus is a heterogeneous nucleus characterized in the adult by diverse neuroendocrine cell types (Dierickx and Vandesande, 1979; Johansson et al., 1984; Lechan and Fekete, 2006). Various chemoarchitectonic mappings of its components suggest an organization into core and shell domains (Arcc; Arcs; Fuxe et al., 1985; Zoli et al., 1986). Though losing in this way a part of its population, the ABa itself remains well populated, at least up to E15.5. Expression data for *Sst* at the Allen Atlas suggest that the ABa population diminishes at later stages, a pattern indicating that perhaps most of its elements finally translocate ventralward. The conjecture that we deal here with a tangential migratory process is based on the temporal sequence of observations, the relative density of *Sst* cells at the cited locations at different stages and the unlikeness of the possibility that this phenomenon can be explained by a radial migration. In particular, the population of *Sst* cells at the Arc nucleus is non-existent before the *Otp*/*Sst*-positive cells translocating from the ABa reach it. At subsequent stages, the number of these Arc cells increases spectacularly, possibly also due to retarded differentiation of early *Otp*-positive/*Sst*-negative elements into *Sst* neurons. It should be noted that another cell population is known to first develop at the ABa, and then becomes displaced ventralward into the Arcs and VMHs. We refer to *proopiomelanocortin* neurons found later at the adult Arc (Shimogori et al., 2010; look up *Pomc* in the Allen Developing Mouse Brain Atlas). It remains to be studied whether there is any causal relationship between these two neuropeptidergic cell types with a parallel developmental pattern.

Tangential migration of SST cells has been reported in other areas of the brain, such as in the case of SST cells originated from the basal telencephalon that contribute via tangential migration to *Sst*-positive GABAergic interneurons of the striatum and cerebral cortex (Anderson et al., 2001; Nery et al., 2002). Tangential migration recently is appearing not to be exceptional, as it occurs either strictly inside the developing hypothalamus (Alvarez-Bolado et al., 2000) or transferring cells from nearby or remote regions outside the hypothalamus into it (Schwanzel-Fukuda and Pfaff, 1989; Wray et al., 1989; Zhao et al., 2008). Cell populations migrating from the diencephalon – the prethalamus – into the hypothalamus were recently identified by genetic labeling of the *Foxb1* cell lineage (Zhao et al., 2008). According to the published images, a prethalamic *Foxb1* migratory stream contributes to the preoptic area and alar hypothalamic domains (their "anterior portion of the lateral hypothalamic area").

Sparse *Sst*-positive cells were detected from the earliest stages examined, though more prominently from E13.5 onward, in a ventral portion of the alar *Dlx5*-expressing RSPa domain, mixed with sparse *Otp*-expressing cells. Theoretically, these cells may have been produced locally in the SPa domain, or may have migrated from elsewhere. The molecular background of the SPa is quite different from that of the Pa, since its derivatives basically express *Dlx5* and *Arx*; DLX function conditions differentiation into GABAergic neurons (Stühmer et al., 2002). In contrast, the Pa derivatives largely differentiate as neurohormonal neuronal types of various sorts, none of which seems to be GABAergic. On the other hand, the ABa population expresses distinctively the basal marker *Nkx2.1*, not present in general in the Pa or SPa, and the CSPa population of *Sst*-expressing cells coincides topographically with a line of *Nkx2.1*-positive cells (Bardet, 2007; Shimogori et al., 2010). This might support a tangential migration from the underlying ABa (CSPa; **Figure 7**), but present evidence does not allow discarding the possibilities of a locally generated character of this *Sst* population at the SPa, or a tangential migration from the CPa. In contrast, the RPa seems to generate the sizeable rostral migratory *Otp*/*Sst*-positive population that bypasses laterally the suprachiasmatic nucleus as it traverses dorsoventrally the RSPa to reach finally the suboptic surface, transforming into the suboptic *Sst* cells (SbO; **Figure 7**). This would imply a sequence of tangential plus radial migration.

Apart of the instances where tangential migration seems to happen, we also noted examples of significant radial migration of *Sst* cells. This occurs particularly at the CPa area, where results at E13.5 and E15.5 indicated radial translocation of *Sst* cells into intermediate levels of the corresponding part of the lateral hypothalamus. These intermediate cells aggregate either at the lateral paraventricular nucleus or at a specific perifornical population. Since the fornix tract courses dorsoventrally across the entire PHy, adjacent to the intrahypothalamic boundary, it is associated not to a single perifornical nucleus, as suggested in the conventional structural schema of the hypothalamus, but to a series of perifornical populations belonging to the diverse molecular domains (**Figures 1B,C**). The *Sst*-positive one is therefore just one component of the whole perifornical complex. We also detected that *Sst* cells developing at the same progenitor area (CPa) reach superficially an entopeduncular position, which implies a longer range of radial migration. While the ABa-generated *Sst* cells do not seem to migrate radially at all, some of the *Sst* cells formed at the RPM do migrate radially, but do not reach the brain surface, and seem to stop deep to the cerebral peduncular tract, caudal to the subthalamic nucleus.

In conclusion, our data show novel aspects such as the detection of the first *Sst*-positive cells at the ABa, a population apparently distributing *Sst* cells to neighboring basal populations, followed by analogous cells developing separately within a ventral subdomain of the Pa area (RPaV, CPaV) and at the subjacent CSPa alar domain, or, separately, at the basal periretromamillary area. All these sources are characterized by the expression of the OTP transcription factor, and the absence of *Dlx5* expression. The alar versus basal sources seem to be distinguished by the presence of *Nkx2.1* as a widespread basal marker, though this is also associated to the small contingent of *Sst* cells developing at the SPa. Various radially migrated *Sst* cell groups were described. Moreover, our results suggest the existence of diverse *Sst*-expressing cell populations that migrate tangentially within the hypothalamus, contributing to its structural and genoarchitectonic complexity. Our conjectures in this regard predict observations that may be checked experimentally, using *Sst* mouse lines to trail the *Sst* cell lineage in combination with specific developmental and neuronal and/or glial markers. The temporal distribution of *Sst* expression observed is more complex than previously reported, particularly at the basal hypothalamus. Analysis of the final distribution of *Sst* cells will require a correlation of present results with perinatal developmental stages, since several well-known adult components are not yet differentiated at E15.5.

ACKNOWLEDGMENTS

This work was funded by the Local Government of Castilla-La Mancha grant PII1I09-0065-8194 (Carmen Díaz), the Spanish Ministry of Science and Innovation grant BFU2008-04156 and SENECA Foundation contract 04548/GERM/06-10891 (Luis Puelles). Nicanor Morales-Delgado is a Ph.D. student at Castilla-La Mancha University under contract from the BFU2008-04156 grant, and Paloma Merchan is a postdoctoral fellow of NIH grant 1-R01-MH070370-01A2 (Luis Puelles). Infrastructural support provided by the Centre for Biomedical Research and Institute for Research in Neurological Disabilities (Castilla-La Mancha) is acknowledged.

REFERENCES

Acampora, D., Postiglione, M. P., Avantaggiato, V., Di Bonito, M., and Simeone, A. (2000). The role of Otx and Otp genes in brain development. *Int. J. Dev. Biol.* 44, 669–677.

Acampora, D., Postiglione, M. P., Avantaggiato, V., Di Bonito, M., Vaccarino, F. M., Michaud, J., and Simeone A. (1999). Progressive impairment of developing neuroendocrine cell lineages in the hypothalamus of mice lacking the Orthopedia gene. *Genes Dev.* 13, 2787–2800.

Altman, J., and Bayer, S. A. (1978). Development of the diencephalon in the rat. I. Autoradiographic study of the time of origin and settling patterns of neurons of the hypothalamus. *J. Comp. Neurol.* 182, 945–971.

Altman, J., and Bayer, S. A. (1986). The development of the rat hypothalamus. *Adv. Anat. Embryol. Cell Biol.* 100, 1–178.

Altman, J., and Bayer, S. A. (1995). *Atlas of Prenatal Rat Brain Development.* Boca Raton: CRC Press.

Alvarez-Bolado, G., Zhou, X., Cecconi, F., and Gruss, P. (2000). Expression of Foxb1 reveals two strategies for the formation of nuclei in the developing ventral diencephalon. *Dev. Neurosci.* 22, 197–206.

Anderson, S. A., Marín, O., Horn, C., Jennings, K., and Rubenstein, J. L. (2001). Distinct cortical migrations from the medial and lateral ganglionic eminences. *Development* 128, 353–363.

Bardet, S. M. (2007). *Organización morfológica y citogenética del hipotálamo del pollo sobre base de mapas moleculares.* Doctoral thesis, Neuroscience Programme, University of Murcia, Spain.

Bardet, S. M., Cobos, I., Puelles, E., Martínez de-la-Torre, M., and Puelles, L. (2006). The chicken lateral septal organ and other circumventricular organs form in the striatal domain, abutting the molecular striatopallidal border. *J. Comp. Neurol.* 499, 745–767.

Bardet, S. M., Martinez-de-la-Torre, M., Northcutt, R. G., Rubenstein, J. L., and Puelles, L. (2008). Conserved pattern of OTP-positive cells in the paraventricular nucleus and other hypothalamic sites of tetrapods. *Brain Res. Bull.* 75, 231–235.

Bendotti, C., Hohmann, C., Forloni, G., Reeves, R., Coyle, J. T., and Oster-Granite, M. L. (1990). Developmental expression of somatostatin in mouse brain. II. In situ hybridization. *Brain Res. Dev. Brain Res.* 53, 26–39.

Bertrand, N., and Dahmane, N. (2006). Sonic hedgehog signaling in forebrain development and its interactions with pathways that modify its effects. *Trends Cell Biol.* 16, 597–605.

Blechman, J., Borodovsky, N., Eisenberg, M., Nabel-Rosen, H., Grimm, J., and Levkowitz, G. (2007). Specification of hypothalamic neurons by dual regulation of the homeodomain protein Orthopedia. *Development* 134, 4417–4426.

Brazeau, P., Vale, W., Burgus, R., Ling, N., Butcher, M., Rivier, J., and Guillemin, R. (1973). Hypothalamic polypeptide that inhibits the secretion of immunoreactive pituitary growth hormone. *Science* 179, 77–79.

Bulfone, A., Puelles, L., Porteus, M. H., Frohman, M. A., Martin, G. R., and Rubenstein, J. L. (1993). Spatially restricted expression of Dlx-1, Dlx-2 (Tes-1), Gbx-2, and Wnt-3 in the embryonic day 12.5 mouse forebrain defines potential transverse and longitudinal segmental boundaries. *J. Neurosci.* 13, 3155–3172.

Caqueret, A., Yang, C., Duplan, S., Boucher, F., and Michaud, J. L. (2005). Looking for trouble: a search for developmental defects of the hypothalamus. *Horm. Res.* 64, 222–230.

Cobos, I., Shimamura, K., Rubenstein, J. L., Martinez, S., and Puelles, L. (2001). Fate map of the avian anterior forebrain at the four-somite stage, based on the analysis of quail-chick chimeras. *Dev. Biol.* 239, 46–67.

Cotter, J. R., and Laemle, L. K. (1987). Distribution of somatostatinlike immunoreactivity in the brain of the little brown bat (*Myotis lucifugus*). *Am. J. Anat.* 180, 280–294.

Dale, J. K., Vesque, C., Lints, T. J., Sampath, T. K., Furley, A., Dodd, J., and Placzek, M. (1997). Cooperation of BMP7 and SHH in the induction of forebrain ventral midline cells by prechordal mesoderm. *Cell* 90, 257–269

Dierickx, K., and Vandesande, F. (1979). Immunocytochemical localization of somatostatin-containing neurons in the rat hypothalamus. *Cell Tissue Res.* 201, 349–359.

Ericson, J., Muhr, J., Jessell, T. M., and Edlund, T. (1995). Sonic hedgehog: a common signal for ventral patterning along the rostrocaudal axis of the neural tube. *Int. J. Dev. Biol.* 39, 809–816.

Fan, C.-M., Kuwana, E., Bulfone, A., Fletcher, C. F., Copeland, N., Jenkins, A., Crews, S., Martinez, S., Puelles, L., Rubenstein, J. L. R., and Tessier-Lavigne, M. (1996). Expression patterns of two murine homologs of *Drosophila* single-minded suggest possible roles in embryonic patterning and in the pathogenesis of Down syndrome. *Mol. Cell. Neurosci.* 7, 1–16.

Flames, N., Pla, R., Gelman, D. M., Rubenstein, J. L. R., Puelles, L., and Marín, O. (2007). Delineation of multiple subpallial progenitor domains by the combinatorial expression of transcriptional codes. *J. Neurosci.* 27, 9682–9695.

Forloni, G., Hohmann, C., and Coyle, J. T. (1990). Developmental expression of somatostatin in mouse brain. I. Immunocytochemical studies. *Brain Res. Dev. Brain Res.* 53, 6–25.

Fuxe, K., Agnati, L. F., Kalia, M., Goldstein, M., Andersson, K., and Härfstrand, A. (1985). "The dopaminergic systems in the brain and in the pituitary," in *Basic and Clinical Aspects of Neuroscience,* eds E. Fluckiger, E. Muller, and M. Thorner (Amsterdam: Springer Press), 11–25.

García-Moreno, F., Pedraza, M., Di Giovannantonio, L. G., Di Salvio, M., López-Mascaraque, L., Simeone, A., and De Carlos, J. A. (2010). A neuronal migratory pathway crossing from diencephalon to telencephalon populates amygdala nuclei. *Nat. Neurosci.* 13, 680–689.

Geng, X., Speirs C., Lagutin O., Inbal A., Liu W., Solnica-Krezel L., Jeong Y., Epstein D., and Oliver G. (2008). Haploinsufficiency of Six3 fails to activate Sonic hedgehog expression in the ventral forebrain and causes holoprosencephaly. *Dev. Cell* 15, 236–247.

Goshu E., Jin H., Lovejoy J., Marion J.-F., Michaud J. L., and Fan C. -M. (2004). Sim2 contributes to neuroendocrine hormone gene expression in the anterior hypothalamus. *Mol. Endocrinol.* 18, 1251–1262.

Gross, D. S., and Longer, J. D. (1979). Developmental correlation between hypothalamic somatostatin and hypophysial growth hormone. *Cell Tissue Res.* 202, 251–261.

Hallonet, M., Hollemann, T., Wehr, R., Jenkins, N. A., Copeland, N. G., Pieler, T., and Gruss, P. (1998). Vax1 is a novel homeobox-containing gene expressed in the developing anterior ventral forebrain. *Development* 125, 2599–2610.

Hidalgo-Sánchez, M., Martínez-de-la-Torre, M., Alvarado-Mallart, R. M., and Puelles, L. (2005). Distinct preisthmic domain, defined by overlap of Otx2 and Pax2 expression domains in the chicken caudal midbrain. *J. Comp. Neurol.* 483, 17–29.

Hoffman, G. E., and Hayes, T. A. (1979). Somatostatin neurons and their projections in dog diencephalon. *J. Comp. Neurol.* 186, 371–391.

Johansson, O., Hökfelt, T., and Elde, R. P. (1984). Immunohistochemical distribution of somatostatin-like immunoreactivity in the central nervous system of the adult rat. *Neuroscience* 13, 265–339.

Kimura, S., Hara, Y., Pineau, T., Fernandez-Salguero, P., Fox, C. H., Ward, J. M., and Gonzalez, F. J. (1996). The T/ebp null mouse: thyroid specific enhancer-binding protein is essential for the organogenesis of the thyroid, lung, ventral forebrain, and pituitary. *Genes Dev.* 10, 60–69.

Lagutin, O. V., Zhu, C. C., Kobayashi, D., Topczewski, J., Shimamura, K., Puelles, L., Russell, H. R. C., McKinnon, P. J., Solnica-Krezel, L., and Oliver, G. (2003). Six3 repression of Wnt signaling in the anterior neuroectoderm is essential for vertebrate forebrain development. *Genes Dev.* 17, 368–379.

Lechan, R. M., and Fekete, C. (2006). The TRH neuron: a hypothalamic integrator of energy metabolism. *Prog. Brain Res.* 153, 209–235.

Le Verche, V., Kaindl, A. M., Verney, C., Csaba, Z., Peineau, S., Olivier, P., Adle-Biassette, H., Leterrier, C., Vitalis, T., Renaud, J., Dargent, B., and Gressens, P. (2009). The somatostatin 2A receptor is enriched in migrating neurons during rat and human brain development and stimulates migration and axonal outgrowth. *PLoS ONE* 4, e5509. doi: 10.1371/journal.pone.0005509

Martí, E., Takada, R., Bumcrot, D. A., Sasaki, H., and McMahon, A. P. (1995). Distribution of Sonic hedgehog peptides in the developing chick and mouse embryo. *Development* 121, 2537–2547.

Michaud, J. L. (2001). The developmental program of the hypothalamus and its disorders. *Clin. Genet.* 60, 255–263.

Nery, S., Fishell, G., and Corbin, J. G. (2002). The caudal ganglionic eminence is a source of distinct cortical and subcortical cell populations. *Nat. Neurosci.* 5, 1279–1287.

Nieuwenhuys, R. (2009). The structural organization of the forebrain: a commentary on the papers presented at the 20th Annual Karger Workshop 'Forebrain Evolution in Fishes'. *Brain Behav. Evol.* 74, 77–85.

Nieuwenhuys, R., Voogd, J., and van Huijzen, C. (2008). "Development," in *The Human Central Nervous System*, 4th Edn. (Berlin/Heidelberg: Springer), 55–56.

Pabst, O., Herbrand, H., Takuma, N., and Arnold, H. H. (2000). NKX2 gene expression in neuroectoderm but not in mesendodermally derived structures depends on sonic hedgehog in mouse embryos. *Dev. Genes Evol.* 210,47–50.

Pera, E. M., and Kessel, M. (1997). Patterning of the chick forebrain anlage by the prechordal plate. *Development* 124, 4153–4162.

Puelles, L. (1995). A segmental morphological paradigm for understanding vertebrate forebrains. *Brain Behav. Evol.* 46, 319–337.

Puelles, L. (2001). Brain segmentation and forebrain development in amniotes. *Brain Res. Bull.* 55, 695–710.

Puelles, L., Amat, J. A., and Martínez-De-la-Torre, M. (1987). Segment-related, mosaic neurogenetic pattern in the forebrain and mesencephalon of early chick embryos. I. Topography of AChE-positive neuroblasts up to stage HH18. *J. Comp. Neurol.* 266, 147–268.

Puelles, L., Kuwana, E., Puelles, E., Bulfone, A., Shimamura, K., Keleher, J., Smiga, S., and Rubenstein, J. L. (2000). Pallial and subpallial derivatives in the embryonic chick and mouse telencephalon, traced by the expression of the genes Dlx-2, Emx-1, Nkx-2.1, Pax-6, and Tbr-1. *J. Comp. Neurol.* 424, 409–438.

Puelles, L., Martinez, S., Martinez-De-La-Torre, M., and Rubenstein, J. L. (2004). "Gene maps and related histogenetic domains in the forebrain and midbrain," in *The Rat Nervous System*, 3rd Edn., ed. G. Paxinos (San Diego: Elsevier), 3–25.

Puelles, L., Martínez-de-La-Torre, M., Paxinos, G., Watson, C., and Martinez, S. (2007). *The Chick Brain in Stereotaxic Coordinates. An Atlas Featuring Neuromeric Subdivisions and Mammalian Homologies.* San Diego: Academic Press-Elsevier.

Puelles, L., and Rubenstein, J. L. (2003). Forebrain gene expression domains and the evolving prosomeric model. *Trends Neurosci.* 26, 469–476.

Rubenstein, J. L., Shimamura, K., Martinez, S., and Puelles, L. (1998). Regionalization of the prosencephalic neural plate. *Annu. Rev. Neurosci.* 21, 445–477.

Scanlan, N., Dufourny, L., and Skinner, D. C. (2003). Somatostatin-14 neurons in the ovine hypothalamus: colocalization with estrogen receptor alpha and somatostatin-28(1-12) immunoreactivity, and activation in response to estradiol. *Biol. Reprod.* 69, 1318–1324.

Schwanzel-Fukuda, M., and Pfaff, D. W. (1989). Origin of luteinizing hormone-releasing hormone neurons. *Nature* 338, 161–164.

Shimada, M., and Nakamura, T. (1973). Time of neuron origin in mouse hypothalamic nuclei. *Exp. Neurol.* 41, 163–173.

Shimamura, K., Hartigan, D. J., Martinez, S., Puelles, L., and Rubenstein, J. L. (1995). Longitudinal organization of the anterior neural plate and neural tube. *Development* 121, 3923–3933.

Shimamura, K., and Rubenstein, J. L. (1997). Inductive interactions direct early regionalization of the mouse forebrain. *Development* 124, 2709–2718.

Shimogori. T., Lee, D. A., Miranda-Angulo, A., Yang, Y., Wang, H., Jiang, L., Yoshida, A. C., Kataoka, A., Mashiko, H., Avetisyan, M., Qi, L., Qian, J., and Blackshaw, S. (2010). A genomic atlas of mouse hypothalamic development. *Nat. Neurosci.* 13, 767–775.

Shiosaka, S., Takatsuki, K., Sakanaka, M., Inagaki, S., Takagi, H., Senba, E., Kawai, Y., Iida, H., Minagawa, H., Hara, Y., Matsuzaki, T., and Tohyama, M. (1982). Ontogeny of somatostatin-containing neuron system of the rat: immunohistochemical analysis. II. Forebrain and diencephalon. *J. Comp. Neurol.* 204, 211–224.

Shiosaka, S., Takatsuki, K., Sakanaka, M., Inagaki, S., Takagi, H., Senba, E., Kawai, Y., and Tohyama, M. (1981). Ontogeny of somatostatin-containing neuron system of the rat: immunohistochemical observations. I. Lower brainstem. *J. Comp. Neurol.* 203, 173–188.

Stühmer, T., Anderson, S. A., Ekker, M., and Rubenstein, J. L. R. (2002). Ectopic expression of the Dlx genes induces glutamic acid decarboxylase and Dlx expression. *Development* 129, 245–252.

Vale, W., Rivier, C., Brown, M., and Rivier, J. (1977). Pharmacology of thyrotropin releasing factor (TRF), luteinizing hormone releasing factor (LRF), and somatostatin. *Adv. Exp. Med. Biol.* 87, 123–156.

Viollet, C., Lepousez, G., Loudes, C., Videau, C., Simon, A., and Epelbaum, J. (2008). Somatostatinergic systems in brain: networks and functions. *Mol. Cell. Endocrinol.* 286, 75–87.

Wang, W., and Lufkin, T. (2000). The murine Otp homeobox gene plays an essential role in the specification of neuronal cell lineages in the developing hypothalamus. *Dev. Biol.* 227, 432–449.

Wray, S., Grant, P., and Gainer, H. (1989). Evidence that cells expressing luteinizing hormone-releasing hormone mRNA in the mouse are derived from progenitor cells in the olfactory placode. *Proc. Natl. Acad. Sci. U.S.A.* 86, 8132–8136.

Yacubova, E., and Komuro, H. (2002). Stage-specific control of neuronal migration by somatostatin. *Nature* 415, 77–81.

Yee, C. L., Wang, Y., Anderson, S., Ekker, M., and Rubenstein, J. L. (2009). Arcuate nucleus expression of NKX2.1 and DLX and lineages expressing these transcription factors in neuropeptide Y(+), proopiomelanocortin(+), and tyrosine hydroxylase(+) neurons in neonatal and adult mice. *J. Comp. Neurol.* 517, 37–50.

Zhao, T., Szabó, N., Ma, J., Luo, L., Zhou, X., and Alvarez-Bolado, G. (2008). Genetic mapping of Foxb1-cell lineage shows migration from caudal diencephalon to telencephalon and lateral hypothalamus. *Eur. J. Neurosci.* 28, 1941–1955.

Zoli, M., Fuxe, K., Agnati, L. F., Härfstrand, A., Terenius, L., Toni, R., and Goldstein, M. (1986). "Computer-assisted morphometry of transmitter-identified neurons: new opening for understanding of peptide-monoamine interactions in the mediobasal hypothalamus," in *Neurohistochemistry. Modern Methods and Applications*, eds P. Panula, H. Päivarinta, and S. Soimila (New York: Alan R. Liss), 137–174.

Conflict of Interest Statement: The authors declare that the research was conducted in the absence of any commercial or financial relationships that could be construed as a potential conflict of interest.

8

Development and organization of the lamprey telencephalon with special reference to the GABAergic system

Manuel A. Pombal*, Rosa Álvarez-Otero, Juan Pérez-Fernández, Cristina Solveira and Manuel Megías

Neurolam Group, Department of Functional Biology and Health Sciences, Faculty of Biology, University of Vigo, Vigo, Spain

Edited by:
Agustín González, Universidad Complutense de Madrid, Spain

Reviewed by:
Nerea Moreno, University Complutense of Madrid, Spain
Sylvie Retaux, Centre National de la Recherche Scientifique, France

***Correspondence:**
Manuel A. Pombal, Neurolam Group, Department of Functional Biology and Health Sciences, Faculty of Biology, University of Vigo, 36310 Vigo, Spain.
e-mail: pombal@uvigo.es

Lampreys, together with hagfishes, represent the sister group of gnathostome vertebrates. There is an increasing interest for comparing the forebrain organization observed in lampreys and gnathostomes to shed light on vertebrate brain evolution. Within the prosencephalon, there is now a general agreement on the major subdivisions of the lamprey diencephalon; however, the organization of the telencephalon, and particularly its pallial subdivisions, is still a matter of controversy. In this study, recent progress on the development and organization of the lamprey telencephalon is reviewed, with particular emphasis on the GABA immunoreactive cell populations trying to understand their putative origin. First, we describe some early general cytoarchitectonic events by searching the classical literature as well as our collection of embryonic and prolarval series of hematoxylin-stained sections. Then, we comment on the cell proliferation activity throughout the larval period, followed by a detailed description of the early events on the development of the telencephalic GABAergic system. In this context, lampreys apparently do not possess the same molecularly distinct subdivisions of the gnathostome basal telencephalon because of the absence of a *Nkx2.1*-expressing domain in the developing subpallium; a fact that has been related to the absence of a medial ganglionic eminence as well as of its derived nucleus in gnathostomes, the pallidum. Therefore, these data raise interesting questions such as whether or not a different mechanism to specify telencephalic GABAergic neurons exists in lampreys or what are their migration pathways. Finally, we summarize the organization of the adult lamprey telencephalon by analyzing the main proposed conceptions, including the available data on the expression pattern of some developmental regulatory genes which are of importance for building its adult shape.

Keywords: pallium, subpallium, cell proliferation, evolution, olfactory bulbs, preoptic region, agnathans, cyclostomes

INTRODUCTION

The lamprey is an interesting animal model due to the position that occupies in the phylogeny, being considered, together with myxines, the sister out-group of the gnathostomes. Many outstanding developmental studies on the lamprey were carried out by the end of the ninetieth and the beginning of the twentieth centuries (reviewed in Nieuwenhuys and Nicholson, 1998; Richardson and Wright, 2003; Richardson et al., 2010). Some of them described in detail the early developmental stages of its central nervous system (CNS). At the time, a number of valuable accounts also addressed the organization of the adult lamprey brain (reviewed in Nieuwenhuys and Nicholson, 1998; Pombal et al., 2009). In the last two decades, there is a growing interest in the molecular genetics of these animals because of their phylogenetic position (reviewed in Kuratani et al., 2002; Murakami et al., 2005; Osório and Rétaux, 2008; Murakami and Watanabe, 2009; Nikitina et al., 2009), as well as on the cytoarchitectonic, chemical, and hodological characterization of their CNS (reviewed in Nieuwenhuys and Nicholson, 1998; Pombal and Puelles, 1999; Weigle and Northcutt, 1999; Osório and Rétaux, 2008; Pombal and Megías, in press). In this paper, we provide an overview and literature survey on the earliest development of the lamprey telencephalon, including some additional information from our own collection of paraffin and semithin serial sections of different developmental stages (including embryonic, prolarvae, larvae, postmetamorphic, and adult animals). In addition, we review the existing data concerning cell proliferation on the lamprey brain with special emphasis on the GABAergic system and add some new data from our experimental material.

Lampreys have a very small brain, as compared with most gnathostomes, and their telencephalon, in particular, is very tiny. The telencephalic hemispheres arise as an unpaired and solid rudiment, which later divides into two portions (Scott, 1887). After hatching, as it occurs for the rest of the brain, they develop slowly throughout the prolarval and larval stages, which can last more than 5 years due to the extremely long larval period of these animals (reviewed in Hardisty and Potter, 1971). Then, the whole brain suffers a dramatic transformation during metamorphosis and practically doubles its size (Healey, 1972). The shape of the brain do not change so much through the adult period, but continues increasing in size.

STAGING AND LAMPREY DEVELOPMENT

In our laboratory, sea lamprey (*Petromyzon marinus*) embryos and prolarvae are grown from *in vitro* fertilized eggs. Sexual mature adult animals of both sexes were handnetted directly from their nests in tributaries of Miño River (NW of Spain) during the breeding season (from May to July). After collection, they are transported to the laboratory to perform the fertilization. Then, the eggs are reared in polypropylene tanks with a circulating water system under appropriate conditions of darkness and temperature (18 ± 0.5°C; Piavis, 1961, 1971). Under these conditions hatching occurs at 10–13 days post-fertilization (dpf).

The most common used staging series of early development for the sea lamprey is that of Piavis (1961, 1971). In his studies, Piavis subdivided the early development into 19 stages, from the ovulated but unfertilized egg to the first stage of larva (or ammocoete), which occurs approximately at 33–40 dpf. Therefore, we will follow this classification by indicating the relative stage (from P10 to P18, where P refers to Piavis), and referring to the age of the animal as days after fertilization (from 4 to 33 dpf) or to the length in millimeters, when known. Although in several recent works the different stages of this developmental period are considered as embryonic, we consider that only those until hatching should be referred to as embryonic, whereas those from hatching to the onset of filter feeding should be regarded as prolarvae. Moreover, as the age of larvae collected in the river is unknown, we will use their total body length in millimeters as reference.

As commented above, there are in the "old" literature a number of high quality reports on lamprey development focusing on the CNS. However, a direct comparison of these reports is sometimes difficult because of variations between species (*P. marinus*, *L. fluviatilis*, and *L. japonica* are the most common species in the literature; see review by Richardson et al., 2010), and/or between the experimental conditions used in each case to raise the animals. An illustrative example concerns the temperature, which can dramatically affects the survival rate and the growth during the early stages of development (Piavis, 1961; Rodríguez-Muñoz et al., 2001). Therefore, the time to hatch and body length of the hatching prolarva can vary in relation to the temperature of incubation of the fertilize eggs (when known): *P. marinus* (hatching at 11–13 dpf and 3–5 mm in size at 18.4°C; Piavis, 1961, 1971), *L. tridentata*, Pacific lamprey and *L. richardsoni*, western brook lamprey (hatching at 15 dpf and about 4.5 mm in size at 14°C; Meeuwig et al., 2006), and *L. reissneri* (hatching at 11–12 dpf and up to 4 mm body length at 16°C; Tahara, 1988).

EARLY DEVELOPMENT OF THE CNS

The CNS of all chordates develops from the neural plate, a thickened and elongated paramedian zone of the ectoderm, which in lampreys is first seen at about 4.5 dpf (Shipley, 1887; von Kupffer, 1906). Then the edges of the neural plate fuse to form a solid cord of neuroectoderm [a neural rod as described by Damas (1944), and Shipley, (1887)], which cavitates to form a hollow neural tube when neurulation has been completed (reviewed in Nieuwenhuys and Nicholson, 1998; Osório and Rétaux, 2008). Initially, the lateral walls of the neural tube consist of a pseudostratified epithelium of elongated cells that soon widens to form a thicker ventricular matrix layer (stratified epithelium), with the first neuroblasts appearing at its external border before hatching. At these earliest stages of development, the cells are filled with yolk platelets (Damas, 1944; Scott, 1887; Shipley, 1887; reviewed in Richardson et al., 2010).

According to Ahlborn (1883), two portions can be distinguished in the lamprey neural tube soon after fecundation (4–5 dpf, P10; Sterzi, 1907): prechordal and chordal (epichordal), which correspond to the archencephalon and deuterencephalon of von Kupffer (1906), respectively; however, the exact rostral ending of the notochord has clearly been unresolved for a long time and the possibility that the entire neural tube is epichordal has been recently proposed (see Pombal et al., 2009). At this stage, the lateral walls consist of a stratum of few cells in thickness whereas the dorsal (roof) and ventral (floor) midlines are formed by a single cell layer epithelium of elongated cells (Sterzi, 1907; Damas, 1944). The nasal epithelium starts its differentiation in a relatively ventral position at this stage, when the cranial flexure attains its maximum (Scott, 1887; Shipley, 1887); shortly after, an ingrowth of ectodermic cells represents the primordium of the nasohypophyseal duct and sac (**Figure 1**). With development, however, the primordium of the olfactory epithelium shifts toward anterior, with the nasal opening (a single and medial small pore) finally arriving to a dorsal position in the top of the head of late prolarvae (about 8 mm length, 26–29 dpf, P17 stage; **Figure 1D**; reviewed in Kuratani et al., 2001; Richardson et al., 2010). This shifting of the olfactory apparatus is conditioned by the enlargement of the upper lip (reviewed in Kuratani et al., 2001; see also their Figures 6 and 10), and by the correction of the cephalic flexure due to a partial rotation of the rostral neural tube (Scott, 1887; Sterzi, 1907; Källén, 1951). It is noteworthy that this rotation implies a simultaneous and remarkable topographical rotation of the most rostral nuclei and regions of the forebrain (rostral to the pretectum), which should be taken into account when interpreting experimental results at these developmental stages.

By the stage P12 (7–8 dpf, 3 mm length), the rostralmost portion of the neural tube that corresponds to the primordium of the evaginated portion of the telencephalon bulges out laterally (i.e., it begins to enlarge and thicken), and a dorsal evagination (the rudiment of the pineal vesicle) also appears in the dorsal midline (Scott, 1887; Shipley, 1887; von Kupffer, 1906; Sterzi, 1907; reviewed in Meléndez-Ferro et al., 2002b; Villar-Cheda et al., 2002). At Piavis developmental stage 13 (P13, prehatching), two diverticula are giving off, which constitute the primordial of the optic stalk and the optic vesicle (**Figure 2A**), and immediately after (4 mm embryo), the optic chiasma is observable at the rostral midline (Shipley, 1887; von Kupffer, 1906; Sterzi, 1907; Damas, 1944; see **Figure 2E**). At this level, an increasing number of fibers subsequently cross the midline to originate a conspicuous postoptic commissure (**Figure 2C**), which can be later subdivided into dorsal and ventral postoptic commissures (Pombal and Puelles, 1999).

At hatching (P14; 10–13 dpf), the lamprey brain is somehow poorly developed, and its lateral walls are thin and mostly formed by spindle shaped cells. According to von Kupffer (1906), it is in this stage when a sulcus intraencephalicus anterior is identified for the first time running dorsoventrally from the vicinity of the habenular commissure down to the preoptic recess (**Figures 2A–D**). Later, Sterzi (1907) made a graphical reconstruction of this sulcus in the 9, 16.5, and 35 mm stages, which, until nowadays, has been commonly used in the literature as a reference for the boundary between the telencephalon and the diencephalon (Nieuwenhuys and Nicholson, 1998; Meléndez-Ferro et al., 2002a; Villar-Cheda et al., 2006). The ontogeny of this and other prosencephalic sulci as well as their interpretation by different workers was addressed in detail by Källén (1951).

After hatching, the number of cells increase and the walls of the brain become thicker, with the first fibers appearing in its ventrolateral margins (**Figure 2B**). In addition, some migrating cells start to

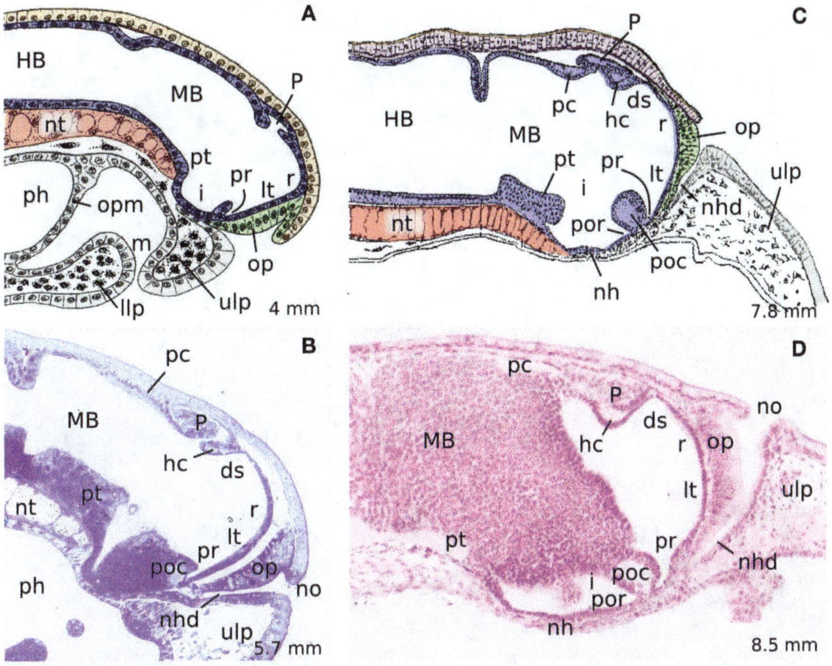

FIGURE 1 | Midsagittal schematic drawings (A,C) and hematoxylin-stained sections (B,D) of different developmental stages of *P. marinus* illustrating the identifiable structures at the midline as well as the variations on the cephalic flexure and the shifting from ventral to dorsal of the olfactory placode and the nasal opening. **(A)** 4 mm embryo, **(B)** 18 dpf prolarvae, **(C)** 7.8 mm prolarvae, **(D)** 29 dpf prolarvae. **(A,C)** are reproduced from Sterzi (1907). Rostral is to the right. ds, dorsal sac; HB, hindbrain; hc, habenular commissure; i, infundibulum; llp, lower lip; lt, lamina terminalis; m, mouth; MB, midbrain; nh, neurohypophysis; nhd, nasohypophyseal duct; no, nasal opening; nt, notochord; op, olfactory placode; opm, oropharyngeal membrane; P, pineal organ; pc, posterior commissure; ph, pharynx; poc, postoptic commissure; por, postoptic recess; pr, preoptic recess; pt, posterior tuberculum; r, neuroporic recess; ulp, upper lip.

colonize the primordium of the cerebral hemispheres. At this stage (which corresponds to P15 stage), the olfactory bulbs are no yet differentiated (Scott, 1887), and were first identified by Bergquist and Källén (1953) in a 12-mm larva; they are, at first, smaller than the telencephalic hemispheres, but grow considerably, probably due to the conspicuous increasing in size and complexity of the olfactory apparatus during metamorphosis, to become larger in the adult (Scott, 1887; VanDenbossche et al., 1995; Pombal et al., 2002; reviewed in Kleerekoper, 1982; Ren et al., 2009). Although Scott (1887) and Shipley (1887) were not able to observe any trace of the lateral ventricles in late prolarvae, in our material the anlage of the hemispheric evagination (foramen interventricular) is already detected around day 32 after fertilization [P17; **Figure 2F**; 7.5 mm stage for Bergquist (1952), and Källén (1951) or 7.8 mm larva according to Sterzi (1907)].

At the rostral end of the neural tube, the walls of the telencephalon impar are connected by the lamina terminalis (**Figures 1 and 2D–F**), which is slowly widened ventrally to form the bed of the anterior commissure (commissure of the lamina terminalis of Pombal and Puelles, 1999). The lamina terminalis continues dorsally with the rostralmost portion of the roof plate represented by the neuroporic recess (**Figure 1**). This recess is followed by the telencephalic commissural plate, which is mostly formed by the interbulbar (dorsal or pallial) commissure; this commissure was recently interpreted as the homolog of the septal commissural plate of gnathostomes, and might include a primordium of the anterior commissure and of a hippocampal commissure at its rostral and caudal ends, respectively (Pombal et al., 2009). Of note, both the commissure of the lamina terminalis and the interbulbar commissure are not yet distinguished in late prolarvae (see **Figures 1 and 2E**). From small larvae (16.5 mm for Sterzi, 1907), the interbulbar commissure increases considerably in size throughout development. Though it was represented in schematic drawings of prolarval lampreys by different authors (Burckhardt, 1894; von Kupffer, 1906; see also Figure 1C from Sterzi, 1907), the commissure of the lamina terminalis, however, cannot be readily identified until after midlarval stages (Scott, 1887). This commissure is also tiny and poorly developed in adult specimens, even in the anadromous *P. marinus* that have the largest brain, where it is formed by a thin commissural lamina that is undoubtedly distinguished only when some of the few fibers crossing through it are specifically labeled (Pombal and Puelles, 1999).

The telencephalic commissural plate continues with a choroidal epithelium constituted by a rostral part (lamina supraneuroporica) and a caudal part (dorsal choroid sac) separated by an inward velum transversum fold (von Kupffer, 1906; Sterzi, 1907; Johnston, 1912; see also Pombal et al., 2009). These structures continue caudally with the epithalamic roof area consisting of the highly asymmetric habenula with a thick habenular commissure and the pineal and parapineal complex (**Figures 1 and 2B,C,E**). Immediately caudal to a small recess of the third ventricle, the pineal recess, there appears the thickest commissure of the prosencephalic roof plate, the posterior commissure (**Figures 1 and 2E**). This last commissure is, in fact, the first to appear during development [around 16 dpf prolarvae

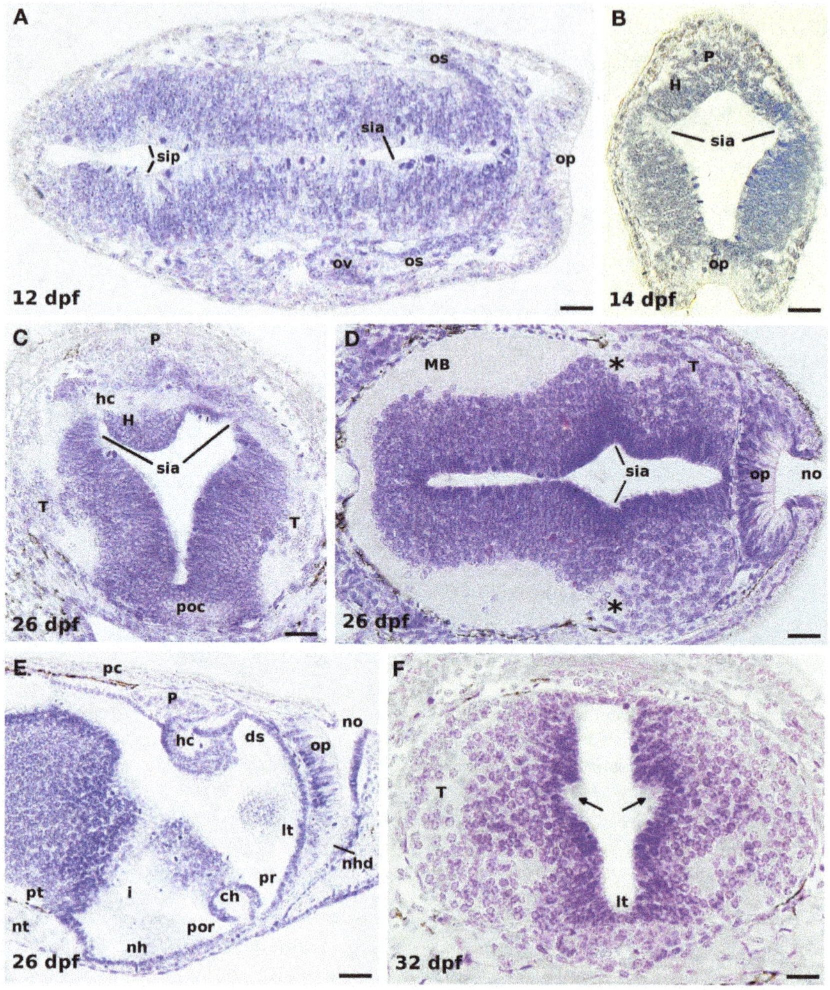

FIGURE 2 | Horizontal (A,D), transverse (B,C,F), and sagittal (E) hematoxylin-stained sections of different developmental stages of *P. marinus*. (A) Early formation of the optic vesicles by bilateral evagination of the rostral neural tube in a 12-dpf embryo. **(B)** Section through the habenula, pineal gland, and the olfactory placode of a 14-dpf prolarvae. **(C)** Section of a 26-dpf prolarvae at the level of the habenular commissure dorsally and the postoptic commissure ventrally. Note the trajectory of numerous axons emerging from the telencephalic hemispheres (primordium of the stria medullaris) coursing to the contralateral side through the habenular commissure. **(D)** Section illustrating the growing telencephalic hemispheres with the projecting axons grouping in its caudodorsal portion (asterisks). **(E)** Sagittal section of a 26-dpf prolarvae showing the midline prosencephalic structures. **(F)** Section through the telencephalon of a late prolarvae showing at both sides the incipient anlage of the interventricular foramen (arrows). In **(A,D,E)** rostral is to the right. ds, dorsal sac; H, habenula; hc, habenular commissure; i, infundibulum; lt, lamina terminalis; MB, midbrain; nh, neurohypophysis; nhd, nasohypophyseal duct; no, nasal opening; nt, notochord; os, optic stalk; ov, optic vesicle; op, olfactory placode; P, pineal organ; pc, posterior commissure; poc, postoptic commissure; por, postoptic recess; pr, preoptic recess; pt, posterior tuberculum; sia, sulcus intraencephalicus anterioris; sip, sulcus intraencephalicus posterioris; T, telencephalon. Scale bars: **(A,C,F)** = 20 μm, **(D)** = 30 μm, **(B,E)** = 40 μm.

or P15; 4 mm length for von Kupffer (1906), 4.5 mm for Damas (1944), and 5 mm length for Sterzi (1907); see **Figures 1 and 2E**], whereas the primordium of the superior (habenular) commissure is distinguished somehow later [about 18 dpf; see **Figures 1 and 2C,E**; 23 dpf for Shipley (1887), and 5 mm length for Sterzi (1907), but earlier (4 mm length) for Damas (1944)]. Lampreys also possess a relatively conspicuous postoptic commissure that is first observed at P15 (about 13–15 dpf). A remarkable number of telencephalic contralateral projections, however, cross through the habenular (superior) commissure (Polenova and Vesselkin, 1993; Yáñez and Anadón, 1994; Northcutt and Wicht, 1997). Curiously enough, the first projecting axons of the primordial telencephalic hemispheres joint together in its dorsocaudal portion, in a topographical location immediately rostral to the habenular commissure, as observed in transverse sections of late prolarvae (**Figure 2C**). This is because the extremely large portion of neural tube located between them in adult animals, i.e., the prethalamic eminence of Pombal et al., (2009), is underdeveloped at these early stages (Bergquist and Källén, 1953; see below). Therefore, at this stage of development, the proximity of the habenular commissure to the telencephalic hemispheres could account for the developing projecting fibers to cross the midline through it. In fact, Shipley (1887), as well as Damas (1944), was of opinion that the superior (habenular) commissure is the first to be recognized in the dorsal midline, just before differentiation of the habenula: "The first transverse commissure to appear is situated just in front of the stalk of the pineal gland. It forms the superior commissure of Osborn. Afterwards the ganglion cells thicken round it and form the asymmetrical ganglia habenulae." (Shipley, 1887, p. 368).

OF CELL PROLIFERATION AND DEVELOPMENT

In the first stages of development there is a remarkable enlargement of the neural tube, and numerous mitotic figures can be readily detected by simple searching of paraffin sections treated with a general staining such as hematoxylin (see **Figure 2**). They are observed exclusively in the proximity of the ventricular surface intermingled with the ependymal and subependymal cells, where they become spherical before division (von Kupffer, 1906; Damas, 1944; Pfister, 1971a; reviewed in Nieuwenhuys and Nicholson, 1998; Villar-Cheda et al., 2006). Afterward, the development of the lamprey brain is a very long process with slow histological differentiation (Schultze, 1856), mainly due to the extremely long larval period (more than 5 years for *P. marinus*) of these animals. In this connection, it may be significant that the same occurs for the body of the larva, which gradually increases in length from around 5 mm at hatching up to 180 mm before metamorphosis, though there is an astonishing variation in growth rates (reviewed in Hardisty and Potter, 1971). During the transformation from ammocoete to adult, a period of only a few months, there is an initial increase of proliferating cell nuclear antigen (PCNA)-labeling that disappears progressively in late metamorphic stages (Villar-Cheda et al., 2006); during this period, however, in *P. marinus* there is a remarkable increase of the brain size that nearly doubles its width and height (see Healey, 1972), most likely as a consequence of the enlargement of pre-existing neurons, glial cells, and their processes, as suggested by Rovainen (1982). In anadromous lampreys, the brain continues enlarging during the parasitic period to reach the final size in adult breeding animals. According with the studies of Villar-Cheda et al. (2006), no PCNA-ir cells were observed in young postmetamorphic animals, and only a few were present in the habenula of adult, sexually mature specimens. Therefore, these data suggest that the brain growth during this last period of its life cycle is also mostly due to an increase in size of existing nervous cells. Contrary to this, it has been shown that, at least, in the spinal cord of *P. marinus* there is an increase in the number of GABAergic cells from postmetamorphic animals to adults (Ruiz et al., 2004).

Neurogenesis is a common feature of vertebrate CNS, but the rate and places of neuron generation vary between species and depend on the stage of developmental (see Ruiz et al., 2004, and references herein). In 2004 it was pointed out, however, that 5′-bromo-2-deoxyuridine (BrdU)-labeled new generated cells in the lamprey rhombencephalon and spinal cord are not neurons but glial cells (Vidal-Pizarro et al., 2004). Several technical reasons may explain this apparent discrepancy: by one hand, the number of BrdU-labeled cells obtained by these authors appears to be rather low compared with those obtained by Villar-Cheda et al. (2006) and ourselves (present results), which may be due to differences in the efficiency of the protocols employed (exposition to BrdU versus injection of 20 µl/g of body weight of 10 mM BrdU into the body cavity posterior to the last gill); on the other hand, almost all the BrdU-labeled cells described by Vidal-Pizarro et al. (2004; their Figure 9) are located periventricularly and, therefore, may not yet started (or are just starting) the differentiation processes (see also Villar-Cheda et al., 2006), which may preclude labeling with neuronal markers. Moreover, the LCM-3 antibody (a lamprey NF-specific monoclonal antibody), used as specific neuronal marker, does not seems to label most of the neuronal cell bodies in the gray matter spinal cord (see their Figures 10A,D where only two dorsal cells are weakly labeled with this marker). In addition, there are several reports using different technical approaches that clearly support neurogenesis in several parts of the lamprey brain (see for example: Pombal et al., 1994; Rodicio et al., 1995; Meléndez-Ferro et al., 2002a; Ruiz et al., 2004; Villar-Cerviño et al., 2008, 2009). Furthermore, several genes involved in neurogenesis (Ngn1, NeuroD2, and Id2/3), and regionalization and patterning (LIM-kinase 2 and several Sox genes) where reported to be expressed in late embryos and early prolarvae (Guérin et al., 2009).

In the literature, there are several experimental studies reporting cell proliferation during lamprey forebrain development, which include the analysis of two markers: PCNA (Meléndez-Ferro et al., 2002a,b; Villar-Cheda et al., 2002), and BrdU (Tobet et al., 1996; Álvarez-Otero et al., 2002; Vidal-Pizarro et al., 2004; Villar-Cheda et al., 2006; reviewed in Osório and Rétaux, 2008). From these studies it was concluded that the presence of proliferation discontinuities in the ventricular zone of PCNA-labeled sections could be interpreted as putative neuroanatomical limits throughout the lamprey brain (Villar-Cheda et al., 2006); this proliferating marker is, therefore, of help to study and compare the evolution of the nuclear organization and topographical extension of different neuronal entities in the developing brain. In addition, these authors also stressed that the cell cycle in lampreys is very long, and this feature was considered the reason why the nervous system grows slowly throughout the extremely long larval period. Very recently, the expression pattern of a number of genes involved in the control of proliferation, neurogenesis, regionalization, and cell signaling in the forebrain of gnathostomes was also reported in lampreys (Guérin et al., 2009), part of which appears to participate in the morphogenesis of the telencephalon.

In our laboratory, short incubation times (4 days) with BrdU of larvae of different body length revealed a number of labeled cells in a periventricular position (**Figures 3A,B,D,E**). In addition, differences are observed between particular ventricular zones in terms of proliferation; so that, in general, the proliferation is higher in some of them such as in the subpallium, being more prominent in the proximities of the lamina terminalis and close to the preoptic recess. At the dorsomedial level, there is a particularly strong proliferation activity in the primordium of the prethalamic eminence (the classical medial pallium) of the different larval sizes analyzed (**Figures 3D,E**). In general, these results are in agreement with those previously reported after 7 days of BrdU incubation (Villar-Cheda et al., 2006).

When increasing the exposition time to BrdU to 16 days (**Figures 3C,F**), the number of BrdU-labeled cells increase in most portions of the lamprey telencephalon. In some regions such as the septum or the olfactory bulb practically all the periventricular cells are labeled, whereas in other regions the labeled cells are more or less homogeneously dispersed. In animals exposed 25 days to BrdU virtually all the periventricular cells are labeled, with

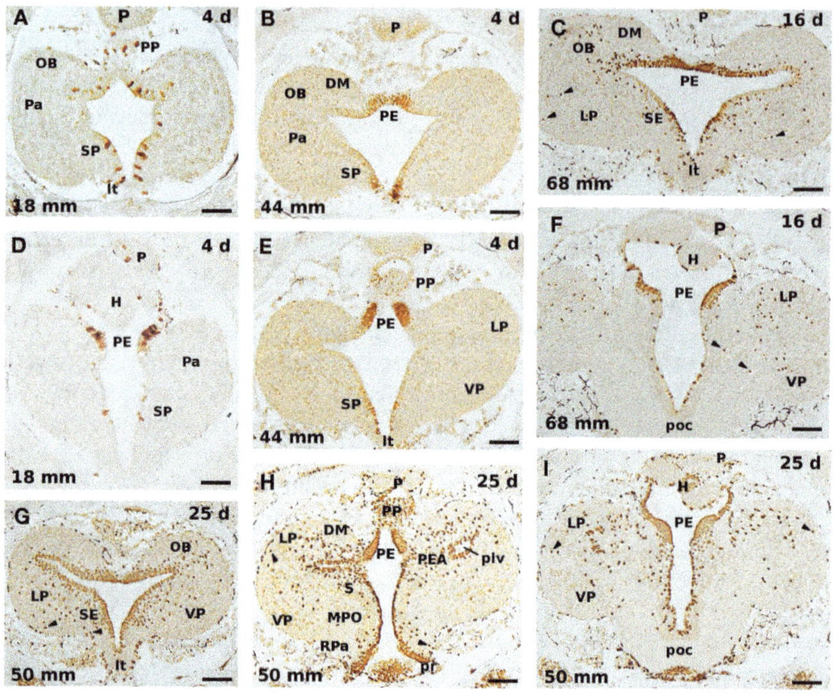

FIGURE 3 | Cell proliferation in transverse sections of the developing sea lamprey forebrain after incubation of 4 (A,B,D,E), 16 (C,F), and 25 (G–I) days in BrdU. (A–C), and **(G)**, as well as **(D–F)**, and **(I)**, illustrate comparable rostrocaudal levels in larvae of different size, whereas **(H)** is intermediate between **(G)** and **(I)**. There is a general increase of immunolabeled cells with the increase of the BrdU exposure time. Note also that numerous migrating labeled cells are detected after 16 days of incubation with this marker **(C,F)**, and that its number increases with longer incubations (25 days; **G–I**); most of them are located at dorsal (pallial) levels. In addition, a prominent BrdU labeling is present in the periventricular portion of the still small prethalamic eminence in all cases. Arrowheads point to laterally displaced labeled cells. OB, olfactory bulb; DM, dorsomedial neuropile; H, habenula; LP, lateral pallium; lt, lamina terminalis; MPO, medial preoptic nucleus; P, pineal organ; Pa, pallium; PE, prethalamic eminence; PEA, pallial extended amygdala; plv, posterior lateral ventricle; poc, postoptic commissure; PP, parapineal; pr, preoptic recess; RPa, rostral paraventricular area; S, striatum; SE, septum; SP, subpallium; VP, ventral pallium. Scale bars: **(A,D,G)** = 60 μm; **(B,C,E,F,H,I)** = 80 μm.

thicker proliferation strata in those regions where more staining was already present with shorter exposition times (**Figures 3G–I**). Curiously enough, the prethalamic eminence area is completely full of BrdU-labeled cells, which means that almost all, if not all, cells in this structure appear to still be proliferating cells in larvae of middle size (50 mm larvae; **Figures 3H,I**). Although anatomically expected due to the large increase of this structure during the larval period, the physiological purpose of this very high and prolonged mitotic activity in this structure is not understood. These results are in agreement with those reported by Pfister (1971b,c), who claimed that the telencephalic primordium hippocampi (our prethalamic eminence), as well as the optic tectum, continues to proliferate for a particularly long time.

These results, as pointed out by Villar-Cheda et al. (2006), show that there is an important proliferation activity in the ventricular zone that last for several years. The presence of a conspicuous postembryonic neurogenesis in lampreys is, most likely, related to the slow and gradual development of these animals with some systems, such as the olfactory, visual, or oculomotor systems (Kleerekoper, 1982; de Miguel et al., 1990; Rubinson, 1990; Pombal et al., 1994; Rodicio et al., 1995; Zielinski et al., 2005), developing throughout the larval and metamorphic periods. A heavy PCNA expression was also observed around the ventricular zone of early prolarvae (Guérin et al., 2009).

Another conspicuous morphological feature of lampreys is that they possess a laminar brain, which means that there is little cellular migration, with most cells located in a more or less continuous and relatively thick periventricular stratum (Nieuwenhuys and Nicholson, 1998; Osório and Rétaux, 2008; Pombal and Megías, in press). However, a number of neurons and neuronal populations migrate away from the central gray zone and are embedded in the white matter. Actually, the telencephalon is one of the brain parts where more cells migrate away from the ventricular proliferative epithelium. The migration process starts early on during development and is particularly evident at pallial levels (see **Figures 2C,D,F**). After incubation with BrdU during 4 days, however, no labeled cell was observed outside the periventricular proliferating epithelium. In a previous study (Villar-Cheda et al., 2006), practically all the BrdU-labeled nuclei were located within or very close to the ventricular zone after a week of exposure to BrdU. These results indicate that the time for the differentiating neuroblast to migrate outside of the ventricular zone is higher than 7 days. In larvae exposed to the BrdU during 16 days (**Figures 3C,F**), a considerable number of BrdU-labeled cells appear laterally displaced in the neural tube, with some of them located far away from the ventricular surface (arrowheads in **Figures 3C,F**). This fact implies that 16 days is enough time for those cells that enter their differentiation to get out of the central matrix and populate the lateral (marginal) zone. When the animals are exposed 25 days to BrdU, the number of migratory postmitotic labeled cells is much higher, with some spreading in the whole extension of the periventricular cell strata, whereas others can be observed nearly to the outer surface of the brain (arrowheads in **Figures 3G–I**). These migrating cells are particularly abundant in the evaginated portion of the telencephalon, being more numerous in the lateral pallium. In this portion of the brain, the wall is slightly thicker and contains a higher number of laterally displaced (migrated) cells in adult specimens. In a previous study in the lamprey rhombencephalon and spinal cord with BrdU labeling, however, in addition to the non-neuronal identification of the labeled cells, it was concluded that there is no migration of BrdU-labeled cells even when the animals were killed 52 days after the injection of the cell proliferation marker (Vidal-Pizarro et al., 2004). Although our largest incubation time in BrdU was 25 days, there is a clear pattern of cellular migration showing a correlation between exposition time and traveled distance from the ependymal zone, as well as a gradual increase in the number of lateral displaced labeled cells (see **Figure 3**). This disparity may, in part, be explained by dilutional effects of multiple mitoses on labeling due to the different protocol employed (see above).

It is noteworthy that the majority of the neurons in the brain of myxines migrate away from the proliferative periventricular area, and, in the pallium, in particular, most cells are clearly segregated in several layers, thus being laminated in appearance (reviewed in Ronan and Northcutt, 1998; Wicht and Nieuwenhuys, 1998; Pombal and Megías, in press); up to now, however, there is no clear correspondence between the different pallial subdivisions recognized in either myxines or lampreys with those established in amniote vertebrates. In addition, it is not known whether the situation in lampreys is an ancestral or a derived character.

GABAergic SYSTEM

In adult lampreys there are many GABA-ir cells throughout the brain and the spinal cord, part of which are of cerebrospinal fluid-contacting type cells (CSF-c; see Robertson et al., 2007, for a review). Concerning the adult lamprey telencephalon, the presence of GABA-ir cells has been previously reported by different authors (Pombal et al., 1997; Meléndez-Ferro et al., 2001; Robertson et al., 2007), which are located in the olfactory bulbs, the pallium, and the subpallium (**Figures 4A–C**). In a detailed study of the olfactory bulbs, Meléndez-Ferro et al. (2001) identified several GABAergic cell populations, including periglomerular cells located around the olfactory glomeruli, cells in the inner cellular layer, some CSF-c at the ventricular level, as well as some cells at the entrance of the olfactory nerve and in the interbulbar commissure. At pallial level, GABA-ir cells were observed inside the limits of the lateral, dorsal, and medial pallia (**Figures 4A–C**; Pombal and Puelles, 1999; Robertson et al., 2007), with the last two corresponding to our pallial extended amygdala and prethalamic eminence, respectively (see Pombal et al., 2009; Martínez-de-la-Torre et al., 2011; Pombal and Megías, in press). In the subpallium, GABA-ir cells distribute in the nucleus of the anterior commissure, the septum, and the striatum (**Figure 4A**; Pombal et al., 1997; Robertson et al., 2007). In these subpallial nuclei there are many CSF-c cells bearing an apical dendrite that ends at the ventricular surface. Additionally, it was recently shown that a number of GABAergic cells located in the caudal part of the medial pallium (our prethalamic eminence) project to the lamprey optic tectum (Robertson et al., 2006). Furthermore, some GABA-ir neurons within the same area as well as a few located in the ventral part of the lateral pallium (our ventral pallium) project to the mesencephalic locomotor region (MLR) of the isthmic region (Ménard et al., 2007). Based on the presence of GABA-ir projection neurons, these authors suggested that the two pallial areas of the lamprey could be considered analogous to the amygdala and/or pallidum of tetrapods (Ménard et al., 2007). An interesting aspect, however, is how this adult GABAergic system is acquired during development? By using immunohistochemical methods, we have studied in detail the early development of the lamprey GABAergic system in both transverse and sagittal semithin sections of the lamprey prosencephalon to get insight on the differentiation and evolution of its GABAergic system.

The first telencephalic immunolabeled cells appear after hatching (by 18 dpf prolarvae), in the outer part of the periventricular proliferating layer of the primordial hemispheres (**Figure 4D**). They are few in number, locate slightly rostral to the small primordium of the optic chiasma, and have short processes running laterally. These GABA-ir cells must correspond to the primordium of the subpallium and, at least part of them are of CSF-c type; it should be noted, however, that at this stage there is no recognizable morphological landmark indicating the boundary between the pallial and non-pallial telencephalic portions. Two days later (20 dpf; **Figures 4E,H**), the number of GABA-ir cells increase considerably in the subpallium with some of them laterally migrated, at the time that the first immunoreactive cells and processes appear more rostrally (and dorsally) in the primordial telencephalic hemispheres. In sagittal sections, a few GABA-ir cells are seen inside the presumptive pallial primordium (**Figure 4H**).

In 23 dpf prolarvae (**Figures 4F,I**), the number of GABA-ir cells continues increasing as do the labeled processes in the ventrolateral margin of the neural tube at the subpallium. Many of these cells distribute in the dorsorostral portion of the telencephalic hemispheres, at the time that the cephalic flexure is partially reduced because of the dorsal shift of the rostral neural tube (see above and **Figure 1**). At this stage, two GABAergic cell populations can be distinguished: a prominent ventral (subpallial) population and a less conspicuous dorsal (pallial) population; both of them are formed by a relatively compact mass of GABA-ir cells in the lateral portion of the matrix zone, with some cells displaced laterodorsally (**Figure 4F**). At the external surface, a slight depression indicates the approximate boundary between the pallial and subpallial portions. The dorsalization of the labeled cells is better observed in sagittal sections (compare **Figures 4H,I**), where those locate in the dorsal (pallial) portion of the telencephalic hemispheres appear as slightly larger and more intense labeled. In addition, at the rostral end of the neural tube numerous CSF-c GABA-ir cells of the subpallial population locate medially close to the lamina terminalis (**Figure 4F**).

By 29 dpf prolarvae (**Figure 4G**), the shape of the evaginated portion of the telencephalon is better discernible from the impar non-evaginated portion. In this stage, the primordium of the septum and the striatum is now better differentiated from the GABA-ir population located close by to the optic chiasma mostly composed of CSF-c neurons (**Figure 4G**). Both populations of labeled cells are separated by a GABA negative portion that is

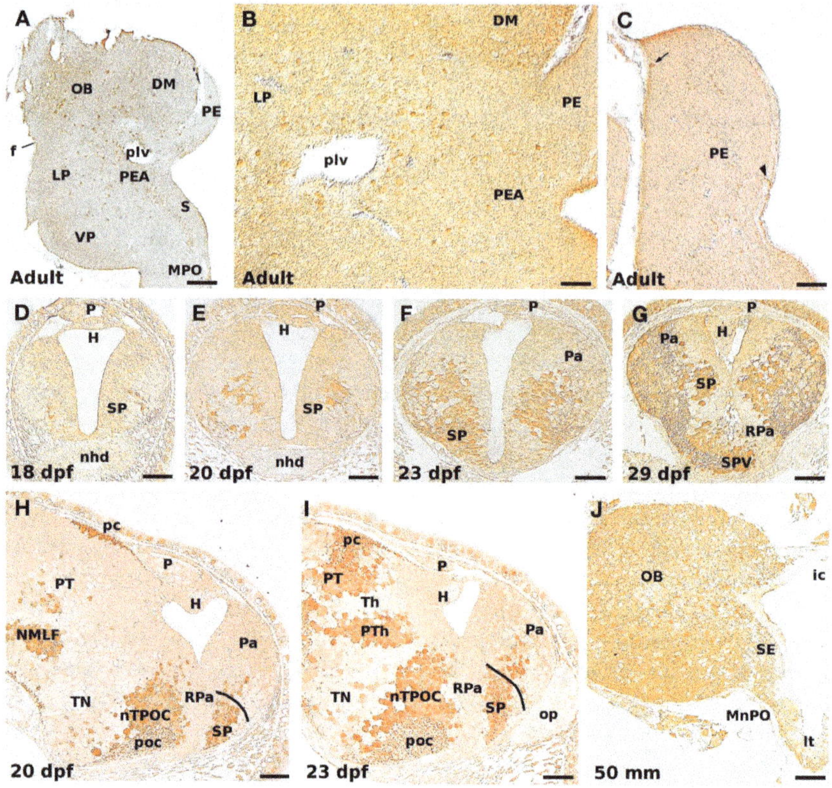

FIGURE 4 | GABA-ir cells in the adult (A–C), developing prolarvae (D–I), and midlarval lamprey telencephalon (J). (A) Transverse section illustrating GABA-ir cells in the olfactory bulb, lateral and ventral pallium, pallial extended amygdala, striatum, and medial preoptic nucleus. **(B)** GABA-ir cells in the lateral pallium, and the pallial extended amygdala. **(C)** GABA-ir cells in the prethalamic eminence. Most of its GABA-ir cells are dispersed at intermediate levels, but a few can be observed at either the medial (ventricular; arrowhead) or lateral (superficial; arrow) borders. Transverse **(D–G)**, and sagittal **(H,I)** sections of prolarvae of different size illustrating the early development of the telencephalic GABAergic cells. Note the increase in the number of GABA-ir cells as well as the progressive colonization of dorsal (pallial) areas. **(J)** GABA-ir cells in the olfactory bulb, septum, and median preoptic nucleus of a 50-mm larva. In sagittal sections **(H,I)**, rostral is to the right. OB, olfactory bulb; DM, dorsomedial neuropile; f, fissura circularis; H, habenula; ic, interbulbar commissure; LP, lateral pallium; lt, lamina terminalis; MnPO, median preoptic nucleus; MPO, medial preoptic nucleus; nhd, nasohypophyseal duct; NMLF, nucleus of the medial longitudinal fascicle; nTPOC, nucleus of the tract of the postoptic commissure; op, olfactory placode; P, pineal organ; Pa, pallium; pc, posterior commissure; PE, prethalamic eminence; PEA, pallial extended amygdala; plv, posterior lateral ventricle; poc, postoptic commissure; PT, pretectum; PTh, prethalamus; RPa, rostral paraventricular area; S, striatum; SE, septum; SP, subpallium; SPV, subparaventricular area; Th, thalamus; TN, tuberal nucleus; VP, ventral pallium. Scale bars: **(A)** = 100 μm; **(B)** = 50 μm; **(C)** = 60 μm; **(D–G,I)** = 30 μm; **(H)** = 40 μm; **(J)** = 70 μm.

now conceived as the anlage of the rostral paraventricular nucleus (Pombal et al., 2009; reviewed in Pombal and Megías, in press), and corresponds to the classical preoptic magnocellular nucleus. Therefore, according to present-day definition of the preoptic area in tetrapods, both portions, the anlage of the rostral paraventricular nucleus and the immediately ventral GABA-ir band do not belong to the telencephalon. Of note, this pattern of GABA-ir cells is in neatly agreement with both the *Dlx* expression in embryonic and early prolarval stages (Murakami et al., 2001; Myojin et al., 2001; Neidert et al., 2001; Kuraku et al., 2010), and DLL (a homeobox transcription factor)-ir in midlarval stages (Martínez-de-la-Torre et al., 2011).

In medium-sized larvae, the pattern of GABA-ir cells is similar to that reported for adult specimens (**Figure 4J**; Meléndez-Ferro et al., 2002a; Robertson et al., 2007); at this stage, however, there are no GABA-ir cells in the prethalamic eminence (the classical medial pallium; see below). This is because this structure is basically undifferentiated with practically all of its cells actively proliferating, as commented above (see also **Figure 3**). In addition, it is worth noting that the pattern of DLL positive cells in larvae of similar size is consistent with a possible tangential migration from the proliferating periventricular subpallium to the pallium (Martínez-de-la-Torre et al., 2011), as reported for several gnathostome species (Dirksen et al., 1993; Cobos et al., 2001; Brox et al., 2003; Carrera et al., 2008; Moreno et al., 2008; reviewed in Puelles et al., 2000; Marín and Rubenstein, 2001, 2003).

These results mostly agree with those previously published on the ontogeny of the GABA-ir populations in the forebrain and midbrain of the sea lamprey (Meléndez-Ferro et al., 2002a), with some minor differences that may be due to the temperature used to raise embryos and prolarvae (18°C versus 16°C).

In the last years, the expression patterns of several regulatory genes were studied during the embryonic and early prolarval development showing striking similarities with those reported in gnathostomes, but also some differences. Therefore, although the developmental program for the brain appears to be quite conservative, there are also some differences concerning the mechanisms of brain patterning and organization. One of these differences concerns the specification of the GABAergic cells in the lamprey telencephalon (reviewed in Osório and Rétaux, 2008; Watanabe et al., 2008). Analysis of the expression pattern of *Hh* (a *Shh* homolog) and *Nkx2.1* (*TTF-1*) in early developing lampreys revealed the presence of two basal plate domains located in the hypothalamus and the ventral aspect of the neural tube including the zona limitans intrathalamica, but the lack of expression in the subpallium (Murakami et al., 2001, 2005; Ogasawara et al., 2001; Uchida et al., 2003; Kluge et al., 2005; Osório et al., 2005; Kano et al., 2010; reviewed in Kuratani et al., 2002; Murakami et al., 2005; Osório and Rétaux, 2008; Watanabe et al., 2008; Murakami and Watanabe, 2009). This fact raised the question on the existence in lampreys of a homolog of the medial ganglionic eminence (MGE) of gnathostome vertebrates, which, in these animals, represents the major source of cortical (pallial) interneurons by originating a conspicuous tangential migratory stream of GABAergic cells that enter several pallial portions (Moreno et al., 2008; reviewed in Marín and Rubenstein, 2001, 2003). The first GABA-ir cells in the lamprey subpallium are observed by Piavis stage 17 (18 dpf; Meléndez-Ferro et al., 2002a; present results), which is slightly latter than the stages analyzed for *Hh* and *Nkx2.1*. In this scenario, there are, at least, three different interpretations or possibilities for the origin of the GABA-ir telencephalic cells in lampreys: (1) they do have a true homolog of the MGE of gnathostomes but the expression of *Hh* and *Nkx2.1* is somehow delayed during development, as it is for the histological differentiation. A significant delay, as compared with gnathostomes, on the telencephalic expression has also been observed for *Fgf8/17* (Guérin et al., 2009); (2) the pallial GABA-ir cells of these animals are originated exclusively from a hypothetical homolog of the gnathostome lateral ganglionic eminence (LGE; see also Watanabe et al., 2008), which has also been reported to contribute to the GABAergic pallial interneurons (see Rubin et al., 2010 and references herein); (3) alternatively, the lamprey GABA-ir pallial neurons could be originated through a different specification mechanism from those known in gnathostomes, as already suggested by Osório and Rétaux (2008). Needless to say that a combination of these options is also possible.

STRUCTURE AND REGIONALIZATION OF THE LAMPREY TELENCEPHALON

The lamprey telencephalon, which is now considered to be the most rostrodorsal portion of the alar plate of the secondary prosencephalon (Pombal et al., 2009; Pombal and Megías, in press), comprises three main parts: the olfactory bulbs, the cerebral hemispheres, and the telencephalon medium (the unevaginated portion; Nieuwenhuys and Nicholson, 1998). The dorsocaudal limit of the telencephalon varied considerably across the literature (**Figure 5**), and some recent changes have also been introduced on its ventral limit, as already commented.

The internal organization of the olfactory bulbs is quite similar to that of other anamniote vertebrates (Heier, 1948; Schnitzlein, 1982; Iwahori et al., 1987; reviewed in Ren et al., 2009). It is noteworthy that the olfactory bulbs of these animals are larger than the cerebral hemispheres from which they are externally demarcated by a shallow groove, the circular fissura. Both of them are hollow structures with their ventricles connected with the median third (diencephalic) ventricle through a common interventricular foramen (or foramen of Monroe).

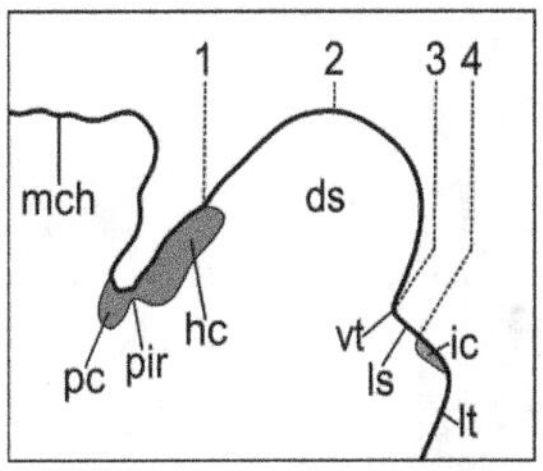

FIGURE 5 | Midsagittal section of the prosencephalic roof plate in *P. marinus* illustrating the dorsal telencephalic/diencephalic limit in either the columnar or the segmental conceptions of the neural tube. 1, Edinger (1888), von Kupffer (1906), Heier (1948), Schöber (1964), Nieuwenhuys and Nicholson (1998); 2, Burckhardt (1894); 3, Sterzi (1907), Pombal and Puelles (1999); 4, Ahlborn (1883), Pombal et al. (2009), Martínez-de-la-Torre et al. (2011). ds, dorsal sac; hc, habenular commissure; ic, interbulbar commissure; ls, lamina supraneuroporica; lt, lamina terminalis; mch, mesencephalic choroidal plexus; pc, posterior commissure; pir, pineal recess; vt, velum transversum.

The cerebral hemispheres and the telencephalon medium can be subdivided into a dorsal pallial region and a ventral subpallial region, with the later including the septum, striatum, and preoptic region. The organization of the lamprey pallium is still a matter of discussion, and different conceptions have been postulated in the last decades (**Figure 6**). Most of the classical studies considered four main subdivisions: primordium hippocampi (or medial pallium) of Johnston (1912), primordium pallii dorsalis (or dorsal pallium), primordium piriforme (or lateral pallium), and lobus (lobulus) subhippocampalis (or subhippocampal lobe) of Herrick and Obenchain (1913) (Heier, 1948; Schöber, 1964; reviewed in Nieuwenhuys and Nicholson, 1998; Pombal et al., 2009). A major difference concerns the interpretation of the subhippocampal lobe as the homolog of the dorsal pallium of tetrapods, as well as the consideration of the evaginated portion as a lateral pallium homolog, which was further subdivided into dorsal and ventral parts (Northcutt and Puzdrowski, 1988). With the postulation of the lamprey prosomeric model (Pombal and Puelles, 1999), the homology of the dorsal pallium was initially rejected and its previous name (subhippocampal lobe) adopted again. Finally, the most recent conception has recognized a putative ventral pallium homolog in the ventral part of the evaginated portion, whereas the subhippocampal lobe was interpreted as a portion of the amygdala, the pallial extended amygdala (Pombal et al., 2009; Martínez-de-la-Torre et al., 2011; Pombal and Megías, in press). A primordial amygdala was first recognized by Schnitzlein (1982), who described this structure as a mass of scattered cells at the ventromedial border of the primordial piriform. In addition, the classical primordium hippocampi of Johnston (1912) or medial pallium was considered as homolog of the prethalamic eminence (as already considered by several earlier authors; reviewed in Pombal et al., 2009). This interpretation is consistent with its topological position in relation with both, the interventricular

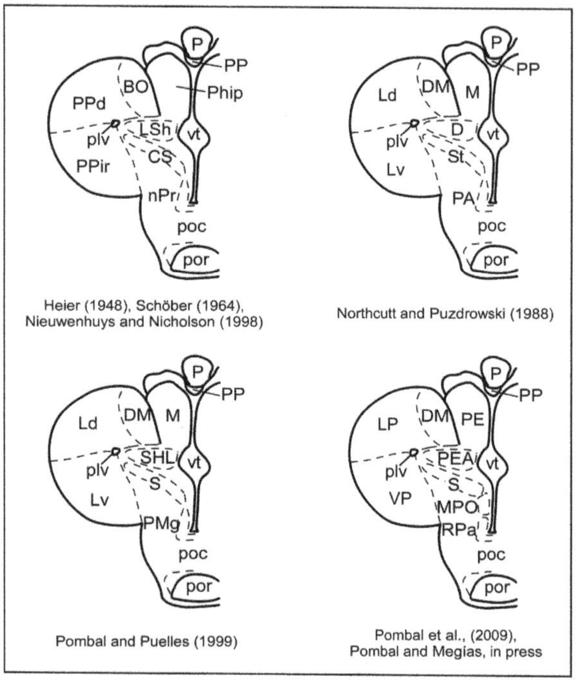

FIGURE 6 | Schematic drawings of a transverse section through the adult lamprey telencephalon and rostral hypothalamus showing the evolution of the nomenclature of the different nuclei and areas. BO, bulbus olfactorius; CS, corpus striatum; D, dorsal pallium; DM, dorsomedial telencephalic neuropile; Ld, lateral pallium, dorsal part; LP, lateral pallium; LSh; lobulus subhippocampalis; M, medial pallium; Lv, lateral pallium, ventral part; MPO, medial preoptic nucleus; nPr, nucleus preopticus; P, pineal organ; PA, preoptic area; PE, prethalamic eminence; PEA, pallial extended amygdala; Phip, primordium hippocampi; plv, posterior lateral ventricle; PMg, magnocellular preoptic nucleus; poc, postoptic commissure; por, postoptic recess; PP, parapineal; PPd, primordium pallium dorsalis; PPir, primordium piriforme; RPa, rostral paraventricular area; S, striatum; SHL, subhippocampal lobe; St, striatum; VP, ventral pallium; vt, impar telencephalic ventricle.

foramen and the velum transversum, as well as with the presence of *Lhx1/5* mRNA (Osório et al., 2006), a marker of the prethalamic eminence in tetrapods (Moreno et al., 2004). Moreover, the presence of a number of GABA-ir cells in this structure in adult lampreys (see **Figure 4C**) could be equally explained for both conceptions (it should be keep in mind that in gnathostome vertebrates GABAergic cells were reported in both of them): they could be originated as part of those migrating from the subpallium (medial pallium conception), or from the alar portion of the prethalamus, which also has *Dlx* expressing cells (Murakami et al., 2001; Myojin et al., 2001; Neidert et al., 2001; Kuraku et al., 2010) and DLL-ir cells (Martínez-de-la-Torre et al., 2011; prethalamic eminence conception).

Some progress regarding the regionalization of the adult lamprey forebrain has been recently achieved based on the specific presence of neurotransmitters or related neurochemicals, of neuroanatomical connections as well as of the expression pattern of a number of developmental regulatory genes. Some of them, such as *Pax6*, *Dlx1/6*, and *Lhx1/5*, are useful markers of different interprosomeric boundaries or their internal subdivisions. Concerning the telencephalon, *Pax6* is expressed in its dorsal (pallial) portion (Murakami et al., 2001; Derobert et al., 2002; Uchida et al., 2003; Osório et al., 2005; reviewed in Kuratani et al., 2002; Murakami et al., 2005; Murakami and Watanabe, 2009), whereas *Dlx1/6* is expressed ventrally (subpallium; Murakami et al., 2001; Myojin et al., 2001; Neidert et al., 2001; Kuraku et al., 2010; reviewed in Kuratani et al., 2002; Murakami et al., 2005; Murakami and Watanabe, 2009), therefore the boundary of their expressing areas do correspond to the pallial/subpallial boundary. This limit is also recognized with an antibody against the *Drosophila* distal-less protein (Martínez-de-la-Torre et al., 2011). In addition, *Emx* (a marker of the dorsal, medial, and lateral pallia in gnathostomes) is expressed in the dorsalmost portion of the primordial pallium in late embryos and early prolarvae (Myojin et al., 2001; reviewed in Kuratani et al., 2002; Murakami et al., 2005; Murakami and Watanabe, 2009). Though that more data are necessary, these results suggest that some of the major subdivisions of the gnathostome telencephalon are also present in lampreys.

CONCLUDING REMARKS

The lamprey forebrain undergoes some important topographical rearrangements during early postembryonic development, and, after that, it grows slowly through an extremely large larval period, with new born cells being added at different rates in virtually all the telencephalic subdivisions. Our detailed study on the distribution and morphological developmental pattern of the GABA-ir cells in the telencephalon of prolarvae reinforce the previously postulated subpallial/pallial migratory pathway in lampreys (Meléndez-Ferro et al., 2002a; Martínez-de-la-Torre et al., 2011), and also suggested for sharks (Carrera et al., 2008); therefore, the characteristic tangential neuronal migration from the subpallium to the pallium described in tetrapods is likely to be already present in agnathans and elasmobranch fishes.

Concerning the general telencephalic organization in lampreys, there is now a general agreement on the subpallial areas, with the recently included preoptic area, but less at pallial level, with new ideas and propositions coming out with the increasing amount of experimental data. In the recently proposed prosomeric model for lampreys, the alar plate of the secondary prosencephalon includes the new conception of the telencephalon, which encompasses the preoptic area, and the alar hypothalamus; in addition, the alar plate of p3 becomes quite enlarged due to the consideration of the classical medial pallium as part of the prethalamic eminence. The available results indicate that the lamprey telencephalon possess a more complex organization than previously though. The increasing data on gene expression, and their combination with chemoarchitectural and hodological techniques, will be useful tools for unraveling the characterization of the telencephalic regions and nuclei in lampreys, providing better comparisons with their counterparts in other vertebrates, in order to clarify the basic molecular mechanisms necessary to originate brain compartments as well as their evolution.

ACKNOWLEDGMENTS

This work was supported by Spanish MEC-FEDER (grant number BFU2006-14127), Spanish MICINN-FEDER (grant number BFU2009-13369), and University of Vigo (grant number 07V1A12).

REFERENCES

Ahlborn, F. (1883). Untersuchungen über das Gehirn der Petromyzonten. *Z. Wissensch. Zool.* XXXIX, 191–294.

Álvarez-Otero, R., Megías, M., and Pombal, M. A. (2002). "Postembryonic cell proliferation in the sea lamprey central nervous system," in *FENS Forum, Paris* (Abstr. A 137.1, 171).

Bergquist, H. (1952). Studies on the cerebral tube in vertebrates. The neuromeres. *Acta Zool.* 33, 117–187.

Bergquist, H., and Källén, B. (1953). Studies on the topography of the migration areas in the vertebrate brain. *Acta Anat. (Basel)* 17, 353–369.

Brox, A., Puelles, L., Ferreiro, B., and Medina, L. (2003). Expression of the genes GAD67 and Distal-less-4 in the forebrain of *Xenopus laevis* confirms a common pattern in tetrapods. *J. Comp. Neurol.* 461, 370–393.

Burckhardt, R. (1894). Zur Homologieen des Zwischenhirndaches und ihre Bedeutung für die Morphologie des Hirns bei niedern Vertebraten. *Anat. Anz.* IX, 152–155.

Carrera, I., Ferreiro-Galve, S., Sueiro, C., Anadón, R., and Rodríguez-Moldes, I. (2008). Tangentially migrating GABAergic cells of subpallial origin invade massively the pallium in developing sharks. *Brain Res. Bull.* 75, 405–409.

Cobos, I., Puelles, L., and Martínez, S. (2001). The avian telencephalic subpallium originates inhibitory neurons that invade tangentially the pallium (dorsal ventricular ridge and cortical areas). *Dev. Biol.* 239, 30–45.

Damas, H. (1944). Recherches sur le développement de *Lampetra fluviatilis* L. Contribution à l'étude de la céphalogenèse des vertébrés. *Arch. Biol.* 25, 1–284.

de Miguel, E., Rodicio, M. C., and Anadón, R. (1990). Organization of the visual system in larval lampreys: an HRP study. *J. Comp. Neurol.* 302, 529–542.

Derobert, Y., Baratte, B., Lepage, M., and Mazan, S. (2002). Pax6 expression patterns in *Lampetra fluviatilis* and *Scyliorhinus canicula* embryos suggest highly conserved roles in the early regionalization of the vertebrate brain. *Brain Res. Bull.* 57, 277–280.

Dirksen, M. L., Mathers, P., and Jamrich, M. (1993). Expression of a *Xenopus* distal-less homeobox gene involved in forebrain and cranio-facial development. *Mech. Dev.* 41, 121–128.

Edinger, L. (1888). Untersuchungen über die vergleichende Anatomie des Gehirns. I. Das Vorderhir*n*. *Abhandlungen der Senckenbergischen Naturforschenden Gesellschaft. Bd.* XV, 91–122.

Guérin, A., d'Aubenton-Carafa, Y., Marrakchi, E., Da Silva, C., Wincker, P., Mazan, S., and Rétaux, S. (2009). Neurodevelopment genes in lampreys reveal trends for forebrain evolution in craniates. *PLoS ONE* 4, e5374. doi: 10.1371/journal.pone.0005374

Hardisty, M. W., and Potter, I. C. (1971). "The behaviour, ecology and growth of larval lampreys," in *The Biology of Lampreys*, Vol. 1, eds M. W. Hardisty and I. C. Potter (London: Academic Press), 85–125.

Healey, E. G. (1972). "The central nervous system," in *The Biology of Lampreys*, Vol. 2, eds M. W. Hardisty and I. C. Potter (London: Academic Press), 307–372.

Heier, P. (1948). Fundamental principles in the structure of the brain. *Acta Anat.* VII, 1–213.

Herrick, C. J., and Obenchain, J. B. (1913). Notes on the anatomy of a cyclostome brain: ichthyomyzon concolor. *J. Comp. Neurol.* 23, 635–675.

Iwahori, N., Kiyota, E., and Nakamura, K. (1987). A Golgi study on the olfactory bulb in the lamprey, *Lampetra japonica*. *Neurosci. Res.* 5, 126–139.

Johnston, J. B. (1912). The telencephalon in cyclostomes. *J. Comp. Neurol.* 22, 341–404.

Källén, B. (1951). Contributions to the ontogeny of the nuclei and the ventricular sulci in the vertebrate forebrain. *Kungl. Fysiogr. Sällsk. Lund Handl. N. F.* 62, 5–34.

Kano, S., Xiao, J., Osório, J., Ekker, M., Hadzhiev, Y., Müller, F., Casane, D., Magdelenat, G., and Rétaux, S. (2010). Two lamprey hedgehog genes share non-coding regulatory sequences and expression patterns with gnathostome hedgehogs. *PLoS ONE* 5, e13332. doi: 10.1371/journal.pone.0013332

Kleerekoper, H. (1982). "The sense organs," in *The Biology of Lampreys*, Vol. 2, eds M. W. Hardisty and I. C. Potter (London: Academic Press), 373–404.

Kluge, B., Renault, N., and Rohr, K. B. (2005). Anatomical and molecular reinvestigation of lamprey endostyle development provides new insight into thyroid gland evolution. *Dev. Genes Evol.* 215, 32–40.

Kuraku, S., Takio, Y., Sugahara, F., Takechi, M., and Kuratani, S. (2010). Evolution of oropharyngeal patterning mechanisms involving Dlx and endothelins in vertebrates. *Dev. Biol.* 341, 315–323.

Kuratani, S., Kuraku, S., and Murakami, Y. (2002). Lamprey as an evo-devo model: lessons from comparative embryology and molecular phylogenetics. *Genesis* 34, 175–183.

Kuratani, S., Nobusada, Y., Horigome, N., and Shigetani, Y. (2001). Embryology of the lamprey and evolution of the vertebrate jaw: insights from molecular and developmental perspectives. *Philos. Trans. R. Soc. Lond., B, Biol. Sci.* 356, 1615–1632.

Marín, O., and Rubenstein, J. L. R. (2001). A long, remarkable journey: tangential migration in the telencephalon. *Nat. Rev. Neurosci.* 2, 780–790.

Marín, O., and Rubenstein, J. L. R. (2003). Cell migration in the forebrain. *Annu. Rev. Neurosci.* 26, 441–483.

Martínez-de-la-Torre, M., Pombal, M. A., and Puelles, L. (2011). Distal-less-like protein distribution in the larval lamprey forebrain. *Neuroscience* 178, 270–284.

Meeuwig, M. H., Bayer, J. M., and Reiche, R. A. (2006). Morphometric discrimination of early life stage *Lampetra tridentata* and *L. richardsoni* (Petromyzonidae) from the Columbia River Basin. *J. Morphol.* 267, 623–633.

Meléndez-Ferro, M., Pérez-Costas, E., Rodríguez-Muñoz, R., Gómez-López, M. P., Anadón, R., and Rodicio, M. C. (2001). GABA immunoreactivity in the olfactory bulbs of the adult sea lamprey *Petromyzon marinus* L. *Brain Res.* 893, 253–260.

Meléndez-Ferro, M., Pérez-Costas, E., Villar-Cheda, B., Abalo, X. M., Rodríguez-Muñoz, R., Rodicio, M. C., and Anadón, R. (2002a). Ontogeny of gamma-aminobutyric acid-immunoreactive neuronal populations in the forebrain and midbrain of the sea lamprey. *J. Comp. Neurol.* 446, 360–376.

Meléndez-Ferro, M., Villar-Cheda, B., Abalo, X. M., Pérez-Costas, E., Rodríguez-Muñoz, R., Degrip, W. J., Yáñez, J., Rodicio, M. C., and Anadón, R. (2002b). Early development of the retina and pineal complex in the sea lamprey: comparative immunocytochemical study. *J. Comp. Neurol.* 442, 250–265.

Ménard, A., Auclair, F., Bourcier-Lucas, C., Grillner, S., and Dubuc, R. (2007). Descending GABAergic projections to the mesencephalic locomotor region in the lamprey *Petromyzon marinus*. *J. Comp. Neurol.* 501, 260–273.

Moreno, N., Bachy, I., Rétaux, S., and González, A. (2004). LIM-homeodomain genes as developmental and adult genetic markers of *Xenopus* forebrain functional subdivisions. *J. Comp. Neurol.* 472, 52–72.

Moreno, N., González, A., and Rétaux, S. (2008). Evidences for tangential migrations in *Xenopus* telencephalon: developmental patterns and cell tracking experiments. *Dev. Neurobiol.* 68, 504–520.

Murakami, Y., Ogasawara, M., Sugahara, F., Hirano, S., Satoh, N., and Kuratani, S. (2001). Identification and expression of the lamprey Pax6 gene: evolutionary origin of the segmented brain of vertebrates. *Development* 128, 3521–3531.

Murakami, Y., Uchida, K., Rijli, F. M., and Kuratani, S. (2005). Evolution of the brain developmental plan: insights from agnathans. *Dev. Biol.* 280, 249–259.

Murakami, Y., and Watanabe, A. (2009). Development of the central and peripheral nervous systems in the lamprey. *Dev. Growth Diff.* 51, 197–205.

Myojin, M., Ueki, T., Sugahara, F., Murakami, Y., Shigetani, Y., Aizawa, S., Hirano, S., and Kuratani, S. (2001). Isolation of Dlx and Emx gene cognates in an agnathan species, *Lampetra japonica*, and their expression patterns during embryonic and larval development: conserved and diversified regulatory patterns of homeobox genes in vertebrate head evolution. *J. Exp. Zool.* 291, 68–84.

Neidert, A. H., Virupannavar, V., Hooker, G. W., and Langeland, J. A. (2001). Lamprey Dlx genes and early vertebrate evolution. *Proc. Natl. Acad. Sci. U.S.A.* 98, 1665–1670.

Nieuwenhuys, R., and Nicholson, C. (1998). "Lampreys, Petromyzontidae," in *The Central Nervous System of Vertebrates*, Vol. 1, eds R. Nieuwenhuys, H. J. ten Donkelaar, and C. Nicholson (Berlin: Springer-Verlag), 297–495.

Nikitina, N., Bronner-Fraser, M., and Sauka-Spengler, T. (2009). The sea lamprey *Petromyzon marinus*: a model for evolutionary and developmental biology. *Cold Spring Harb. Protoc.* 2009, pdb.emo113.

Northcutt, R. G., and Puzdrowski, R. L. (1988). Projections of the olfactory bulb and nervus terminalis in the silver lamprey. *Brain Behav. Evol.* 32, 96–107.

Northcutt, R. G., and Wicht, H. (1997). Afferent and efferent connections of the lateral and medial pallia of the silver lamprey. *Brain Behav. Evol.* 49, 1–19.

Ogasawara, M., Shigetani, Y., Suzuki, S., Kuratani, S., and Satoh, N. (2001). Expression of thyroid transcription factor-1 (TTF-1) gene in the ventral forebrain and endostyle of the agnathan vertebrate, *Lampetra japonica*. *Genesis* 30, 51–58.

Osório, J., Mazan, S., and Rétaux, S. (2005). Organisation of the lamprey (*Lampetra fluviatilis*) embryonic brain: insights from LIM-homeodomain, Pax and hedgehog genes. *Dev. Biol.* 288, 100–112.

Osório, J., Megías, M., Pombal, M. A., and Rétaux, S. (2006). Dynamic expression of the LIM-homeodomain gene Lhx15 through larval brain development of the sea lamprey (*Petromyzon marinus*). *Gene Expr. Patterns* 6, 873–878.

Osório, J., and Rétaux, S. (2008). The lamprey in evolutionary studies. *Dev. Genes. Evol.* 218, 221–235.

Pfister, C. (1971a). Die Matrix im Gehirn von Neunaugenembryonen (*Lampetra planeri*) (Bloch 1874). *Z. Mikrosk. Anat. Forsch.* 84, 485–492.

Pfister, C. (1971b). Die Matrixentwicklung in Tel- und Diencephalon von *Lampetra planeri* (Bloch) (Cyclostomata) im Verlaufe de Individualklus. *J. Hirnforsch.* 13, 363–375.

Pfister, C. (1971c). Die Matrixentwicklung in Mes- und rhombencephalon von *Lampetra planeri* (Bloch) (Cyclostomata) im Verlaufe de Individualzyklus. *J. Hirnforsch.* 13, 377–383.

Piavis, G. W. (1961). Embryological stages in the sea lamprey and effects of temperature on development. *U.S. Fish Wildl. Serv. Fish. Bull.* 61, 111–143.

Piavis, G. W. (1971). "Embryology," in *The Biology of Lampreys*, Vol. 1, eds M. W. Hardisty and I. C. Potter (London: Academic Press), 361–400.

Polenova, O. A., and Vesselkin, N. P. (1993). Olfactory and nonolfactory projections in the river lamprey (*Lampetra fluviatilis*) telencephalon. *J. Hirnforsch.* 34, 261–279.

Pombal, M. A., de Arriba, M. C., Sampedro, C., Alvarez, R., and Megías, M. (2002). Immunocytochemical localization of calretinin in the olfactory system of the adult lamprey, *Lampetra fluviatilis. Brain Res. Bull.* 57, 281–283.

Pombal, M. A., El Manira, A., and Grillner, S. (1997). Organization of the lamprey striatum – transmitters and projections. *Brain Res.* 766, 249–254.

Pombal, M. A., and Megías, M. (in press). "Functional morphology of the brain of agnathans," in *Encyclopedia of Fish Physiology: From Genome to Environment*, ed. T. Farrel (San Diego: Academic Press).

Pombal, M. A., Megías, M., Bardet, S. M., and Puelles, L. (2009). New and old thoughts on the segmental organization of the forebrain in lampreys. *Brain Behav. Evol.* 74, 7–19.

Pombal, M. A., and Puelles, L. (1999). Prosomeric map of the lamprey forebrain based on calretinin immunocytochemistry, Nissl stain, and ancillary markers. *J. Comp. Neurol.* 414, 391–422.

Pombal, M. A., Rodicio, M. C., and Anadón, R. (1994). Development and organization of the ocular motor nuclei in the larval sea lamprey, *Petromyzon marinus* L.: an HRP study. *J. Comp. Neurol.* 341, 393–406.

Puelles, L., Kuwana, E., Puelles, E., Bulfone, A., Shimamura, K., Keleher, J., Smiga, S., and Rubenstein, J. L. (2000). Pallial and subpallial derivatives in the embryonic chick and mouse telencephalon, traced by the expression of the genes Dlx-2, Emx-1, Nkx-2.1, Pax-6, and Tbr-1. *J. Comp. Neurol.* 424, 409–438.

Ren, X., Chang, S., Laframboise, A., Green, W., Dubuc, R., and Zielinski, B. (2009). Projections from the accessory olfactory organ into the medial region of the olfactory bulb in the sea lamprey (*Petromyzon marinus*): a novel vertebrate sensory structure? *J. Comp. Neurol.* 516, 105–116.

Richardson, M. K., Admiraal, J., and Wright, G. M. (2010). Developmental anatomy of lampreys. *Biol. Rev. Camb. Philos. Soc.* 85, 1–33.

Richardson, M. K., and Wright, G. M. (2003). Developmental transformations in a normal series of embryos of the sea lamprey *Petromyzon marinus* (Linnaeus). *J. Morphol.* 257, 348–363.

Robertson, B., Auclair, F., Ménard, A., Grillner, S., and Dubuc, R. (2007). GABA distribution in lamprey is phylogenetically conserved. *J. Comp. Neurol.* 503, 47–63.

Robertson, B., Saitoh, K., Ménard, A., and Grillner, S. (2006). Afferents of the lamprey optic tectum with special reference to the GABA input: combined tracing and immunohistochemical study. *J. Comp. Neurol.* 499, 106–119.

Rodicio, M. C., Pombal, M. A., and Anadón, R. (1995). Early development and organization of the retinopetal system in the larval sea lamprey, *Petromyzon marinus* L. An HRP study. *Anat. Embryol. (Berl.)* 192, 517–526.

Rodríguez-Muñoz, R., Nicieza, A., and Braña, F. (2001). Effects of temperature on developmental performance, survival and growth of sea lamprey embryos. *J. Fish. Biol.* 58, 475–486.

Ronan, M., and Northcutt, R. G. (1998). "The central nervous system of hagfishes," in *The Biology of Hagfishes*, eds J. M. Jorgensen, J. P. Lomholt, R. E. Weber, and H. Malte (London: Chapman & Hall), 452–479.

Rovainen, C. M. (1982). "Neurophysiology," in *The Biology of Lampreys*, Vol. 4, eds M. W. Hardisty and I. C. Potter (London: Academic Press), 1–136.

Rubin, A. N., Alfonsi, F., Humphreys, M. P., Choi, C. K. P., Rocha, S. F., and Kessaris, N. (2010). The germinal zones of the basal ganglia but not the septum generate GABAergic interneurons for the cortex. *J. Neurosci.* 30, 12050–12062.

Rubinson, K. (1990). The developing visual system and metamorphosis in the lamprey. *J. Neurobiol.* 21, 1123–1135.

Ruiz, Y., Pombal, M. A., and Megías, M. (2004). Development of GABA-immunoreactive cells in the spinal cord of the sea lamprey, *P. marinus. J. Comp. Neurol.* 470, 151–163.

Schnitzlein, H. N. (1982). "Cyclostomes," in *Comparative Correlative Neuroanatomy of the Vertebrate Telencephalon*, eds E. C. Crosby and H. N. Schnitzlein (New York: Macmillan Press), 4–26.

Schöber, W. (1964). Vergleichend-anatomische Untersuchungen am Gehirn der Larven und adulten Tiere von *Lampetra fluvialis* (Linné, 1758) und *Lampetra planeri* (Bloch, 1984). *J. Hirnforsch.* 7, 107–209.

Schultze, M. S. (1856). *Die Entwickelungs-Geschichte von Petromyzon planeri.* Harlem: Loosjes.

Scott, W. B. (1887). Notes on the development of Petromyzon. *J. Morphol.* 1, 253–310.

Shipley, A. E. (1887). On some points in the development of *Petromyzon fluviatilis. Q. J. Microsc. Sci.* 27, 325–370.

Sterzi, G. (1907). *Il Sistema Nervoso Centrale dei Vertebrati. Ricerche Anatomiche ed Embriologiche, Vol.* 1. *Ciclostomi.* Padova: Angelo Draghi.

Tahara, Y. (1988). Normal stages of development in the lamprey, *Lampetra reissneri* (Dybowski). *Zool. Sci.* 5, 109–118.

Tobet, S. A., Chickering, T. W., King, J. C., Stopa, E. G., Kim, K., Kuo-Leblank, V., and Schwarting, G. A. (1996). Expression of gamma-aminobutyric acid and gonadotropin-releasing hormone during neuronal migration through the olfactory system. *Endocrinology* 137, 5415–5420.

Uchida, K., Murakami, Y., Kuraku, S., Hirano, S., and Kuratani, S. (2003). Development of the adenohypophysis in the lamprey: evolution of epigenetic patterning programs in organogenesis. *J. Exp. Zool. B Mol. Dev. Evol.* 300, 32–47.

VanDenbossche, J., Seelye, J. G., and Zielinski, B. S. (1995). The morphology of the olfactory epithelium in larval, juvenile and upstream migrant stages of the sea lamprey, *Petromyzon marinus. Brain Behav. Evol.* 45, 19–24.

Vidal-Pizarro, I., Swain, G. P., and Selzer, M. E. (2004). Cell proliferation in the lamprey central nervous system. *J. Comp. Neurol.* 469, 298–310.

Villar-Cerviño, V., Barreiro-Iglesias, A., Anadón, R., and Rodicio, M. C. (2009). Development of glycine immunoreactivity in the brain of the sea lamprey: comparison with gamma-aminobutyric acid immunoreactivity. *J. Comp. Neurol.* 512, 747–767.

Villar-Cerviño, V., Holstein, G. R., Martinelli, G. P., Anadón, R., and Rodicio, M. C. (2008). Glycine-immunoreactive neurons in the developing spinal cord of the sea lamprey: comparison with the gamma-aminobutyric acidergic system. *J. Comp. Neurol.* 508, 112–130.

Villar-Cheda, B., Pérez-Costas, E., Meléndez-Ferro, M., Abalo, X. M., Rodríguez-Muñoz, R., Anadón, R., and Rodicio, M. C. (2002). Proliferating cell nuclear antigen (PCNA) immunoreactivity and development of the pineal complex and habenula of the sea lamprey. *Brain Res. Bull.* 57, 285–287.

Villar-Cheda, B., Pérez-Costas, E., Meléndez-Ferro, M., Abalo, X. M., Rodríguez-Muñoz, R., Anadón, R., and Rodicio, M. C. (2006). Cell proliferation in the forebrain and midbrain of the sea lamprey. *J. Comp. Neurol.* 494, 986–1006.

von Kupffer, K. (1906). "Die Morphogenie des Centralnervensystems," in *Handbuch der Vergleichenden und Experimentellen Entwicklungslehre der Wirbeltiere*, Vol. 2, Part III, ed. O. Hertwig (Jena: Fisher), 1–272.

Watanabe, A., Hirano, S., and Murakami, Y. (2008). Development of the lamprey central nervous system, with reference to vertebrate evolution. *Zool. Sci.* 25, 1020–1027.

Weigle, C., and Northcutt, R. G. (1999). The chemoarchitecture of the forebrain of lampreys: evolutionary implications by comparisons with gnathostomes. *Eur. J. Morphol.* 37, 122–125.

Wicht, H., and Nieuwenhuys, R. (1998). "Hagfishes (Myxinoidea)," in *The Central Nervous System of Vertebrates*, Vol. 1, eds R. Nieuwenhuys, H. J. ten Donkelaar, and C. Nicholson. (Berlin: Springer-Verlag), 497–549.

Yáñez, J., and Anadón, R. (1994). Afferent and efferent connections of the habenula in the larval sea lamprey (*Petromyzon marinus* L.): an experimental study. *J. Comp. Neurol.* 345, 148–160.

Zielinski, B. S., Fredricks, K., McDonald, R., and Zaidi, A. U. (2005). Morphological and electrophysiological examination of olfactory sensory neurons during the early developmental prolarval stage of the sea lamprey *Petromyzon marinus* L. *J. Neurocytol.* 34, 209–216.

Conflict of Interest Statement: The authors declare that the research was conducted in the absence of any commercial or financial relationships that could be construed as a potential conflict of interest.

9

GABAergic projections to the oculomotor nucleus in the goldfish (*Carassius auratus*)

M. Angeles Luque, Julio Torres-Torrelo, Livia Carrascal, Blas Torres, Luis Herrero*

Department of Physiology and Zoology, University of Seville, Seville, Spain

Edited by:
Fernando Martinez-Garcia, Universidad de Valencia, Spain

Reviewed by:
Hans Straka, Ludwig Maximilian University Munich, Germany
Julian Yañez, University of A Coruña, Spain

***Correspondence:**
Luis Herrero, Departamento de Fisiología y Zoología, Facultad de Biología, Avenida Reina Mercedes 6, 41012 Sevilla, Spain.
e-mail: lherrero@us.es

The mammalian oculomotor nucleus receives a strong γ-aminobutyric acid (GABA)ergic synaptic input, whereas such projections have rarely been reported in fish. In order to determine whether this synaptic organization is preserved across vertebrates, we investigated the GABAergic projections to the oculomotor nucleus in the goldfish by combining retrograde transport of biotin dextran amine, injected into the antidromically identified oculomotor nucleus, and GABA immunohistochemistry. The main source of GABAergic afferents to the oculomotor nucleus was the ipsilateral anterior octaval nucleus, with only a few, if any, GABAergic neurons being located in the contralateral tangential and descending nuclei of the octaval column. In mammals there is a nearly exclusive ipsilateral projection from vestibular neurons to the oculomotor nucleus *via* GABAergic inhibitory inputs; thus, the vestibulooculomotor GABAergic circuitry follows a plan that appears to be shared throughout the vertebrate phylogeny. The second major source of GABAergic projections was the rhombencephalic reticular formation, primarily from the medial area but, to a lesser extent, from the inferior area. A few GABAergic oculomotor projecting neurons were also observed in the ipsilateral nucleus of the medial longitudinal fasciculus. The GABAergic projections from neurons located in both the reticular formation surrounding the abducens nucleus and the nucleus of the medial reticular formation have primarily been related to the control of saccadic eye movements. Finally, all retrogradely labeled internuclear neurons of the abducens nucleus, and neurons in the cerebellum (close to the caudal lobe), were negative for GABA. These data suggest that the vestibuloocular and saccadic inhibitory GABAergic systems appear early in vertebrate phylogeny to modulate the firing properties of the oculomotor nucleus motoneurons.

Keywords: oculomotor system, vestibuloocular reflex, saccadic eye movements, GABA immunohistochemistry, fish

INTRODUCTION

Based on immunohistochemical studies, the mammalian oculomotor nucleus has been reported to receive a strong γ-aminobutyric acid (GABA)ergic synaptic input (de la Cruz et al., 1992; Spencer et al., 1992; Wentzel et al., 1996). Electrophysiological investigations have demonstrated an ipsilateral disynaptic inhibition from the labyrinth to the oculomotor nucleus motoneurons; this inhibitory postsynaptic potential is blocked by the GABA antagonists bicuculline and picrotoxin (Ito et al., 1970; Highstein, 1973; Precht et al., 1973; Uchino and Suzuki, 1983). These data, together with those showing a high density of GABA-immunoreactive vestibular neurons (Highstein and Holstein, 2006), suggest that this neurotransmitter plays a key role in mediating the vertical vestibuloocular reflex (Highstein and McCrea, 1988). It has also been proposed that GABA is utilized as an inhibitory neurotransmitter by premotor neurons related to the control of horizontal and vertical saccadic eye movements (de la Cruz et al., 1992; Spencer and Wang, 1996; Horn et al., 2003). The oculomotor system in the goldfish provides a suitable model for comparative research as these animals exhibit compensatory eye movements in response to head and visual-field displacements, together with a marked pattern of spontaneous saccades in the horizontal plane (Easter, 1971; Pastor et al., 1992; Keng and Anastasio, 1997; Mensh et al., 2004). The motoneurons innervating the eye muscles in the goldfish lie in similar locations to those found in other vertebrates (Graf and McGurk, 1985), and their firing properties resemble those reported in both cats and monkeys (Delgado-Garcia et al., 1986a; Fuchs et al., 1988; de la Cruz et al., 1989). Furthermore, the extraocular motor nuclei in the goldfish show GABAergic innervation, and the stimulation of the vestibular nerve produces ipsilateral inhibitory postsynaptic potentials (Graf et al., 1997). Finally, the structures projecting to the ocular motor nuclei in the goldfish are similar to those reported in mammals (Allum et al., 1981; Torres et al., 1992, 1995). Based on these similarities, the present study was designed to investigate the GABAergic projections to the oculomotor nucleus in the goldfish, in order to determine if this inhibitory circuitry is preserved throughout vertebrate phylogeny.

MATERIALS AND METHODS

Experiments were carried out in 10–15 cm long goldfish (*Carassius auratus*), which were obtained from local suppliers. All studies were performed in accordance with the European Community Directive 2003/65, as well as with the Spanish Royal Decree 120/2005 and University of Seville regulations on the care of laboratory animals. Under general anesthesia (tricaine methanesulfonate, MS222, 1:2000 wt/vol, Sigma-Aldrich), the animal was clamped between two sponge rubber pads inside a home-made Perspex water chamber. The mouth was fitted to a plastic tube connected to a well aerated recirculating system propelled by a pump to ensure a constant flow over the gills. The cranial bones and the tissues overlying the tectal and telencephalic lobes were gently removed to avoid bleeding, after which an insulated silver (250 μm diameter) bipolar electrode was implanted in the left oculomotor nerve with a micromanipulator (**Figure 1A**). The final location of the stimulating electrode was such that a single short pulse (50 μs) of low current strength (<100 μA) evoked a twitch of the medial rectus muscle, leading to a nasally directed eye movement. The left oculomotor nucleus was identified by recording the antidromic field potential (**Figure 1B**) with a 2-M NaCl-filled glass micropipette (1–5 MΩ). This microelectrode was then exchanged for a glass micropipette (10–15 μm tip diameter) filled with 10% biotin dextran amine (BDA, Invitrogen) in phosphate buffered saline (PBS, 0.1 M, pH = 7.4). The micropipette was driven to the oculomotor nucleus, which was again identified based on the antidromic field potential. Cathodal pulses (10 s on followed by 5 s off) of 5–7 μA were delivered over a period of 15–20 min. After injection, the piece of bone removed during surgery was restored and fixed in place.

Following 7–10 days of postoperative survival time, the fish was again anesthetized in MS222, then transcardially perfused with 100 ml teleost Ringer's solution, followed by 200 ml of a fixative solution (4% paraformaldehyde, 0.08% glutaraldehyde, and 15% picric acid in 0.1M phosphate buffer, pH = 7.4). The brain was removed from the skull and cut serially in a cryostat into 50 μm transverse sections. Free-floating sections were washed in PBS and incubated for 1 h at room temperature in 10% normal goat serum (Sigma-Aldrich). They were then exposed to rabbit anti-GABA (1:1000, Sigma-Aldrich) overnight at room temperature and to goat anti-rabbit IgG-Cy3 (1:400, Jackson Immunoresearch) for 2 h. To visualize the BDA tracer, the sections were treated with 2% fetal bovine serum for 1 h, before being incubated with antibiotin-FITC (1:120, Sigma-Aldrich) for 2 h. To reveal the location of the injection site in relation to the oculomotor nucleus, the motoneurons were immunohistochemically stained for choline acetyl transferase (ChAT). Transverse mesencephalic sections were incubated with 3% rabbit serum for 1 h, followed by a solution of goat anti-ChAT antibody (1:100, Millipore) overnight at room temperature, and rabbit anti-goat IgG-Cy3 (1:200, Jackson ImmunoResearch Labs.) for 2 h. All solutions were prepared in a PBS solution containing 0.3% Triton X-100. Furthermore, the specificity of the immunolabeling was tested by incubating some sections without the primary antibody. Additional information about the specificity of the primary antibody used in the present study was provided by Sigma; that is, rabbit anti-GABA shows positive binding with GABA, in a dot blot assay, and negative binding with BSA. Finally, the sections were placed on gelatinized glass slides and coverslipped with fluorescent mounting medium (Dako Cytomation). Sections were first analyzed using a fluorescence microscope (Olympus BX61), then photographed in a confocal microscope (Leica TCS-SP2). Data were collected from six experiments in which the central core of the injection site lay in the oculomotor nucleus, the BDA retrograde transport was deemed to be effective because stained cells were located as distant as the inferior rhombencephalic reticular formation, and GABA showed good penetration (>60% of the section thickness). Both retrogradely labeled and GABA-positive cells were scored (stated as mean ± SE) and mapped onto transverse schematics. Ipsilateral and contralateral neurons were depicted relative to the injection side. The average somal diameter (long axis + short axis/2) was measured. The nomenclature adopted in this study was that used by McCormick and Bradford (1994) and Meek and Nieuwenhuys (1998).

RESULTS

The location of the injection site within the oculomotor nucleus was first determined by the antidromic field potential evoked following the electrical microstimulation of the third nerve (**Figure 1A**). This field potential was characterized by a prominent negative voltage wave with a latency of less than 1 ms from the stimulus onset to the negative peak. The amplitude of the negative peak increased toward the center of the oculomotor nucleus (**Figure 1B**). In all cases (n = 6), the antidromic potential was recorded along 300–600 μm in the dorso-ventral axis and exhibited a negative peak larger than 0.4 mV. The injection site was also characterized by the extent of the central core and spread area of the BDA tracer in relation to the labeling of the motoneurons (revealed by ChAT immunohistochemistry). The central core of the injection site was confined to the oculomotor cellular column close to the midline (**Figures 1C,D**), extending from the rostral to the caudal pole of the nucleus (~500 μm). In other words, the region of effective BDA uptake included all motoneuronal pools (that is, the motoneurons innervating the ipsilateral medial rectus, the inferior rectus, and the inferior oblique eye muscles) of the oculomotor nucleus in the goldfish (Graf and McGurk, 1985). In the contralateral (non-injected) oculomotor nucleus, some cell bodies positive for both ChAT and BDA were observed (see arrow in **Figure 1D**); these probably correspond to the motoneurons innervating the contralateral superior rectus and/or superior oblique eye muscles. However, the vast majority of the cells in the non-injected nucleus (see arrowheads in **Figure 1D**) were only positive for ChAT, even though they were located close to the midline. The spread area of the injection site reached the dorso-lateral aspects of the oculomotor nucleus (where some of the motoneurons innervating the ipsilateral inferior rectus and inferior oblique eye muscles are located), the ipsilateral medial longitudinal fasciculus and, to a lesser extent, the contralateral oculomotor nucleus.

Retrogradely labeled GABA-positive neurons were more numerous in the octaval column nuclei, less abundant within the rhombencephalic reticular formation, and very scarce within the nucleus of the medial longitudinal fasciculus (**Figure 2**). Within the nuclei of the octaval column, GABAergic neurons projecting to the oculomotor nucleus were located almost exclusively in the ipsilateral anterior octaval nucleus, and only occasionally in the contralateral tangential and descending nuclei. A group of labeled neurons (31.7 ± 3.4) was found in the ipsilateral anterior octaval nucleus and, of these cells, a high proportion were also positive for GABA (~45%; **Figures 2C,D and 3A**). Single- and double-labeled cells, the somata of which were spherical or multipolar (19.6 ± 3.4 μm), were arranged in a rounded cluster, located in the cerebellar peduncle rostral to the entry of the eighth nerve. The axons of these cells traveled toward the ipsilateral medial longitudinal fasciculus, and in some cases were also positive for GABA (**Figure 3B**). In addition, a few stained neurons were located in

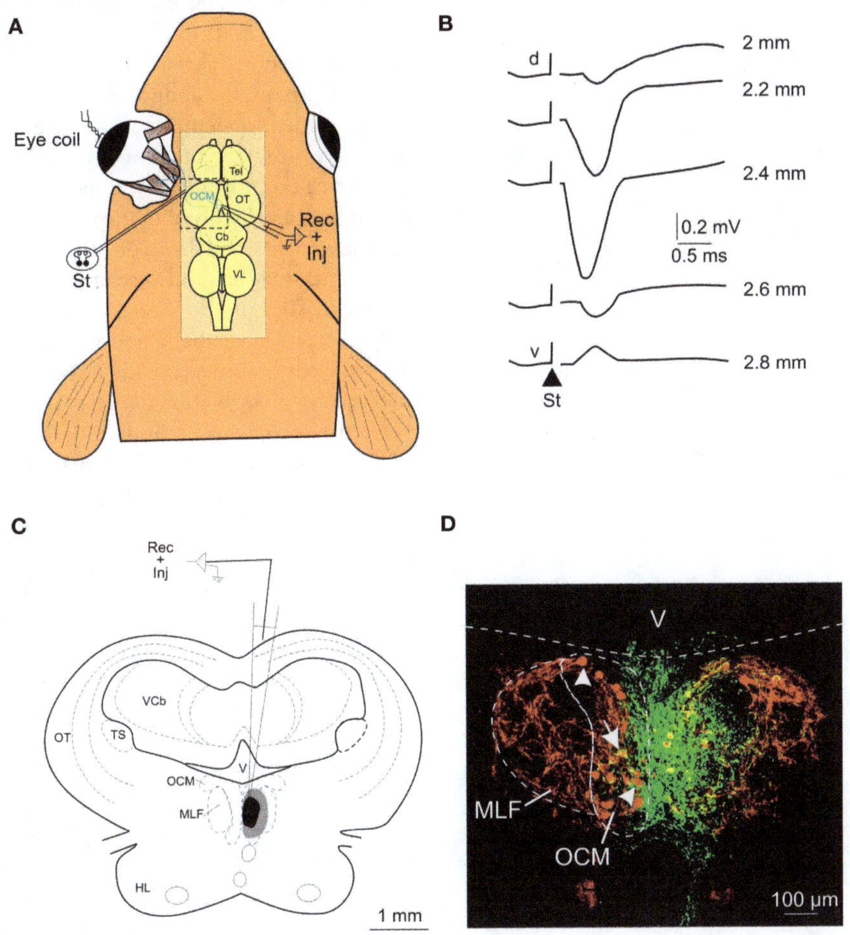

FIGURE 1 | Electrophysiological identification of the oculomotor nucleus and location of the injection site. (A) Schematic representation of the experimental design for the antidromic identification of the oculomotor nucleus following electrical stimulation (St) of the third cranial nerve. The location of the oculomotor nucleus and the trajectory of the third nerve are schematically illustrated in blue. **(B)** Antidromic field potentials recorded in the oculomotor nucleus following oculomotor nerve stimulation (St; triangle shows the onset of the stimulus). Recordings were obtained at several depths (indicated in mm) as the electrode was driven from the dorsal (d) to the ventral (v) part of the nucleus. **(C)** Schematic drawing showing the location of the BDA injection site at the level of the oculomotor nucleus; the central core is shown in black and the spread area of the injection site in gray. **(D)** Confocal photomicrograph of the injection site. The green area corresponds to the deposit of BDA and the motoneurons are stained in red after immunohistochemistry against ChAT. Some ChAT-positive motoneurons (arrowheads) and a double-labeled motoneuron (arrow) can be seen contralateral to the injected oculomotor nucleus. Anatomical abbreviations in **Figure 2**.

the contralateral anterior octaval nucleus (6.6 ± 1.9) and in the contralateral magnocellular nucleus (5.1 ± 3.1), but none of these was positive for GABA (**Figures 2C,D**). Caudal to the anterior octaval nucleus, labeled neurons were observed in the contralateral tangential (31.4 ± 7.3) and descending (33.5 ± 5.7) octaval nuclei. Although a few (<5 per experiment) of the cells in these two nuclei were also positive for GABA, such double-labeled cells were only observed in two of the six cases analyzed. The somata of these double-labeled neurons were spherical (18.6 ± 1.7 µm) and fusiform (18.1 ± 2.1 µm), respectively, in the tangential and descending nuclei.

Retrogradely labeled neurons, some of which were positive for GABA (<25%, for each side), were also found in the rhombencephalic reticular formation (**Figures 2E–I**), distributed bilaterally in relation to the injection site, but with contralateral predominance. These cells, which were mainly multipolar (21.5 ± 3.4 µm; **Figures 3C,D**), were located throughout the medial reticular area (contralateral, 25.2 ± 6.7; ipsilateral, 15.3 ± 5.8), and in the rostral pole of the inferior reticular area (contralateral, 12.8 ± 3.2; ipsilateral, 5.1 ± 1.9). Occasionally (three of six experiments), neurons were also observed in the caudal pole of the superior reticular area. In addition, neurons projecting to the oculomotor nucleus were bilaterally placed in the nucleus of the medial longitudinal fasciculus or close to it (ipsilateral, 7.5 ± 3.2; contralateral 3.3 ± 3.2); a few of these cells (<2 per experiment), lying ipsilateral to the injection site, were also positive for GABA. Finally, GABA-negative neurons (putative eurydendroid cells) were found just above the granular cell layer of the cerebellar vestibulolateral lobe (23.2 ± 4.1; **Figures 2C,D**) and close to the contralateral caudal abducens nucleus (putative abducens internuclear neurons). These latter neurons were distributed in two separated clusters: one close to the caudal abducens nucleus (18.1 ± 5.1, **Figure 2F**) and the other one posterior to it (17.2 ± 6.7, not illustrated).

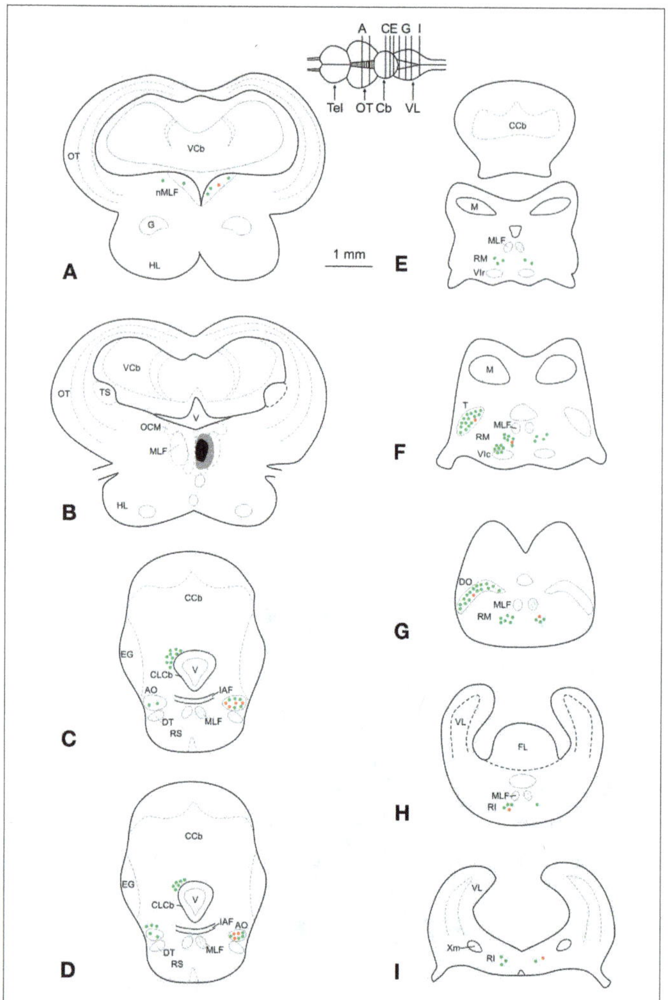

FIGURE 2 | (A–I) Schematic maps of transverse sections through the mesencephalon and the rhombencephalon in a representative experiment, illustrating the injection site, as well as the location of retrogradely labeled GABA-immunonegative (green dots) and GABA-immunoreactive (red dots) neurons. Each dot corresponds to two labeled neurons. Abbreviations: AO, anterior octaval nucleus; Cb, cerebellum; CCb, corpus cerebelli; CLCb, caudal lobe of the cerebellum; DO, descending octaval nucleus; DT, descending trigeminal tract; EG, eminentia granularis; FL, facial lobe; G, nucleus glomerulosus; HL, hypothalamic lobe; IAF, internal arcuate fibers; M, nucleus medialis; MLF, medial longitudinal fasciculus; nMLF, nucleus of the medial longitudinal fasciculus; OCM, oculomotor nucleus; OT, optic tectum; RI, inferior rhombencephalic reticular formation; RM, medial rhombencephalic reticular formation; RS, superior rhombencephalic reticular formation; T, tangential nucleus; Tel, telencephalon; TS, torus semicircularis; V, ventricle; VCb, cerebellar valvula; VIc, caudal subdivision of the abducens nucleus; VIr, rostral subdivision of the abducens nucleus; VL, vagal lobe; Xm, vagal motor nucleus.

DISCUSSION

The present study demonstrates for the first time that the teleost oculomotor nucleus receives GABAergic projections from neurons lying in the nuclei of the octaval column, in the rhombencephalic reticular formation, and in the nucleus of the medial longitudinal fasciculus. In contrast, all of the retrogradely labeled neurons that we observed in the contralateral abducens nucleus and the vestibulolateral lobe of the cerebellum were GABA negative. These results are discussed in the context of available information in mammals and interpreted in a functional context.

In mammals, the abducens nucleus is formed by motoneurons and internuclear neurons which project to the ipsilateral lateral rectus eye muscle and to the contralateral medial rectus population of the oculomotor nucleus, respectively. The abducens nucleus is physiologically involved in the generation of conjugate horizontal eye movements, which are produced by the contraction of the lateral rectus muscle in one eye and the medial rectus muscle in the other eye. The burst-tonic activity in abducens motoneurons drives the contraction of the lateral rectus muscle, while the abducens internuclear neurons provide a similar signal to the contralateral medial rectus population of the oculomotor nucleus, which innervates the medial rectus muscle (Delgado-Garcia et al., 1986a,b; Fuchs et al., 1988). The abducens internuclear synaptic endings labeled by anterograde transport are immunoreactive for glutamate and/or aspartate, which is consistent with the physiological and morphological features of the excitatory inputs to the medial rectus motoneurons (Nguyen and Spencer, 1999). The abducens internuclear neurons have already been proposed in the goldfish by retrograde labeling studies (Cabrera et al., 1992). This proposal is supported by the present findings which demonstrate that the abducens internuclear neurons in goldfish are not inhibitory, at least not *via* GABAergic input to the oculomotor nucleus. The vestibulolateral lobe, consisting of the eminentia granularis and the caudal lobe, is one of the cerebellar subdivisions in teleosts. Various findings have implicated the vestibulateral lobe in the teleost oculomotor system network: electrical microstimulation of this region elicits ipsiversive horizontal eye movements, and its Purkinje cells exhibit eye-velocity-related activity (Pastor et al., 1997). Furthermore, the eminentia granularis receives mechano- or vestibulo-sensitive inputs from numerous hindbrain sources, and Purkinje cells directly project from the caudal lobe to the vestibular nuclei (Straka et al., 2006). Another source of direct cerebellar output is provided by the eurydendroid cells (Finger, 1978; Ikenaga et al., 2005), which are equivalent to mammalian deep cerebellar nucleus neurons. Eurydendroid cells could underlie the efferent output from the cerebellar vestibulolateral lobe to the oculomotor nucleus, given the similarity of their somato-dendritic morphology (Torres et al., 1992) and their putative non-inhibitory character (as shown here, labeled cells were negative for GABA). Furthermore, this pathway seems to be particular to fish, as it has not been reported in mammals (Torres et al., 1992).

In mammals, the rostral interstitial nucleus of the medial longitudinal fasciculus and the interstitial nucleus of Cajal are located rostral to the oculomotor nucleus. These two nuclei, which contain premotor neurons that are related to vertical upward, downward, and torsional saccadic eye movements, project to the oculomotor nucleus, predominantly on the ipsilateral side (reviewed in Horn, 2006). Anatomical studies have revealed GABAergic neurons in the rostral interstitial nucleus of the medial longitudinal fasciculus and interstitial nucleus of Cajal projecting to the oculomotor nucleus, and these neurons could contribute to the control of vertical eye movements (Spencer and Wang, 1996; Horn et al., 2003). Studies of the region rostral to the oculomotor nucleus in the goldfish, which includes the nucleus of the medial longitudinal fasciculus,

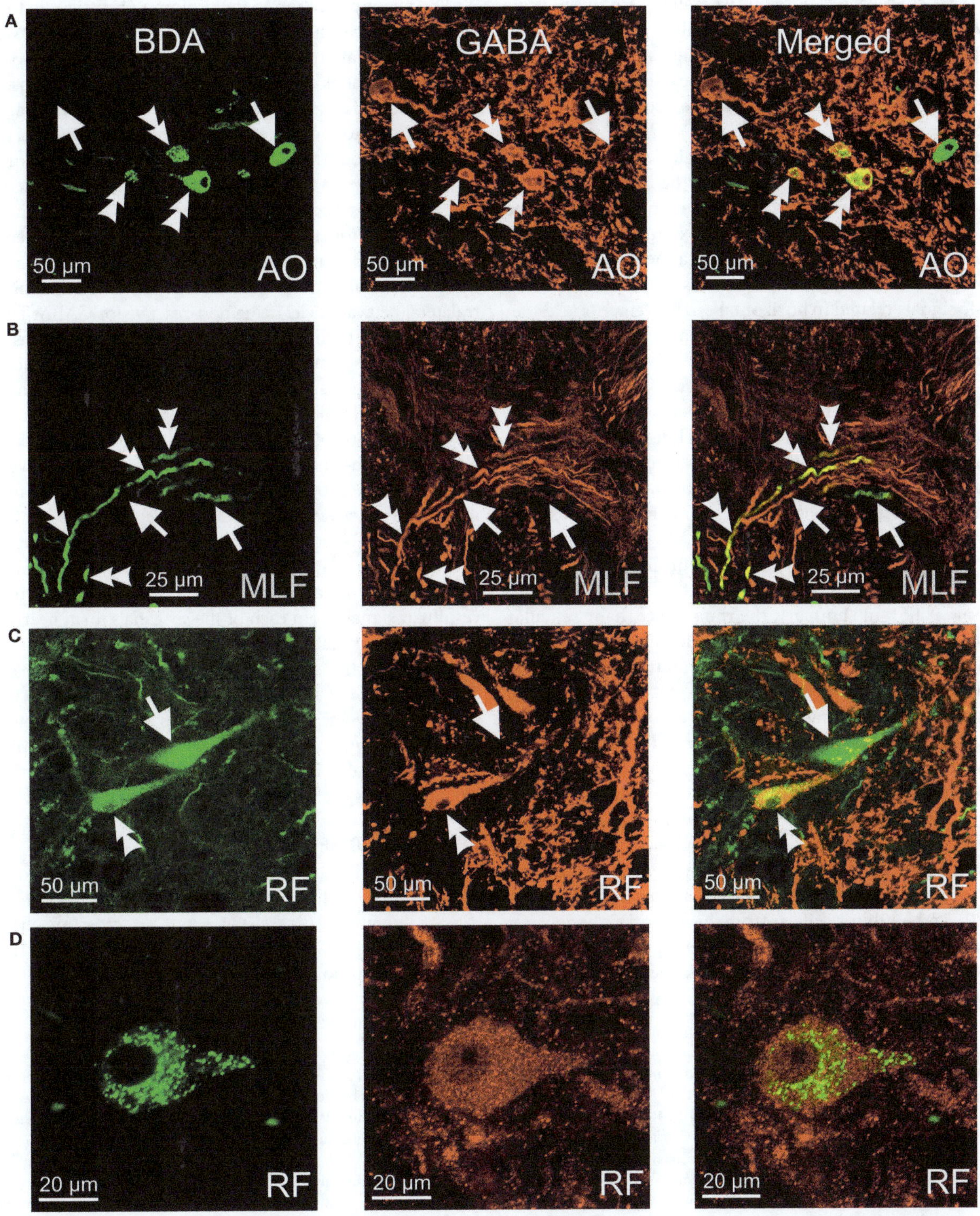

FIGURE 3 | Confocal photomicrographs of retrogradely labeled (green), GABA-immunoreactive (red) and double-labeled (yellow) neurons and fibers. (A) Neurons in the anterior octaval nucleus (AO). **(B)** Axons running from the anterior octaval nucleus to the medial longitudinal fasciculus (MLF). **(C,D)** Neurons in the rhombencephalic reticular formation (RF). Double arrowheads indicate double-labeled cells and fibers; arrows indicate labeled cells/fibers positive for retrograde tracer or for GABA.

have suggested that it is involved in locomotion (Kobayashi et al., 2009) but could also contribute to the encoding of vertical and horizontal saccadic eye movements (Luque et al., 2006). Neurons located within the nucleus of the medial longitudinal fasciculus or close to it were bilaterally labeled, with ipsilateral predominance, following the injection of the BDA into the oculomotor nucleus, and some of these cells (all located ipsilaterally) were also positive for GABA. Based on these findings, the possibility remains that the nucleus of the medial longitudinal fasciculus and its surrounding area in the goldfish could contribute to eye-body movements, similar to those nuclei located rostral to the oculomotor nucleus in mammals.

The second major projection of GABAergic neurons to the oculomotor nucleus in the goldfish was from the rhombencephalic reticular formation. These neurons were mainly located in the medial reticular region and, to a lesser extent, in the inferior reticular region. In functional terms, reticular neurons surrounding the rostral and caudal abducens nucleus exhibit phasic–tonic and phasic signals related to horizontal eye movements (Gestrin and Sterling, 1977). Caudal to the abducens nucleus, the activity of neurons has been correlated with eye-velocity and eye-position, and from a physiological perspective (for the lack of an explicit compelling nomenclature) these neurons are located in the hindbrain nuclei called Area II and Area I, respectively (Pastor et al., 1994; Aksay et al., 2000). On the basis of vestibular synaptic inputs, firing patterns, and embryological evidence, the Area I and Area II have been proposed as functionally analogous (not homologous) to the mammalian prepositus hypoglossi nucleus; but eye-position and eye-velocity related neurons are located into two separate hindbrain nuclei in goldfish (for further details see Straka et al., 2006). In summary, the rhombencephalic reticular formation neurons of goldfish discharge with similar patterns to the mammalian neurons involved in the circuitry for the generation of horizontal saccades (Scudder et al., 2002; Sparks, 2002). Assuming that the retrogradely labeled neurons found in the present study were saccade-related cells, it could be proposed that premotor neurons lying in the reticular formation of the goldfish are involved in the control of eye movements and fixation through a direct connection, in part GABAergic, with the oculomotor nucleus. Consistent with this proposal, monosynaptic inhibitory inputs to the oculomotor nucleus motoneurons from pontine reticular regions have been reported in mammals (Grantyn et al., 1980), and inhibitory effects from the prepositus hypoglossi nucleus upon these motoneurons have been proposed (Lopez-Barneo et al., 1981). This pathway could act concurrently with the abducens internuclear neurons to perform conjugate horizontal movements in vertebrates.

The major projection to the oculomotor nucleus in the goldfish was located in the nuclei of the octaval column. Neurons were found in the ipsilateral anterior octaval nucleus and in the contralateral anterior, tangential, and descending octaval nuclei. This rostro-caudal arrangement of retrogradely labeled neurons in the octaval column is similar to that found in the mammalian vestibular nuclei projection to the oculomotor nucleus, with labeled cells being reported in the ipsilateral superior vestibular nucleus and the contralateral medial, lateral, and descending vestibular nuclei (Highstein and McCrea, 1988). In addition, the most abundant source of GABAergic inputs to the oculomotor nucleus in the goldfish arises from the ipsilateral anterior octaval nucleus, with most of the neurons within the contralateral octaval nuclei being non-reactive for GABA. This pattern is consistent with the available information in the goldfish showing that electrical stimulation of the ipsilateral vestibular nerve evokes inhibitory postsynaptic potentials in the oculomotor motoneurons, whereas the stimulation of the contralateral nerve evokes excitatory postsynaptic potentials (Graf et al., 1997). Studies in frogs also support a push–pull organization of signals reaching vertical and oblique motoneurons in the oculomotor and trochlear nuclei from the second order vestibular neurons. Such organization involves an ipsilateral-GABAergic inhibitory input to the motoneurons (Straka and Dieringer, 2004). The results in fish and frogs resemble those reported in mammals, as a result of which it has been proposed that vestibular signals from each of the six canals form nearly exclusive contralateral/excitatory and ipsilateral/inhibitory three neuron arcs terminating in the appropriate extraocular motoneuron subgroups (Evinger, 1988; Highstein and McCrea, 1988). Therefore, the pattern of connectivity and GABAergic inputs to the oculomotor nucleus reported here supports the proposal by Graf et al. (1997) that homologous structural traits have been essentially preserved in the vestibulooculomotor system throughout vertebrate phylogeny.

ACKNOWLEDGMENTS

The authors wish to thank María Luisa Alvarez Parra for her technical assistance with immunohistochemistry and to Dr. Juan Luis Ribas-Salgueiro for his assistance in the microscopy service of the Seville University (CITIUS). This work was supported by the Spanish Ministerio de Innovacion y Ciencia (Grant BFU 2009-07867) and by Andalusian government grants (Proyecto de Investigacion de Excelencia: P08-CVI-039 and P09-CVI-4617).

REFERENCES

Aksay, E., Baker, R., Seung, H. S., and Tank, D. W. (2000). Anatomy and discharge properties of pre-motor neurons in the goldfish medulla that have eye-position signals during fixations. *J. Neurophysiol.* 84, 1035–1049.

Allum, J. H. J., Greef, N. G., and Tokunaga, A. (1981). "Projections to the rostral and caudal abducens nuclei in the goldfish," in *Progress in Oculomotor Research*, eds A. F. Fuchs and W. Becker (New York: Elsevier), 253–262.

Cabrera, B., Torres, B., Pasaro, R., Pastor, A. M., and Delgado-Garcia, J. M. (1992). A morphological study of abducens nucleus motoneurons and internuclear neurons in the goldfish (*Carassius auratus*). *Brain Res. Bull.* 28, 137–144.

de la Cruz, R. R., Escudero, M., and Delgado-Garcia, J. M. (1989). Behaviour of medial rectus motoneurons in the alert cat. *Eur. J. Neurol.* 1, 288–295.

de la Cruz, R. R., Pastor, A. M., Martinez-Guijarro, F. J., Lopez-Garcia, C., and Delgado-Garcia, J. M. (1992). Role of GABA in the extraocular motor nuclei of the cat: a postembedding immunocytochemical study. *Neuroscience* 51, 911–929.

Delgado-Garcia, J. M., Pozo, F. D., and Baker, R. (1986a). Behavior of neurons in the abducens nucleus of the alert cat. I. Motoneurons. *Neuroscience* 17, 929–952.

Delgado-Garcia, J. M., Pozo, F. D., and Baker, R. (1986b). Behavior of neurons in the abducens nucleus of the alert cat. II. Internuclear neurons. *Neuroscience* 17, 953–973.

Easter, S. S. (1971). Spontaneous eye movements in restrained goldfish. *Vision Res.* 11, 333–342.

Evinger, C. (1988). "Extraocular motor nuclei: location, morphology and afferents," in *Neuroanatomy of the Oculomotor System*, ed. J. A. Büttner-Ennever (New York: Elsevier), 81–117.

Finger, T. E. (1978). Efferent neurons of the teleost cerebellum. *Brain Res.* 153, 608–614.

Fuchs, A. F., Scudder, C. A., and Kaneko, C. R. S. (1988). Discharge patterns and recruitment order of identified motoneurons and internuclear neurons in the monkey abducens nucleus. *J. Neurophysiol.* 60, 1874–1895.

Gestrin, P., and Sterling, P. (1977). Anatomy and physiology of goldfish oculomotor system. II. Firing pattern of neurons in abducens nucleus and surrounding medulla and their relation to eye movements. *J. Neurophysiol.* 40, 573–588.

Graf, W., and McGurk, J. F. (1985). Peripheral and central oculomotor organization in the goldfish, *Carassius auratus*. *J. Comp. Neurol.* 239, 391–401.

Graf, W., Spencer, R., Baker, H., and Baker, R. (1997). Excitatory and inhibitory vestibular pathways to the extraocular motor nuclei in goldfish. *J. Neurophysiol.* 77, 2765–2779.

Grantyn, A., Grantyn, R., Gaunitz, U., and Robiné K. P. (1980). Sources of direct excitatory and inhibitory inputs from the medial rhombencephalic tegmentum to lateral and medial rectus motoneurons in the cat. *Exp. Brain Res.* 39, 49–61.

Highstein, S. M. (1973). Synaptic linkage in the vestibulo-ocular and trochlear reflex pathways in the rabbit. *Exp. Brain Res.* 17, 301–314.

Highstein, S. M., and Holstein, G. R. (2006). "The anatomy of the vestibular nuclei," in *Neuroanatomy of the Oculomotor System*, ed. J. A. Büttner-Ennever (New York: Elsevier), 157–203.

Highstein, S. M., and McCrea, R. A. (1988). "The anatomy of the vestibular nuclei," in *Neuroanatomy of the Oculomotor System*, ed. J. A. Büttner-Ennever (New York: Elsevier), 177–202.

Horn, A. K., Helmchen, C., and Wahle, P. (2003). GABAergic neurons in the rostral mesencephalon of the macaque monkey that control vertical eye movements. *Ann. N. Y. Acad. Sci.* 1004, 19–28.

Horn, A. K. E. (2006). "The reticular formation," in *Neuroanatomy of the Oculomotor System*, ed. J. A. Büttner-Ennever (New York: Elsevier), 127–155.

Ikenaga, T., Yoshida, M., and Uematsu, K. (2005). Morphology and immunohistochemistry of efferent neurons of the goldfish corpus cerebelli. *J. Comp. Neurol.* 487, 300–311.

Ito, M., Highstein, S. M., and Tsuchiya, T. (1970). The postsynaptic inhibition of rabbit oculomotor neurones by secondary vestibular impulses and its blockage by picrotoxin. *Brain Res.* 17, 520–523.

Keng, M. J., and Anastasio, T. J. (1997). The horizontal optokinetic response of the goldfish. *Brain Behav. Evol.* 49, 214–229.

Kobayashi, N., Yoshida, M., Matsumoto, N., and Uematsu, K. (2009). Artificial control of swimming in goldfish by brain stimulation: confirmation of the midbrain nuclei as the swimming center. *Neurosci. Lett.* 452, 42–46.

Lopez-Barneo, J., Ribas, J., and Delgado-Garcia, J. M. (1981). Identification of prepositus neurons projecting to the oculomotor nucleus in the alert cat. *Brain Res.* 214, 174–179.

Luque, M. A., Pérez-Pérez, M. P., Herrero, L., Waitzman, D. M., and Torres, B. (2006). Eye movements evoked by electrical microstimulation of the mesencephalic reticular formation in goldfish. *Neuroscience* 137, 1051–1073.

McCormick, C. A., and Bradford, M. R. (1994). Organization of inner-ear endorgan projection in the goldfish, *Carassius auratus*. *Brain Behav. Evol.* 43, 189–205.

Meek, J., and Nieuwenhuys, R. (1998). "Holosteans and teleosts," in *The Central Nervous System of Vertebrates*, eds R. Nieuwenhuys, H. J. Ten Donkelaar, and C. Nicholson (Berlin: Springer), 759–937.

Mensh, B. D., Aksay, E., Lee, D. D., Seung, H. S., and Tank, D. W. (2004). Spontaneous eye movements in goldfish: oculomotor integrator performance, plasticity, and dependence on visual feedback. *Vision Res.* 44, 711–726.

Nguyen, L. T., and Spencer, R. F. (1999). Abducens internuclear and ascending tract of deiters inputs to medial rectus motoneurons in the cat oculomotor nucleus: neurotransmitters. *J. Comp. Neurol.* 411, 73–86.

Pastor, A. M., de la Cruz, R. R., and Baker, R. (1992). Characterization and adaptive modification of the goldfish vestibuloocular reflex by sinusoidal and velocity step vestibular stimulation. *J. Neurophysiol.* 68, 2003–2015.

Pastor, A. M., de la Cruz, R. R., and Baker, R. (1994). Eye position and eye velocity integrators reside in separate brainstem nuclei. *Proc. Natl. Acad. Sci. U.S.A.* 91, 807–811.

Pastor, A. M., de la Cruz, R. R., and Baker, R. (1997). Characterization of Purkinje cells in the goldfish cerebellum during eye movement and adaptive modification of the vestibulo-ocular reflex. *Prog. Brain Res.* 114, 359–381.

Precht, W., Baker, R., and Okada, Y. (1973). Evidence for GABA as the synaptic transmitter of the inhibitory vestibulo-ocular pathway. *Exp. Brain Res.* 18, 415–428.

Scudder, C. A., Kaneko, C. S., and Fuchs, A. F. (2002). The brainstem burst generator for saccadic eye movements: a modern synthesis. *Exp. Brain Res.* 142, 439–462.

Sparks, D. L. (2002). The brainstem control of saccadic eye movements. *Nat. Rev. Neurosci.* 3, 952–964.

Spencer, R. F., and Wang, S. F. (1996). Immunohistochemical localization of neurotransmitters utilized by neurons in the rostral interstitial nucleus of the medial longitudinal fasciculus (riMLF) that project to the oculomotor and trochlear nuclei in the cat. *J. Comp. Neurol.* 366, 134–148.

Spencer, R. F., Wang, S. F., and Baker, R. (1992). The pathways and functions of GABA in the oculomotor system. *Prog. Brain Res.* 90, 307–331.

Straka, H., Beck, J. C., Pastor, A. M., and Baker, R. (2006). Morphology and physiology of the cerebellar vestibulolateral lobe pathways linked to oculomotor function in the goldfish. *J. Neurophysiol.* 96, 1963–1980.

Straka, H., and Dieringer, N. (2004). Basic organization principles of the VOR: lessons from frogs. *Prog. Neurobiol.* 73, 259–309.

Torres, B., Fernandez, S., Rodriguez, F., and Salas, C. (1995). Distribution of neurons projecting to the trochlear nucleus in goldfish (*Carassius auratus*). *Brain Behav. Evol.* 45, 272–285.

Torres, B., Pastor, A. M., Cabrera, B., Salas, C., and Delgado-García, J. M. (1992). Afferents to the oculomotor nucleus in the goldfish (*Carassius auratus*) as revealed by retrograde labeling with horseradish peroxidase. *J. Comp. Neurol.* 324, 449–461.

Uchino, Y., and Suzuki, S. (1983). Axon collaterals to the extraocular motoneuron pools of inhibitory vestibuloocular neurons activated from the anterior, posterior and horizontal semicircular canals in the cat. *Neurosci. Lett.* 37, 129–135.

Wentzel, P. R., Gerrits, N. M., and de Zeeuw, C. I. (1996). GABAergic and glycinergic inputs to the rabbit oculomotor nucleus with special emphasis on the medial rectus subdivision. *Brain Res.* 707, 314–319.

Conflict of Interest Statement: The authors declare that the research was conducted in the absence of any commercial or financial relationships that could be construed as a potential conflict of interest.

10

Amygdaloid projections to the ventral striatum in mice: direct and indirect chemosensory inputs to the brain reward system

Amparo Novejarque[1†], Nicolás Gutiérrez-Castellanos[2†], Enrique Lanuza[2]* and Fernando Martínez-García[1]*

[1] Departament de Biologia Funcional i Antropologia Física, Facultat de Ciències Biològiques, Universitat de València, València, Spain
[2] Departament de Biologia Cel•lular, Facultat de Ciències Biològiques, Universitat de València, València, Spain

Edited by:
Agustín González, Universidad Complutense de Madrid, Spain

Reviewed by:
Daniel W. Wesson, Case Western Reserve University, USA
James L. Goodson, Indiana University, USA

***Correspondence:**
Enrique Lanuza, Departament de Biologia Cel•lular, Facultat de Ciències Biològiques, Universitat de València, C/Dr. Moliner, 50 ES-46100 Burjassot, València, Spain.
e-mail: enrique.lanuza@uv.es;
Fernando Martínez-García, Departament de Biologia Funcional i Antropologia Física, Facultat de Ciències Biològiques, Universitat de València, C/Dr. Moliner, 50 ES-46100 Burjassot, València, Spain.
e-mail: fernando.mtnez-garcia@uv.es

†Present address:
Amparo Novejarque, Department of Surgery and Cancer, Faculty of Medicine, Imperial College London, Chelsea and Westminster Hospital, London, UK;
Nicolás Gutiérrez-Castellanos, Cerebellar coordination and cognition group, Netherlands Institute for Neuroscience, Amsterdam, Netherlands.

Rodents constitute good models for studying the neural basis of sociosexual behavior. Recent findings in mice have revealed the molecular identity of the some pheromonal molecules triggering intersexual attraction. However, the neural pathways mediating this basic sociosexual behavior remain elusive. Since previous work indicates that the dopaminergic tegmento-striatal pathway is not involved in pheromone reward, the present report explores alternative pathways linking the vomeronasal system with the tegmento-striatal system (the limbic basal ganglia) by means of tract-tracing experiments studying direct and indirect projections from the chemosensory amygdala to the ventral striato-pallidum. Amygdaloid projections to the nucleus accumbens, olfactory tubercle, and adjoining structures are studied by analyzing the retrograde transport in the amygdala from dextran amine and fluorogold injections in the ventral striatum, as well as the anterograde labeling found in the ventral striato-pallidum after dextran amine injections in the amygdala. This combination of anterograde and retrograde tracing experiments reveals direct projections from the vomeronasal cortex to the ventral striato-pallidum, as well as indirect projections through different nuclei of the basolateral amygdala. Direct projections innervate mainly the olfactory tubercle and the islands of Calleja, whereas indirect projections are more widespread and reach the same structures and the shell and core of nucleus accumbens. These pathways are likely to mediate innate responses to pheromones (direct projections) and conditioned responses to associated chemosensory and non-chemosensory stimuli (indirect projections). Comparative studies indicate that similar connections are present in all the studied amniote vertebrates and might constitute the basic circuitry for emotional responses to conspecifics in most vertebrates, including humans.

Keywords: chemosensory amygdala, nucleus accumbens, olfactory tubercle, islands of Calleja, striatal cell bridges, emotional brain

INTRODUCTION

It is generally accepted that the amygdala is a key structure in the generation of emotional behaviors (LeDoux, 2000). Remarkably, in this view of the amygdala as the core of the emotional brain, its chemosensory role is usually neglected (see Aggleton, 2000), despite the fact that one of the major sensory inputs to the amygdala originates in the main and accessory olfactory bulbs, providing directly olfactory and vomeronasal information (Pitkänen, 2000). Chemosensory stimuli have a strong influence on the behavior of rodents, in particular in sociosexual behaviors

Abbreviations: AA, anterior amygdaloid area (AAD: dorsal; AAV: ventral); AB, accessory basal (or basomedial) amygdaloid nucleus (ABa: anterior; ABp: posterior); *ac*, anterior commissure (*aca*: anterior part; *acp*: posterior part); Acb, nucleus accumbens (AcbC: core; AcbSh: shell; LAcbSh: lateral shell; MAcbSh: medial shell); AHA, amygdalohippocampal area (AHAl: lateral division; AHAm: medial division); APir, amygdalopiriform transition area; AStr, amygdalo-striatal transition area; B, basal (or basolateral) amygdaloid nucleus (Ba: anterior; Bp: posterior; Bv: ventral); BAOT, bed nucleus of the accessory olfactory tract; BST, bed nucleus of the *stria terminalis*; CB, cell bridges of the ventral striatum; Ce, central amygdaloid nucleus (CeC: capsular or paracapsular division; CeL: lateral division; CeM: medial division); Cl, claustrum; COAa, anterior cortical amygdaloid nucleus; COApl, posterolateral cortical amygdaloid nucleus; COApm, posteromedial cortical amygdaloid nucleus; CPu, caudate–putamen (dorsal striatum); CxA, cortex–amygdala transition zone; DEn, dorsal endopiriform nucleus; HDB, horizontal limb of the diagonal band nucleus; I, intercalated nuclei of amygdala; ICj, islands of Calleja; ICjM, major island of Calleja; IPAC, interstitial nucleus of the posterior limb of the anterior commissure; L, lateral amygdaloid nucleus (Lvl: ventrolateral, Ldl: dorsolateral, Lm: medial); LGP, lateral globus pallidus; LOT, nucleus of the lateral olfactory tract (1: layer 1; 2: layer 2; 3: layer 3); Me, medial amygdaloid nucleus; MeA, anterior medial amygdala; MeP, posterior medial amygdala (MePV: ventral; MePD: dorsal); Pir, piriform cortex; SI, *substantia innominata*; *st*, *stria terminalis*; Tu, olfactory tubercle; VEn, ventral endopiriform nucleus.

having an important emotional component. In this respect, recent findings in mice have uncovered the molecular identity of two particular pheromonal molecules triggering intersexual attraction (Roberts et al., 2010) and sexual receptivity (Haga et al., 2010). Male-soiled bedding containing some of these pheromones can be used to induce conditioned place preference (Martínez-Ricós et al., 2007) and, therefore, these sexual pheromones should be considered rewarding stimuli. Since the major pathway involved in reward processing is the dopaminergic tegmento-striatal pathway, our group has previously analyzed the role of this projection in pheromonal reward in mice. Neither systemic administration of anti-dopaminergic drugs (Agustín-Pavón et al., 2007), nor lesions of the dopaminergic neurons of the ventral tegmental area (Martínez-Hernández et al., 2006) abolish female preference for male-soiled bedding, thus suggesting that the dopaminergic tegmento-striatal pathway is not involved in pheromone reward.

In mice, at least some male sexual pheromones attractive for females are detected by the vomeronasal system (Martínez-Ricós et al., 2008), and consequently information about these sexual pheromones is processed in the vomeronasal amygdala. There is increasing evidence on the role of the amygdala on reward-related processes (Baxter and Murray, 2002; Everitt et al., 2003), but the role of the amygdala in reward driven by chemosensory stimuli has been rarely explored. The pioneering studies by Everitt, Robbins, and collaborators (Cador et al., 1989; Everitt et al., 1989, 1991; Robbins et al., 1989) indicated that basolateral amygdala projections to the nucleus accumbens mediate reward-related learning. In contrast, much less information is available regarding the projections from the chemosensory amygdala to the nucleus accumbens and other centers of the ventral striatum (McDonald, 1991b; Canteras et al., 1992; Shammah-Lagnado and Santiago, 1999).

The present report explores alternative pathways linking the chemosensory amygdala with the brain reward system by means of tract-tracing experiments studying the projections of different amygdaloid nuclei to the ventral striato-pallidum. To do so, we combine anterograde and retrograde tracing experiments to reveal amygdaloid projections to the nucleus accumbens, olfactory tubercle, and adjoining structures such as the islands of Calleja (ICj). Our results might help to understand the neural pathways mediating the behavioral responses to chemical cues, including rewarding sexual pheromones.

MATERIALS AND METHODS

ANIMALS

For this study, 35 adult, female mice (*Mus musculus,* Harlan, Barcelona, Spain; 25 of the C57BL/J6 strain and 10 of the CD1 strain) were used (17.9–35.1 g). Animals were maintained in cages with food and water *ad libitum*, under natural day/night cycle, at 22–25°C. All experiments were performed in accordance with the guidelines of the European Community Council Directive 86/609/EEC on the treatment of experimental animals, and procedures were approved by the Committee of Ethics on Animal Experimentation of the University of València.

TRACT-TRACING EXPERIMENTS

To study the amygdaloid projections to the ventral striatum in the mouse, we first injected neuroanatomical tracers in different parts of the Acb (medial shell, $n = 4$; lateral shell, $n = 1$; core, $n = 5$; non-restricted injections, $n = 2$) and other regions of the ventral striatum [olfactory tubercle, $n = 6$; major island of calleja (ICjM), $n = 1$], to study the distribution of retrograde labeling in the amygdala. Then, tracers were injected in the different nuclei of the amygdala that showed retrograde labeling in the previous experiments (cortical amygdala, $n = 7$; deep pallial amygdala, $n = 10$) and the resulting anterograde labeling in the ventral striatum was analyzed. In order to study whether the associative nuclei of the deep pallial amygdala (lateral, basal and accessory basal) can indirectly relay chemosensory information to the ventral striatum, we also studied the intra-amygdaloid projections from the cortical (chemosensory) amygdaloid nuclei to the deep pallial amygdala.

In the present work, three different tracers were used: biotinylated dextran amine (BDA, 10,000 and 3,000 MW lysine fixable; Invitrogen, Carlsbad, CA, USA), tetramethylrhodamine-labeled dextran amine (RDA, 10,000 MW, lysine fixable, fluoro-ruby; Invitrogen) and fluorogold (Biotium, Hayward, CA, USA). To minimize the number of animals, each mouse usually received two tracer injections (total number of tracer injections, 46). Therefore, each injection is identified with a letter indicative of the tracer (B for BDA; R for RDA; F for fluorogold) and a number indicative of the specimen.

For surgery, animals were deeply anesthetized with an intraperitoneal injection of 6.5 μl of sodium pentobarbital (11 mg/ml, Sigma-Aldrich, St. Louis, MO, USA) per gram of body weight. Using stereotaxic coordinates (Paxinos and Franklin, 2001), dextran amines (5–10% in 0.01 M phosphate buffer, pH 7.6), and fluorogold (2% in saline solution) were ionophoretically injected through glass micropipettes with an inner diameter tip of 10–20 μm, using positive current (7 s on/off; 3–5 μA) during 10 min. The pipette was left in place for 5 min after injection. To avoid diffusion of the tracer along the pipette track, a mild continuous retention current (−0.9 μA) was applied during entrance and withdrawal of the micropipette. After 7–8 days of survival, animals received an overdose of sodium pentobarbital and were perfused transcardially with phosphate buffered saline (PBS; 0.9% NaCl in 0.1 M PB pH 7.6), followed by fixative (4% paraformaldehyde in 0.1 M PB, pH 7.6). Brains were postfixed for 4 h in the same fixative at 4°C and then immersed in 30% sucrose in 0.1 M PB until they sank. Frontal sections (40 μm) obtained with a freezing microtome were collected into five parallel series.

Before (immuno)histochemical processing, endogenous peroxidase was inhibited with 1% H_2O_2 in 0.05 M TRIS buffer (TB) pH 7.6 plus 0.9% NaCl (TRIS-buffered saline, TBS) for 30 min at room temperature. For BDA detection, sections were incubated in avidin–biotin complex (ABC Elite kit; Vector Laboratories, Burlingame, CA, USA) in TBS with 0.3% Triton X-100, either overnight at 4°C or for 2 h at room temperature, and then the peroxidase activity was revealed with 3,3′-diaminobenzidine (DAB, Sigma; 0.02% in 0.05 M TB, pH 7.6–8.0) and 0.01% H_2O_2. Nickel salts (0.4% nickel ammonium sulfate) were added as an enhancing agent of the reaction product (DAB-Ni).

For immunodetection of tetramethyl rhodamine, sections were incubated in primary antibody against tetramethyl rhodamine (raised in rabbit, Molecular Probes, Cat. # A-6397, Lot: 7051-3), diluted 1:4,000 in TBS with 0.3% Triton X-100, followed by a standard peroxidase–antiperoxidase procedure (goat anti-rabbit IgG,1:100, Nordic Immunological Laboratories, Tilburg, The Netherlands; rabbit PAP, 1:800, Nordic Immunological Labs). The resulting peroxidase label was revealed as above, with or without nickel enhancement.

Fluorogold injections were observed with fluorescence microscopy. Some series were also processed for the immunohistochemical detection of the tracer. To do so, sections were postfixed with 0.1% glutaraldehyde in PBS for 4 h at 4°C, rinsed in TBS and the endogenous peroxidase activity was inhibited with 1% H_2O_2 (30 min). Sections were then sequentially incubated in primary antibody (rabbit anti-FG, Chemicon, Billerica, MA, USA) diluted 1:5,000 in TBS with 0.3% Triton X-100 and 2.5% normal goat serum, overnight at 4°C; secondary antibody (biotinylated goat anti-rabbit IgG, Vector Laboratories, Burlingame, CA, USA) diluted 1:200 in TBS-Tx for 2 h at room temperature; and ABC Elite (2 h, room temperature, Vector Labs) diluted in the same buffer. The resulting peroxidase labeling was visualized as detailed above.

IMAGE ACQUISITION AND PROCESSING

Slides were photographed in a Leitz DMRB microscope equipped with a Leica DC 300 digital camera (Leica Microsystems, Wetzlar, Germany). Digital images were imported into Adobe Photoshop (Adobe Systems, Mountain View, CA, USA), flattened by subtracting background illumination and converted to gray scale. Brightness and contrast were adjusted and resolution was set at 600 dpi. No additional filtering or manipulation of the images was performed. The final figures were composed and labeled with Adobe Photoshop.

Chartings of anterograde labeling in specific sections were drawn for illustration purposes. To do so, low-power photomicrographs of the sections were taken as described and two transparent sheets were created on top of them using Adobe Photoshop. One of them was used to delineate the cytoarchitecture of the section, whereas in the other one a detailed map of the labeling was drawn using some elements of the photograph as spatial landmarks (vessels, ventricles, Nissl staining, etc.) while observing the slides at high magnification through the microscope.

RESULTS

The results of our experiments are described following the nomenclature by Paxinos and Franklin (2001), except for the amygdala, where we have partially adapted the nomenclature of Pitkänen (2000). This terminology has the advantage of avoiding the confusion between the basolateral nucleus and the basolateral division of the amygdala. Briefly, the amygdala consists of a mixture of structures with pallial or subpallial origin (Puelles et al., 2000; see **Figure 1**). The pallial structures of the amygdala give rise to the bulk of the amygdalo-striatal projections, and therefore are the focus of the present investigation. Within the pallial amygdala, we distinguish the cortical nuclei (superficial, olfacto-recipient, and layered) and several non-layered nuclei located topologically deep to them (**Figure 1**). The cortical nuclei include the nucleus of the lateral olfactory tract (LOT, **Figure 1A,A′**), the anterior cortical amygdaloid nucleus (COAa, **Figure 1A–B′**), the posterolateral cortical amygdaloid nucleus (COApl, **Figure 1B–D′**), as well as of two secondary vomeronasal centers, the bed nucleus of the accessory olfactory tract (BAOT, not shown) and the posteromedial cortical amygdaloid nucleus (COApm, **Figure 1C–D′**). In addition, there are several transitional areas interposed between the cortical amygdala and the piriform cortex (cortex–amygdala transition zone,

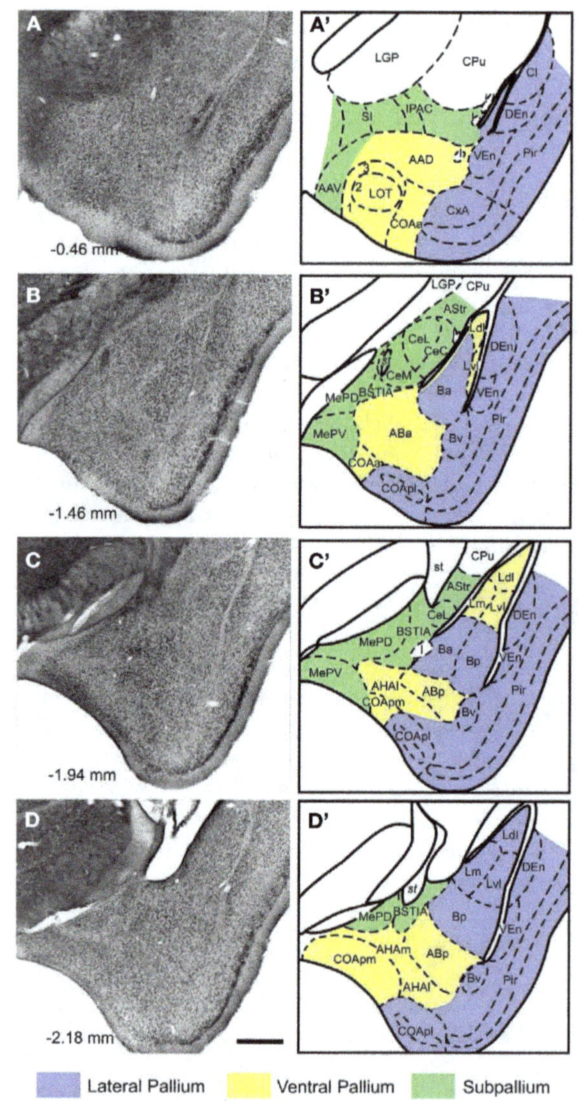

FIGURE 1 | Cytoarchitecture of the amygdaloid complex of the mouse Nissl-stained frontal sections (A–D) through the amygdala of the mouse (A rostral, D caudal) with indication of the antero-posterior level relative to Bregma according to Paxinos and Franklin (2001). In the right panels **(A′–D′)**, the boundaries between the different nuclei and fiber tracts are delineated in schematic drawings of the same sections. The embryological origin (subpallial, lateropallial, ventropallial) of the different amygdaloid structures is also indicated. For abbreviations, see list. Calibration bar = 400 μm.

CxA, **Figure 1A,A′**; amygdalopiriform transition area, APir, not shown). The deep pallial nuclei of the amygdala include the basal (B, or basolateral, **Figure 1B–D′**), the accessory basal (AB, or basomedial, **Figure 1B–D′**), and the lateral (L, **Figure 1B–D′**) amygdaloid nuclei, as well as the amygdalohippocampal area (AHA, **Figure 1C–D′**). According to Paxinos and Franklin (2001), we consider that the B includes anterior (Ba), posterior (Bp), and ventral (Bv) divisions. Within the AB we distinguish anterior (ABa) and posterior (ABp) portions. The L shows ventrolateral (Lvl), dorsolateral (Ldl), and medial (Lm) divisions. Finally, within the AHA we consider medial (AHAm) and lateral (AHAl) subnuclei.

In the ventral striatum we consider the core (AcbC) and shell (AcbSh) of the nucleus accumbens (with its lateral and medial divisions; LAcbSh and MAcbSh respectively) following Paxinos and Franklin (2001). We also include the olfactory tubercle (Tu), the ICj, and the cell bridges of the ventral striatum (CB) since the anterograde labeling in nucleus accumbens after injections in the pallial amygdala was continuous with the one found in these structures (for previous descriptions of the striatal cell bridges in the rat see Seifert et al., 1998; Riedel et al., 2002).

RETROGRADE LABELING ANALYSIS

Retrograde labeling in the amygdala after injections in the nucleus accumbens

We describe in detail the retrograde labeling of representative cases of tracer injections in the Acb (see **Table 1**). Remarkably, all of these injections gave rise to retrograde labeling in the cortical and deep pallial amygdala (see below). In contrast, retrogradely labeled cells were not observed in the central or the medial amygdaloid nuclei (with the exception of one injection involving part of the ventral septum, which gave rise to retrograde labeling in the medial amygdala, see Caffé et al., 1987).

Injections in the accumbens shell. Injections encompassing the MAcbSh rendered retrograde labeling in both the cortical and deep pallial amygdala (see **Table 1**). After these injections (**Figure 2A**), the cortical amygdala displayed a few labeled cells in the deep, lateral edge between the COAa and the CxA (**Figure 2B**) and in the caudal APir (**Figure 2E**). Injections including the rostral edge of the MAcbSh (R0304 and R0301) displayed few labeled neurons in the deep COApm (**Table 1; Figure 2E**). Within the deep pallial amygdala retrograde labeling was abundant in the whole B, including an area ventral to the Ba which we tentatively

Table 1 | Retrogradely labeled neurons in the different areas of the pallial amygdala (columns) after injections in the ventral striatum (rows) graded semi-quantitatively according to the following scores: –, absent; X, scarce; XX, moderate; XXX, dense; B, contralateral labeling.

	Cortical amygdala						Deep pallial amygdala									
	COApm	LOT	COAa	CxA	COApl	APir	Ba	Bp	Bv	ABa	*ABp*	AHAl	AHAm	Lm	Lvl	Ldl
ACCUMBENS SHELL																
R0304 MAcbSh +1.34 mm	X	–	X	–	–	X	XX	XXX B	XX	–	X	X	X	–	–	–
B0419 MAcbSh +0.98 mm	–	–	X	–	–	X	XXX	XXX	XX	–	XX	X	X	–	–	–
R0331 LAcbSh +1.10 mm	–	XX	X	XX	–	X	XXX B	XX	XX	–	XX	X	–	–	XX	–
ACCUMBENS CORE																
B0302 AcbC from +1.34 to +1.10 mm	–	X B	X	X	–	–	XX B	X	XX B	–	XXX B	X B	–	–	X	XXX B
B0309 dorsomedialAcbC +1.18 mm	–	X	–	X	–	–	X	X	–	–	X	–	–	–	–	X
B0321 lateralAcbC +1.18 mm	–	X	–	–	–	–	XX	X	X	–	X	–	–	–	X	XX
OLFACTORY TUBERCLE																
F08100 ICj anteromedial +0.98 mm	XX	XX	XX	X	XX	XX	–	XXX B	X	XX	XXX B	XX	X	–	–	–
NON-RESTRICTED INJECTIONS																
R0301 MAcbSh (+medial AcbC) +1.18 mm	X	–	X	–	–	X	XX	XXX B	XX	–	X B	X	X	–	X	–
R0338 dorsal MAcbSh + AcbC +0.98 mm	X	X	X	–	X	X	XX	XX B	XX	–	XX B	X B	XX	X	X	X
B0312 lateral S + ICjM from +1.34 to +1.10 mm	XXX	X B	X B	X	X	–	X	XX	–	XX B	X	XX	XX	–	X	–

The rostro-caudal extent of the injection site is indicated (coordinates from Bregma). For abbreviations, see list.

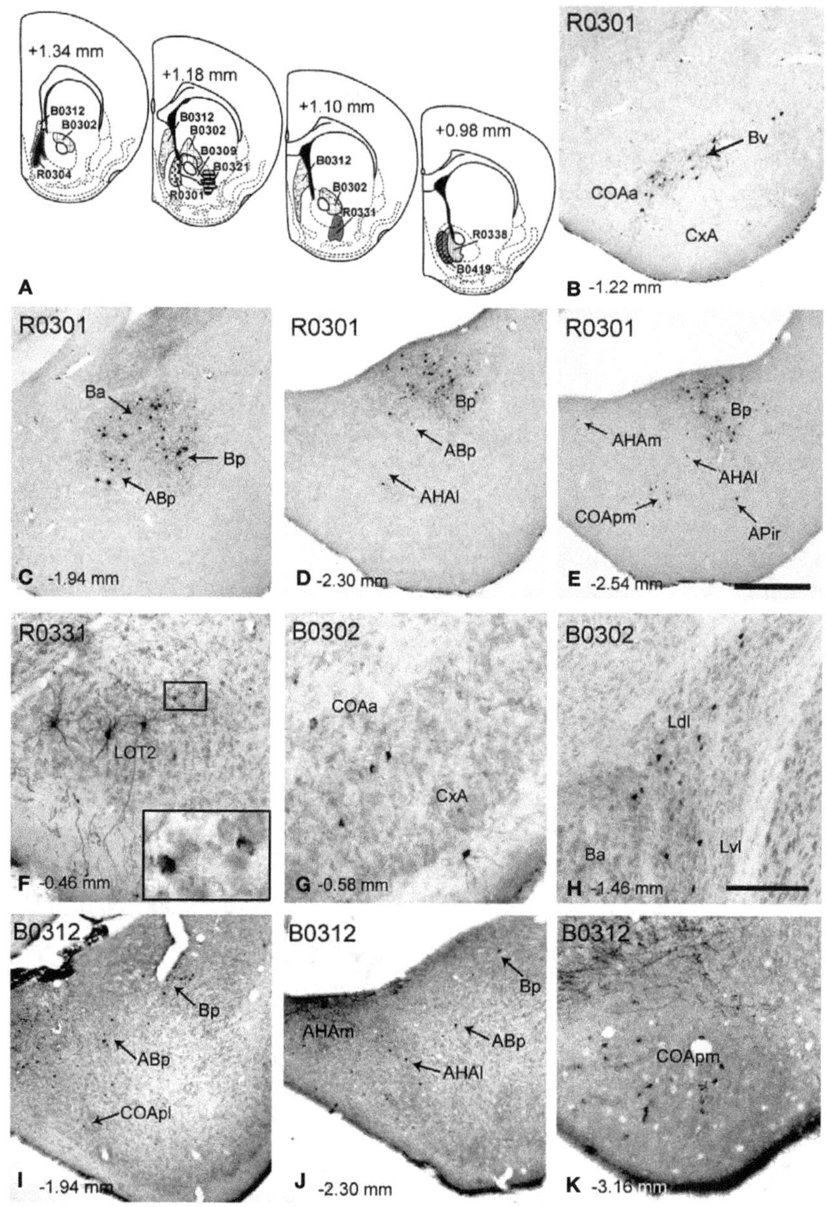

FIGURE 2 | Retrograde labeling in the pallial amygdala after tracer injections in the nucleus accumbens and associated major island of Calleja. (A) Semi-schematic drawings of coronal sections through the ventral striatum of the mouse showing the extent of tracer injections in the Acb and in the major island of Calleja. The antero-posterior coordinate relative to Bregma is indicated in each section as well as in every photograph in the figure. **(B–E)** Retrograde labeling in the pallial amygdala after an RDA injection encompassing the MAcbSh and a small portion of the medial AcbC (R0301). Although most of the labeling is located in the basolateral amygdala, retrogradely labeled cells are also present in deep layers of some cortical nuclei both in the anterior **(B,C)** and posterior amygdala **(D,E)**. **(F)** Retrogradely labeled neurons in the LOT ipsilateral to a tracer injection in the LAcbSh (R0331). Golgi-like labeled cells are clearly visible in layer 2, but layer 3 also displays cells showing granular labeling (inset). **(G,H)** Retrograde labeling in different centers of the pallial amygdala, resulting from a BDA injection in the AcbC (B0302). **(I–K)** Retrogradely labeled neurons in the pallial amygdala after a BDA injection in the ventral septum that encompassed the major island of Calleja (B0312). For abbreviations, see list. Calibration bar in **(E)** = 400 μm [also valid for **(B–D,I,J)**]. Scale bar in **(H)** = 150 μm [also valid for **(F–K)**].

consider as the Bv (**Figure 2B**). In addition, the caudal part of the Ba (**Figure 2C**) and the whole Bp (**Figures 2C–E**) showed many labeled somata. The most rostral injection in the MacbSh (R0304), as well as those injections involving both MAcbSh and AcbC (R0301 and R0338), rendered retrograde labeling in the contralateral Bp (**Table 1**). Moreover, retrogradely labeled cells were found in the posterior part of the AB (**Figures 1C,D**), where labeling was bilateral in the injections encompassing both the MAcbSh and AcbC (see **Table 1**). A few retrograde labeled cells were also present in the medial and lateral AHA (**Table 1; Figures 2D,E**). Finally, injections confined to the MAcbSh showed no labeled cells in the L (**Table 1**).

The injection in the lateral AcbSh (LAcbSh; R0331, **Figure 2A**) resulted in numerous labeled cells in several pallial amygdaloid centers. Within the cortical amygdala, labeled cells were abundant in the CxA but scarce in the COAa (see **Table 1**). At these rostral levels, the LOT showed Golgi-like labeled cells in layer 2 (**Figure 2F**), as well as a number of faintly labeled cell bodies in layer 3 (see inset in **Figure 2F**). At caudal levels, a few somata displayed granular retrograde labeling in the APir (not shown). In the deep pallial amygdala, labeled cells were abundant in all the subnuclei of the B, especially in the Ba, where labeling was bilateral with ipsilateral dominance (**Table 1**). The ABp also showed a moderate-to-high density of retrogradely labeled neurons (**Table 1**). A few labeled cells were also present in the AHAl (**Table 1**). Finally, a population of labeled neurons was confined to the rostral portion of the Lvl (**Table 1**).

Injections in the accumbens core. Two small injections restricted to the AcbC and a larger injection (B0302) including most of the dorsal AcbC plus a small portion of the adjacent caudate–putamen (**Figure 2A**) displayed scarce retrograde labeling (see **Table 1**) within the cortical amygdala. A few labeled cells were found bilaterally in layer 3 of the LOT (**Table 1**) and ipsilaterally in the CxA, especially in its deep portion, adjacent to the COAa (**Figure 2G**). On the other hand, the deep pallial amygdala showed a dense population of retrogradely labeled cells in the most anterior part of the L, especially dense in the Ldl, where labeling was bilateral. Labeled neurons were also observed in the Lvl (**Table 1; Figure 2H**). It is worth noting that this labeling was absent in the injections restricted to the MAcbSh. In addition, many retrogradely labeled neurons were observed in both hemispheres in the caudal aspect of the Ba (**Figure 2H**), in the Bv and in the AHAl. Moreover, some labeled neurons were observed in the rostralmost part of the Bp (not shown) and the ABp showed a dense population of retrogradely labeled cells (**Table 1**).

Injection involving the major island of Calleja. One injection centered in the lateral septum (B0312) extended ventrally to encompass the ICjM, which was the only structure in the ventral striatum affected by the injection (**Figure 2**). This injection gave rise to a high number of retrogradely labeled cells in different amygdaloid pallial centers (**Table 1**). All the nuclei in the cortical amygdala, with the exception of the APir, showed retrograde labeling (**Table 1**), the deep portion of the COApm (mainly its caudal aspect) being the nucleus with the highest density of labeled cells (**Figure 2K**). The COApl also showed some labeled somata in its most rostral and deep aspect (**Figure 2I**). Both the superficial COAa (bilaterally) and the medial CxA showed some labeled neurons (**Table 1**). The LOT also displayed neurons with granular labeling in the layer 2 bilaterally (not shown). In the deep pallial amygdala some neurons were present in the ventral and caudal end of the Ba and a moderate number of labeled cells in the Bp (**Figures 2I,J**). The AB showed some labeled neurons in the ventral region of the caudalmost ABa (bilaterally) and in the ABp (**Table 1; Figures 2I,J**). In the AHA the number of labeled cells was moderate in both subdivisions (**Figure 2J**). Finally, some neurons in the Lvl showed granular labeling (**Table 1**).

Retrograde labeling in the amygdala after injections in the olfactory tubercle

Fluorogold injections involved the olfactory tubercle in six occasions. Retrograde labeling in experiment F08100 is shown as representative example. In this case, the tracer injection was centered in the ventromedial aspect of the olfactory tubercle and encompassed the anteromedial ICj (**Figure 3A**). Retrogradely labeled neurons in the cortical amygdala appeared mainly in the LOT (**Table 1**), COAa (**Figure 3B**), COApm and COApl, (in all three structures located in layers 2 and 3), and in APir (**Figures 3C,D**). A number of labeled somata appeared also in CxA. Of note, labeled cells were also observed in the medial amygdala (subpallium), but only in its anterior part (**Figure 3B**). In the deep pallial amygdala, fluorogold-labeled cells were abundant in the AB (both anterior and posterior parts), B (posterior and ventral parts), and AHA (**Figures 3C,D**). In contrast, virtually no labeling was present in the Ba and very few cells were observed in the caudal L. Outside the amygdala, but worth mentioning given its olfactory nature, dense retrograde labeling was observed in the posterior aspect of the piriform cortex (**Figures 3C,D**).

ANTEROGRADE LABELING ANALYSIS

Anterograde labeling in the ventral striatum after injections in the cortical amygdala

Seven injections were aimed at the cortical portion of the pallial amygdala (**Figure 4**), six of which were centered in the caudal cortical amygdala whereas the other one encompassed the rostral CxA and the COAa (**Figure 4A**). The anterograde labeling observed in the ventral striatum in representative cases (see **Tables 2** and **3**) is described below.

Injections in the posterior cortical amygdala. Injections B0415 and R0341 involved, to different degrees, the COApm and COApl. Case B0415 was a large BDA injection, which mainly affected the COApm but also encompassed the medialmost aspect of the COApl. On the other hand, R0341 was quite a restricted injection in the COApl, but slightly involved the lateralmost COApm (**Figure 4A**). In both cases, the pipette track labeled a few cells in the caudal ABp and AHAl. In addition, cases B0815, B0816, and B0817 were centered in the caudal COApm and case B0880 was centered in the COApl (not shown). In all these cases, labeled fibers arising from the injection site used three different pathways (as defined in the rat by Petrovich et al., 1996) to reach the ventral striatum, namely the *stria terminalis*, the *ansa peduncularis* (running through the interstitial nucleus of the posterior limb of the anterior commissure, IPAC, and substantia innominata, SI) and the longitudinal association bundle (which runs rostral and ventral to reach the Tu, see Johnston, 1923). These pathways gave rise to terminal fields in the midcaudal Acb and Tu.

In the injections centered in the COApm, the AcbC showed labeled fibers in its ventral portion (**Figures 4C–E**). Sparse labeled fibers were present in most of the shell of the Acb, including its rostral tip, whereas dense terminal fields were observed in the periphery of the caudoventral LAcbSh (**Figure 4E**) and in the ventral aspect of the MAcbSh, next to some cell bridges of the ventral striatum (CB, **Figure 4C**; see below). In contrast,

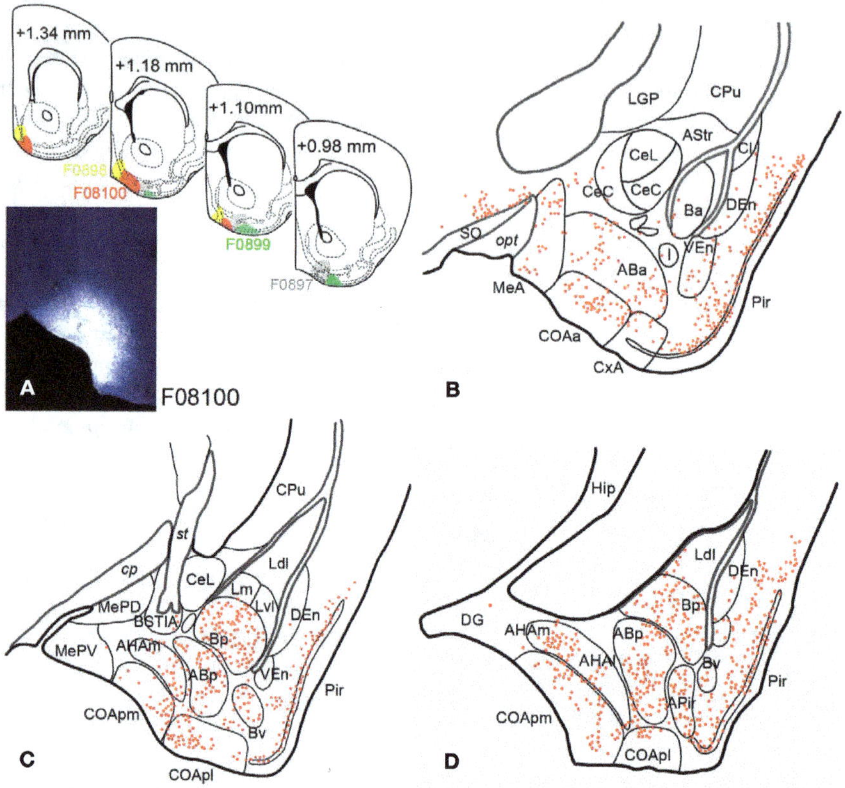

FIGURE 3 | Retrograde labeling in the pallial amygdala after tracer injections in the olfactory tubercle. (A) Semi-schematic drawings of coronal sections through the ventral striatum of the mouse brain showing the extent of fluorogold injections in the Tu, with indication of the antero-posterior coordinate relative to Bregma. The photomicrograph shows the injection site in case F08100, which encompasses the anteromedial island of Calleja. The resulting retrograde labeling is mapped in **(B–D)**. **(B–D)** Camera lucida drawings of frontal sections of the amygdala of a mouse mapping the retrograde labeling observed after an injection of fluorogold in the ventromedial olfactory tubercle (F08100). Note that retrogradely labeled neurons appear both in olfactory and vomeronasal nuclei and also in non-chemosensory amygdaloid structures, such as the basolateral amygdaloid complex.

in injection R0341 (centered in the COApl), the caudal AcbC showed sparse labeled fibers in its medial portion (see pattern in **Figure 9A**) and only a few labeled fibers were present in the AcbSh (**Table 2**).

The injections in COApm and COApl rendered a similar pattern of anterograde labeling in the rest of the ventral striatum, although the labeling resulting from injections in the COApm (e.g., B0415) was always denser than that observed following the injection in the COApl (R0341). After these injections, the densest terminal fields in the ventral striatum were observed in some of the CB (**Figures 4C,D**) and in parts of the caudomedial Tu next to them, where most of the anterograde labeling appeared in layer 3 (inset in **Figure 4D**) in close association with the islands of Calleja dorsal to it (ICj; **Figure 4B** and asterisks in **Figures 4D,E**). Regarding this, a relatively dense terminal field was associated with the lateral aspect of the ICjM (see inset in **Figure 4C**). Therefore, injections involving the caudal cortical amygdala resulted in prominent anterograde labeling in the CB and ICj (including the ICjM, see **Table 3**). Although much less dense, a similar distribution of anterograde labeling was found in the contralateral ventral striatum (**Tables 2–3**), probably connected with a compact bundle of labeled fibers located dorsally in the posterior part of the anterior commissure (*acp*) that appeared after large injections encompassing the COApm/pl.

Injection in the anterior cortical amygdala. Injection B0324 was centered in the caudal aspect of the CxA and the lateral edge of the COAa (**Figure 4A**), but the pipette track also labeled a few cells in the anterior part of the Ba and in the amygdalostriatal transition area (AStr). Labeled fibers arising from the injection site entered the *stria terminalis* to end in the ventral striatum. Moreover, labeled fibers in the *ansa peduncularis* (running through the IPAC) also contributed to the labeling in the LAcbSh and caudal AcbC, whereas labeled fibers that ran through the longitudinal association bundle mainly innervated the olfactory tubercle.

In contrast to the injections in the posterior cortical amygdala, in this case conspicuous anterograde labeling was found throughout the antero-posterior axis of the Acb including its rostral tip (**Table 2**) and even reached the medial anterior olfactory nucleus (not shown). In the AcbSh labeling formed three main

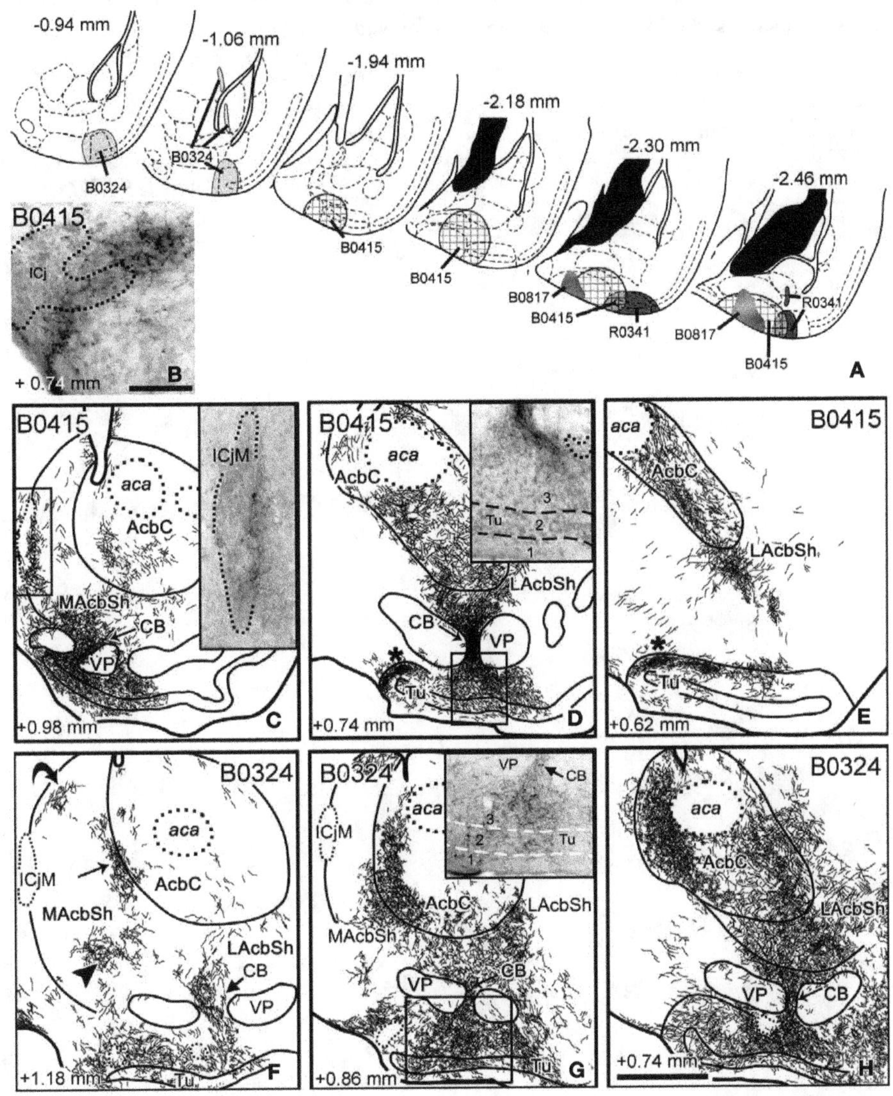

FIGURE 4 | Anterograde labeling in the ventral striatum after tracer injections in the cortical amygdala. (A) Semi-schematic drawings of frontal sections through the amygdala of the mouse showing the extent of the tracer injections in the cortical amygdala indicating the antero-posterior coordinate relative to Bregma. **(B)** High-power microphotograph of a toluidine blue-counterstained section showing the anterograde labeling in the islands of Calleja after an injection of BDA centered in the COApm (B0415). **(C–E)** Anterograde labeling in the ventral striatum resulting from a tracer injection centered in the COApm (B0415). The asterisks in **(D,E)** indicate a labeled terminal field in the caudomedial Tu and adjacent islands of Calleja. Inset in C shows the meshwork of labeled fibers apposed to the medial aspect of the ICjM. Labeling in the CB extends into layer 3 of the Tu [inset in **(D)**]. **(F–H)** Schematic drawings of frontal sections through the ventral striatum of a mouse that received an injection of BDA in the CxA (B0324), showing the resulting anterograde labeling. Three arrows in **(F)** point to the three main terminal fields in the MacbSh, and a fourth arrow remarks the dense innervation of a cell bridge. Labeling in the Tu occupies layers 2 and 3 but also invades the deepest layer 1 [inset in **(G)**]. Arrows in **(G,H)** also point to the innervation of the striatal cell bridges. For abbreviations, see list. Calibration bar in **(B)** = 50 μm. Scale bar in **(H)** = 400 μm [also valid for **(C–G)**].

terminal fields located in the medial (arrowhead and straight arrow in **Figures 4F,G**), ventral (**Figures 4G,H**), and caudolateral shell (**Figure 4H**). In addition, a small group of labeled fibers occupied the boundary between the MAcbSh and the rostral lateral septum (curved arrow in **Figure 4F**). At mid-rostral levels, the dense terminal fields that occupied the ventral portion of the MAcbSh and LAcbSh seemed to be continuous, through the CB, with labeling in the whole mediolateral extension of the Tu. In this injection, anterograde labeling in the Tu was dense in all three layers (maybe slightly denser in layer 3; see inset in **Figure 4G**), but showed no evident association with the ICj (see **Table 3**).

In the caudal AcbC we observed a dense terminal field that extended ventromedially in the rostral direction, innervating the boundary with the MAcbSh (**Figures 4G,H**). In contrast, the ventrolateral AcbC showed less dense anterograde labeling, which appeared continuous with the terminal field found in the LAcbSh (**Figure 4H**).

Table 2 | Semiquantitative rating of the density of the anterograde labeling found in three rostro-caudal levels of the nucleus accumbens shell and core (columns) after different injections in the cortical and deep pallial amygdala (rows).

	MAcbSh			LAcbSh			AcbC		
	r (from +1.78 to +1.54 mm)	i (from +1.42 to +1.18 mm)	c (from +1.10 to +0.86 mm)	r (from +1.34 to +1.18 mm)	i (from +1.10 to +0.98 mm)	c (from +0.86 to +0.74 mm)	r (from +1.94 to +1.70 mm)	i (from +1.54 to +1.34 mm)	c (from +1.18 to +0.98 mm)
CORTICAL AMYGDALA									
R0341 COApl	–	/	/	–	/	X	–	/	X
from −2.30 to −2.46 mm			b			b			b
B0415 COApm + COApl	–	/	/	–	/	XX	–	/	X
from −1.94 to −2.46 mm		b	b		b	b		b	b
B0817 COApm	/	XX	X	–	X	/	–	/	–
from −2.46 to −2.80 mm		b	b		b				
B0324 CxA (+ COAa)	X	XX	XX	X	XX	XX	X	X	XX
from −0.94 to −1.06 mm		B	b			b	b	b	B
DEEP PALLIAL AMYGDALA									
B0310 Ba	XXXX	XXX	XX	XXX	XXX	XXX	XXXX	XXX	XXX
from −1.06 to −1.82 mm		b	b	B	B	B	B	b	b
R0336 Bp	X	XXX	XXX	/	X	XX	XX	XXX	XXXX
from −2.30 to −2.70 mm		b	B			b		B	B
B0311 ABa	/	X	XX	/	/	X	/	/	X
from −0.58 to −0.82 mm			b		b	B		B	B
R0324 ABp	X	XX	XX	X	X	XX	XX	XX	XX
−1.82 mm			b	b	B	B	b		
R0335 ABp		XXX	XXX	XX	XX	XXX	XXX	XXX	XXX
−2.18 mm		B	B	b	B	B	B	B	B
R0311 AHAl	/	X	XX	/	X	X	/	X	XX
from −1.82 to −1.94 mm		b	B			B		b	B
R0305 Lvl	XX	XX	X	XX	XXX	XXX	XXX	XXX	XXX
−1. 82 mm	B	B	B	B	B	B	B	B	B
R0330 Lvl (Ldl + CPu)	XX	XX	XXX	X	XX	XX	XXX	XXX	XXX
−1.70 mm	B	B	B	B	B	B	B	B	B
B0334	X	X	XX	/	X	X	X	XX	XXX
Lvl(+Ldl + Lm + AStr)			b			b		b	b
from −1.70 to −2.30 mm									

The rostro-caudal extent (coordinates from Bregma) of each injection is indicated. The relative density is indicated as follows: –, no labeling; /, very few fibers; X, few fibers; XX moderate density; XXX dense terminal field; XXXX very dense terminal field; XXXXX extremely dense terminal field; B, conspicuous contralateral labeling; b, scarce contralateral labeling. For abbreviations, see list.

In this case, labeling in the Acb, Tu, and CB was bilateral with clear ipsilateral dominance (**Tables 2** and **3**, more evident in the MAcbSh and caudal AcbC, see **Table 2**). Labeled fibers were seen to cross the midline through the *acp* but did not conform conspicuous bundles.

Anterograde labeling in the deep pallial amygdala after injections in the cortical amygdala

To check whether the associative nuclei of the deep pallial amygdala (L, B, and AB) can indirectly relay chemosensory information to the ventral striatum, we studied the intra-amygdaloid projections from the cortical (chemosensory) amygdaloid nuclei to the deep pallial amygdala. Injections in the vomeronasal-recipient COApm gave rise to anterograde labeling in the AB (**Figure 5A**), particularly dense in the posterior part of this nucleus, with sparse fibers observed in the B and L. In contrast, injections in the olfactory-recipient nuclei COApl rendered moderate-to-dense anterograde labeling in the B, mainly in its lateral part, extending into the ventrolateral L (**Figure 5B**). Finally, the injection placed in the CxA (which receives olfactory projections, but also a minor vomeronasal input, Gutiérrez-Castellanos et al., 2010), resulted in abundant anterograde labeling in both the AB and B, which was especially dense in their lateral aspect (**Figure 5C**). In this case, moderately dense anterograde labeling was also observed in the Lvl (**Figure 5C**).

Anterograde labeling in the ventral striatum after injections in the deep pallial amygdala

Ten injections were aimed at the deep pallial amygdala (**Tables 2** and **3**; **Figures 6–8**): three of them were confined to the B, three were located in the AB, one in the AHAl and the last three injections were restricted to the L.

Table 3 | Semiquantitative rating of the density of the anterograde labeling found in three rostro-caudal levels of the olfactory tubercle (Tu; the antero-posterior coordinates to Bregma are indicated), the cell bridges of the ventral striatum (CB), and in association with the islands of Calleja (ICj) and the major island of Calleja (ICjM) (columns), after different injections in the cortical and deep pallial amygdala (rows).

	Tu			CB	ICj	ICjM
	r (from + 1.98 to + 1.42 mm)	i (from + 1.34 to + 0.74 mm)	c (from + 0.62 to + 0.02 mm)			
CORTICAL AMYGDALA						
R0341 COApl	/	X	XX	XX	XX	X
from −2.30 to −2.46 mm		b	b	b		
B0415 COApm + COApl	X	XX	XXX	XXX	XXX	XXX
from −1.94 to −2.46 mm		B	b	B	B	B
B0817 COApm	XX	XXX	/	XXX	XXX	XXX
from −2.46 to −2.80 mm						b
B0324 CxA (+ COAa)	XX	XX	XXX	XXX	/	/
from −0.94 to −1.06 mm		b	b	b		
B0310 Ba	XXXXX	XXXX	XXX	XXXX	X	/
from −1.06 to −1.82 mm	B	B	B	B	B	
R0336 Bp	XX	XXX	XX	XXX	X	X
from −2.30 to −2.70 mm	b	B	B	B	b	b
DEEP PALLIAL AMYGDALA						
B0311 ABa	X	X	X	XX	X	X
from −0.58 to −0.82 mm	b	b	b	b	b	b
R0324 ABp	XX	XX	XX	XX	/	–
−1.82 mm	B	B	B	B	b	
R0335 ABp	XXX	XXX	XXX	XXX	X	/
−2.18 mm	B	B	B	B	b	b
R0311 AHAl	X	XX	XX	X	XX	XX
from −1.82 to −1.94 mm	b	B	B	B	b	B
R0305 Lvl	XXX	XXX	XXX	XXX	X	/
−1. 82 mm	B	B	B	B	B	
R0330 Lvl (Ldl + CPu)	XXX	XX	XX	XXX	X	/
−1.70 mm	B	B	B	B	B	
B0334 Lvl(+Ldl + Lm + AStr)	/	X	X	X	/	/
from −1.70 to −2.30 mm						

The rostro-caudal extent (coordinates from Bregma) of each injection is indicated. The density of labeling is scored according to the following code: –, no labeling; /, very few fibers; X, few fibers; XX, moderate density; XXX, dense terminal field; XXXX, very dense terminal field; XXXXX, extremely dense terminal field; B, conspicuous contralateral labeling; b, scarce contralateral labeling. For abbreviations, see list.

Injections in the basal nucleus. Injection B0310 was restricted to the medial aspect of the Ba, although a few cells in the anterior edge of the AStr were apparently labeled by the pipette track (**Figure 6A**). A bundle of thick, labeled fibers entered the *stria terminalis*, where they could be followed up to the Acb. A different group of labeled fibers ran in the *ansa peduncularis* (through the IPAC and SI) and seemed to be continuous with the labeling in the caudal LAcbSh. Moreover, labeled fibers left the injection site and run rostralwards (through the longitudinal association bundle) to innervate the LOT and, after crossing the ventral anterior amygdala (AAV) gave rise to a dense terminal field in the Tu (**Figures 6B,C**).

The Acb displayed dense fields of anterograde labeling in all its divisions (**Table 2**). In its lateral half, labeling was very dense and showed a complex patchy distribution (**Figure 6C**), whereas in the medial AcbC labeling was mainly composed of sparse labeled fibers except for dense terminal field in its rostral aspect (**Figure 6B**). The MAcbSh displayed patchy, dense fiber labeling mainly confined to its ventral aspect (**Figures 6B,C**). This labeling showed continuity (through the CB, **Figure 6C**) with even denser terminal fields in the medial Tu (**Figures 6B,C**). In contrast, in the dorsal aspect of the MAcbSh only sparse labeled fibers were visible that did not make up well-defined terminal fields (**Figures 6B,C**). The LAcbSh showed a dense terminal field that was also continuous with the extremely dense labeling found in the lateral CB and Tu (**Figure 6C**). In the Tu, the labeling was dense in layer 3 and very dense in layer 2 (**Figures 6B,C** and inset in **Figure 6C**), but showed no clear association with the deep ICj or ICjM. On the contrary, the anterograde labeling in the Tu showed a gap where a superficial ICj was present (**Figure 6C** and inset). However, a few, thick, labeled fibers always reached these superficial ICj (see inset in **Figure 6C**).

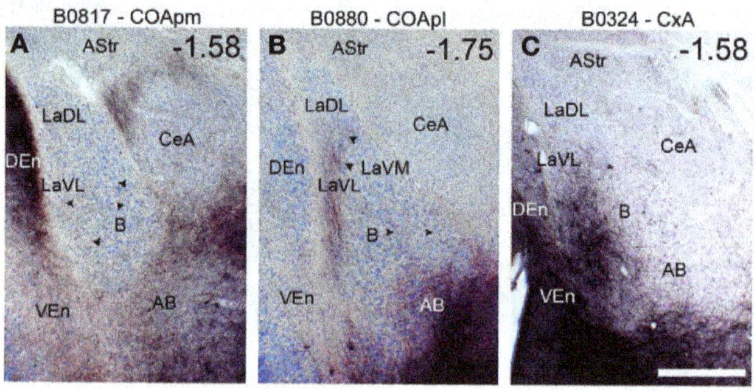

FIGURE 5 | Anterograde labeling in the multimodal amygdaloid nuclei following tracer injections in the chemosensory amygdala. (A) Dense anterograde labeling observed in the accessory basal nucleus of the amygdala following a BDA injection in the COApm, which is the main cortical target of vomeronasal information relayed by the AOB. A few scattered fibers are also present in the basal nucleus of the amygdala (arrowheads). **(B)** Anterograde labeling found in the basolateral complex of the amygdala after a BDA injection in the COApl. Note the band of labeled fibers in the lateral aspect of the B and the ventrolateral L. In addition, scattered fibers are observed throughout the B. **(C)** Anterograde labeling in the basolateral amygdaloid complex following a BDA injection centered in the CxA, which also affected a small portion of the neighboring COAa. Thre resulting anterograde labeling is especially dense in the lateral part of the B and AB, and extends into the ventrolateral L. For abbreviations, see list. Scale bar in **(C)** = 500 μm, valid for the whole figure. The antero-posterior coordinate relative to Bregma is indicated in the upper right corner of each photograph.

In this injection in the Ba, labeled fibers were seen to cross the midline through the *acp*. Dealing with this, the contralateral Acb (especially the LAcbSh and rostral AcbC, **Table 2**) and the rest of the contralateral ventral striatum (**Table 3**) showed a low density of labeled fibers.

Two injections (B0336 and R0336) were located in the Bp. Injection B0336 encompassed the caudolateral Bp, whereas R0336 was a restricted to the caudal portion of the Bp (**Figure 6A**). Although labeled fibers connecting the injection site with the ventral striatum were similar to those found in the previous case, the pattern of anterograde labeling in the ventral striatum differed substantially from that found after injections in the Ba. Thus, the caudomedial AcbC showed extremely dense anterograde labeling (**Figure 6E**) that was apparently connected with a dense terminal field in the bed nucleus of the *stria* terminalis (BST, not shown). Labeling also extended into the MAcbSh where it was very dense (**Figures 6D,E**), with patchy distribution (arrowheads, **Figure 6E**). A few labeled fibers in the periphery of the AcbSh seemed to enter the ICjM (**Figure 6E**). Labeling in the periphery of the MAcbSh could be followed through the medial CB into the medialmost Tu (**Figure 6E**), where labeled fibers were found in deep layer 1 and in layers 2 and 3 (inset in **Figure 6E**). Only a few labeled fibers entered the medial ICj (see inset in **Figure 6E**). In the LAcbSh anterograde labeling was diffuse and its density gradually decreased from caudal to rostral (**Table 2; Figures 6D,E**). In these injections, labeled fibers crossed the midline trough the *acp* and gave rise to scattered but conspicuous anterograde labeling in the contralateral ventral striatum (**Tables 2** and **3**).

Injections in the accessory basal nucleus. Injection B0311 was centered in the rostral tip of ABa, and also affected the deepest aspect of the COAa and the intercalated cell masses of the amygdala (I), as well as a few cells in the AAD and the SI (**Figure 7**). In contrast to injections in B, this case displayed scarce labeling in the Acb and the Tu (**Table 2; Figure 7B**). Three groups of fibers could be tracked from the injection to the ventral striatum. First, thick, labeled fibers ran through the *stria terminalis* up to terminal fields in the BST and dorsolateral, caudal AcbC (not shown). Some labeled fibers followed the *ansa peduncularis* (through the IPAC) to the caudalmost LacbSh and the ventral pallidum (**Figure 7B**). Finally, fibers in the longitudinal association bundle gave rise to a dense terminal meshwork in the horizontal limb of the diagonal band nucleus (HDB) that extended into the medialmost CB (inset in **Figure 7B**) and the medial Tu, where it innervated all three layers. A few labeled fibers apparently entered some ICj (inset in **Figure 7B**), and surrounded the ICjM (**Figure 7B**). Moreover, the ventral MAcbSh displayed scarce fiber labeling apparently connected with the bundles innervating the HDB and/or VP (**Figure 7B**). The contralateral, caudal ventral striatum also showed few labeled fibers (see **Tables 2** and **3**), which were observed to cross the midline through the *acp*.

Two small injections (R0324 and R0335) located in the ABp (with a few labeled cells in the AHAl in case R0335; **Figure 7A**) revealed a pattern of fiber labeling in the ventral striatum substantially more extensive than the one observed following the injection in the ABa (compare the **Figures 7B–D**). The amygdalofugal fibers followed the three pathways described above. First, thin labeled fibers of the *stria terminalis* apparently gave rise to a moderately dense terminal field in the whole AcbC and the ventral MAcbSh (**Figures 7C,D**). Second, labeled fibers in the *ansa peduncularis* gave rise to a terminal field extending from the IPAC to the caudal LAcbSh, where labeling was less dense (**Table 2; Figures 7C,D**). Finally, labeled fibers in the longitudinal association bundle reached the Tu, where they preferentially innervated layers 2, 3, and 1b of its central aspect (inset in **Figure 7D**). Labeling in the Tu was continuous, through the CB, with the one observed in the ventral AcbSh (see arrows in **Figures 7C,D**). Few labeled fibers were associated to the outer edge of most of the ICj (inset in **Figure 7C**) and, to a lesser extent, to the inner margin of the ICjM (arrowhead in **Figure 7C**). In both injections, the contralateral ventral striatum also showed a moderate density of anterograde labeling (**Tables 2** and **3**).

Injection in the amygdalohippocampal area. A small injection (R0311) was restricted to the rostral tip of the AHAl (**Figure 7A**). Labeled fibers in the *stria terminalis* apparently innervated the AcbC (where labeling decreased from caudal to rostral, see **Table 2**), especially its ventral half (**Figures 7E,F**) and the mid-caudal MAcbSh, where labeled fibers were preferentially found in the medial edge of the nucleus (arrow in **Figure 7F**) and next to the core-shell boundary (**Figures 7E,F**). A dense terminal field was closely associated to the inner ICjM (see inset in **Figure 7F**). The labeled bundles in the IPAC/SI could be followed rostrally up to the midcaudal LAcbSh, where sparse anterograde labeling was observed (**Figure 7F**). Finally, labeled fibers running in

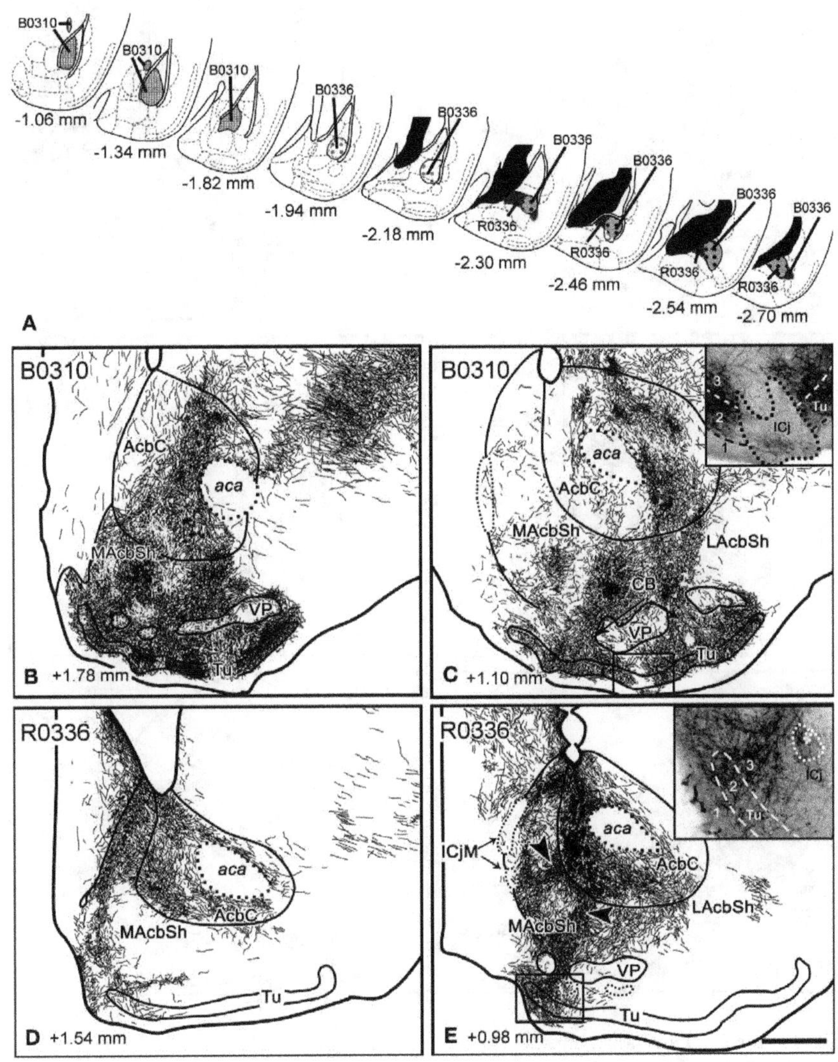

FIGURE 6 | Anterograde labeling in the ventral striatum after tracer injections in the basal nucleus of the amygdala. (A) Semi-schematic drawings of frontal sections showing the extent of the tracer injections in the basal nucleus of the amygdala, with indication of the antero-posterior coordinate relative to Bregma. **(B,C)** Anterograde labeling found in the ventral striatum after a tracer injection in the Ba (B0310). Although the ICj are nearly devoid of labeling, a few thick, labeled fibers enter the clusters of granule cells [see inset in **(C)**]. Labeling in the AcbSh shows continuity with the one in the Tu through the CB. Labeling in the Tu occupies layers 2 and 3, whereas layer 1 is virtually free of labeling [inset in **(C)**]. **(D,E)** Anterograde labeling in the ventral striatum after injection R0336, which involved a large portion of the Bp. Labeling in the core of the Acb apparently shows continuity with the one in MAcbSh [see arrowheads in **(E)**] and, through it, with the labeling in the CB and medial Tu. labeling in the Tu occupies not only layers 2 and 3 but also deep layer 1 [inset in **(E)**]. For abbreviations, see list. Scale bar in **(E)** = 400 μm, valid for the whole figure.

the longitudinal association bundle innervated the HDB and all three layers of Tu, preferentially in its medial half (**Figure 7F**). This terminal field, which was connected with the one in the AcbSh through the CB (see asterisk in **Figures 7E,F**), also included dense labeled fibers in close association with the medial ICj (**Figure 7F**).

Labeled fibers crossed the midline trough the *acp* to innervated some structures of the contralateral, caudal ventral striatum (**Tables 2** and **3**).

Injections in the lateral nucleus. Three injections were aimed at the L (see **Figure 8**). Injection R0330 was centered in the rostral Lvl, although it also encompassed the ventral part of the Ldl and involved a few cells in the caudoventral CPu. Injection R0305 consisted of a small injection restricted to the Lvl at intermediate antero-posterior levels. Finally, a large BDA injection encompassed the whole caudal L (Ldl, Lvl, and Lm) and the AStr (B0334). In these three injections, labeled fibers ran in the *stria terminalis* up to the AcbC, where they gave rise to the densest terminal field in the ventral striatum, which extended to the adjacent, ventralmost CPu (**Table 2; Figures 8B–E**). From the AcbC, anterogradely labeled fibers extended to the ventral AcbSh, where they formed a conspicuous terminal field (**Figures 8B–D**), whereas the dorsal MAcbSh (interposed between the core and the medial

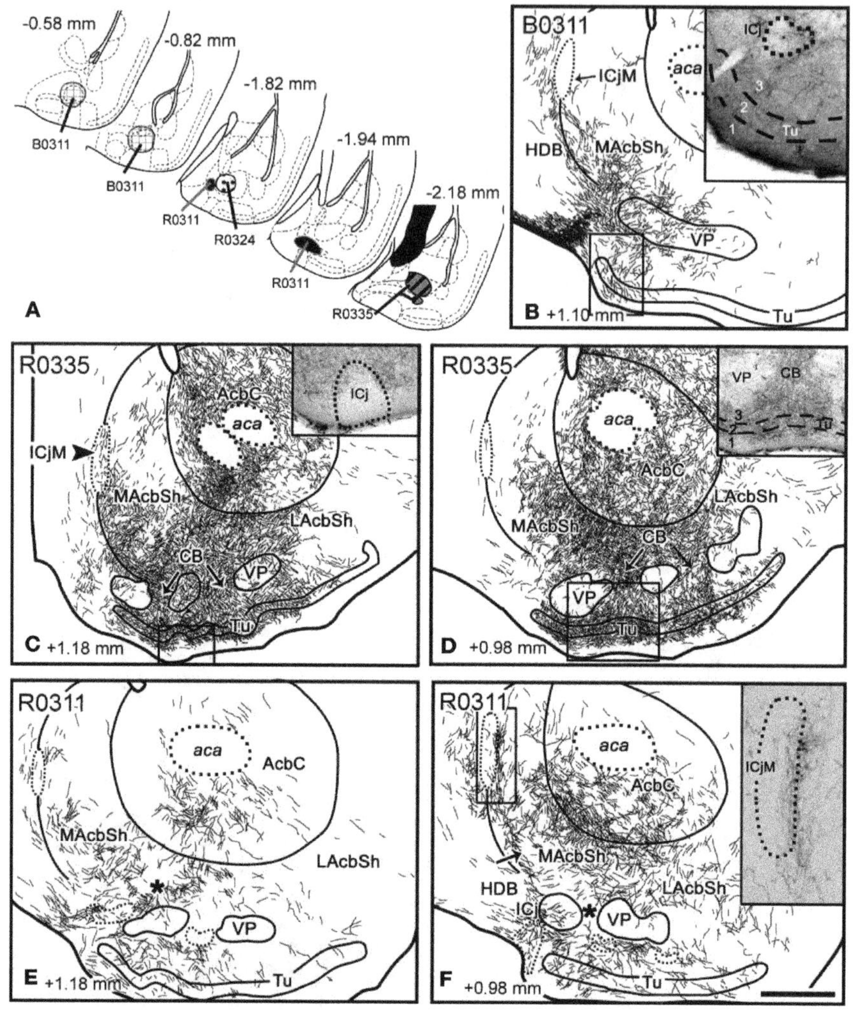

FIGURE 7 | Anterograde transport in the ventral striatum after tracer injections in the accessory basal amygdaloid nucleus and amygdalohippocampal area. (A) Semi-schematic drawings of frontal sections showing the extent of the tracer injections in the accessory basal nucleus of the amygdala. The antero-posterior coordinate relative to Bregma is indicated in each section. **(B)** Anterograde transport in the MAcbSh and medialmost caudal Tu after a tracer injection in the ABa (B0311). Scattered labeled fibers are present in the ICj and in all three layers of the Tu (inset). **(C,D)** Frontal sections through the ventral striatum of a mouse that received an RDA injection in the ABp(R0335; no counterstaining). Besides extensive labeling in the Acb core and shell (especially in the LAcbSh), a labeled terminal field is found next to some of the ICj [inset in **(C)**] and in the ICjM [arrowhead in **(C)**]. In the Tu, anterograde labeling is found in layers 2 and 3 and in deep layer 1 [inset in **(D)**]. **(E,F)** Anterograde labeling in the ventral striatum after an RDA injection restricted to the lateral AHA (R0311) (no counterstaining). Moderately dense labeling occupies the ventral core as well as parts of the medial and lateral shell of the Acb. Scattered labeled fibers are also found in the neighboring CB (asterisks) and in the Tu. In addition, conspicuous terminal fields are found in the medial ICj and, especially, next to the ICjM [see inset in **(F)**]. For abbreviations, see list. Scale bar in **(F)** = 400 μm, valid for the whole figure.

septum), was virtually devoid of labeling (**Figures 8B–D**). Labeling in the ventral AcbSh was continuous, through the CB, with labeling in the Tu (**Figures 8C–E**). Anterogradely labeled fibers displayed a clear association with the most medial ICj (see inset in **Figure 8D**), but not with the ICjM (see **Figure 8D**). After the small injections in the rostral L (R0305, R0330), labeling in the Tu was particularly dense, and preferentially occupied layer 3 and (to a lesser extent) layer 2 (**Figures 8B–D** and inset in **Figure 8B**).

In addition, some labeled fibers ran through the *ansa peduncularis* (through the SI and the IPAC) and gave rise to a moderate-to-dense terminal field in the midcaudal LAcbSh (**Figure 8E**). Finally, a small number of labeled fibers were seen in longitudinal association bundle, apparently giving rise to anterograde labeling in the Tu.

In all the injections encompassing the L, anterograde labeling in the ventral striatum was bilateral with ipsilateral dominance (see **Tables 2** and **3**).

DISCUSSION

Our work combines anterograde and retrograde tracing to analyze the projections of the amygdala to the ventral striatum, with emphasis on the putative pathways allowing the transfer of chemosensory information to the reward system of the brain.

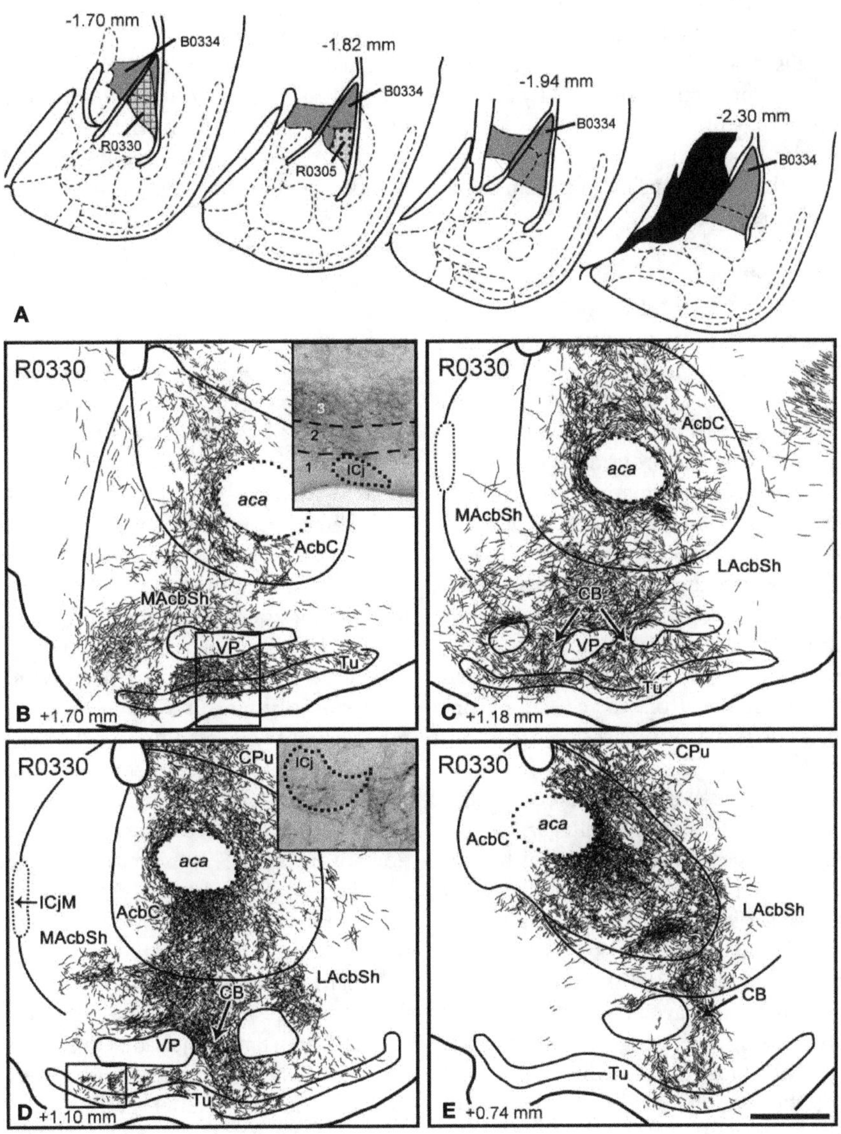

FIGURE 8 | Anterograde labeling in the ventral striatum after tracer injections in the lateral nucleus of the amygdala. (A) Semi-schematic drawings of frontal sections through the amygdala depicting the extent of tracer injections in the lateral nucleus. The antero-posterior coordinate relative to Bregma is indicated in each section. **(B–E)** Semi-schematic drawings of four frontal sections through the brain of a mouse that received an RDA injection in the Lvl and Ldl (R0330), showing the distribution of anterograde labeling in the ventral striatum. Labeling occupies parts of the core and shell of the Acb, a large portion of the Tu [layers 2 and 3, inset in **(B)**] and those CB linking both structures (arrows). In some islands of Calleja a few, thick, labeled fibers are seen in the clusters of granule cells [inset in **(D)**]. For abbreviations, see list. Scale bar in **(E)** = 400 μm, valid for the whole figure.

To properly interpret our results we should first discuss some limitations of the tract-tracing techniques we have used.

METHODOLOGICAL CONSIDERATIONS

In the first part of the study we have used the retrograde transport of fluorogold and biotin- and rhodamine-labeled dextran amines to label the amygdaloid afferents to the ventral striatum. Although dextran amines are generally used as anterograde tracers, in certain conditions they also reliably render retrograde transport (Rajakumar et al., 1993; Reiner et al., 2000; Schofield, 2008) and they have been used as such in mammals (Schofield and Cant, 1996). In fact, our retrograde tracing experiments replicate the results of similar experiments in rats using fluorogold (Brog et al., 1993). In addition, our results of retrograde tracing of the amygdalo-striatal pathways are consistent with those of anterograde tracing of the same projections (see below).

In the second part of the study, we have injected dextran amines in the amygdala to analyze the anterograde transport to the ventral striatum and within the amygdala itself. Since in our experimental conditions dextran amines are transported both retrogradely and anterogradely, in the interpretation of the results we take into account the possibility of fiber labeling due to axon collaterals from retrogradely labeled cells. In addition, in every injection anterogradely labeled fibers can be tracked through previously defined tracts (see below) from the injection site to the terminal fields in the ventral striatum. This indicates that the bulk of the labeling found in the striatum originates in cells located in the injection site in the amygdala. On the other hand, the projections revealed by anterograde labeling in the amygdala have been confirmed by means of retrograde labeling from injections in the striatum, except for a single case, the projection from the lateral nucleus of the amygdala to the olfactory tubercle, as discussed below.

DIRECT AND INDIRECT PATHWAYS THROUGH THE AMYGDALA RELAY CHEMOSENSORY INFORMATION TO THE VENTRAL STRIATUM

Our results demonstrate that both cortical and deep amygdaloid nuclei extensively innervate the ventral striatum. Given that the cortical amygdaloid nuclei (COAa, CxA, COApl, and COApm) receive olfactory and vomeronasal projections from the olfactory bulbs, it is likely that the amygdalo-striatal projections originated in these nuclei convey chemosensory information. In addition, our results show that intra-amygdaloid projections originated from these cortical amygdaloid nuclei innervate the lateral, basal, and accessory basal nuclei of the basolateral complex, which are considered associative nuclei (they receive important projections from unimodal and multimodal areas from the thalamus and cortex, see Turner and Herkenham, 1991; McDonald, 1998; Swanson and Petrovich, 1998). These projections from the chemosensory cortical amygdala to the deep associative nuclei are consistent with previous data reported in rats. The projection from the vomeronasal-recipient COApm to the AB was observed by Canteras et al. (1992) and Kemppainen et al. (2002). Regarding the COApl, it is included as part of the periamygdaloid cortex by several authors (see Pitkänen, 2000), and a number of studies show projections from the periamygdaloid cortex to the L (Ottersen, 1982; Luskin and Price, 1983; Majak and Pitkänen, 2003) and to the B (Ottersen, 1982; Luskin and Price, 1983). Finally, to our knowledge the connections of the CxA have not been previously analyzed, but a previous study using the retrograde transport of HRP in the rat showed retrogradely labeled cells in this area following injections in the L and B (Ottersen, 1982; see his Figures 2D and 5F). None of these intra-amygdaloid projections had been previously shown in mice. Therefore, both the direct projections from the chemosensory cortical amygdala and the indirect projections from the associative amygdaloid nuclei may convey chemosensory information to the ventral striatum.

ORGANIZATION OF AMYGDALO-STRIATAL PATHWAYS IN THE MOUSE

These amygdalo-striatal projections course through three pathways, namely the *stria terminalis*, the *ansa peduncularis*, and the longitudinal association bundle, in agreement with previous descriptions (Johnston, 1923; Kelley et al., 1982; Petrovich et al., 1996). In general, the amygdaloid fibers terminating in the AcbC and dorsomedial AcbSh course through the *stria terminalis* and represent a rostral extension of the terminal fields in the BST. A second amygdalo-striatal pathway courses through the *ansa peduncularis* crossing the SI/IPAC and entering the lateral AcbSh, and maybe the caudolateral AcbC. A third contingent of amygdalo-striatal fibers runs rostralwards through the longitudinal association bundle (Johnston, 1923) thus reaching directly the caudal Tu and adjacent structures. Fibers running in all three pathways might contribute to the innervation of the ventral aspect of the AcbSh and the adjoining CB.

The termination fields of the main amygdaloid projections to the ventral striatum are summarized in **Figure 9**. As it can be observed, virtually all the divisions of the ventral striatum receive inputs from one or several amygdaloid nuclei, thus depicting a complex pattern of amygdalo-striatal projections.

Ventral striatal projections of the cortical amygdaloid nuclei

Our experiments reveal important amygdalo-striatal projections arising from several cortical amygdaloid nuclei which, according to the present results, were probably underestimated in previous studies. The anterior aspect of the cortical amygdala displays substantial projections to the Acb and Tu/CB apparently originated from deep cells in the CxA/COAa boundary (**Figures 2B** and **3B**). This projection was also suggested by previous observations in rats (McDonald, 1991b) and monkeys (Friedman et al., 2002). Regarding the posterior cortical amygdala, our results show that a number of deep cells of the COApm and COApl are retrogradely labeled by injections in the Tu. These projections are confirmed by the anterograde labeling following injections in the COApm and COApl, which reveal a conspicuous projection to the deep Tu, CB, and some ICj (see below; Úbeda-Bañón et al., 2008), as well as sparse projections to the caudal AcbC and AcbLSh (see **Figure 9**), in agreement with previous results in rats (Canteras et al., 1992).

Our injections in the core and lateral shell of the Acb, also showed retrogradely labeled cells in the LOT. The location of these labeled cells depended on the injection site: whereas tracer injections in the LAcbSh rendered retrograde labeling in layers 2 and 3 of the LOT, those in the AcbC only showed labeled cells in layer 3. These data fully fit the results of anterograde tracing in the rat reported by Santiago and Shammah-Lagnado (2004).

Finally, in agreement with the findings by Brog et al. (1993) in the rat, our results of retrograde labeling demonstrate the presence of important projections to the MAcbSh and Tu arising from the APir. Although we have not performed tracer injections in the APir, experiments of anterograde transport carried out in the rat by Shammah-Lagnado and Santiago (1999) confirm this projection. As suggested previously (Luskin and Price, 1983), these projections might be association fibers, originating from pyramidal cells located in layers II and II.

Ventral striatal projections of the deep nuclei of the pallial amygdala

This pattern of amygdalo-striatal projections originated by the deep pallial amygdala displays three main similarities with the results of previous studies in other mammalian species.

Firstly, as described in rats and cats (Krettek and Price, 1978; Groenewegen et al., 1980; Kelley et al., 1982; Russchen and Price, 1984; McDonald, 1991a,b; Brog et al., 1993; Wright et al., 1996) and in monkeys (Russchen et al., 1985; Price et al., 1987; Friedman et al., 2002; Fudge et al., 2002, 2004), the bulk of the amygdalo-Acb projections arises from deep pallial nuclei (B and AB). Secondly, our results indicate that in mice, like in rats and cats (Krettek and Price, 1978; Wright et al., 1996) the projections from the anterior and posterior parts of the B to the Acb display a rough topography according to which the Ba projects mostly to the anterior

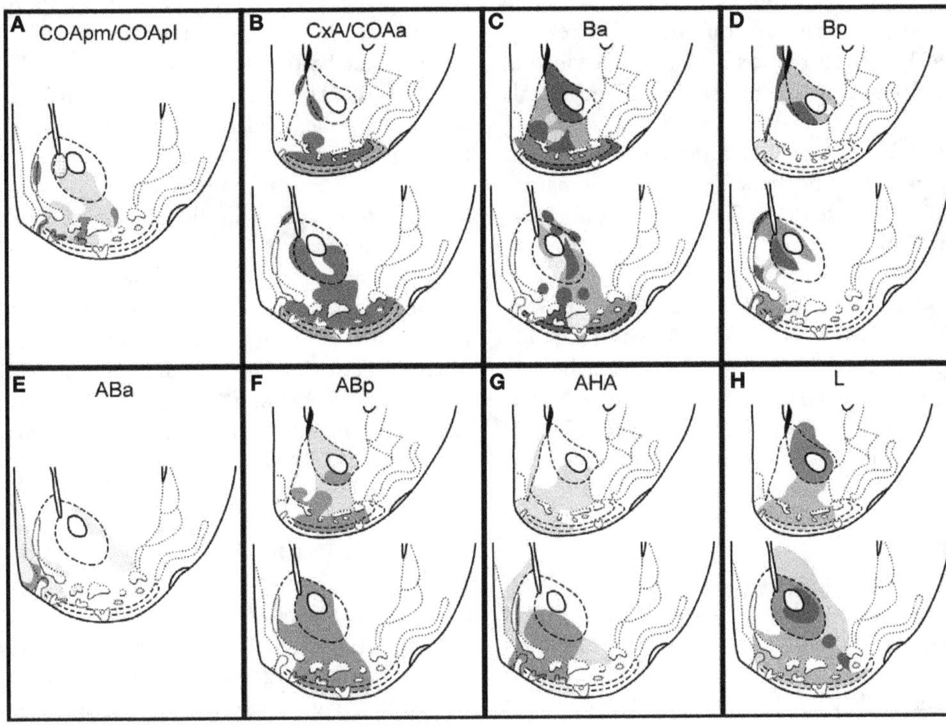

FIGURE 9 | Summary of the projections from pallial amygdala to the ventral striatum in the mouse. Schematic drawings of frontal sections through the ventral striatum of the mouse (rostral on top, caudal bottom), showing the main terminal fields of the projections from the cortical **(A,B)** and deep pallial amygdala **(C–H)** in the ventral striatum. The relative density of the terminal fields, as inferred from our injections, is represented as different gray levels (the darker the denser). The patterned area in the medial AcbC in **(A)** indicates a terminal field that is labeled after the injection in the COApm but not in the injection centered in the COApl. For abbreviations, see list.

and posterolateral Acb/Tu, whereas the Bp projects mainly to the medial posterior Acb/Tu (**Figures 9C,D**). And finally, anterograde transport after injections in B and AB reveal a patchy distribution of labeled fibers in the medial AcbSh (see **Figures 6C,E** and **7B,D**) that recalls the one described in the rat and cat by Krettek and Price (1978). Whether or not these patchy projections are related to inhomogeneities in calbindin-immunoreactivity as reported in the rat (Wright et al., 1996), the similarities in the amygdalo-Acb projections between mice and other mammals are noticeable. This similarity also makes very unlikely that the labeled fibers observed in our material be due to labeling of axonic collaterals from retrogradely labeled cells.

An additional conclusion drawn from our findings is that the AHA and L substantially contribute to the projections from the deep pallial amygdala to the Acb and Tu. Experiments in rats have also demonstrated substantial anterograde transport to the caudal Acb after tracer injections in the AHA (Canteras et al., 1992, posterior amygdala using their nomenclature) and dense retrograde labeling in the AHA following injections in the MAcbSh (McDonald, 1991b; Brog et al., 1993).

Finally, our results clearly indicate that the L, a nucleus usually viewed as the sensory interface of the amygdala (at least in the context of fear conditioning, LeDoux et al., 1990; Pitkänen et al., 1997), shows important projections to the ventral striatum. The existence of this connection has been previously suggested in rats (Kelley et al., 1982; McDonald, 1991b; Brog et al., 1993) and primates (Friedman et al., 2002; Fudge et al., 2002). Our results indicate that these projections mainly arise from the dorsolateral (Ldl) and ventrolateral subnuclei (Lvl, see **Table 1**). This is confirmed by anterograde transport after injections in the L (involving the Lvl and/or Ldl), which display labeled fibers in the midcaudal AcbC (from where they extend into the rostromedial CPu), as well as in the ventral aspect of the MAcbSh and in the LAcbSh (**Figure 9H**). This projection apparently extends into the Tu/CB complex and the ICj, although we could not confirm this observation with retrograde labeling.

Amygdaloid projections to the islands of Calleja and associated territories of the olfactory tubercle

Our tracing experiments reveal not only important amygdaloid projections to the Tu, but also very important connections with other structures including ICj and the CB (see **Figure 9**). The ICj are densely packed groups of small cells that occupy diverse positions within the ventral striatum. Most of them are placed within the Tu, where they are located in layers 2–3 and even impinge upon layer 1 reaching the pial surface. In contrast, the ICjM separates the medial AcbSh from the ventral aspect of the lateral septum. The COApm/COApl and AHA display strong projections to the medial ICjs and ICjM (see **Table 3**). In contrast, the remaining amygdaloid nuclei give rise to limited projections to the ICj, which are relatively rare in the case of the ICjM (see **Table 3**). These results partially agree with previous studies on the ICj connections indicating that the bulk of the amygdaloid projections to the ICj arose from the cortical nuclei (Krettek and Price, 1978; Fallon, 1983). Recent reports have also described in some detail these projections in rats and mice (Úbeda-Bañón et al., 2007, 2008).

The projections to the CB have received minor attention. In this respect, labeling in a portion of the Tu was always accompanied by labeling of those CB adjacent to it (see **Table 3**) suggesting that the Tu and CB are functionally related.

FUNCTIONAL CONSIDERATIONS: ROLE OF AMYGDALO-STRIATAL PATHWAYS IN EMOTIONAL EVALUATION OF CHEMOSENSORY STIMULI

As we have seen, the pallial amygdala projects heavily to the core and shell of the nucleus accumbens, the olfactory tubercle, and the striatal cell bridges linking the ventral Acb with the Tu, and the ICj. The amygdalo-accumbens projection is considered to be involved in reward-related processes (Everitt et al., 1999; Baxter and Murray, 2002; see below). In this respect, our findings lead to two main conclusions.

First of all, the Tu receives massive projections from the pallial amygdala, conveying olfactory and vomeronasal information (from the cortical amygdala) and non-chemosensory information (from the basolateral amygdala). Since these projections mainly terminate in layers 2 and 3, they likely target the cell bodies and proximal dendrites of the principal cells and thus probably have a strong influence on the activity of the Tu. Therefore, the Tu, CB and ICj constitute a portion of the ventral striatum mediating responses to a variety of chemosensory and non-chemosensory stimuli, as suggested by Talbot et al. (1988a,b) on the basis of anatomical and neurochemical studies in different mammals. In this respect, several nuclei of the pallial amygdala project to the ICj. However, the projection from the COApm (the main cortical target of the accessory olfactory bulb, Scalia and Winans, 1975) apparently terminates, in a fairly specific way, in the neuropile-rich core of the ICj, and in the lateral aspect of the ICjM. Although the inner structure and cell composition of the ICj are very complex (Fallon et al., 1978, 1983; Fallon, 1983), the specific input from a vomeronasal relay suggest that some ICj might be specialized structures of the ventral striatum devoted to processing vomeronasal information.

The second conclusion drawn from our findings is that the medial Tu and adjoining structures (CB and ICj) are very likely involved in mediating (affective) reward-related responses to chemical signals. This is supported by the fact that both electrical stimulation in the medial Tu (Prado-Alcala and Wise, 1984) and local administration of addictive drugs (Kornetsky et al., 1991; Ikemoto et al., 2005) are rewarding. Since the medial aspect of the Tu and neighboring CB and ICj, including the ICjM, receive distinct projections from the vomeronasal amygdala (COApm and AHA) and stimulation of the vomeronasal amygdala is rewarding (Kane et al., 1991), it is likely that these amygdalo-striatal projections mediate reward responses to (among other stimuli) vomeronasal-and/or olfactory-detected chemosignals (see also Úbeda-Bañón et al., 2007, 2008).

Regarding the projections from the basolateral amygdala to the ventral striatum, they are involved in the expression of reward-related behaviors toward secondary reinforcers (Cador et al., 1989; Everitt et al., 1989). In fact, Pavlovian second-order conditioning is impaired by lesions of either the accumbens (Parkinson et al., 1999) or the basolateral amygdala (Hatfield et al., 1996; Blundell et al., 2001). These findings indicate that the learning processes occurring in the basolateral amygdala endow neutral stimuli with appetitive properties by means of their association with primary reinforcers. Through its projections to the ventral striatum, the basolateral amygdala would mediate goal-directed responses to these newly attractive stimuli.

In this respect, it has been shown in female mice that odorants are not innately attractive but become so after their association with non-volatile (e.g., vomeronasal), innately rewarding male pheromones (Moncho-Bogani et al., 2002; Martínez-Ricós et al., 2007, 2008; Roberts et al., 2010). This association of olfactory and vomeronasal stimuli might occur in the basolateral amygdala, since the cortical amygdala, and piriform cortex (present results; McDonald, 1998) display convergent projections to deep amygdaloid nuclei (Canteras et al., 1992; Pitkänen, 2000; Lanuza et al., 2008). This hypothesis is consistent with the expression of c-fos in the basolateral amygdala of female mice induced by male odors before and after olfactory–vomeronasal associative learning (Moncho-Bogani et al., 2005). A similar role has been proposed for the basolateral amygdala in olfactory–gustatory associative learning mediating go–no go appetitive responses (Schoenbaum et al., 1999).

EVOLUTION OF THE EMOTIONAL BRAIN

Comparative studies (Bruce and Neary, 1995; Martínez-García et al., 2002, 2007) indicate that reptiles possess a well-developed pallial amygdala composed of chemosensory cortical structures (superficial, layered) and multimodal deep nuclei. Anatomical and neurochemical data in different reptiles and in birds strongly suggest that the projections from the pallial amygdala to the ventral striatum were already present in the ancestral amniote and underwent a conservative evolution (Novejarque et al., 2004; Martínez-García et al., 2007). In this respect, our finding that parts of the cortical amygdala of mammals display substantial projections to the ventral striatum fit the results of similar studies in non-mammals. Thus, the vomeronasal cortex of squamate reptiles (the nucleus sphericus), like its mammalian counterpart, the COApm, projects massively to a portion of the ventral striatum located between the nucleus accumbens and the olfactory tubercle. In snakes this portion of the ventral striatum is called the olfactostriatum (Lanuza and Halpern, 1997), and displays characteristic neurochemical features (Martínez-Marcos et al., 2005). Together with recent data in rats (Úbeda-Bañón et al., 2008), the present results suggest that the "olfactostriatum" would be represented in the mammalian brain by the anteromedial cell bridges and ICj, plus portions of the adjacent Tu that receive the projection from the COApm. In fact, like the ophidian olfactostriatum (Martínez-Marcos et al., 2005) the medial portions of the CB, the ICj, and the Tu display a moderate-to-dense innervation of neuropeptide Y-immunoreactive fibers (Riedel et al., 2002; Úbeda-Bañón et al., 2008). In addition, cells in the Tu and the ICj express 5-hydroxytryptamine-2A receptors (Mijnster et al., 1997; Jansson et al., 2001). Although these data support this homology, it is noteworthy that the CB, the ICj, and the Tu show a high density of TH-immunoreactive axons (Seifert et al., 1998; Riedel et al., 2002; Úbeda-Bañón et al., 2008), whereas the ophidian olfactostriatum displays a comparatively sparser innervation of TH-immunoreactive fibers (Martínez-Marcos et al., 2005).

Anatomical, neurochemical, and functional data suggest that the telencephalon of the ancestral amniote possessed an amygdalo-striatal system. The fact that this circuitry has remained well conserved indicates that its function is crucial for survival and reproduction. Indeed, the amygdala receives multimodal sensory information and controls the expression of basic emotional behaviors, namely reward/attraction (throughout its projections to ventral striatum) or fear/anxiety/aversion (throughout its projections to the central extended amygdala). Therefore, in the ancestral amniote, the amygdalo-striatal system constituted part of the primordial emotional brain, since it probably allowed not only the appropriate behavioral response toward unconditioned attractive (rewarding) stimuli, but also learning from these events by means of the emotional tagging of neutral sensory stimuli.

ACKNOWLEDGMENTS

Funded by the Spanish Ministry of Education and Science-FEDER (BFU2007-67912-C02-01/BFI and BFU2010-16656), Generalitat Valenciana (ACOMP/2010/127) and the Junta de Comunidades de Castilla-La Mancha (PEIC11-0045-4490).

REFERENCES

Aggleton, J. P. (ed.). (2000). *The Amygdala. A Functional Analysis*, 2nd Edn. Oxford: Oxford University Press.

Agustín-Pavón, C., Martínez-Ricós, J., Martínez-García, F., and Lanuza, E. (2007). Effects ofdopaminergic drugs on innate pheromone-mediated reward in female mice: a new case of dopamine-independent "liking". *Behav. Neurosci.* 121, 920–932.

Baxter, M. G., and Murray, E. A. (2002). The amygdala and reward. *Nat. Rev. Neurosci.* 3, 563–573.

Blundell, P., Hall, G., and Killcross, S. (2001). Lesions of the basolateral amygdala disrupt selective aspects of reinforcer representation in rats. *J. Neurosci.* 21, 9018–9026.

Brog, J. S., Salyapongse, A., Deutch, A. Y., and Zahm, D. S. (1993). The patterns of afferent innervation of the core and shell in the "accumbens" part of the rat ventral striatum: immunohistochemical detection of retrogradely transported fluoro-gold. *J. Comp. Neurol.* 338, 255–278.

Bruce, L. L., and Neary, T. J. (1995). The limbic system of tetrapods: a comparative analysis of cortical and amygdalar populations. *Brain Behav. Evol.* 46, 224–234.

Cador, M., Robbins, T. W., and Everitt, B. J. (1989). Involvement of the amygdala in stimulus-reward associations: interaction with the ventral striatum. *Neuroscience* 30, 77–86.

Caffé, A. R., van Leeuwen, F. W., and Luiten, P. G. (1987). Vasopressin cells in the medial amygdala of the rat project to the lateral septum and ventral hippocampus. *J. Comp. Neurol.* 261, 237–252.

Canteras, N. S., Simerly, R. B., and Swanson, L. W. (1992). Connections of the posterior nucleus of the amygdala. *J. Comp. Neurol.* 324, 143–179.

Everitt, B. J., Cador, M., and Robbins, T. W. (1989). Interactions between the amygdala and ventral striatum in stimulus-reward associations: studies using a second-order schedule of sexual reinforcement. *Neuroscience* 30, 63–75.

Everitt, B. J., Cardinal, R. N., Parkinson, J. A., and Robbins, T. W. (2003). Appetitive behavior: impact of amygdala-dependent mechanisms of emotional learning. *Ann. N. Y. Acad. Sci.* 985, 233–250.

Everitt, B. J., Morris, K. A., O'Brien, A., and Robbins, T. W. (1991). The basolateral amygdala-ventral striatal system and conditioned place preference: further evidence of limbic-striatal interactions underlying reward-related processes. *Neuroscience* 42, 1–18.

Everitt, B. J., Parkinson, J. A., Olmstead, M. C., Arroyo, M., Robledo, P., and Robbins, T. W. (1999). Associative processes in addiction and reward. The role of amygdala- ventral striatal subsystems. *Ann. N. Y. Acad. Sci.*877, 412–438.

Fallon, J. H. (1983). The islands of Calleja complex of rat basal forebrain II: connections of medium and large sized cells. *Brain Res. Bull.* 10, 775–793.

Fallon, J. H., Loughlin, S. E., and Ribak, C. E. (1983). The islands of Calleja complex of rat basal forebrain. III. Histochemical evidence for a striatopallidal system. *J. Comp. Neurol.* 218, 91–120.

Fallon, J. H., Riley, J. N., Sipe, J. C., and Moore, R. Y. (1978). The islands of Calleja: organization and connections. *J. Comp. Neurol.* 181, 375–395.

Friedman, D. P., Aggleton, J. P., and Saunders, R. C. (2002). Comparison of hippocampal, amygdala, and perirhinal projections to the nucleus accumbens: combined anterograde and retrograde tracing study in the Macaque brain. *J. Comp. Neurol.* 450, 345–365.

Fudge, J. L., Breitbart, M. A., and McClain, C. (2004). Amygdaloid inputs define a caudal component of the ventral striatum in primates. *J. Comp. Neurol.* 476, 330–347.

Fudge, J. L., Kunishio, K., Walsh, P., Richard, C., and Haber, S. N. (2002). Amygdaloid projections to ventromedial striatal subterritories in the primate. *Neuroscience* 110, 257–275.

Groenewegen, H. J., Becker, N. E., and Lohman, A. H. (1980). Subcortical afferents of the nucleus accumbens septi in the cat, studied with retrograde axonal transport of horseradish peroxidase and bisbenzimid. *Neuroscience* 5, 1903–1916.

Gutiérrez-Castellanos, N., Martínez-Marcos, A., Martínez-García, F., and Lanuza, E. (2010). Chemosensory function of the amygdala. *Vitam. Horm.* 83, 165–196.

Haga, S., Hattori, T., Sato, T., Sato, K., Matsuda, S., Kobayakawa, R., Sakano, H., Yoshihara, Y., Kikusui, T., and Touhara, K. (2010). The male mouse pheromone ESP1 enhances female sexual receptive behaviour through a specific vomeronasal receptor. *Nature* 466, 118–122.

Hatfield, T., Han, J. S., Conley, M., Gallagher, M., and Holland, P. (1996). Neurotoxic lesions of basolateral, but not central, amygdala interfere with Pavlovian second-order conditioning and reinforcer devaluation effects. *J. Neurosci.* 16, 5256–5265.

Ikemoto, S., Qin, M., and Liu, Z.-H. (2005). The functional divide for primary reinforcement of D-amphetamine lies between the medial and lateral ventral striatum: is the division of the accumbens core, shell, and olfactory tubercle valid? *J. Neurosci.* 25, 5061–5065.

Jansson, A., Tinner, B., Bancila, M., Verge, D., Steinbusch, H. W., Agnati, L. F., and Fuxe, K. (2001). Relationships of 5-hydroxytryptamine immunoreactive terminal-like varicosities to 5-hydroxytryptamine-2A receptor-immunoreactive neuronal processes in the rat forebrain. *J. Chem. Neuroanat.* 22, 185–203.

Johnston, J. B. (1923). Further contributions to the study of the evolution of the forebrain. *J. Comp. Neurol.* 35, 337–481.

Kane, F., Coulombe, D., and Miliaressis, E. (1991). Amygdaloid self-stimulation: a movable electrode mapping study. *Behav. Neurosci.* 105, 926–932.

Kelley, A. E., Domesick, V. B., and Nauta, W. J. H. (1982). The amygdalostriatal projection in the rat – an anatomical study by anterograde and retrograde tracing methods. *Neuroscience* 7, 615–630.

Kemppainen, S., Jolkkonen, E., and Pitkänen, A. (2002). Projections from the posterior corticalnucleus of the amygdala to the hippocampal formation and parahippocampal regionin rat. *Hippocampus* 12, 735–755.

Kornetsky, C., Huston-Lyons, D., and Porrino, L. J. (1991). The role of the olfactory tubercle in the effects of cocaine, morphine and brain-stimulation reward. *Brain Res.* 541, 75–81.

Krettek, J. E., and Price, J. L. (1978). Amygdaloid projections to subcortical structures within the basal forebrain and brainstem in the rat and cat. *J. Comp. Neurol.* 178, 225–254.

Lanuza, E., and Halpern, M. (1997). Afferent and efferent connections of the nucleus sphericus in the snake Thamnophis sirtalis: convergence of olfactory and vomeronasal information in the lateral cortex and the amygdala. *J. Comp. Neurol.* 385, 627–640.

Lanuza, E., Novejarque, A., Martínez-Ricós, J., Martínez-Hernández, J., Agustín-Pavón, C., and Martínez-García, F. (2008). Sexual pheromones and the evolution of the reward system of the brain: the chemosensory function of the amygdala. *Brain Res. Bull.* 75, 460–466.

LeDoux, J. E. (2000). Emotion circuits in the brain. *Annu. Rev. Neurosci.* 23, 155–184.

LeDoux, J. E., Cicchetti, P., Xagoraris, A., and Romanski, L. M. (1990). The lateral amygdaloid nucleus: sensory interface of the amygdala in fear conditioning. *J. Neurosci.* 10, 1062–1069.

Luskin, M. B., and Price, J. L. (1983). The topographic organization of associational fibers ofthe olfactory system in the rat, including centrifugal fibers to the olfactorybulb. *J. Comp. Neurol.* 216, 264–291.

Majak, K., and Pitkänen, A. (2003). Projections from the periamygdaloid cortex to theamygdaloid complex, the hippocampal formation, and the parahippocampal region: a PHA-L study in the rat. *Hippocampus* 13, 922–942.

Martínez-García, F., Martínez-Marcos, A., and Lanuza, E. (2002). The pallial amygdala of amniote vertebrates: evolution of the concept, evolution of the structure. *Brain Res. Bull.* 57, 463–469.

Martínez-García, F., Novejarque, A., and Lanuza, E. (2007). "Evolution of the amygdala in vertebrates"in *Evolution of Nervous Systems*, ed. J. H. Kaas (Oxford: Academic Press), 255–334.

Martínez-Hernández, J., Lanuza, E., and Martínez-García, F. (2006). Selective dopaminergic lesions of the ventral tegmental area impair preference for sucrose but not formale sexual pheromones in female mice. *Eur. J. Neurosci.* 24, 885–893.

Martínez-Marcos, A., Úbeda-Bañón, I., Lanuza, E., and Halpern, M. (2005). Chemoarchitecture and afferent connections of the "olfactostriatum": a specialized vomeronasal structure within the basal ganglia of snakes. *J. Chem. Neuroanat.* 29, 49–69.

Martínez-Ricós, J., Agustín-Pavón, C., Lanuza, E., and Martínez-García, F. (2007). Intraspecific communication through chemical signals in female mice: reinforcing properties of involatile male sexual pheromones. *Chem. Senses* 32, 139–148.

Martínez-Ricós, J., Agustín-Pavón, C., Lanuza, E., and Martínez-García, F. (2008). Role of the vomeronasal system in intersexual attraction in female mice. *Neuroscience* 153, 383–395.

McDonald, A. J. (1991a). Organization of amygdaloid projections to the prefrontal cortex and associated striatum in the rat. *Neuroscience* 44, 1–14.

McDonald, A. J. (1991b). Topographical organization of amygdaloid projections to the caudatoputamen, nucleus accumbens, and related striatal-like areas of the rat brain. *Neuroscience* 44, 15–33.

McDonald, A. J. (1998). Cortical pathways to the mammalian amygdala. *Prog. Neurobiol.* 55, 257–332.

Mijnster, M. J., Raimundo, A. G., Koskuba, K., Klop, H., Docter, G. J., Groenewegen, H. J., and Voorn, P. (1997). Regional and cellular distribution of serotonin 5-hydroxytryptamine 2a receptor mRNA in the nucleus accumbens, olfactory tubercle, and caudate putamen of the rat. *J. Comp. Neurol.* 389, 1–11.

Moncho-Bogani, J., Lanuza, E., Hernández, A., Novejarque, A., and Martínez-García, F. (2002). Attractive properties of sexual pheromones in mice. Innate or learned? *Physiol. Behav.* 77, 167–176.

Moncho-Bogani, J., Martínez-García, F., Novejarque, A., and Lanuza, E. (2005). Attraction to sexual pheromones and associated odorants in female mice involves activation of the reward system and basolateral amygdala. *Eur. J. Neurosci.* 21, 2186–2198.

Novejarque, A., Lanuza, E., and Martínez-García, F. (2004). Amygdalostriatal projections in reptiles: a tract-tracing study in the lizard Podarcis hispanica. *J. Comp. Neurol.* 479, 287–308.

Ottersen, O. P. (1982). Connections of the amygdala of the rat. IV: corticoamygdaloid andintraamygdaloid connections as studied with axonal transport of horseradishperoxidase. *J. Comp. Neurol.* 205, 30–48.

Parkinson, J. A., Olmstead, M. C., Burns, L. H., Robbins, T. W., and Everitt, B. J. (1999). Dissociation in effects of lesions of the nucleus accumbens core and shell on appetitive pavlovian approach behavior and the potentiation of conditioned reinforcement and locomotor activity by D-amphetamine. *J. Neurosci.* 19, 2401–2411.

Paxinos, G., and Franklin, K. B. J. (2001). *The Mouse Brain in Stereotaxic Coordinates*, 2nd Edn. San Diego: Academic Press.

Petrovich, G. D., Risold, P. Y., and Swanson, L. W. (1996). Organization of projections from the basomedial nucleus of the amygdala: a PHAL study in the rat. *J. Comp. Neurol.* 374, 387–420.

Pitkänen, A. (2000). "Connectivity of the rat amygdaloid complex"in *The Amygdala. A functional analysis*, 2nd Edn, ed. J. P. Aggleton (Oxford: Oxford University Press), 31–115.

Pitkänen, A., Savander, V., and Ledoux, J. E. (1997). Organization of intra-amygdaloid circuitries in the rat: an emerging framework for understanding functions of the amygdala. *Trends Neurosci.* 20, 517–523.

Prado-Alcala, R., and Wise, R. A. (1984). Brain stimulation reward and dopamine terminal fields. I. Caudate-putamen, nucleus accumbens and amygdala. *Brain Res.* 297, 265–273.

Price, J. L., Russchen, F. T., and Amaral, D. G. (1987). "The limbic region. II: the amygdaloid complex" in *Handbook of Chemical Neuroanatomy, Vol. 5, Integrated Systems*, eds T. Hökfelt, A. Björklund, and L. W. Swanson (Amsterdam: Elsevier), 279–338.

Puelles, L., Kuwana, E., Puelles, E., Bulfone, A., Shimamura, K., Keleher, J., Smiga, S., and Rubenstein, J. L. (2000). Pallial and subpallial derivatives in the embryonic chick and mouse telencephalon, traced by the expression of the genes Dlx-2, Emx-1, Nkx- 2.1, Pax-6, and Tbr-1. *J. Comp. Neurol.* 424, 409–438.

Rajakumar, N., Elisevich, K., and Flumerfelt, B. A. (1993). Biotinylated dextran: a versatile anterograde and retrograde neuronal tracer. *Brain Res.* 607, 47–53.

Reiner, A., Veenman, C. L., Medina, L., Jiao, Y., Del Mar, N., and Honig, M. G. (2000). Pathway tracingusing biotinylated dextran amines. *J. Neurosci. Methods* 103, 23–37.

Riedel, A., Hartig, W., Seeger, G., Gartner, U., Brauer, K., and Arendt, T. (2002). Principles of rat subcortical forebrain organization: a study using histological techniques and multiple fluorescence labeling. *J. Chem. Neuroanat.* 23, 75–104.

Robbins, T. W., Cador, M., Taylor, J. R., and Everitt, B. J. (1989). Limbic-striatal interactions in reward-related processes. *Neurosci. Biobehav. Rev.* 13, 155–162.

Roberts, S. A., Simpson, D. M., Armstrong, S. D., Davidson, A. J., Robertson, D. H., McLean, L., Beynon, R. J., and Hurst, J. L. (2010). Darcin: a male pheromone that stimulates female memory and sexual attraction to an individual male's odour. *BMC Biol.* 8, 75. doi: 10.1186/1741-7007-8-75

Russchen, F. T., Bakst, I., Amaral, D. G., and Price, J. L. (1985). The amygdalostriatal projections in the monkey. An anterograde tracing study. *Brain Res.* 329, 241–257.

Russchen, F. T., and Price, J. L. (1984). Amygdalostriatal projections in the rat. Topographical organization and fiber morphology shown using the lectin PHA-L as an anterograde tracer. *Neurosci. Lett.* 47, 15–22.

Santiago, A. C., and Shammah-Lagnado, S. J. (2004). Efferent connections of the nucleus of the lateral olfactory tract in the rat. *J. Comp. Neurol.* 471, 314–332.

Scalia, F., and Winans, S. S. (1975). The differential projections of the olfactory bulb and accessory olfactory bulb in mammals. *J. Comp. Neurol.* 161, 31–55.

Schoenbaum, G., Chiba, A. A., and Gallagher, M. (1999). Neural encoding in orbitofrontal cortex and basolateral amygdala during olfactory discrimination learning. *J. Neurosci.* 19, 1876–1884.

Schofield, B. R. (2008). Retrograde axonal tracing with fluorescent markers. *Curr. Protoc. Neurosci.* Chapter 1, Unit 1.17.

Schofield, B. R., and Cant, N. B. (1996). Origins and targets of commissural connections between the cochlear nuclei in guinea pigs. *J. Comp. Neurol.* 375, 128–146.

Seifert, U., Hartig, W., Grosche, J., Bruckner, G., Riedel, A., and Brauer, K. (1998). Axonal expression sites of tyrosine hydroxylase, calretinin- and calbindin-immunoreactivity in striato-pallidal and septal nuclei of the rat brain: a double-immunolabelling study. *Brain Res.* 795, 227–246.

Shammah-Lagnado, S. J., and Santiago, A. C. (1999). Projections of the amygdalopiriform transition area (APir). A PHA-L study in the rat. *Ann. N. Y. Acad. Sci.* 877, 665–660.

Swanson, L. W., and Petrovich, G. D. (1998). What is the amygdala? *Trends Neurosci.* 21, 323–331.

Talbot, K., Woolf, N. J., and Butcher, L. L. (1988a). Feline islands of Calleja complex: I. Cytoarchitectural organization and comparative anatomy. *J. Comp. Neurol.* 275, 553–579.

Talbot, K., Woolf, N. J., and Butcher, L. L. (1988b). Feline islands of Calleja complex: II. Cholinergic and cholinesterasic features. *J. Comp. Neurol.* 275, 580–603.

Turner, B. H., and Herkenham, M. (1991). Thalamoamygdaloid projections in the rat: a test of the amygdala's role in sensory processing. *J. Comp. Neurol.* 313, 295–325.

Úbeda-Bañón, I., Novejarque, A., Mohedano-Moriano, A., Pro-Sistiaga, P., de la Rosa-Prieto, C., Insausti, R., Martinez-Garcia, F., Lanuza, E., and Martinez-Marcos, A. (2007). Projections from the posterolateral olfactory amygdala to the ventral striatum: neural basis for reinforcing properties of chemical stimuli. *BMC Neurosci.* 8, 103. doi: 10.1186/1471-2202-8-103

Úbeda-Bañón, I., Novejarque, A., Mohedano-Moriano, A., Pro-Sistiaga, P., Insausti, R., Martinez-Garcia, F., Lanuza, E., and Martinez-Marcos, A. (2008). Vomeronasal inputs to the rodent ventral striatum. *Brain Res. Bull.* 75, 467–473.

Wright, C. I., Beijer, A. V. J., and Groenewegen, H. J. (1996). Basal amygdaloid complex afferents to the rat nucleus accumbens are compartmentally organized. *J. Neurosci.* 16, 1877–1893.

Conflict of Interest Statement: The authors declare that the research was conducted in the absence of any commercial or financial relationships that could be construed as a potential conflict of interest.

11

Pyramidal cells in prefrontal cortex of primates: marked differences in neuronal structure among species

Guy N. Elston[1]*, Ruth Benavides-Piccione[2], Alejandra Elston[1], Paul R. Manger[3] and Javier DeFelipe[2]

[1] Centre for Cognitive Neuroscience, Sunshine Coast, QLD, Australia
[2] Laboratorio de Circuitos Corticales (CTB), Universidad Politécnica de Madrid, Instituto Cajal (CSIC), Centro de Investigación Biomédica en Red sobre Enfermedades Neurodegenerativas (CIBERNED), Madrid, Spain
[3] School of Anatomical Sciences, Faculty of Health Sciences, University of the Witwatersrand, Johannesburg, South Africa

Edited by:
Agustín González, Universidad Complutense de Madrid, Spain

Reviewed by:
Kathleen S. Rockland, Massachusetts Institute of Technology, USA
Patrick R. Hof, Mount Sinai School of Medicine, USA

***Correspondence:**
Guy N. Elston, Centre for Cognitive Neuroscience, 60 Duke Road, Doonan, Sunshine Coast, QLD 4562, Australia.
e-mail: guyelston@yahoo.com

The most ubiquitous neuron in the cerebral cortex, the pyramidal cell, is characterized by markedly different dendritic structure among different cortical areas. The complex pyramidal cell phenotype in granular prefrontal cortex (gPFC) of higher primates endows specific biophysical properties and patterns of connectivity, which differ from those in other cortical regions. However, within the gPFC, data have been sampled from only a select few cortical areas. The gPFC of species such as human and macaque monkey includes more than 10 cortical areas. It remains unknown as to what degree pyramidal cell structure may vary among these cortical areas. Here we undertook a survey of pyramidal cells in the dorsolateral, medial, and orbital gPFC of cercopithecid primates. We found marked heterogeneity in pyramidal cell structure within and between these regions. Moreover, trends for gradients in neuronal complexity varied among species. As the structure of neurons determines their computational abilities, memory storage capacity and connectivity, we propose that these specializations in the pyramidal cell phenotype are an important determinant of species-specific executive cortical functions in primates.

Keywords: macaque, baboon, human, guenon, spine, primate, cognition, connectivity

INTRODUCTION

Pyramidal cell structure is remarkably heterogeneous in the primate cerebral cortex. Estimates of the total number of spines (putative excitatory inputs) in the dendritic trees of pyramidal cells reveal more than a 30-fold difference between populations of cells sampled in different cortical areas (Elston et al., 2001, 2005c). Moreover, there are systematic trends for increasingly more complex phenotypes through a series of functionally related cortical areas. For example, neurons become progressively larger, more branched and more spinous with anterior progression through the dorsal and ventral visual pathways (Elston and Rosa, 1997, 1998, 2000; Elston et al., 1999a, 2005b,d,e,h; Elston, 2003b). There is a progressive systematic increase in the complexity of pyramidal cell structure through somatosensory areas 3b, 1, 2, 5, and 7 (Elston and Rockland, 2002; Elston et al., 2005g,j), which continues with anterior progression through cingulate areas 23 and 24 to granular prefrontal cortex (gPFC; Elston et al., 2001, 2005a,f,i).

Pyramidal cells are the most common neuron in the cerebral cortex. They are the major source of intrinsic excitatory cortical synapses, and their dendritic spines are the main postsynaptic target of excitatory synapses. Moreover, they form most intra-areal projections and nearly all interareal projections (DeFelipe and Fariñas, 1992). Therefore, they are considered the principal neuronal building blocks of the cerebral cortex. Thus, specializations in their structure are likely to influence cortical function at the subcellular, cellular, and systems levels (Elston, 2002, 2003a; Jacobs and Scheibel, 2002; Passingham et al., 2002; Roth and Dicke, 2005; Treves, 2005). More specifically, complexity in dendritic structure determines their biophysical properties thus influencing their functional capacity and potential for plastic changes (Koch, 1999; Mel, 1999; Jan and Jan, 2001; Chklovskii et al., 2004; London and Häusser, 2005). These specializations in neuron structure in the gPFC are thought to subserve executive functions (Funahashi and Kubota, 1994; Courtney et al., 1998; Duncan and Owen, 2000; Goldman-Rakic, 2000; Miller, 2000; Rolls, 2000; Fuster, 2001; Wang, 2001; Treves, 2005); however, pyramidal cell structure has been quantified in only few of the many cortical areas within gPFC.

Broadly speaking, prefrontal cortex has been divided into the lateral, medial, and orbital regions, which are believed to be involved in different types of processing (Goldman-Rakic, 1987, 2000; Funahashi and Kubota, 1994; Fuster, 1997, 2002; Cavada et al., 2000; Miller, 2000; Passingham et al., 2000; Petrides, 2000; Roberts and Wallis, 2000; Rolls, 2000; Funahashi and Takeda, 2002). Various gradients in patterns of connectivity and function have been reported within these three regions (Petrides, 1987, 1991; Wilson et al., 1993; Ó Scalaidhe et al., 1997; Hirsch et al., 2001; Denys et al., 2004; Barbas et al., 2005; Hagler and Sereno, 2006; Nelissen et al., 2005; Noppeney et al., 2005). However, there are no standardized quantitative data on pyramidal cell structure within these different gradients in the gPFC. Here we studied cells in multiple cortical areas in the lateral, medial, and orbital gPFC of the macaque monkey to enable comparisons between these regions. In particular, we injected pyramidal cells in layer III of areas 9d, 10, 12vl, 13, and 46vr.

Recently we have demonstrated that pyramidal cells have markedly different dendritic structure in the gPFC of the macaque monkey, vervet monkey, and baboon, and that there appears to be a parallel trend for increasing size of the gPFC and increasingly more spinous pyramidal cells (Elston et al., 2006). However, it remains to be determined whether this trend is common to all cortical areas within the gPFC. To investigate this we studied layer III pyramidal

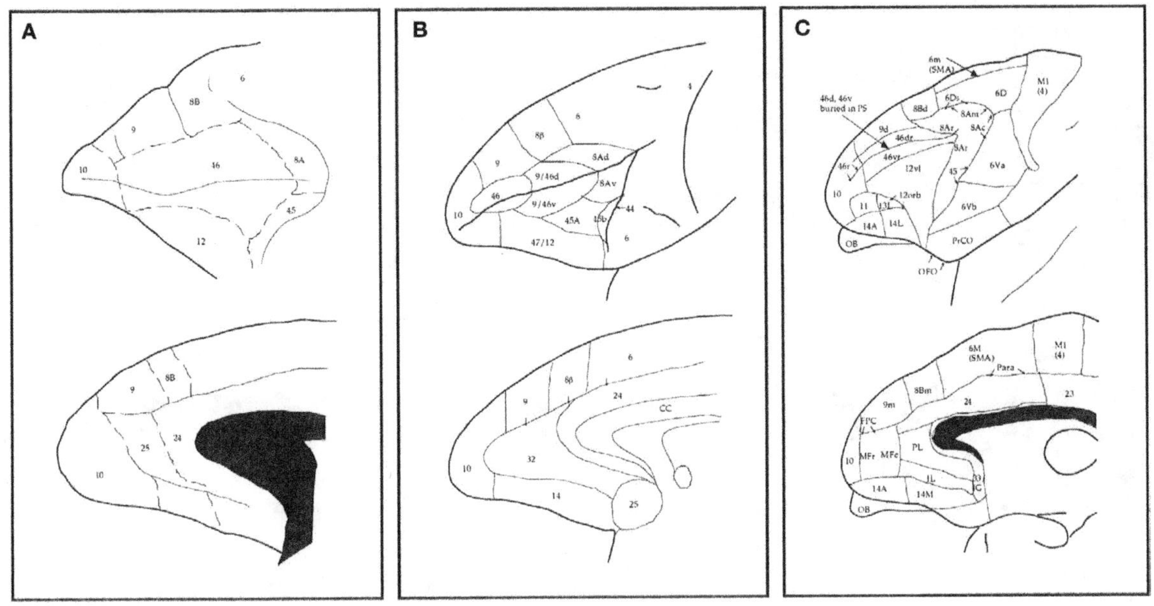

FIGURE 1 | Schematic illustrating some different interpretations of the number, size, and location of cortical areas in prefrontal cortex of the macaque monkey. (A) Modified from Walker (1940), **(B)** Petrides and Pandya (1999) and **(C)** Preuss and Goldman-Rakic (1991a).

cell structure in lateral, medial, and orbital gPFC of the vervet monkey and baboon for comparison with those studied in the macaque monkey. These species were included as they represented closely related primates of similar and different brain size (Gould, 2002). We found that, in general, pyramidal cells in the gPFC were characterized by highly complex structure as compared with those in other cortical regions. In addition we found regional variation in pyramidal cell structure within the gPFC in all three species; however, the topography of the gradients differed between species. We also found marked interindividual variation in pyramidal cell structure in the gPFC in all three species of an order not observed in visual, somatosensory, motor, or cingulate cortex.

MATERIALS AND METHODS

Two adult macaque monkeys (*Macaca fascicularis*; 4.5 years old; MF1 ≈ 5 kg, MF2 ≈ 4.5 kg), two adult vervet monkeys (*Cercopithecus pygerythrus*; age unknown; VM1 = 6.1 kg, VM2 = 5.5 kg), and two adult baboons (*Papio ursinus*; age unknown; B1 = 23.1 kg, B2 = 23.1 kg) were used in the present study. Based on weight, musculature and appearence of the vervet monkeys and baboons we estimate that they were mature but not adolescent nor elderly. All animals were males. All tissue was sampled from the left hemisphere. Macaque tissue was taken from the anterior lateral portion of the superior frontal gyrus (corresponding to Walker's and Petrides and Pandya's area 9 or Preuss and Goldman-Rakic's area 9d) (Walker, 1940; Preuss and Goldman-Rakic, 1991a,b,c; Petrides and Pandya, 2001), the anterior medial portion of the superior frontal gyrus (area 9m of Preuss and Goldman-Rakic, corresponding to Walker's area 9), the medial frontal gyrus (corresponding to Walker's and Petrides and Pandya's area 46 or Preuss and Goldman-Rakic's area 46vr), the inferior frontal gyrus (corresponding to Walker's area 46, Petrides and Pandya's area 45A or Preuss and Goldman-Rakic's area 12vl), the medial portion of the frontal pole anterior to the rostral sulcus (corresponding to area 10 of Walker, Preuss and Goldman-Rakic and Petrides and Pandya), the end of the orbital cortex between the medial orbital sulcus and the lateral orbital sulcus, inferior to the intermediate orbital sulcus (area 12orb of Preuss and Goldman-Rakic, corresponding to Walker's area 13 and Petrides and Pandya's area 14) of the left hemisphere (**Figure 2**). Likewise, tissue from the vervet monkey and baboon was sampled from dorsolateral, medial, and orbital gPFC (**Figure 2**). Specifically, prefrontal areas 9d, 10, 46d, 12vl, and 13 were studied in the baboon and prefrontal areas 9m, 9d, 10, 13, and cingulate area 32, were studied in the vervet monkey. The homology of the specific areas included for analyses remains to be determined.

Methodology used in the present study has been outlined in detail in previous studies (Buhl and Schlote, 1987; Elston and Rosa, 1997; Elston, 2001). Briefly, the animals were deeply anesthetized by intramuscular injection of a mixture of ketamine hydrochloride (100 mg/ml) and xylazine (50 mg/ml) (2:1, 0.1 ml/kg), then an i.v. dose of sodium pentabarbitone (200 mg/kg) in accordance with protocols approved by the University of Queensland and University of the Witwatersrand Animal Ethics Committees and regulations for the care and use of animals set out by the NIH (publication No. 86-23, revised 1985). The animals were then perfused intracardially and the brain removed. The white matter was trimmed from the blocks and the remaining gray matter was "unfolded" and postfixed overnight between glass slides in a solution of 4% paraformaldehyde in 0.1 M phosphate buffer (PB). Serial thick sections (250 μm) were cut tangential to the cortical surface with the aid of a vibratome. Individual sections were incubated in a solution containing 10^{-5} mol/L of the fluorescent dye 4′,6-diamidino-2-phenylindole (DAPI; Sigma D9542, St Louis,

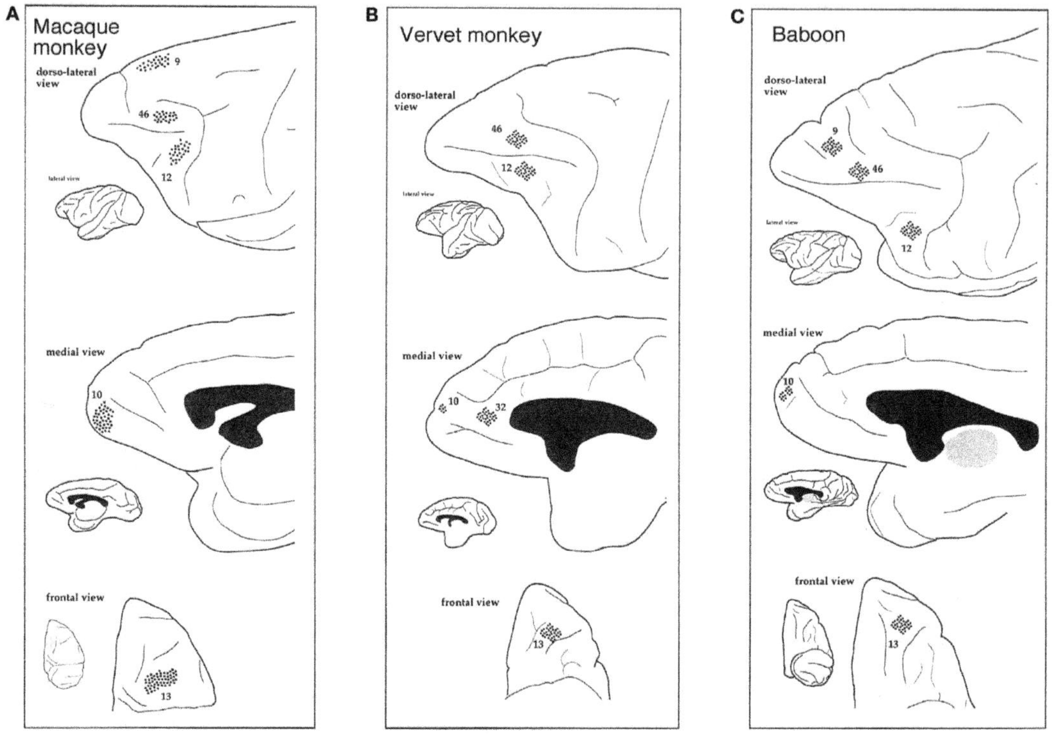

FIGURE 2 | Schematic illustrating where neurons were sampled (dots) in the dorsolateral, medial, and orbital prefrontal cortex of the macaque monkey (A), vervet monkey (B), and baboon (C).

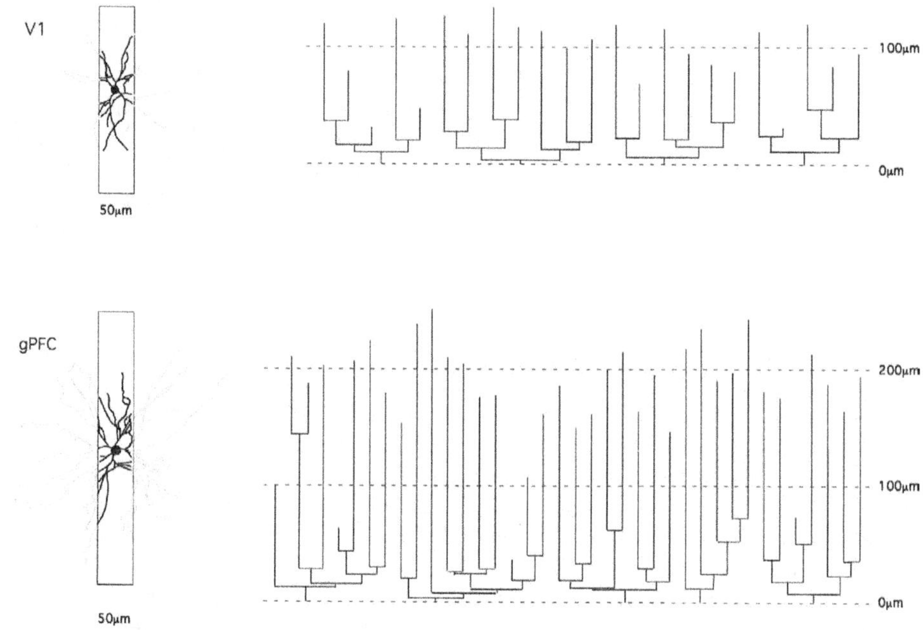

FIGURE 3 | Schematic illustrating how the study of pyramidal cell morphology in the transverse plane may bias for uniformity in structure. Illustrated are two cells sampled from the primary visual area (V1) and granular prefrontal cortex (gPFC) of the macaque monkey. At left are the basal dendritic trees of the two cells as seen in the tangential plane. In black is the part of the dendritic tree that would be seen in a 50-μm transverse section (of the type used in many Golgi studies). The portion of the dendrites extending beyond the section is illustrated in gray. Note the relative similarity in structure of the part of the dendritic tree revealed in the 50-μm transverse sections. At right are illustrated the dendrograms of each of the two cells, which resulted from reconstruction of the complete basal dendritic tree as seen in the tangential plane. Based on our observations, transverse sections would have to be of the order of 1 mm thick to include all dendrites (e.g., human temporal lobe; Elston et al., 2001).

USA) in PB at room temperature for approximately 10 min and mounted between Millipore filters (AABG02500, Bedford, USA). The slice preparation was then mounted in a perspex dish on a Zeiss fixed stage microscope and the preparation visualized with UV excitation (341–343 nm).

In the present study we focused on cells at the base of layer III, enabling comparison with data obtained at the base of layer III in visual, somatosensory, motor, and cingulate cortex of these an other species. Layer III was easily identified in the DAPI-labeled sections immediately above the neuron-dense granular layer. Even in tangential sections it is easy to distinguish the transition from layer III to layer IV due to the change in density and size of somata (see Figure 3 of Elston and Rosa, 1997). Neurons were injected in tangential sections so as to be able to reconstruct the entire basal dendritic tree. Such an approach has been central to the demonstration of regional and species specializations in pyramidal cell dendritic structure as the entire tangential extent of the basal dendritic tree is revealed, unlike in most previous studies in transverse sections in which many of the basal dendrites are truncated thus selecting for uniformity (**Figure 3**). In addition, by injecting neurons in the tangential plane aspects of their structure can be related directly with features reported elsewhere such as intrinsic axon patches and receptive fields (Levitt et al., 1993; Kritzer and Goldman-Rakic, 1995; Pucak et al., 1996; Melchitzky et al., 1998, 2001; González-Burgos et al., 2000). However, unfortunately, it is difficult to inject large numbers of cells under visual control in sections thick enough to contain the entire dendritic arborization (both apical and basal). Thus, we have focused on one dendritic "compartment" of a select group of pyramidal cells (those in layer III). It remains to be determined to what extent regional and species variation in the basal dendritic trees reflects any potential variation in their apical dendrites, and how this may differ from patterns of connectivity in other cortical areas/species (Binzegger et al., 2004).

4′,6-Diamidino-2-phenylindole(DAPI)-labeled neurons were injected under visual guidance with continuous current (up to 100 nA). Cell bodies were impaled not at the cut surface of the sections, but some tens of micrometers below the surface so that pyramidal neurons could be identified by the presence of the proximal part of their apical dendrite. Once a suitable number of neurons had been injected, the slice was processed for a light-stable reaction product (see Elston and Rosa, 1997). Briefly, the sections were processed in a solution containing 1:400,000 anti-Lucifer Yellow in stock solution [2% bovine serum albumin (Sigma A3425), 1% Triton X-100 (BDH 30632), and 5% sucrose in PB] for 5 days at room temperature, washed three times in PB, then incubated in biotinylated anti-rabbit (1:200 Amersham RPN 1004) in stock solution for 2 h, washed another three times before being processed for a further 2 h in streptavidin biotin horseradish peroxidase (1:200, Amersham RPN1051) in PB. 3,3′-diamino-benzidine (DAB; Sigma D 8001; 1:200 in PB) was used as the chromogen (**Figure 4**).

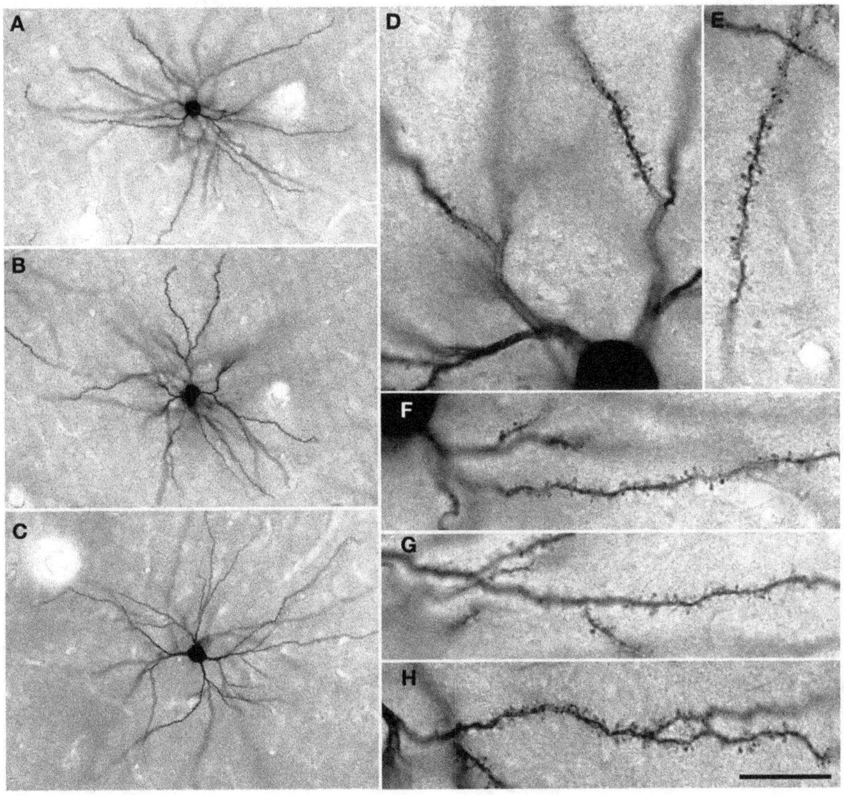

FIGURE 4 | (A–C) Low power photomicrographs of Lucifer Yellow-injected layer III pyramidal cells in tangential sections taken from the granular prefrontal cortex of the macaque monkey (area 12vl). **(D–H)** Higher power photomicrographs of these same neurons as viewed through a ×100 oil-immersion Zeiss objective, revealing aspects of their fine structure including dendritic spines. Scale bar = 100 μm in **(A–C)** and 20 μm in **(D–H)**.

Cells were only included for analysis if they had an unambiguous apical dendrite, had their complete basal dendritic tree contained within the section, and were well filled. We focused our analyses on the basal dendritic trees of supragranular pyramidal cells for several reasons. Of particular interest to us are horizontally projecting intrinsic axonal patches that arise from these cells and project to the basal dendritic trees of neighboring pyramidal cells (Gilbert and Wiesel, 1979, 1983; Rockland and Lund, 1982, 1983; Rockland et al., 1982; Livingstone and Hubel, 1984; Martin and Whitteridge, 1984; Rockland, 1985; Kisvárday et al., 1986; McGuire et al., 1991; Fujita and Fujita, 1996). As many as 80–95% of the horizontal projection synapses of individual supragranular pyramidal cells are formed with other nearby supragranular pyramidal cells (Kisvárday et al., 1986; McGuire et al., 1991) in reciprocally connected patches (Kisvárday and Eysel, 1992). These reciprocal patches have been reported in many different cortical areas in the primate brain, and are believed to provide an anatomical basis for functional domains among the patches (Mitchison and Crick, 1982; Matsubara et al., 1985; T'so et al., 1986; T'so and Gilbert, 1988; Gilbert and Wiesel, 1989; Malach et al., 1993; Malonek et al., 1994). By focusing on the basal dendritic trees of layer III pyramidal cells we are revealing relevant information on the connectivity of these intrinsic circuits and how they may vary among cortical areas. Moreover, we have focused on these dendritic trees here so as to be able to make direct comparisons with our previous data sampled from the basal dendritic trees of layer III pyramidal cells in visual, somatosensory, auditory, motor, and cingulate cortex of thee same species.

Neurons were drawn, and their dendritic field areas determined with NIH Image by tracing a convex hull around the outermost distal dendrites (see Elston and Rosa, 1997). Sholl (1953) analyses were performed on the 2D drawings, with concentric circles of increasing radii (25 μm increments) centered on the cell body. Spine densities were calculated by drawing the entire dendrite of randomly selected cells with the aid of a Zeiss ×100 oil-immersion objective and counting the number of spines per 10 μm segment from the cell body to the distal tip (Eayrs and Goodhead, 1959; Valverde, 1967). Horizontally projecting dendrites were selected to avoid trigonometric error. All spines were drawn and no distinction was made between different spine types. In Golgi studies it is common to apply correction factors when attempting to quantify spine density as spines issuing from under the dendrite may be obscured (Feldman and Peters, 1979). No such correction factors were applied here as the DAB reaction product is more transparent than the Golgi precipitate and allows direct visualization of spines through the dendrite. Furthermore, the basal dendrites have a diameter smaller than the neck length of many spines, and any possible error that may arise because some populations of cells have thicker basal dendrites than others would only reduce the extent of differences we report for cells among cortical areas (i.e., more spinous cells have, on average, thicker parent dendrites than the less spinous cells). Estimates of the total number of spines found within the basal dendritic arbor of the "average" cell in each cortical area were made by summing the product of the average number of dendrites by the average spine density for corresponding segments along the dendrites – from the cell body to the distal tips of the dendrites (Elston, 2001). Cell bodies were drawn by tracing the outermost perimeter, excluding the proximal basal dendrites, while viewed through a Zeiss ×100 oil objective and their areas were determined with NIH Image. Statistical comparisons were made using SPSS (SPSS Inc., IL, USA). One-way ANOVAS were used where there was a single data point for each cell, such as the size of the cell bodies of the size of the dendritic trees. When there were multiple data points for each cell, e.g., branching structure or spine density sampled radially from cell body to the distal tips of the dendrites, repeated measures ANOVAs were used.

RESULTS

A total of 854 layer III pyramidal cells were included for analyses as they satisfied the criteria for inclusion (see Materials and Methods). Over 80,000 individual dendritic spines were drawn and tallied. Data on the size, branching complexity, and spine density of the basal dendritic trees are reported for each cortical area of both animals studied from each of the three species, as are data on cell body size and our estimates of the number of spines in the basal dendritic tree of the "average" neuron in each area.

MACAQUE MONKEYS (AREAS 9d, 10, 12vl, 13, AND 46vr)

Basal dendritic field areas

Qualitative observation revealed variation in the size of the dendritic trees of pyramidal cells among prefrontal areas 9d, 10, 12vl, 13, and 46vr in both MF1 and MF2 (**Figure 5A**; **Table 1**). Statistical analysis (one-way ANOVAs) revealed these differences to be significant ($p < 0.05$) in both MF1 ($F_{(4)} = 8.92$) and MF2 ($F_{(4)} = 15.33$). *Post hoc* Scheffe tests revealed 3 of 10 possible between-area comparisons to be significantly different in MF1 and 4 of 10 in MF2 (**Table 2**).

Branching patterns of the basal dendritic arbors

Plots of the branching patterns of the basal dendritic arbors of pyramidal neurons, as determined by Sholl analysis, are shown in **Figure 5B**. From the figure it can be seen that the branching structure of cells in prefrontal areas 9d, 10, 12vl, 13, and 46vr was not uniform. Repeated measures ANOVAs (5 × 12 design) revealed significant differences ($p < 0.05$) in the branching patterns in both MF1 ($F_{(1,4)} = 11.27$) and MF2 ($F_{(1,4)} = 6.78$). *Post hoc* Scheffe tests revealed 4 of 10 possible between-area comparisons to be significantly different in MF1 and 3 of 10 in MF2 (**Table 2**).

Spine densities of the basal dendrites

From **Figure 5C**, it can be seen that plots of the average spine density, as a function of distance from the soma to the distal tips, were similar among cortical areas. Repeated measures ANOVAs revealed no significant difference in spine density for neurons in either MF1 ($F_{(1,4)} = 1.00$) and MF2 ($F_{(1,4)} = 2.58$). The total number of dendritic spines in the basal dendritic arbor of the "average" pyramidal neuron in each area was calculated by combining data from the Sholl analyses with that of spine densities (see Materials and Methods). These estimates revealed up to >50% difference in of the number of spines in the "average" neuron among prefrontal areas (**Figure 6**; **Table 3**).

Somal areas

Individual cell bodies were drawn, in the plane tangential to the cortical layers, and plotted in **Figure 5D** (see also **Table 4**). One-way ANOVAs revealed significant differences in cell body size between neurons in the different cortical areas in both MF1 ($F_{(4)} = 5.10$) and MF2 ($F_{(4)} = 26.13$). *Post hoc* Scheffe tests revealed 2 of 10 possible between-area comparisons to be significantly different in MF1 and 6 of 10 in MF2 (**Table 2**).

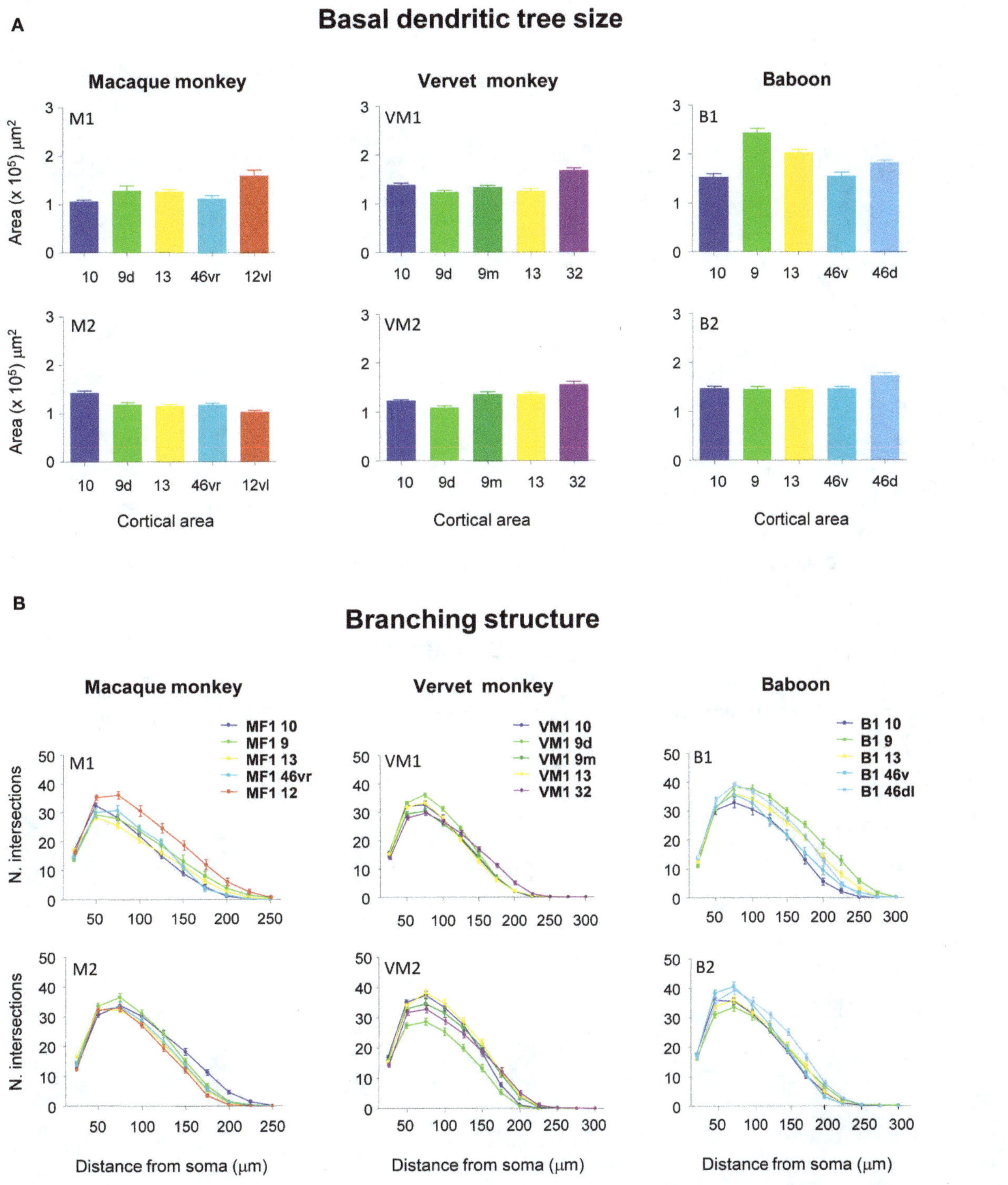

FIGURE 5 | *(Continued)*

VERVET MONKEYS (AREAS 9d, 9m, 10 AND 13, AND 32)

Basal dendritic field areas

Qualitative observation of pyramidal cells revealed that cells in cingulate area 32 were larger than those in prefrontal areas 9d, 9m, 10 and 13 in both VM1 and VM2 (**Figure 5A**; **Table 5**). Statistical analysis (one-way ANOVAs) revealed a significant difference ($p < 0.05$) in the size of the dendritic trees of neurons in both VM1 ($F_{(4)} = 16.81$) and VM2 ($F_{(4)} = 18.14$). *Post hoc* Scheffe tests revealed that cells in cingulate area 32 had significantly larger dendritic trees than those in prefrontal areas in both VM1 and

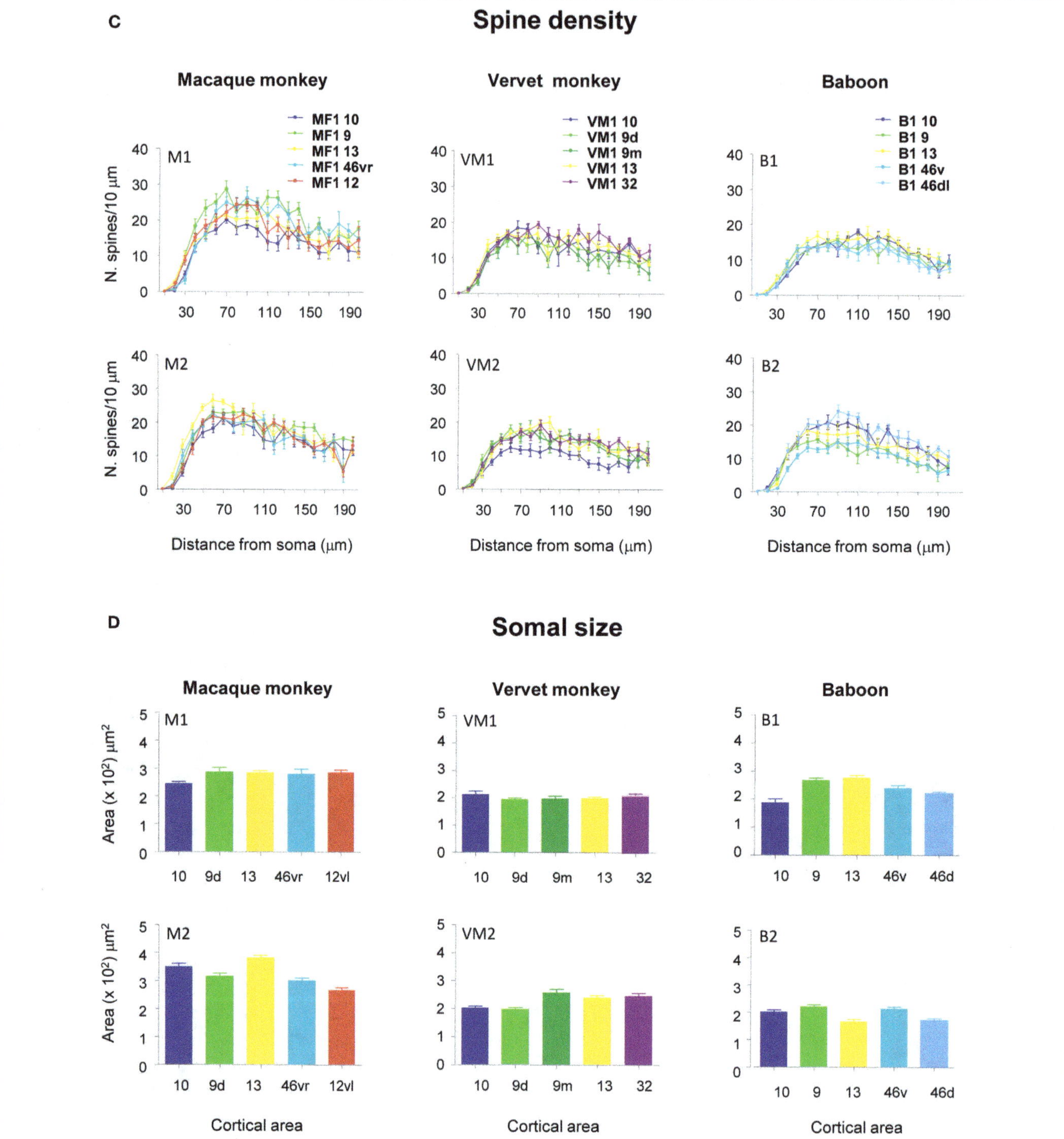

FIGURE 5 | Frequency histograms and plots of the (A) size, **(B)** branching patterns, **(C)** spine density of the basal dendritic trees, and **(D)** cell body size, of layer III pyramidal neurons sampled in granular prefrontal cortex of the macaque monkey (M1 and M2), vervet monkey (VM1 and VM2) and baboon (B1 and B2). Error bars = standard errors.

VM2, except for area 9m in VM2. None of the six possible pair-wise comparisons between prefrontal areas were significantly different in VM1, two of the six pair-wise comparisons between prefrontal areas were significantly different in VM2 (**Table 6**).

Branching patterns of the basal dendritic arbors

Branching patterns of the basal dendritic arbors of pyramidal neurons are illustrated in **Figure 5B**. Repeated measures ANOVAs (5×13 design) revealed a significant difference ($p < 0.05$) in

Table 1 | Number, size [mean, standard deviation (SD), standard error of the mean (SEM), minimum, and maximum] of the basal dendritic trees of layer III pyramidal cells in cortical areas 9, 10, 12vl, 13, and 46 in the prefrontal cortex of the macaque monkey.

Cortical area	*n*	Mean (×10⁴μm²)	SD (×10⁴)	SEM (×10⁴)	Minimum (×10⁴ μm²)	Maximum (×10⁴ μm²)
MF1						
9d	11	12.86	3.21	0.97	9.78	17.44
10	33	10.62	2.14	0.37	7.37	14.81
12vl	20	15.96	5.44	1.21	8.29	28.90
13	23	12.58	2.33	0.47	8.48	17.06
46	11	11.36	1.89	0.57	8.60	15.35
MF2						
9d	26	11.89	2.13	0.42	7.81	17.90
10	35	14.25	2.63	0.44	9.12	20.77
12vl	34	10.26	1.90	0.33	6.69	14.89
13	39	11.54	1.94	0.31	6.47	15.09
46	35	11.79	2.18	0.37	7.07	16.40

n, Number of neurons.

Table 2 | Summary of *post hoc* pair-wise Scheffe comparisons of morphological parameters of neurons in the gPFC of the macaque monkey.

	Area 9d	Area 10	Area 12vl	Area 13
MF1				
10				
12vl	b	a,b,d		
13		d	a,b	
46			a,b	
MF2				
10	a			
12vl	b,d	a,d		
13	b,d	a	d	
46	b	a,d		d

a – Significant difference in the size of the basal dendritic trees.
b – Significant difference in the branching structure of the basal dendritic trees.
c – Significant difference in the spine density of the basal dendritic trees.
d – Significant difference in the size of the cell bodies.
Significance determined as $p < 0.05$.

the branching patterns in both VM1 ($F_{(1,4)} = 3.05$) and VM2 ($F_{(1,4)} = 10.12$). *Post hoc* Scheffe tests revealed no significant difference in branching structure, except in VM2 where cells in area 9d differed to those in all other cortical areas (**Table 6**).

Spine densities of the basal dendrites

The mean and standard deviation in spine density per 10 μm (as a function of distance from the soma to the distal tips of 10 randomly selected horizontally projecting basal dendrites of different cells in each cortical area) are plotted in **Figure 5C**. Repeated measures ANOVAs revealed a significant difference ($p < 0.05$) in the distribution of spines along the dendrites cells between cortical areas in both VM1 ($F_{(1,4)} = 4.23$) and VM2 ($F_{(1,4)} = 7.53$). *Post hoc* Scheffe tests revealed that spine density in area 32 was significantly different to that in areas 9d and 9m in VM1 and

Table 3 | Estimates of the total number of spines in the basal dendritic tree of the "average" layer III pyramidal cell in prefrontal areas of the macaque monkey.

	Area 13	Area 9d	Area 46vr	Area 12vl	Area 10
MF1	5504	7676	6621	8507	6887
MF2	7393	7599	6548	5454	6090

Table 4 | Number, size [mean, standard deviation (SD), standard error of the mean (SEM), minimum, and maximum] of the somata of layer III pyramidal cells (in the tangential plane) in cortical areas 9, 10, 12vl, 13, and 46 in the prefrontal cortex of the macaque monkey.

Cortical area	*n*	Mean (μm²)	SD	SEM	Minimum (μm²)	Maximum (μm²)
MF1						
9d	11	285.99	50.49	15.22	197.95	376.8
10	33	243.38	35.44	6.17	168.50	316.20
12vl	20	282.68	38.42	8.59	221.29	361.68
13	23	281.80	32.58	6.79	207.02	361.69
46	11	278.31	58.89	17.76	178.78	364.52
MF2						
9d	26	316.16	48.84	9.58	225.68	428.06
10	35	349.56	61.80	10.45	246.31	558.86
12vl	34	265.53	46.81	8.03	168.20	346.97
13	39	381.12	52.11	8.34	232.23	494.49
46	35	300.43	50.24	8.49	218.40	437.77

n, Number of neurons.

Table 5 | Number, size [mean, standard deviation (SD), standard error of the mean (SEM), minimum, and maximum] of the basal dendritic trees of layer III pyramidal cells in cortical areas 10, 13, 9 (medial and dorsal), and 32 in the vervet monkey.

Cortical area	*n*	Mean (×10⁴ μm²)	SD (×10⁴)	SEM (×10⁴)	Minimum (×10⁴ μm²)	Maximum (×10⁴ μm²)
VM1						
10	24	13.80	2.14	0.44	8.17	16.90
13	43	12.56	3.09	0.47	8.96	22.31
9m	26	13.33	1.99	0.39	9.23	19.12
9d	41	12.40	2.15	0.21	8.44	16.90
32	31	16.75	2.56	0.46	11.87	22.03
VM2						
10	45	12.28	1.57	0.23	9.03	15.48
13	33	13.61	2.17	0.38	8.90	18.45
9m	14	13.83	2.11	0.56	10.88	17.25
9d	30	10.85	1.96	0.36	7.09	14.55
32	19	15.74	3.19	0.73	8.09	20.81

n, Number of neurons.

area 10 in VM2. None of the six possible pair-wise comparisons between prefrontal areas were significantly different in VM1. Three of the six pair-wise comparisons between prefrontal areas were significantly different in VM2 (**Table 6**). There was a >50% difference in our estimates of the total number of dendritic spines in the basal dendritic arbor of the "average" pyramidal neuron in areas of the gPFC (**Figure 7**; **Table 7**).

Table 6 | Summary of *post hoc* pair-wise Scheffe comparisons of morphological parameters of neurons in the vervet monkey.

	Area 9m	Area 9d	Area 10	Area 13
VM1				
9d				
10				
13				
32	a,c	a,c	a	a
VM2				
9d	a,b,d			
10	c,d	b,c		
13		a,b,d	c,d	
32		a,b,d	a,c,d	a

a – Significant difference in the size of the basal dendritic trees.
b – Significant difference in the branching structure of the basal dendritic trees.
c – Significant difference in the spine density of the basal dendritic trees.
d – Significant difference in the size of the cell bodies.
Significance determined as $p < 0.05$.

Somal areas

Frequency distributions of the size of the cell bodies of pyramidal cells are plotted in **Figure 5D** and listed in **Table 8**. One-way ANOVAs revealed a significant difference in the size of the somata among neurons in VM2 ($F_{(4)} = 13.51$) but not VM1 ($F_{(4)} = 1.39$). *Post hoc* Scheffe tests revealed that cells in cingulate area 32 in VM2 had significantly larger cell bodies than those in areas 9d and 10. Four of the six possible pair-wise comparisons between prefrontal areas in VM2 were significantly different (**Table 6**).

BABOONS (AREAS 9d, 10, 13 46v AND 46d)

Basal dendritic field areas

The size of the dendritic arbors was calculated and frequency distributions are plotted in **Figure 5A** (see also **Table 9**). Statistical analysis (one-way ANOVAs) revealed a significant difference in the size of the dendritic trees of neurons in both B1 ($F_{(95)} = 20.99$) and B2 ($F_{(176)} = 6.50$). *Post hoc* Scheffe tests revealed that 6 and 4 of all possible 10 pair-wise comparisons were significant in B1 and B2 (respectively; **Table 10**).

Branching patterns of the basal dendritic arbors

Sholl analysis was performed and the branching profiles of the basal dendritic arbors of pyramidal neurons are illustrated in **Figure 5B**. Statistical analysis (repeated measures ANOVAs) revealed a significant difference ($p < 0.05$) in the branching patterns of cells between cortical areas in both B1 ($F_{(1,4)} = 7.86$) and B2 ($F_{(1,4)} = 3.27$). *Post hoc* Scheffe tests revealed that 3 of all 10 pair-wise between-area comparisons were significant in B1 and 1 of all 10 comparisons was significant in B2 (**Table 10**).

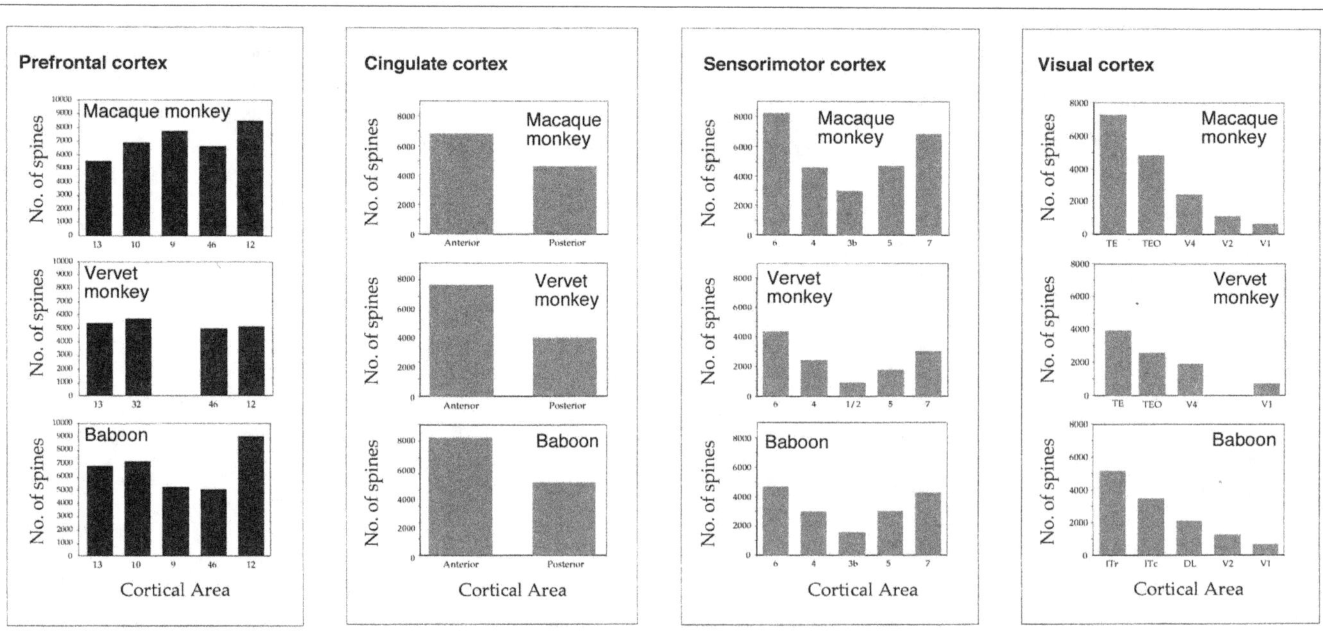

FIGURE 6 | Plots of our estimates of the total number of dendritic spines in the basal dendritic tree of the "average" layer III pyramidal cell in visual, sensorimotor, cingulate, and prefrontal cortex of the macaque monkey, vervet monkey, and baboon. Note the remarkable similarity in the trends of these estimates in visual, sensorimotor, and limbic cortex of both animals. Note, however, the differences in these estimates in the granular prefrontal cortex among species. V1 = primary visual, V2 = second visual, V4 = fourth visual, 3b = primary somatosensory, 1/2/5/7 = somatosensory association, 4 = primary motor, 6 = premotor, 23 = posterior cingulate, 24 = anterior cingulate, 9/10/12/13/46 = prefrontal areas, 32 = cingulate.

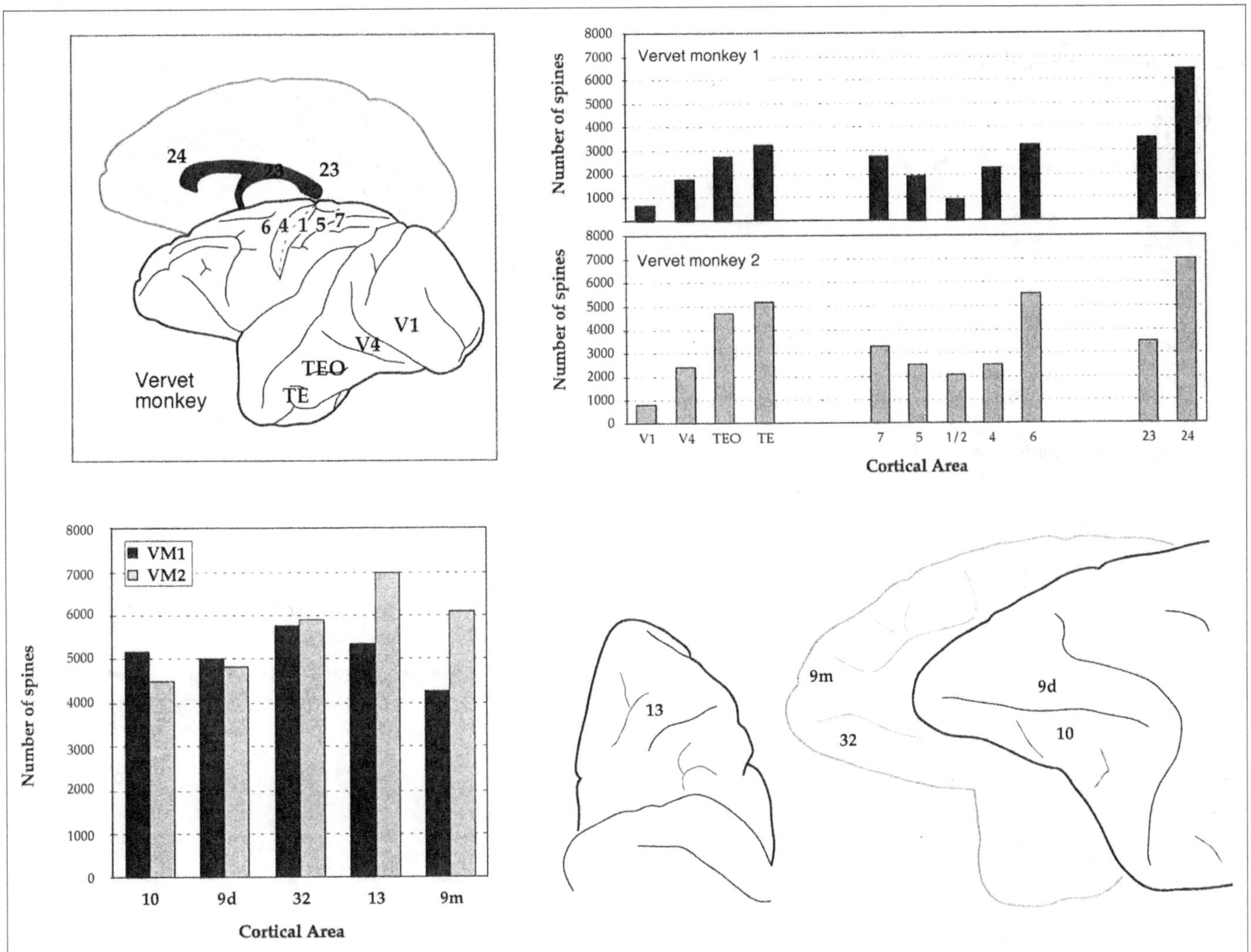

FIGURE 7 | Plots of our estimates of the total number of dendritic spines in the basal dendritic tree of the "average" layer III pyramidal cell in visual, somatosensory, motor, limbic, and prefrontal cortex of the vervet monkey. Sampling from the same cortical regions in the two animals (stylized at top right) resulted in remarkably similar trends in these estimates in visual, somatosensory, motor, and limbic cortex of both animals (top right). In granular prefrontal cortex (gPFC), however, we found unprecedented differences in our estimates of the total number of dendritic spines in the basal dendritic tree of the "average" layer III pyramidal cell among cortical areas (bottom left), despite standardizing the regions sampled between cases (bottom right). V1 = primary visual, V2 = second visual, V4 = fourth visual, 3b = primary somatosensory, 1/2/5/7 = somatosensory association, 4 = primary motor, 6 = premotor, 23 = posterior cingulate, 24 = anterior cingulate, 9/10/12/13/46 = prefrontal areas, 32 = cingulate.

Spine densities of the basal dendrites

The spine density, as a function of distance from the cell body to the distal tips of the dendrites, is plotted in **Figure 5C**. Repeated measures ANOVAs (cortical area × distance from soma × spine density) revealed a significant difference ($p < 0.001$) in the distribution of spines between cortical areas in B2 ($F_{(1,4)} = 13.51$), but not B1 ($F_{(1,4)} = 3.32$). *Post hoc* Scheffe tests revealed a significance ($p < 0.05$) between cells in orbital and dorsolateral gPFC in B2 (**Table 10**). Estimates in the number of spines in the basal dendritic tree of the "average" layer III pyramidal cell revealed a >60% difference between cortical areas (**Figure 6**; **Table 11**).

Somal areas

Frequency distributions of the size of the cell bodies of layer III pyramidal cells, in the plane tangential to the cortical surface, are plotted in **Figure 5D** (see also **Table 12**). Variance in the size of the cell bodies between cortical areas did not always coincide with that observed for the size of their dendritic trees (**Figures 5A–D**). One-way ANOVAs revealed significant differences ($p < 0.05$) in the size of the cell bodies of neurons between cortical areas in both B1 ($F_{(95)} = 13.87$) and B2 ($F_{(176)} = 13.33$). *Post hoc* Scheffe tests revealed that 5 of all 10 pair-wise between-area comparisons were significant in B1 and 6 of all 10 comparisons were significant in B2 (**Table 10**).

DISCUSSION

In the present investigation we studied pyramidal cell structure in the gPFC of the macaque monkey, the vervet monkey, and the baboon. We focused on the gPFC because of its involvement in executive functions such as conceptual thinking, prioritizing, and planning. The aim of the study was to determine whether there exists any appreciable variation in pyramidal cell structure

Table 7 | Estimates of the total number of spines in the basal dendritic tree of the "average" layer III pyramidal cell in prefrontal areas of the vervet monkey.

	Area 10	Area 13	Area 9m	Area 9d	Area 32
VM1	5152	5345	4240	4982	5724
VM2	4475	6976	6079	4790	5877

Table 8 | Somata of layer III pyramidal cells (in the tangential plane) sampled in the prefrontal cortex of the vervet monkey.

Cortical area	*n*	Mean (×10⁴ μm²)	SD (×10⁴)	SEM (×10⁴)	Minimum (×10⁴ μm²)	Maximum (×10⁴ μm²)
VM1						
10	24	211.11	57.39	11.70	136.89	449.08
13	43	196.71	28.97	4.42	142.93	258.96
9m	26	196.15	43.19	8.47	108.71	278.25
9d	41	192.75	31.50	4.92	138.56	287.64
32	31	207.79	30.50	5.48	133.74	261.12
VM2						
10	45	201.55	36.66	5.46	141.39	301.52
13	33	238.14	36.26	6.31	171.12	315.14
9m	14	256.78	43.43	11.61	195.23	324.12
9d	30	196.45	31.94	5.83	140.04	282.30
32	19	244.18	39.42	9.04	165.21	310.46

n, Number of neurons.

Table 9 | Size of the basal dendritic trees of layer III pyramidal cells in baboon gPFC.

Cortical area	*n*	Mean (×10⁴)	SD (×10⁴)	SEM (×10⁴)	Minimum (×10⁴)	Maximum (×10⁴)
B1						
13	24	20.26	3.30	0.67	14.75	28.93
10	14	15.20	2.73	0.73	11.53	19.21
9d	18	24.28	3.59	0.85	18.53	29.78
46d	21	18.38	2.82	0.62	10.53	23.15
12vl	23	15.65	4.31	0.90	7.84	23.97
B2						
13	30	14.47	2.47	0.45	10.31	18.93
10	44	14.71	2.95	0.45	7.75	21.88
9d	41	14.56	3.32	0.52	7.97	22.01
46d	28	14.62	2.29	0.43	8.76	19.67
12vl	38	17.32	3.20	0.52	11.04	25.84

n, Number of neurons.

Table 10 | Summary of *post hoc* pair-wise Scheffe comparisons of morphological parameters of neurons in the gPFC of the baboon.

	Area 9d	Area 10	Area 13	Area 12vl
B1				
10	a,b,d			
13	a	a,d		
12vl	a,b	d	a	
46	a,d	b	d	
B2				
10	c			
13	d	d		
12vl	a,b,c,d	a,d	a	
46		c	c,d	a,c,d

a – Significant difference in the size of the basal dendritic trees.
b – Significant difference in the branching structure of the basal dendritic trees.
c – Significant difference in the spine density of the basal dendritic trees.
d – Significant difference in the size of the cell bodies.
Significance determined as $p < 0.05$.

Table 11 | Estimates of the total number of spines in the basal dendritic tree of the "average" layer III pyramidal cell in prefrontal areas of the Chacma baboon.

	Area 9d	Area 46d	Area 12vl	Area 10	Area 13
B1	7203	5604	6268	4792	7630
B2	5247	5049	8977	7101	6780

Table 12 | Size of the cell bodies of layer III pyramidal cells (in the tangential plane) in the baboon gPFC.

Cortical area	*n*	Mean (μm²)	SD	SEM	Minimum (μm²)	Maximum (μm²)
B1						
13	24	273.86	42.69	8.71	201.70	370.16
10	14	185.77	49.88	13.33	92.08	249.85
9d	18	266.14	30.46	7.18	220.59	320.15
46d	21	218.68	26.49	5.78	147.96	263.77
12vl	23	236.99	48.30	10.07	161.88	355.10
B2						
13	30	164.64	40.61	7.41	107.13	235.68
10	44	200.72	42.12	6.35	105.85	278.77
9d	41	219.32	40.01	6.25	126.30	316.06
46d	28	211.63	29.86	5.64	147.74	273.71
12vl	38	169.14	44.31	7.19	90.14	251.80

n, Number of neurons.

within the gPFC, and compare any such variation across species. The results reveal significant differences in pyramidal cell structure among cortical areas within the gPFC in all animals studied. Moreover, the extent and topology of these trends differed between animals. However, it remains unclear whether regional variation in pyramidal cell structure reported here represent species specializations or interindividual variation. In either event, the extent of variation observed in the gPFC is unparalleled in any other cortical regions studied (visual, somatosensory, motor, and cingulate cortex) in all cases examined. Evolutionary, developmental, and functional implications of these findings are discussed below.

NEURONAL HETEROGENEITY IN GRANULAR PREFRONTAL CORTEX

The gPFC has been divided into several cortical areas, the number, and location of which varies between studies (Vogt and Vogt, 1919; Walker, 1940; Petrides and Pandya, 1988, 1999, 2001; Barbas and Pandya, 1989; Preuss and Goldman-Rakic, 1991a,b,c; Carmichael and Price, 1996; Petrides, 1998; Barbas et al., 1999; Barbas, 2000; Pandya and Yeterian, 2000). While these studies have been instrumental in characterizing regional and species differences in the gPFC, they provide limited quantitative data on cortical microcircuitry. Examination of the present results (**Figure 5**) reveals new findings on the cortical microstructure not predictable from these cytological and connectional data. Namely, cortical pyramidal cells of similar size cell bodies may be characterized by dendritic trees of different size, branching structure, and spine density. *Vice versa*, pyramidal cells of different cell body size may have dendritic trees of similar size, branching structure or spine density. This lack of correspondence between cell body size and the structure of the dendritic tree has been reported in other cortical regions in primates, including the sensorimotor and cingulate cortex (Elston and Rockland, 2002; Elston et al., 2005a,f,g,i,j). Thus, while cytoarchitecture is an excellent means of detecting differences in areal and laminar structure in the cerebral cortex, it provides little insight into regional differences in patterns of connectivity and the integrative capabilities of the component neurons.

Previously we published a report in which pyramidal cell structure was compared in areas 10, 11, and 12 of the macaque monkey, and revealed quantifiable differences in cell morphology among these regions (Elston, 2000). The present data confirm and extend this original observation. In particular, previously we reported up to a 20% difference in our estimates of the numbers of spines in the dendritic tree of the average cell in areas 10 and 12 of the macaque monkey. Here we found up to a 22% difference in these estimates between areas within the gPFC of the macaque monkey (12vl and 46vr in case MF1). We found up to a 27% difference in these estimates in the vervet monkey (areas 9d and 9m in case VM1) and a 70% difference in the baboon (areas 9d and 12vl of case B2). Furthermore, as discussed above, we found different trends in the gradients of neuronal complexity among cortical areas within the gPFC within and between species. In future studies it will be worthwhile to study age, hemisphere, and sex effects to better understand the extent of heterogeneity in pyramidal cell structure in the gPFC.

INTERINDIVIDUAL VARIATION IN THE PYRAMIDAL CELL PHENOTYPE

While we would expect to find some degree of interindividual variation in cell structure, that observed in the gPFC is unprecedented. We found, for example, a 56% difference in our estimates of the total number of dendritic spines in the basal dendritic tree of the average neuron in area 12vl between the two macaque monkeys. Likewise we found a 43% difference in our estimates of the total number of dendritic spines in the basal dendritic tree of the average neuron in area 9m between the two vervet monkeys and a 48% difference in area 10 between the two baboons. These percentages are considerably higher than those reported in visual somatosensory, motor, and cingulate cortex of these same animals, or, indeed all other species studied. For example, the maximum interindividual difference in our estimates of the total number of dendritic spines in the basal dendritic tree of the average neuron observed in the primary visual cortex was 16%, 25% in primary motor cortex and less than 9% in cingulate cortex (Elston and Rosa, 1997; Elston et al., 2005g,h,i). Moreover, trends for increasing complexity in the dendritic trees of pyramidal cells in visual somatosensory, motor, and cingulate cortex have always been consistent between individuals of any given species, where as this is not the case in the gPFC (**Figure 7**). The large number of pyramidal neurons included in these studies (**Table 13**) makes it unlikely that this observation is attributable to different numbers of cells included for analyses in each region. However, differences in sulcal patterns and sampling of different locations within a given cortical area (e.g., dorsal vs. ventral) are likely to have contributed to these apparent interindividual differences. For example, differences in pyramidal cell structure have been reported in layer III within V1 according to visuotopy and within inferotemporal cortex according to gross location (cf. Elston and Rosa, 1997; Elston et al., 1999a,b). A better understanding of these apparent interindividual differences will require that more individuals are included for analyses. It should be noted that these differences in our estimates of the total number of dendritic spines in the basal dendritic trees of layer III pyramidal cells in the gPFC equate to four times those reported in the entire basal dendritic trees in V1.

PHENOTYPIC SPECIALIZATION OF THE PYRAMIDAL CELL WITHIN THE gPFC

Here we found differences in the relative trends in morphological complexity among cortical areas in the gPFC between individuals. For example, cells in the dorsolateral gPFC were the most spinous in both the macaque monkey and baboon, but those in the orbital and medial gPFC were the most spinous in the vervet monkeys. These differences may be attributable to the selection of cortical areas included for analyses in each of the different species, but it is worthwhile noting that no such interspecies differences have been observed in visual, somatosensory, motor, or limbic cortex of these same species. Instead, trends reported in the visual, somatosensory, motor, and limbic cortex of the macaque monkey are the same as those reported in the vervet monkey and baboon (**Figure 6**). Moreover, trends reported in these cortical areas in the macaque monkey, vervet monkey, and baboon are similar to those reported in all other primate species studied to date (Elston et al., 2005a,b,c,g,h,i,j).

Table 13 | Number of layer III pyramidal cells included for study in the granular prefrontal (gPFC), cingulate, sensorimotor, and visual cortex of the animals studied here.

	gPFC	Cingulate	Sensorimotor	Visual	Total
Baboon	281	44	141	161	627
Macaque monkey	267	120	161	120	668
Vervet monkey	306	94	273	269	942
Total	854	258	575	550	2237

Animals include baboons 1 and 2 (B1 and B2), macaque monkeys MF1 and MF2 and vervet monkeys 1 and 2 (VM1 and VM2).

Another possibility is that the different trends reflect species differences. The lineage leading to modern day vervet monkeys diverged from that leading to modern day baboons and macaque monkeys approximately 10 million years ago. The lineage leading to modern day baboons diverged from that leading to macaque monkeys about 7 million years ago (Gould, 2002). Thus, it is tempting to conclude that highly complex pyramidal cells in the dorsolateral gPFC is a characteristic of the latter species, which may differ from that in other primates that diverged earlier, such as New World monkeys and the great apes. Alternatively, the apparent species differences may reflect regional variation in neuronal maturation rates (Jacobs and Scheibel, 1993; Jacobs et al., 1995, 1997; Page et al., 2002; Duan et al., 2003; Elston et al., 2009, 2010a,b) or arise through sampling different subsets of projection neurons in the different cortical areas, which have been shown to differ in both their morphology (Schofield et al., 1987; Hallman et al., 1988; Hübener and Bolz, 1988; de Lima et al., 1990; Hübener et al., 1990; Einstein, 1996; Matsubara et al., 1996; Duan et al., 2002; Soloway et al., 2002; Elston and Rosa, 2006) and density (Jones and Powell, 1970; Barbas, 1992; Young, 1992; Pandya and Yeterian, 2000; Petrides, 2000; Collins et al., 2005) in different cortical areas. In either case, the result is consistent with our main conclusion that pyramidal cells develop differently among cortical areas and mature into specialized circuits. Clearly, more comparative and developmental data on pyramidal cell structure are required to reveal a more complete picture.

Not withstanding these limitations on the interpretation of the trends for regional variation in pyramidal cell structure within the gPFC, the present results confirm previous findings that pyramidal cells in the gPFC are characterized by a highly complex structure (Lund et al., 1993; Elston, 2000; Elston et al., 2001; Jacobs et al., 2001). However, previously it was reported that pyramidal cells in the gPFC have a more complex phenotype than those in the visual, somatosensory, and motor and cingulate cortex (Elston and Rosa, 1997, 1998, 2000; Elston and Rockland, 2002). The present data reveal that, in the macaque monkey, cells in inferotemporal and anterior cingulate cortex were more spinous than those area 12vl (case MF2; Elston et al., 1999a, 2005a; present results). Likewise, cells in the anterior cingulate gyrus in both the vervet monkey and baboon have larger, more branched and more spinous dendritic trees than those in some cortical areas within the gPFC (Elston et al., 2005f,i). Therefore, the present data reveal that some *but not all* pyramidal cells in the gPFC have a more complex structure than those in other cortical regions. More specifically, those in the gPFC have the most complex branching structure and the highest spine density while those in the anterior cingulate gyrus and inferotemporal cortex may have the largest dendritic trees. As discussed below, these different morphological parameters are likely to influence different aspects of cellular and systems function.

FORM SERVES FUNCTION

As reviewed in detail elsewhere (Elston, 2002, 2003a; Jacobs and Scheibel, 2002) differences in the size, branching complexity, spine density in the dendritic trees may influence various aspects of function at the subcellular, cellular, and systems levels. For example, differences in the size of the dendritic trees may influence the sampling geometry of neurons, the topographic relationship between the pattern of inputs and the size of the dendritic tree influencing receptive field properties (Lund et al., 1993; Malach, 1994). Differences in the diameter and total length of the dendrites determines their electrotonic properties (Rall, 1959, 1989; Mainen and Sejnowski, 1986; Rothnie et al., 2005). Differences in the number of branches in the dendritic tree may influence the potential to compartmentalize the processing of inputs within the arbor and, thus, the functional capacity of the neurons, as well as the decay of the backpropagating potentials believed to be important in Hebbian type reinforcement of inputs (Rall et al., 1992; Stuart et al., 1997; Segev and Rall, 1998; Mel, 1999; Spruston et al., 1999; Vetter et al., 2001; Elston, 2007). Differences in the number and density of spines along the dendrites may influence the potential for local summation and/or the inhibitory vetoing of inputs (White, 1989; Koch, 1999). In addition, as each dendritic spine in mature cortex receives at least one asymmetrical synapse (Arellano et al., 2007), which have been demonstrated to contain the excitatory transmitter glutamate (DeFelipe et al., 1988; Petralia et al., 1994a,b,c), differences in the total number of spines in the dendritic tree likely reflect differences in the number of excitatory inputs to the neuron: highly spinous cells receiving more excitatory inputs than less spinous cells (Elston, 2002, 2003a).

These differences in the density and distribution of inputs throughout the dendritic trees, and the spatial distribution of the dendritic tree, have been shown to influence both the functional capacity of neurons and the memory storage capacity of cortical circuits they comprise (Poirazi and Mel, 2001; Stepanyants et al., 2002; Losonczy et al., 2008; Spruston, 2008). The dramatic differences in the branching structure of, and number of spines in, the dendritic trees of neurons in the gPFC of primates (Elston et al., 2006) makes it implausible that function in this region of the brain is the same across species. Indeed, modeling studies have demonstrated a difference of up to two orders of magnitude in the memory capacity of cortical circuitry attributable to differences in the branching structure and number/distribution of inputs throughout the dendritic trees of the component pyramidal cells (Mel, 2002; Chklovskii et al., 2004).

Perhaps not surprisingly, differences in discharge properties of cortical neurons have also been reported among cortical regions. For example, neurons in the gPFC are characterized by tonic discharge properties that are sustained despite interruption from distractors, those in association cortex are characterized by tonic discharge properties that may be interrupted by distractors and those in and primary sensory cortex are characterized by phasic activity (Fuster and Alexander, 1971; Fuster, 1973; Fuster et al., 1982; Fuster and Jervey, 1983; Ashford and Fuster, 1985; Funahashi et al., 1989, 1993; Miller et al., 1993, 1996; Constantinidis and Steinmetz, 1996; Sakai et al., 2002; Shinomoto et al., 2005).

Finally, from the intrinsic point of view of cortical organization, there are also significant differences in the distribution of GABAergic interneurons in different cortical areas of primates (Lewis and Lund, 1990; Gabbott et al., 1997; DeFelipe et al., 1999; Elston and González-Albo, 2003; Ballesteros-Yánez et al., 2005; Benavides-Piccione and DeFelipe, 2007; Inda et al., 2007; Blazquez-Llorca et al., 2010). Since GABAergic neurons are involved in the shaping the activity of pyramidal neurons, it is likely that the different intrinsic functional attributes of the cortical regions examined depends on all these features or in a combination of them. Further correlative physiological and microanatomical/neurochemical studies would be necessary to perform to find out the role of each cortical component on the processing of information characteristic of the different cortical areas.

CONCLUSION

Here we found significant differences in pyramidal cell structure among cortical areas within the gPFC of the macaque monkeys, vervet monkeys, and baboons. Moreover we found species differences when comparing pyramidal cell structure between homologous/corresponding cortical areas. The data suggest regional as well as interindividual and species differences in the functional capabilities of pyramidal cells in different cortical areas of the gPFC of cercopithecid primates. Because pyramidal cells comprise >70% of neurons within the gPFC, differences in the number of dendritic spines (putative excitatory inputs) found within their dendritic trees suggest that cortical areas within the gPFC are characterized by different patterns of connectivity. As patterns of connectivity determine the computational abilities cortical circuits, the present data suggest regional and species differences in computations performed in the gPFC of macaque monkeys, vervet monkeys, and baboons. Functions often ascribed to the gPFC, such as planning, prioritizing, and conceptualization, are likely then to be influenced by specialization in the pyramidal cell phenotype.

ACKNOWLEDGMENTS

Supported by grants from the National Health and Medical Research Council of Australia (Guy N. Elston), the McDonnell Foundation (Guy N. Elston), the Japanese Science and Technology Corporation (Guy N. Elston), Hear and Say Australia (Guy N. Elston), CIBERNED CB06/05/0066 (Javier DeFelipe), Fundación CIEN (Javier DeFelipe), and the Spanish Ministry of Education, Science and Innovation SAF2009-09394 (Javier DeFelipe), and the South African National Research Foundation (Paul R. Manger). Thanks to Brendan Zietsch and Laura Ferris for technical help.

REFERENCES

Arellano, J. I., Espinosa, A., Fairen, A., Yuste, R., and DeFelipe, J. (2007). Nonsynaptic dendritic spines in neocortex. *Neuroscience* 145, 464–469.

Ashford, J. W., and Fuster, J. M. (1985). Occipital and inferotemporal responses to visual signals in the monkey. *Exp. Neurol.* 90, 444–446.

Ballesteros-Yánez, I., Muñoz, A., Contreras, J., Gonzalez, J., Rodriguez-Veiga, E., and DeFelipe, J. (2005). The double bouquet cell in the human cerebral cortex and a comparison with other mammals. *J. Comp. Neurol.* 486, 344–360.

Barbas, H. (1992). Architecture and cortical connections of the prefrontal cortex in the rhesus monkey. *Adv. Neurol.* 57, 91–115.

Barbas, H. (2000). Connections underlying the synthesis of cognition, memory, and emotion in primate prefrontal cortices. *Brain Res. Bull.* 52, 319–330.

Barbas, H., Ghashghaei, H., Dombrowski, S. M., and Rempel-Clower, N. L. (1999). Medial prefrontal cortices are unified by common connections with superior temporal cortices and distinguished by input from memory-related areas in the rhesus monkey. *J. Comp. Neurol.* 410, 343–367.

Barbas, H., Hilgetag, C. C., Saha, S., Dermon, C. R., and Suski, J. L. (2005). Parallel organization of contralateral and ipsilateral prefrontal cortical projections in the rhesus monkey. *BMC Neurosci.* 6, 32. doi: 10.1186/1471-2202-6-32

Barbas, H., and Pandya, D. N. (1989). Architecture and intrinsic connections of the prefrontal cortex in the rhesus monkey. *J. Comp. Neurol.* 286, 353–375.

Benavides-Piccione, R., and DeFelipe, J. (2007). Distribution of neurons expressing tyrosine hydroxylase in the human cerebral cortex. *J. Anat.* 211, 212–222.

Binzegger, T., Douglas, R. J., and Martin, K. A. (2004). A quantitative map of the circuit of cat primary visual cortex. *J. Neurosci.* 24, 8441–8453.

Blazquez-Llorca, L., Garcia-Marin, V., and DeFelipe, J. (2010). GABAergic complex basket formations in the human neocortex. *J. Comp. Neurol.* 518, 4917–4937.

Buhl, E. H., and Schlote, W. (1987). Intracellular Lucifer yellow staining and electronmicroscopy of neurons in slices of fixed epitumourous human cortical tissue. *Acta Neuropathol.* 75, 140–146.

Carmichael, S. T., and Price, J. L. (1996). Connectional networks within the orbital and medial prefrontal cortex of macaque monkeys. *J. Comp. Neurol.* 371, 179–207.

Cavada, C., Compañy, T., Tejedor, J., Cruz-Rizzolo, R. J., and Reinoso-Suárez, F. (2000). The anatomical connections of the macaque orbitofrontal cortex. *Cereb. Cortex* 10, 220–242.

Chklovskii, D. B., Mel, B. W., and Svoboda, K. (2004). Cortical rewiring and information storage. *Nature* 431, 782–788.

Collins, C. E., Lyon, D. C., and Kaas, J. H. (2005). Distribution across cortical areas of neurons projecting to the superior colliculus in new world monkeys. *Anat. Rec.* 285, 619–627.

Constantinidis, C., and Steinmetz, M. A. (1996). Neuronal activity in posterior parietal area 7a during the delay periods of a spatial memory task. *J. Neurophysiol.* 76, 1352–1355.

Courtney, S. M., Petit, L., Haxby, J. V., and Ungerlieder, L. G. (1998). The role of prefrontal cortex in working memory: examining the contents of consciousness. *Philos. Trans. R. Soc. Lond., B, Biol. Sci.* 353, 1819–1828.

de Lima, A. D., Voigt, T., and Morrison, J. H. (1990). Morphology of the cells within the inferior temporal gyrus that project to the prefrontal cortex in the macaque monkey. *J. Comp. Neurol.* 296, 159–172.

DeFelipe, J., Conti, F., Van Eyck, S. L., and Manzoni, T. (1988). Demonstration of glutamate-positive axon terminals forming asymmetric synapses in cat neocortex. *Brain Res.* 455, 162–165.

DeFelipe, J., del Río, M. R., González-Albo, M. C., and Elston, G. N. (1999). Distribution and patterns of connectivity of interneurons containing calbindin, calretinin and parvalbumin in visual areas of the occipital and temporal lobes of the macaque monkey. *J. Comp. Neurol.* 412, 515–526.

DeFelipe, J., and Fariñas, I. (1992). The pyramidal neuron of the cerebral cortex: morphological and chemical characteristics of the synaptic inputs. *Prog. Neurobiol.* 39, 563–607.

Denys, K., Vanduffel, W., Fize, D., Nelissen, K., Sawamura, H., Georgieva, S., Vogels, R., Van Essen, D., and Orban, G. A. (2004). Visual activation in prefrontal cortex is stronger in monkeys than in humans. *J. Cogn. Neurosci.* 16, 1505–1516.

Duan, H., Wearne, S., Morrison, J., and Hof, P. (2002). Quantitative analysis of the dendritic morphology of corticocortical projection neurons in the macaque monkey association cortex. *Neuroscience* 114, 349–359.

Duan, H., Wearne, S. L., Rocher, A. B., Macedo, A., Morrison, J. H., and Hof, P. R. (2003). Age-related dendritic and spine changes in corticocortically projecting neurons in macaque monkeys. *Cereb. Cortex* 13, 950–961.

Duncan, J., and Owen, A. (2000). Common regions of human frontal lobe recruited by diverse cognitive demands. *Trends Neurosci.* 23, 475–483.

Eayrs, J. T., and Goodhead, B. (1959). Postnatal development of the cerebral cortex in the rat. *J. Anat.* 93, 385–402.

Einstein, G. (1996). Reciprocal projections of cat extrastriate cortex: I. Distribution and morphology of neurons projecting from posterior medial lateral suprasylvian sulcus to area 17. *J. Comp. Neurol.* 376, 518–529.

Elston, G. N. (2000). Pyramidal cells of the frontal lobe: all the more spinous to think with. *J. Neurosci.* 20, RC95.

Elston, G. N. (2001). Interlaminar differences in the pyramidal cell phenotype in cortical areas 7m and STP (the superior temporal polysensory area) of the macaque monkey. *Exp. Brain Res.* 138, 141–152.

Elston, G. N. (2002). Cortical heterogeneity: implications for visual processing and polysensory integration. *J. Neurocytol.* 31, 317–335.

Elston, G. N. (2003a). Cortex, cognition and the cell: new insights into the pyramidal neuron and prefrontal function. *Cereb. Cortex* 13, 1124–1138.

Elston, G. N. (2003b). Pyramidal cell heterogeneity in the visual cortex of the nocturnal New World owl monkey

(*Aotus trivirgatus*). *Neuroscience* 117, 213–219.

Elston, G. N. (2007). "Specializations in pyramidal cell structure during primate evolution," in *Evolution of Nervous Systems*, eds J. H. Kaas and T. M. Preuss (Oxford: Academic Press), 191–242.

Elston, G. N., Benavides-Piccione, R., and DeFelipe, J. (2001). The pyramidal cell in cognition: a comparative study in human and monkey. *J. Neurosci.* 21, RC163.

Elston, G. N., Benavides-Piccione, R., and DeFelipe, J. (2005a). A study of pyramidal cell structure in the cingulate cortex of the macaque monkey with comparative notes on inferotemporal and primary visual cortex. *Cereb. Cortex* 15, 64–73.

Elston, G. N., Elston, A., Casagrande, V. A., and Kaas, J. (2005b). Areal specialization in pyramidal cell structure in the visual cortex of the tree shrew: a new twist revealed in the evolution of cortical circuitry. *Exp. Brain Res.* 163, 13–20.

Elston, G. N., Elston, A., Casagrande, V. A., and Kaas, J. (2005c). Pyramidal neurons of granular prefrontal cortex the galago: complexity in the evolution of the psychic cell in primates. *Anat. Rec.* 285, 610–618.

Elston, G. N., Elston, A., Kaas, J., and Casagrande, V. A. (2005d). Regional specialization in pyramidal cell structure in the visual cortex of the galago: an intracellular injection study with comparative notes on New World and Old World monkeys. *Brain Behav. Evol.* 66, 10–21.

Elston, G. N., Benavides-Piccione, R., Elston, A., DeFelipe, J., and Manger, P. (2005e). Pyramidal cell specialization in the occipitotemporal cortex of the Chacma baboon (*Papio ursinus*). *Exp. Brain Res.* 167, 496–503.

Elston, G. N., Benavides-Piccione, R., Elston, A., DeFelipe, J., and Manger, P. (2005f). Specialization in pyramidal cell structure in the cingulate cortex of the Chacma baboon (*Papio ursinus*): an intracellular injection study of the posterior and anterior cingulate gyrus with comparative notes on the macaque and vervet monkeys. *Neurosci. Lett.* 387, 130–135.

Elston, G. N., Benavides-Piccione, R., Elston, A., DeFelipe, J., and Manger, P. (2005g). Specialization in pyramidal cell structure in the sensory–motor cortex of the vervet monkey (*Cercopithecus pygerythrus*). *Neuroscience* 134, 1057–1068.

Elston, G. N., Benavides-Piccione, R., Elston, A., Manger, P., and DeFelipe, J. (2005h). Pyramidal cell specialization in the occipitotemporal cortex of the vervet monkey (*Cercopithecus pygerythrus*). *Neuroreport* 16, 967–970.

Elston, G. N., Benavides-Piccione, R., Elston, A., Manger, P., and DeFelipe, J. (2005i). Regional specialization in pyramidal cell structure in the limbic cortex of the vervet monkey (*Cercopithecus pygerythrus*): an intracellular injection study of the anterior and posterior cingulate gyrus. *Exp. Brain Res.* 167, 315–323.

Elston, G. N., Benavides-Piccione, R., Elston, A., Manger, P., and DeFelipe, J. (2005j). Specialization in pyramidal cell structure in the sensory–motor cortex of the Chacma baboon (*Papio ursinus*) with comparative notes on the macaque monkey. *Anat. Rec.* 286A, 854–865.

Elston, G. N., Benavides-Piccione, R., Elston, A., Zietsch, B., DeFelipe, J., Manger, P., Casagrande, V., and Kaas, J. H. (2006). Specializations of the granular prefrontal cortex of primates: implications for cognitive processing. *Anat. Rec.* 288A, 26–35.

Elston, G. N., and González-Albo, M. C. (2003). Parvalbumin-, calbindin- and calretinin-immunoreactive neurons in the prefrontal cortex of the owl monkey (*Aotus trivirgatus*): a standardized quantitative comparison with sensory and motor cortex. *Brain Behav. Evol.* 62, 19–30.

Elston, G. N., Oga T., and Fujita I. (2009). Spinogenesis and pruning scales across functional hierarchies. *J. Neurosci.* 29, 3271–3275.

Elston, G. N., Oga, T., Okamoto, T., and Fujita, I. (2010a). Spinogenesis and pruning from early visual onset to adulthood: an intracellular injection study of layer III pyramidal cells in the ventral visual cortical pathway of the macaque monkey. *Cereb. Cortex* 20, 1398–1408.

Elston, G. N., Okamoto, T., Oga, T., Dornan, D., and Fujita, I. (2010b). Spinogenesis and pruning in the primary auditory cortex of the macaque monkey (*Macaca fascicularis*): an intracellular injection study of layer III pyramidal cells. *Brain Res.* 1316, 35–42.

Elston, G. N., and Rockland, K. (2002). The pyramidal cell of the sensorimotor cortex of the macaque monkey: phenotypic variation. *Cereb. Cortex* 10, 1071–1078.

Elston, G. N., and Rosa, M. G. P. (1997). The occipitoparietal pathway of the macaque monkey: comparison of pyramidal cell morphology in layer III of functionally related cortical visual areas. *Cereb. Cortex* 7, 432–452.

Elston, G. N., and Rosa, M. G. P. (1998). Morphological variation of layer III pyramidal neurones in the occipitotemporal pathway of the macaque monkey visual cortex. *Cereb. Cortex* 8, 278–294.

Elston, G. N., and Rosa, M. G. P. (2000). Pyramidal cells, patches, and cortical columns: a comparative study of infragranular neurons in TEO, TE, and the superior temporal polysensory area of the macaque monkey. *J. Neurosci.* 20, RC117.

Elston, G. N., and Rosa, M. G. P. (2006). Ipsilateral corticocortical projections to the primary and middle temporal visual areas of the primate cerebral cortex: area-specific variations in the morphology of connectionally identified pyramidal cells. *Eur. J. Neurosci.* 23, 3337–3345.

Elston, G. N., Tweedale, R., and Rosa, M. G. P. (1999a). Cortical integration in the visual system of the macaque monkey: large scale morphological differences of pyramidal neurones in the occipital, parietal and temporal lobes. *Proc. R. Soc. Lond., B, Biol. Sci.* 266, 1367–1374.

Elston, G. N., Tweedale, R., and Rosa, M. G. P. (1999b). Cellular heterogeneity in cerebral cortex. A study of the morphology of pyramidal neurones in visual areas of the marmoset monkey. *J. Comp. Neurol.* 415, 33–51.

Feldman, M. L., and Peters, A. (1979). A technique for estimating total spine numbers on Golgi-impregnated dendrites. *J. Comp. Neurol.* 188, 527–542.

Fujita, I., and Fujita, T. (1996). Intrinsic connections in the macaque inferior temporal cortex. *J. Comp. Neurol.* 368, 467–486.

Funahashi, S., Bruce, C. J., and Goldman-Rakic, P. S. (1989). Mnemonic coding of visual space in the monkey's dorsolateral prefrontal cortex. *J. Neurophysiol.* 61, 331–349.

Funahashi, S., Chafee, M. V., and Goldman-Rakic, P. S. (1993). Prefrontal activity in rhesus monkeys performing a delayed anti-saccad task. *Nature* 365, 753–756.

Funahashi, S., and Kubota, K. (1994). Working memory and prefrontal cortex. *Neurosci. Res.* 21, 1–11.

Funahashi, S., and Takeda, K. (2002). Information processes in the primate prefrontal cortex in relation to working memory processes. *Nat. Rev. Neurosci.* 13, 313–345

Fuster, J. M. (1973). Unit activity in prefrontal cortex during delayed-response performance: neuronal correlates of transient memory. *J. Neurophysiol.* 36, 61–78.

Fuster, J. M. (1997). *The Prefrontal Cortex: Anatomy, Physiology, and Neuropsychology of the Frontal Lobe.* Philadelphia: Lippincott-Raven.

Fuster, J. M. (2001). The prefrontal cortex – an update; time is of the essence. *Neuron* 30, 319–333.

Fuster, J. M. (2002). Frontal lobe and cognitive development. *J. Neurocytol.* 31, 373–385.

Fuster, J. M., and Alexander, G. E. (1971). Neuron activity related to short-term memory. *Science* 173, 652–654.

Fuster, J. M., Bauer, R. H., and Jervey, J. P. (1982). Cellular discharge in the dorsolateral prefrontal cortex of the monkey in cognitive tasks. *Exp. Neurol.* 77, 679–694.

Fuster, J. M., and Jervey, J. P. (1983). Neuronal firing in the inferotemporal cortex of the monkey in a visual memory task. *J. Neurosci.* 2, 361–375.

Gabbott, P. L., Jays, P. R., and Bacon, S. J. (1997). Calretinin neurons in human prefrontal cortex (areas 24, 32 and 25). *J. Comp. Neurol.* 381, 389–410.

Gilbert, C. D., and Wiesel, T. N. (1979). Morphology and intracortical projections of functionally characterised neurones in the cat visual cortex. *Nature* 280, 120–125.

Gilbert, C. D., and Wiesel, T. N. (1983). Clustered intrinsic connections in cat visual cortex. *J. Neurosci.* 3, 1116–1133.

Gilbert, C. D., and Wiesel, T. N. (1989). Columnar specificity of intrinsic horizontal and corticocortical connections in the cat visual cortex. *J. Neurosci.* 9, 2432–2442.

Goldman-Rakic, P. S. (1987). "Circuitry of primate prefrontal cortex and regulation of behavior by representational memory," in *Handbook of Physiology: The Nervous System*, Vol. 5, ed. F. Plum (Bethesda: American Physiological Society), 373–417.

Goldman-Rakic, P. S. (2000). "The prefrontal landscape: implications of functional architecture for understanding human mentation and the central executive," in *The Prefrontal Cortex. Executive and Cognitive Functions*, eds A. C. Roberts, T. W. Robbins, and L. Weiskrantz (Oxford: Oxford University Press), 87–102.

González-Burgos, G., Barrionuevo, G., and Lewis, D. A. (2000). Horizontal synaptic connections in monkey prefrontal cortex: an in vitro electrophysiological study. *Cereb. Cortex* 10, 82–92.

Gould, S. J. (2002). *The Structure of Evolutionary Theory*. Cambridge, MA: Harvard University Press.

Hagler, D. J., and Sereno, M. I. (2006). Spatial maps in frontal and prefrontal cortex. *Neuroimage* 29, 567–577.

Hallman, L. E., Schoefield, B. R., and Lin, C.-S. (1988). Dendritic morphology and axon collaterals of corticotectal, corticopontine, and callosal neurons in layer V of the primary visual cortex of the hooded rat. *J. Comp. Neurol.* 272, 149–160.

Hirsch, J., Rodriguez Moreno, D., and Kim, K. H. S. (2001). Interconnected large-scale systems for three fundamental cognitive tasks revealed by functional MRI. *J. Cogn. Neurosci.* 13, 389–405.

Hübener, M., and Bolz, J. (1988). Morphology of identified projection neurons in layer 5 of rat visual cortex. *Neurosci. Lett.* 94, 76–81.

Hübener, M., Schwarz, C., and Bolz, J. (1990). Morphological types of projection neurons in layer 5 of cat visual cortex. *J. Comp. Neurol.* 301, 655–674.

Inda, M. C., Defelipe, J., and Munoz, A. (2007). The distribution of chandelier cell axon terminals that express the GABA plasma membrane transporter GAT-1 in the human neocortex. *Cereb. Cortex* 17, 2060–2071.

Jacobs, B., Chugani, H. T., Allada, V., Chen, S., Phelps, M. E., Pollack, D. B., and Raleigh, M. J. (1995). Developmental changes in brain metabolism in sedated rhesus macaques and vervet monkeys revealed by positron emission tomography. *Cereb. Cortex.* 5, 222–233.

Jacobs, B., Larsen-Driscoll, L., and Schall, M. (1997). Lifespan dendritic and spine changes in areas 10 and 18 of human cortex: a quantitative Golgi study *J. Comp. Neurol.* 386, 661–680.

Jacobs, B., Schall, M., Prather, M., Kapler, L., Driscoll, L., Baca, S., Jacobs, J., Ford, K., Wainwright, M., and Treml, M. (2001). Regional dendritic and spine variation in human cerebral cortex: a quantitative study. *Cereb. Cortex* 11, 558–571.

Jacobs, B., and Scheibel, A. B. (1993). A quantitative analyses of Wernicke's area in humans. I. Lifespan changes. *J. Comp. Neurol.* 327, 83–96.

Jacobs, B., and Scheibel, A. B. (2002). "Regional dendritic variation in primate cortical pyramidal cells," in *Cortical Areas: Unity and Diversity*, eds A. Schüz and R. Miller (London: Taylor and Francis), 111–131.

Jan, Y.-N., and Jan, L. Y. (2001). Dendrites. *Genes Dev.* 15, 2627–2641.

Jones, E. G., and Powell, T. P. S. (1970). An anatomical study of converging sensory pathways within the cerebral cortex of the monkey brain. *Brain* 93, 793–820.

Kisvárday, Z. F., and Eysel, U. T. (1992). Cellular organization of reciprocal patchy networks in layer III of cat visual cortex (area 17). *Neuroscience* 46, 275–286.

Kisvárday, Z. F., Martin, K. A. C., Freund, T. F., Magloczky, Z., Whitteridge, D., and Somogyi, P. (1986). Synaptic targets of HRP-filled layer III pyramidal cells in the cat striate cortex. *Exp. Brain Res.* 64, 541–552.

Koch, C. (1999). *Biophysics of Computation. Information Processing in Single Neurons.* New York: Oxford University Press.

Kritzer, M., and Goldman-Rakic, P. S. (1995). Intrinsic circuit organization of the major layers and sublayers of the dorsolateral prefrontal cortex in monkeys. *J. Comp. Neurol.* 359, 131–143.

Levitt, J. B., Lewis, D. A., Yoshioka, T., and Lund, J. S. (1993). Topography of pyramidal neuron intrinsic connections in macaque monkey prefrontal cortex (areas 9 and 46). *J. Comp. Neurol.* 338, 360–376.

Lewis, D. A., and Lund, J. S. (1990). Heterogeneity of chandelier neurons in monkey neocortex: corticotropin-releasing factor and parvalbumin immunoreactive populations. *J. Comp. Neurol.* 293, 599–615.

Livingstone, M. S., and Hubel, D. H. (1984). Anatomy and physiology of a color system in the primate visual cortex. *J. Neurosci.* 4, 309–356.

London, M., and Häusser, M. (2005). Dendritic computation. *Annu. Rev. Neurosci.* 28, 503–532.

Losonczy, A., Makara, J. K., and Magee, J. C. (2008). Compartmentalized dendritic plasticity and input feature storage in neurons. *Nature* 452, 436–441.

Lund, J. S., Yoshioka, T., and Levitt, J. B. (1993). Comparison of intrinsic connectivity in different areas of macaque monkey cerebral cortex. *Cereb. Cortex* 3, 148–162.

Mainen, Z. F., and Sejnowski, T. J. (1986). Influence of dendritic structure on firing pattern in model neocortical neurons. *Nature* 382, 363–366.

Malach, R. (1994). Cortical columns as devices for maximizing neuronal diversity. *Trends Neurosci.* 17, 101–104.

Malach, R., Amir, Y., Harel, M., and Grinvald, A. (1993). Relationship between intrinsic connections and functional architecture revealed by optical imaging and in vivo targeted biocytin injections in primate striate cortex. *Proc. Natl. Acad. Sci. U.S.A.* 90, 10469–10473.

Malonek, D., Tootell, R. B. H., and Grinvald, A. (1994). Optical imaging reveals the functional architecture of neurons processing shape and motion in owl monkey area MT. *Proc. R. Soc. Lond., B, Biol. Sci.* 258, 109–119.

Martin, K. A. C., and Whitteridge, D. (1984). Form, function and intracortical projections of spiny neurones in the striate visual cortex of the cat. *J. Physiol.* 353, 463–504.

Matsubara, J., Cynader, M., Swindale, N. V., and Stryker, M. P. (1985). Intrinsic projections within visual cortex: evidence for orientation-specific local connections. *Proc. Natl. Acad. Sci. U.S.A.* 82, 935–939.

Matsubara, J. A., Chase, R., and Thejomayen, M. (1996). Comparative morphology of three types of projection-identified pyramidal neurons in the superficial layers of cat visual cortex. *J. Comp. Neurol.* 366, 93–108.

McGuire, B. A., Gilbert, C. D., Rivlin, P. K., and Wiesel, T. N. (1991). Targets of horizontal connections in macaque primary visual cortex. *J. Comp. Neurol.* 305, 370–392.

Mel, B. (1999). "Why have dendrites? A computational perspective," in *Dendrites*, eds G. Stuart, N. Spruston, and M. Häusser (New York: Oxford University Press), 271–289.

Mel, B. W. (2002). Have we been Hebbing down the wrong path? *Neuron* 34, 175–177.

Melchitzky, D. S., González-Burgos, G., Barrionuevo, G., and Lewis, D. A. (2001). Synaptic targets of the intrinsic axon collaterals of supragranular pyramidal neurons in monkey prefrontal cortex. *J. Comp. Neurol.* 430, 209–221.

Melchitzky, D. S., Sesack, S. R., Pucak, M. L., and Lewis, D. A. (1998). Synaptic targets of pyramidal neurons providing intrinsic horizontal connections in monkey prefrontal cortex. *J. Comp. Neurol.* 390, 211–224.

Miller, E. K. (2000). The prefrontal cortex and cognitive control. *Nat. Neurosci.* 1, 59–65.

Miller, E. K., Erickson, C. A., and Desimone, R. (1996). Neural mechanisms of visual working memory in prefrontal cortex of the macaque. *J. Neurosci.* 16, 5154–5167.

Miller, E. K., Li, L., and Desimone, R. (1993). Activity of neurons in anterior inferior temporal cortex during a short-term memory task. *J. Neurosci.* 13, 1460–1478.

Mitchison, G., and Crick, F. H. C. (1982). Long axons within the striate cortex: their distribution, orientation and patterns of connection. *Proc. Natl. Acad. Sci. U.S.A.* 79, 3661–3665.

Nelissen, K., Luppino, G., Vanduffel, W., Rizzolatti, G., and Orban, G. A. (2005). Observing others: multiple action representation in the frontal lobe. *Science* 310, 332–336.

Noppeney, U., Price, C. J., Penny, W. D., and Friston, K. J. (2005). Two distinct neural mechanisms for category-selective responses. *Cereb. Cortex* 16, 437–445.

Ó Scalaidhe, S. P., Wilson, F. A. W., and Goldman-Rakic, P. S. (1997). Areal segregation of face-processing neurons in prefrontal cortex. *Science* 278, 1135–1138.

Page, T. L., Einstein, M., Duan, H., He, Y., Flores, T., Rolshud, D., Erwin, J. M., Wearne, S. L., Morrison, J. H., and Hof, P. R. (2002). Morphological alterations in neurons forming corticocortical projections in the neocortex of aged Patas monkeys. *Neurosci. Lett.* 317, 37–41.

Pandya, D. N., and Yeterian, E. H. (2000). "Comparison of prefrontal architecture and connections," in *The Prefrontal Cortex*, eds A. C. Roberts, T. W. Robbins, and L. Weiskrantz (Oxford: Oxford University Press), 51–66.

Passingham, R., Stephan, K. E., and Kötter, R. (2002). The anatomical basis of functional localization in the cortex. *Nat. Neurosci.* 3, 606–616.

Passingham, R. E., Toni, I., and Rushworth, M. F. S. (2000). Specialisation within the prefrontal cortex: the ventral prefrontal cortex and associative learning. *Exp. Brain Res.* 133, 103–113.

Petralia, R. S., Yokotani, N., and Wenthold, R. J. (1994a). Light and electron microscope distribution of the NMDA receptor subunit NMDAR1 in the rat nervous system using a selective antipeptide antibody. *J. Neurosci.* 14, 667–696.

Petralia, R. S., Wang, Y. X., and Wenthold, R. J. (1994b). The NMDA receptor subunits NR2A and NR2B show histological and ultrastructural localization patterns similar to those of NR1. *J. Neurosci.* 14, 6102–6120.

Petralia, R. S., Wang, Y.-X., and Wenthold, R. J. (1994c). Histological and ultrastructural localization of kainate receptor subunits, KA2 and GluR6/7, in the rat nervous system using selective antipeptide antibodies. *J. Comp. Neurol.* 349, 85–110.

Petrides, M. (1987). "Conditional learning and the primate prefrontal cortex," in *The Frontal Lobes Revisited*, ed. E. Perecman (New York, IRBN Press), 91–108.

Petrides, M. (1991). Functional specialization within the dorsolateral prefrontal cortex for serial order memory. *Proc. R. Soc. Lond., B, Biol. Sci.* 246, 299–306.

Petrides, M. (1998). "Specialised systems for the processing of mnemonic information within the primate frontal cortex," in *The Prefrontal Cortex*, eds A. C. Roberts, T. W. Robbins, and L. Weiskrantz (Oxford: Oxford University Press), 103–106.

Petrides, M. (2000). "Mapping prefrontal cortical systems for the control of cognition," in *Brain Mapping: The Systems*, eds A. W. Toga and J. C. Mazziotta (San Diego: Academic), 159–176.

Petrides, M., and Pandya, D. N. (1988). Association fiber pathways to the frontal cortex from the superior temporal region in the rhesus monkey. *J. Comp. Neurol.* 273, 52–66.

Petrides, M., and Pandya, D. N. (1999). Dorsolateral prefrontal cortex: comparative cytoarchitectonic analysis in the human and the macaque monkey brain and corticocortical connection patterns. *Eur. J. Neurosci.* 11, 1011–1036.

Petrides, M., and Pandya, D. N. (2001). Comparative cytoarchitectonic analysis of the human and the macaque dorsolateral prefrontal cortex and corticocortical connection patterns in the monkey. *Eur. J. Neurosci.* 16, 291–310.

Poirazi, P., and Mel, B. (2001). Impact of active dendrites and structural plasticity on the storage capacity of neural tissue. *Neuron* 29, 779–796.

Preuss, T. M., and Goldman-Rakic, P. S. (1991a). Architectonics of the parietal and temporal association cortex in the strepsirhine primate Galago compared to the anthropoid *Macaca. J. Comp. Neurol.* 310, 475–506.

Preuss, T. M., and Goldman-Rakic, P. S. (1991b). Ipsilateral cortical connections of granular frontal cortex in the strepsirhine primate Galago, with comparative comments on anthropoid primates. *J. Comp. Neurol.* 310, 507–549.

Preuss, T. M., and Goldman-Rakic, P. S. (1991c). Myelo- and cytoarchitecture of the granular frontal cortex and surrounding regions in the strepshrine primate Galago and the anthropoid primate Macaca. *J. Comp. Neurol.* 310, 429–474.

Pucak, M. L., Levitt, J. B., Lund, J. S., and Lewis, D. A. (1996). Patterns of intrinsic and associational circuitry in monkey prefrontal cortex. *J. Comp. Neurol.* 376, 614–630.

Rall, W. (1959). Branching dendritic trees and motorneuron membrane resistivity. *Exp. Neurol.* 1, 491–527.

Rall, W. (1989). "Cable theory for dendritic neurons," in *Methods in Neuronal Modeling: From Synapses to Networks*, eds C. Koch and I. Segev (Cambridge, MA: MIT), 9–62.

Rall, W., Burke, R. E., Holmes, W. R., Jack, J. J. B., Redman, S. R., and Segev, I. (1992). Matching dendritic neuron models to experimental data. *Physiol. Rev.* 72, 159–186.

Roberts, A. C., and Wallis, J. D. (2000). Inhibitory control and affective processing in the prefrontal cortex: neuropsychological studies in the common marmoset. *Cereb. Cortex* 10, 252–262.

Rockland, K. S. (1985). A reticular pattern of intrinsic connections in primate area V2 (area 18). *J. Comp. Neurol.* 235, 467–478.

Rockland, K. S., and Lund, J. S. (1982). Widespread periodic intrinsic connections in the tree shrew visual cortex. *Science* 215, 1532–1534.

Rockland, K. S., and Lund, J. S. (1983). Intrinsic laminar lattice connections in primate visual cortex. *J. Comp. Neurol.* 216, 303–318.

Rockland, K. S., Lund, J. S., and Humphrey, A. L. (1982). Anatomical banding of intrinsic connections in striate cortex of tree shrews (*Tupaia glis*). *J. Comp. Neurol.* 209, 41–58.

Rolls, E. T. (2000). "The orbitofrontal cortex," in *The Prefrontal Cortex*, eds A. C. Roberts, T. W. Robbins, and L. Weiskrantz (Oxford: Oxford University Press), 67–86.

Roth, G., and Dicke, U. (2005). Evolution of the brain and intelligence. *Trends Cogn. Sci.* 9, 250–257.

Rothnie, P., Kabaso, D., Hof, P. R., Henry, B. I., and Wearne, S. L. (2005). Functionally relevant measures of spatial complexity in neuronal dendritic arbors. *J. Theor. Biol.* 238, 505–526.

Sakai, K., Rowe, J. B., and Passingham, R. E. (2002). Active maintenance in prefrontal area 46 creates distractor-resistant memory. *Nat. Neurosci.* 5, 479–484.

Schofield, B. R., Hallman, L. E., and Lin, C.-S. (1987). Morphology of corticotectal cells in the primary visual cortex of hooded rats. *J. Comp. Neurol.* 261, 85–97.

Segev, I., and Rall, W. (1998). Excitable dendrites and spines: earlier theoretical insights elucidate recent direct observations. *Trends Neurosci.* 21, 453–460.

Shinomoto, S., Miyazaki, Y., Tamura, H., and Fujita, I. (2005). Regional and laminar differences in in vivo firing patterns of primate cortical neurons. *J. Neurophysiol.* 94, 567–575.

Sholl, D. A. (1953). Dendritic organization in the neurons of the visual and motor cortices of the cat. *J. Anat.* 87, 387–406.

Soloway, A. S., Pucak, M. L., Melchitzky, D. S., and Lewis, D. A. (2002). Dendritic morphology of callosal and ipsilateral projection neurons in monkey prefrontal cortex. *Neuroscience* 109, 461–471.

Spruston, N. (2008). Pyramidal neurons: dendritic structure and synaptic integration. *Nat. Rev. Neurosci.* 9, 206–221.

Spruston, N., Stuart, G., and Häusser, M. (1999). "Dendritic integration," in *Dendrites*, eds G. Stuart, N. Spruston, and M. Häusser (New York: Oxford University Press), 231–270.

Stepanyants, A., Hof, P. R., and Chklovskii, D. B. (2002). Geometry and structural plasticity of synaptic connectivity. *Neuron* 34, 275–288.

Stuart, G. J., Spruston, N., Sackman, B., and Häusser, M. (1997). Action potential initiation and backpropagation in neurons of the mammalian CNS. *Trends Neurosci.* 20, 125–131.

Treves, A. (2005). Frontal latching networks: a possible neural basis for infinite recursion. *Cogn. Neuropsychol.* 22, 276–291.

T'so, D. Y., and Gilbert, C. D. (1988). The organization of chromatic and spatial interactions in the primate striate cortex. *J. Neurosci.* 8, 1712–1727.

T'so, D. Y., Gilbert, C. D., and Wiesel, T. N. (1986). Relationships between horizontal interactions and functional architecture in the cat striate cortex as revealed by cross-correlation analysis. *J. Neurosci.* 6, 1160–1170.

Valverde, F. (1967). Apical dendritic spines of the visual cortex and light deprivation in the mouse. *Exp. Brain Res.* 3, 337–352.

Vetter, P., Roth, A., and Häusser, M. (2001). Propagation of action potentials in dendrites depends on dendritic morphology. *J. Neurophysiol.* 85, 926–937.

Vogt, C., and Vogt, O. (1919). Allgemeine ergebnisse unserer hirnforschung. *J. Psychol. Neurol.* 25, 279–462.

Walker, A. E. (1940). A cytoarchitectural study of the prefrontal areas of the macaque monkey. *J. Comp. Neurol.* 73, 59–86.

Wang, X.-J. (2001). Synaptic reverberation underlying mnemonic persistent activity. *Trends Neurosci.* 24, 455–463.

White, E. L. (1989). *Cortical Circuits: Synaptic Organization of the Cerebral Cortex. Structure, Function and Theory.* Boston: Birkhaüser.

Wilson, F. A. W., Ó Scalaidhe, S. P., and Goldman-Rakic, P. S. (1993). Dissociation of object and spatial processing domains in primate prefrontal cortex. *Science* 260, 1955–1958.

Young, M. P. (1992). Objective analysis of the topological organization of the primate cortical visual system. *Nature* 358, 152–154.

Conflict of Interest Statement: The authors declare that the research was conducted in the absence of any commercial or financial relationships that could be construed as a potential conflict of interest.

12

Regionalization of the shark hindbrain: a survey of an ancestral organization

Isabel Rodríguez-Moldes[1]*, Ivan Carrera[1], Sol Pose-Méndez[1], Idoia Quintana-Urzainqui[1], Eva Candal[1], Ramón Anadón[1], Sylvie Mazan[2] and Susana Ferreiro-Galve[1]

[1] Department of Cell Biology and Ecology, University of Santiago de Compostela, Santiago de Compostela, Spain
[2] UMR 7150, Centre National de la Recherche Scientifique, Université Pierre et Marie Curie and Université Européene de Bretagne, Station Biologique de Roscoff, Roscoff, France

Edited by:
Luis Puelles, University of Murcia, Spain

Reviewed by:
Faustino Marin, University of Murcia, Spain
Luis Puelles, University of Murcia, Spain

****Correspondence:***
Isabel Rodríguez-Moldes, Department of Cell Biology and Ecology, University of Santiago de Compostela, Building CIBUS, South Campus, 15782 Santiago de Compostela, Spain
e-mail: isabel.rodriguez-moldes@usc.es

Cartilaginous fishes (chondrichthyans) represent an ancient radiation of vertebrates currently considered the sister group of the group of gnathostomes with a bony skeleton that gave rise to land vertebrates. This out-group position makes chondrichthyans essential in assessing the ancestral organization of the brain of jawed vertebrates. To gain knowledge about hindbrain evolution we have studied its development in a shark, the lesser spotted dogfish *Scyliorhinus canicula* by analyzing the expression of some developmental genes and the origin and distribution of specific neuronal populations, which may help to identify hindbrain subdivisions and boundaries and the topology of specific cell groups. We have characterized three developmental periods that will serve as a framework to compare the development of different neuronal systems and may represent a suitable tool for comparing the absolute chronology of development among vertebrates. The expression patterns of *Pax6*, *Wnt8*, and *HoxA2* genes in early embryos of *S. canicula* showed close correspondence to what has been described in other vertebrates and helped to identify the anterior rhombomeres. Also in these early embryos, the combination of Pax6 with protein markers of migrating neuroblasts (DCX) and early differentiating neurons (general: HuC/D; neuron type specific: GAD, the GABA synthesizing enzyme) revealed the organization of *S. canicula* hindbrain in both transverse segmental units corresponding to visible rhombomeres and longitudinal columns. Later in development, when the interrhombomeric boundaries fade away, accurate information about *S. canicula* hindbrain subdivisions was achieved by comparing the expression patterns of Pax6 and GAD, serotonin (serotoninergic neurons), tyrosine hydroxylase (catecholaminergic neurons), choline acetyltransferase (cholinergic neurons), and calretinin (a calcium-binding protein). The patterns observed revealed many topological correspondences with other vertebrates and led to reconsideration of the current view of the elasmobranch hindbrain segmentation as peculiar among vertebrates.

Keywords: rhombomeres, *HoxA2*, *Wnt8*, calretinin, cartilaginous fishes, shark embryo, development, evolution

INTRODUCTION

In elasmobranchs, as in other vertebrates, two prominent external constrictions divide the early developing brain (neural tube) into the three neural vesicles giving rise to the basic regions of the adult brain: forebrain (or prosencephalon), midbrain (or mesencephalon), and hindbrain (or rhombencephalon). These vesicles represent the fundamental antero-posterior (i.e., rostrocaudal) subdivisions that later on may become subdivided into more or less evident transverse bands or neuromeres, which have defined relations with other structures of the head and the peripheral nervous system, being very useful in comparative studies. In the hindbrain, these transverse units, called rhombomeres, exhibit a segmental organization and appear as prominent ventricular outpouchings separated by constrictions. Coinciding with the emergence of rhombomeres, longitudinal zones with distinct morphological and functional identity become organized along the brain and spinal cord. Four columns separated by ventricular sulci have been commonly recognized in the adult shark hindbrain: ventral and ventrolateral columns (derived from the basal plate), and dorsolateral and dorsal columns (derived from the alar plate). These columns represent the classical four functional zones (Gaskell, 1886, 1889; Herrick, 1918): the alar plate-derived somato- and viscerosensory columns and the basal plate-derived viscero- and somatomotor columns. Taking into account this developmental pattern, the different hindbrain regions and nuclei have been usually assigned to longitudinal bands and segmental units. However, this classic

Abbreviations: AOL, octavolateral area; br1–br4, branchial arches; c1–c2, pharyngeal clefts 1–2; cer, cerebellum; H, hypophysis; IIIm, oculomotor nucleus; IIIn, oculomotor nerve; IVm, trochlear motor nucleus; IXm, glossopharyngeal motor nucleus; IXn, glossopharyngeal nerve; LC, locus coeruleus; Mes, mesencephalon; mlf, medial longitudinal fascicle; n, notochord; Oli, inferior olive; os, optic stalk; ot, otic placode; p1–p3, prosomeres; ph1–ph3, pharyngeal pouches; Pal, pallium; Pros, prosencephalon; R, Rathke's pouch; r1–r8, rhombomeres; Ra, raphe (medial) cells of the reticular formation; Re, reticular (lateral) cells of the reticular formation; Rh, rhombencephalon; Sc, nucleus subcoeruleus; Sp, subpallium; spc, spinal cord; SV, saccus vasculosus; VIIIm, magnocellular octaval nucleus; VIIIn, octaval nerve; VIIm, facial motor nucleus; VIIn, facial nerve; VIM, visceromotor area; VIm, abducens nucleus; VIn, abducens nerve; VIS, viscerosensory lobe; Vm, trigeminal motor nucleus; Vn, trigeminal nerve; Xm, vagal motor nucleus; Xn, vagal nerve.

conception is under revision after the identification of molecular markers that revealed distinct longitudinal subdivisions in these columns (Briscoe et al., 2000; Sieber et al., 2007) and because of the existence of migratory processes in basal plate-born motoneurons that reached the alar plate (Ju et al., 2004).

Understanding brain segmentation has become essential for comparative neuroanatomical studies. In particular, studies in different vertebrate groups have revealed that the segmental organization of rhombencephalic structures is rather well conserved in evolution (Gilland and Baker, 1993, 2005; Marín and Puelles, 1995; Pritz, 1999; Cambronero and Puelles, 2000; Straka et al., 2002). Comparative studies have also pointed some variations among vertebrates in the organization of individual hindbrain segments (Gilland and Baker, 1993, 2005), but their evolutionary significance has not been cleared yet. Some neurochemical markers were found helpful in studies about hindbrain organization, since they can identify neuronal populations that show segmental patterns. Among them, calretinin (CR, a calcium-binding protein) has proven to be a useful tool to identify hindbrain subpopulations (Marín and Puelles, 1995; Pritz, 1999; Díaz-Regueira and Anadón, 2000; Castro et al., 2006; Morona and González, 2009). Other markers such as choline acetyltransferase (ChAT), serotonin (5-HT), or tyrosine hydroxylase (TH) have also been used to examine the segmental organization of the hindbrain in different vertebrate species, including elasmobranchs (Anadón et al., 2000; Carrera et al., 2005, 2008).

Our present aim is to contribute to knowledge about hindbrain regionalization in a small shark, the lesser spotted dogfish *Scyliorhinus canicula*, by highlighting some aspects of its development. This common coastal dogfish is becoming the prevailing chondrichthyan model in comparative neurobiology and developmental studies (Coolen et al., 2009). The fairly transparent eggs can be easily maintained in the laboratory until hatching, which occurs 6 months after fertilization. The protracted development and the relatively large size of the embryonic brain allow a detailed analysis of developmental processes. To know how regionalization is achieved, we have analyzed the expression of some developmental genes involved in the transverse segmentation of the anterior hindbrain. In particular, we have used HoxA2 and Wnt8 because the former is the only *Hox* gene expressed in rhombomere 2 (r2; Tümpel et al., 2008; Alexander et al., 2009) and the latter seems to be responsible for the determination of rhombomere 4 (r4) identity (Bouillet et al., 1996). Furthermore, we have analyzed the development of specific neuronal populations using markers that proved to be very useful to identify topographically restricted neuronal populations relative to brain subdivisions and/or segmental boundaries. We have constrained the characterization of transverse and longitudinal subdivisions of *S. canicula* hindbrain at early and intermediate embryonic stages. The results of this study bear on how the hindbrain of cartilaginous fish becomes organized and about possible ancestral features of hindbrain regionalization. The results described are consistent with the model that advocates the evolutionary conservation of the segmental rhombencephalic entities (Gilland and Baker, 1993, 2005; Marín and Puelles, 1995; Pritz, 1999; Cambronero and Puelles, 2000; Straka et al., 2002) which is useful for comparative purposes. This helps understanding how hindbrain development evolved during phylogeny.

MATERIALS AND METHODS

EXPERIMENTAL ANIMALS

Embryos of the lesser spotted dogfish (*S. canicula*) were provided by the Oceanário in Lisbon (Portugal), and the Aquarium Finisterrae in A Coruña (Spain). Additional embryos were supplied by the Station Biologique de Roscoff (France). Embryos of *S. canicula* were staged according to Ballard et al. (1993). The following stages were analyzed: stage 20 (four pairs of unopened pharyngeal pouches visible by translucence), stage 22 (two pairs of pharyngeal clefts open), stage 23 (three pairs of pharyngeal clefts open), stage 24 (diamond-shaped mouth), stage 25 (four pairs of open pharyngeal clefts), stages 26 (five pairs of open pharyngeal clefts, simple gill bars), stage 27 (diamond-shaped mouth and primordial gill filaments), stage 28 (transverse oval mouth, gills with external filaments), stage 29 (mandibular arches crowded into the mouth opening and initial eye pigmentation), stages 30 (eyeballs circled with black pigment), stage 31 (detectable rostrum and long branchial filaments), stage 32 (regression of branchial filaments), stages 33 and 34 (prehatching).

TISSUE PREPARATION

All procedures conformed to the guidelines established by the European Communities Council Directive of 24 November 1986 (86/609/EEC) and by the Spanish Royal Decree 1201/2005 for animal experimentation and were approved by the Ethics Committee of the University of Santiago de Compostela. Embryos were anesthetized with 0.5% tricaine methane sulfonate (MS-222; Sigma, St. Louis, MO, USA) in seawater and fixed in 4% paraformaldehyde (PFA) in elasmobranch phosphate buffer containing urea for 48–72 h depending on the stage, as described by Carrera et al. (2008). Parallel series of 14–18 μm thick sections were obtained after cryostat sectioning of specimens in sagittal, transverse, or horizontal planes in relation to the main body axis.

IN SITU HYBRIDIZATION

We applied *in situ* hybridization for ScPax6 (Derobert et al., 2002), ScWnt8 (Coolen et al., 2007), and ScHoxA2 (Oulion et al., 2010). These probes were selected from a collection of *S. canicula* embryonic cDNA library (mixed stages, S9 to 22), submitted to high throughput EST sequencing (coord. S. Mazan).Sense and antisense digoxigenin-UTP-labeled RNA probes were synthesized directly by *in vitro* transcription using as templates linearized recombinant plasmid DNA (Pax6 probe) or cDNA fragments prepared by PCR amplification of the recombinant plasmids (ScWnt8 and ScHoxA2 probes).

Whole-mount *in situ* hybridization was carried out in S20, S22, and S24 embryos following standard protocols (Coolen et al., 2007). Briefly, embryos were permeabilized with proteinase K, hybridized with sense or antisense probes overnight at 70°C and incubated with the alkaline phosphatase-coupled anti-digoxigenin antibody (1:2000, Roche Applied Science, Mannheim, Germany) overnight at 4°C. The color reaction was performed in the presence of BM-Purple (Roche). Control sense probes did not lead to any detectable signal.

IMMUNOHISTOCHEMISTRY

Sections were processed for the ABC method (single labeling) or for double immunofluorescence following Ferreiro-Galve et al. (2010). As primary antibodies we used polyclonal rabbit anti-Pax6 (Covance; dilution 1:400) or polyclonal goat anti-Pax6 (Novus Biologicals; dilution: 1:200), polyclonal rabbit anti-sonic hedgehog

(Shh; Santa Cruz Biotech.; dilution 1:300) polyclonal rabbit anti-CR (Swant; dilution 1:250-500), polyclonal rabbit anti-serotonin (5-HT; Diasorin/Immunostar; dilution 1:5,000); polyclonal rabbit anti-doublecortin (DCX; Cell Signaling; dilution 1:300–500) or polyclonal goat anti-DCX (Santa Cruz Biotech.; dilution 1:100); monoclonal mouse anti-TH (Millipore; dilution 1:500-1,000), monoclonal mouse anti-proliferating cell nuclear antigen (PCNA; Sigma; dilution 1:200), monoclonal mouse anti-HuC/D (Molecular Probes; dilution 1:200), and polyclonal sheep anti-GAD65/67 (GAD 1440; kindly provided by Dr. E. Mugnaini; dilution 1:20,000).

For single immunoperoxidase labeling, sections were pretreated to remove the endogenous biotin-like and peroxidase activities, as described by Sueiro et al. (2004). As secondary antibody we used a biotinylated goat anti-rabbit or anti-mouse antiserum, appropriately to the primary antibody employed (Dako; dilution 1:500), followed by incubation with the preformed avidin-biotinylated horseradish peroxidase complex (Vector Laboratories). The immunoreaction was finally developed, either with 0.25 mg/ml diaminobenzidine tetrahydrochloride (DAB; Sigma) containing 2.5 mg/ml nickel ammonium sulfate and 0.00075% H_2O_2 (blue precipitate), or with SIGMAFAST™ 3,3′-DAB tablets (brown precipitate).

For double immunofluorescence, the following secondary antibodies were used: Alexa Fluor 488-conjugated donkey anti-rabbit immunoglobulin (Molecular Probes; diluted 1:200) and FluoProbes 546-conjugated donkey anti-mouse (Interchim; diluted 1:100), TRITC-conjugated swine anti-rabbit immunoglobulin (Dako; diluted 1:100), Alexa Fluor 488-conjugated donkey anti-sheep immunoglobulin (Molecular Probes; diluted 1:100). Sections were photographed with a fluorescence microscope fitted with an Olympus DP 70 color digital camera and a Leica Spectral Confocal Laser Scanning Microscope (TCS-SP2).

Embryos processed *in toto* for *in situ* hybridization with ScWnt8 were sectioned on cryostat in sagittal plane at 18–20 μm thick and then sections were treated for immunohistochemistry for rabbit anti-DCX as described previously for immunoperoxidase labeling.

RESULTS AND DISCUSSION

PERIODS OF BRAIN DEVELOPMENT IN THE LESSER SPOTTED DOGFISH

In order to establish an outline for comparative studies, we distinguished three periods in the development of the lesser spotted dogfish, based on the histogenetic stage of the brain walls (**Table 1**). During the *first period* (from embryo stages 17–26), the neural walls mainly consist of a thick proliferating neuroepithelium. Late during this period, radially migrating neuroblasts are first noticed and a primordial mantle layer appears. During the *second period* (from embryo stages 27–31) the brain walls are subdivided radially into the standard three primary layers or zones (ventricular, mantle/intermediate, marginal/subpial). During this period, cell proliferation, migration, and differentiation are very active and lead to the topological organization of most neuronal systems and the differentiation of the major pathways. The majority of brain catecholaminergic and serotoninergic cell populations develop during this time (Carrera et al., 2005, 2008). During this second period the morphological differentiation of the main brain centers occurs. The *third period* is the longest one (3 months, just a half of the embryonic period) and corresponds to the prehatching period of Ballard et al. (1993). It starts at stage 32, when the embryo looks like a small juvenile with an attached yolk sac. In the brain, cell proliferation is still very active in some ventricular regions, and migrating neuroblasts are also present in some regions; but most neurons have already migrated away from the ventricular zone. Distinct cells groups are hardly recognized with conventional staining, because of the considerable dispersion of mantle cells, but boundaries can be discerned by their neurochemical content. During this stage, most neuronal populations observed in juveniles and adults are established, although morphogenesis continues in some brain regions. The third period thus can be considered as a period of brain maturation.

Since a similar histogenetic sequence occurs in the brain of all vertebrates, the corresponding relative timing of periods can be used as a framework for comparative studies. The three developmental periods described in *S. canicula* can be roughly recognized in other vertebrates, although the time of occurrence varies largely as a result of sizeable differences in the length of the embryonic period (**Table 1**).

REGIONALIZATION OF THE HINDBRAIN IN EARLY EMBRYOS (FIRST DEVELOPMENTAL PERIOD)

Transverse segmental regions

During *S. canicula* development, as in other vertebrates, prominent ventricular ridges divide the rhombencephalon into transverse segmental units exhibiting shallow ventricular outpouchings and corresponding outer bulges, the rhombomeres. Six apparently interrhombomeric limits can be clearly identified in the hindbrain of early *S. canicula* embryos.

Table 1 | Correspondence among embryonic developmental stages of different vertebrate embryos according to the three development periods defined in *S. canicula* and some external features.

	First period Brain walls formed by a pseudo-stratified neuroepithelium	Second period Layering of the brain walls and development of mantle zone structures	Third period Development of nuclei from layers and migrated cells
DOGFISH[1]	S17–S26	S27–S31	S32–S34 (hatching)
CHICK[2]	HH9–HH18	HH19–HH30	HH31–HH45 (hatching at HH46)
MOUSE	E8.5–E10.5	E10.5–E14.5	E14.5-birth
ZEBRAFISH	12–24 hpf	24–48 hpf	48–72 hpf (hatching)

[1] *Stages from Ballard et al. (1993).*
[2] *Stages from Hamburger and Hamilton (1951).*

The analysis of the expression of the *ScHoxA2* gene has revealed an interesting finding. In the early *S. canicula* embryos analyzed this gene was expressed along several rhombomeres with a sharp anterior limit of expression at the level of a conspicuous interrhombomeric boundary (**Figures 1A–C**). Assuming that in dogfish, as in other vertebrates (Prince et al., 1998; Glover, 2001; Tümpel et al., 2008), the anterior limit of HoxA2 expression coincides with the r1/r2 boundary, we could identify the rhombomeres 1 and 2 (r1 and r2)

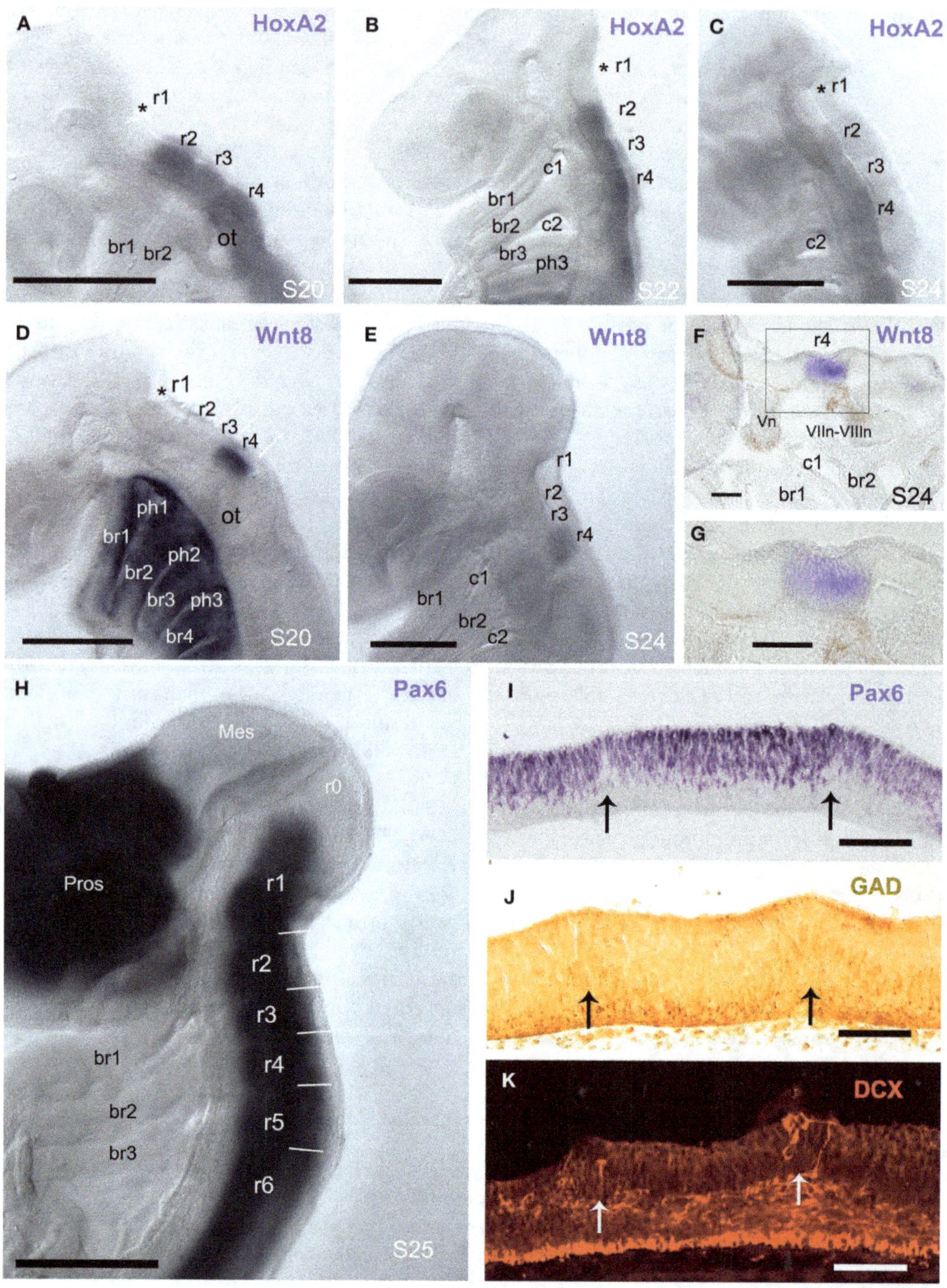

FIGURE 1 | Rhombomeres are visible in early embryos as the interrhombomeric limits are evident. (A–H) Whole-mount *in situ* hybridization for ScHoxA2 **(A–C)**, ScWnt8 **(D–G)**, and ScPax6 **(H)** in the early developing embryo in lateral view at the indicated developmental stages. Asterisks in **(A–D)** label the rostralmost intrarhombomeric ventricular ridge at r1. **(F,G)** are panoramic and detail of a sagittal section of a S24 embryo whole-mount processed for *in situ* hybridization showing ScWnt8 expression in r4 (in blue) where DCX-immunoreactive fibers of the acoustic-facial nerve roots emerge. **(I–K)** Parasagittal sections immunolabeled for Pax6 **(I)**, GAD **(J)**, and DCX **(K)** showing ventricular ridges that coincide with interrhombomeric limits. At these boundaries low density of Pax6 cells **(I)**, radially oriented GAD-ir **(J)** and DCX **(K)** cells are observed. Scale bars: 500 μm **(A–E, H)**; 100 μm **(F,G, I,J)**.

of *S. canicula* as showed in **Figures 1A–C**. As the anterior limit of expression of ScHoxA2 coincides with the r1/r2 boundary, and the position of the rostralmost ScHoxA2-expression rhombomere is adjacent to the position of the trigeminal ganglion (see Figure 3 of O'Neill et al., 2007), we have identified the rhombomere 2 of *S. canicula* as the rostralmost rhombomere expressing HoxA2 (**Figures 1A–C**). Interestingly, we have noted that in *S. canicula* the r1/r2 boundary is not the rostralmost ventricular ridge since an intrarhombomeric ventricular ridge is recognized anteriorly (asterisks in **Figures 1A–C**). Considering the actual extension of r1 inferred by the lack of HoxA2 expression, we questioned the identification of rhombomeres in *S. canicula* embryos on the basis of the expression of the Ephrin receptor EphA4 described by Freitas and Cohn (2004), in particular the rhombomere 3 (compare their Figure 2d with our **Figure 1B**, both from stage 22).

The expression pattern of the *ScWnt8* gene in early embryos has allowed to identify unequivocally rhombomeres 3 and 4. In early pharyngula stages (S20), the expression of this gene was very intense and exclusively of one rhombomere, which was caudal but not adjacent to r2. Later in development (S24, late pharyngula) ScWnt8 expression was maintained in the same rhombomere but with a weaker signal. Considering that the rhombomere 4 in mouse shows the latest detectable expression of Wnt8 (Bouillet et al., 1996), we postulate that in *S. canicula* embryos the ScWnt8-expressing rhombomere also corresponds to r4. Moreover, in whole-stained embryos the position of rhombomeres 2 and 4 showed a correspondence with the position of branchial arches (**Figures 1B,D–F**). In addition, sections of ScWnt8-hybridized embryos and immunohistochemically stained with the anti-DCX antibody revealed that the roots of the VII–VIII nerves (which in all vertebrates studied exit from r4, see below) emerge from the ScWnt8-expressing rhombomere (**Figures 1F–G**).

Pax6-expressing cells formed a continuous column along the basal rhombencephalon and the spinal cord. As in other gnathostomes, the expression of Pax6 is observed in all *S. canicula* rhombomeres (**Figure 1H**) even at very early stages, in contrast with agnathans, in which Pax6 expression in rhombomere 4 is delayed in relation to other rhombomeres (Murakami et al., 2001; Derobert et al., 2002).

Transverse segmental bands that match with morphologically noticeable rhombomeres were observed in parasagittal sections of S26 embryos stained to show the distribution of Pax6-positive cells and GABAergic cells (**Figures 1I,J**). Interrhombomeric limits appeared as a series of small ventricular ridges corresponding laterally with Pax6-poor gaps separating Pax6-rich bulges. The similarity between the hindbrain ventricular profiles of *S. canicula* embryos at stage 26 and those reported in chick embryos at stage HH18 (Heyman et al., 1993) supports our proposal of equivalences in developmental periods in various vertebrates (see **Table 1**). There was a markedly lower density of Pax6-positive cells at the ventricular ridges (arrows in **Figure 1I**), which was more notable at later stages. The distribution of GABAergic cells in relation to the interrhombomeric boundaries is also of interest (**Figure 1J**). Numerous GABAergic cells adopting a fan-shaped alignment formed wedge-shaped crests in the mantle layer, which pointed toward the ventricular surface. Within these crests, apical GABAergic cells showed a short apical process and displayed the appearance of radially migrating cells, while the rest of GABAergic cells at the intermediate layer sent longer processes into the marginal layer. In addition, migrating neuroblasts identified by their immunolabeling for DCX were observed in these areas (**Figure 1K**).

Although in early embryos the interrhombomeric constrictions only allowed to distinguish clearly rhombomeres 1–6 (r1–r6), we have also contemplated the existence of additional rhombomeres flanking them rostrally (r0) and caudally (r7 and r8; **Figure 2**).

The rhombomere 0 (r0; Puelles, 2001; Aroca and Puelles, 2005) is the rostralmost rhombencephalic segment, and corresponds to the isthmic territory. The continuous column of Pax6-immunoreactive cells observed in the rhombencephalon of early *S. canicula* embryos does not extend to the constriction that marks the midbrain–hindbrain boundary, i.e., the midbrain-r0 boundary, thus suggesting that the Pax6-free region observed caudally to the midbrain–hindbrain boundary may represent the isthmus or r0 hindbrain division (**Figures 1H and 3A**). The anterior limit of the rhombencephalic expression of Pax6 in *S. canicula* does not overlap with the FGF8 expression domain that, as in other vertebrates, largely corresponds to the isthmus (unpublished observations). Accordingly, the anterior limit of the rhombencephalic Pax6-positive domain roughly coincides with the r0–r1 boundary. In this region, there is a population of dorsoventrally oriented GABAergic cells, some of them being DCX positive (**Figures 3B–F**).

The segmental organization of the elasmobranch rhombencephalon has been considered peculiar in relation to the exit of the trigeminal (V) nerve root. In the late pharyngula stage of *S. torazame* and other elasmobranch species (Kuratani and Horigome, 2000; Gilland and Baker, 2005; and references therein), the V nerve root has been described located in r3, close to the "acoustic-facial" (VII–VIII) nerve roots fixed in r4 (**Figures 2 and 4A–D**), instead than in r2 as in other vertebrates (reviewed by Gilland and Baker, 2005). It has been argued that the unusual localization of the dogfish V nerve root is acquired secondarily because it appears to enter in r2 in early pharyngula stages of *S. torazame* (Kuratani

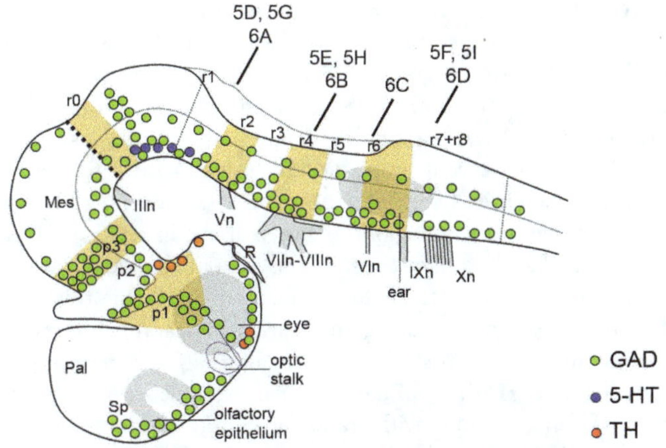

FIGURE 2 | Schematic representation of the embryonic brain at stage 26 showing the distribution of GAD-ir (green dots), 5-HT-ir (dark blue dots), and TH-ir (red dots) cells and the relation to transverse segments. The dotted line indicates the alar–basal boundary. The vertical bars indicate the approximate levels of sections of **Figures 5 and 6.** For abbreviations, see list.

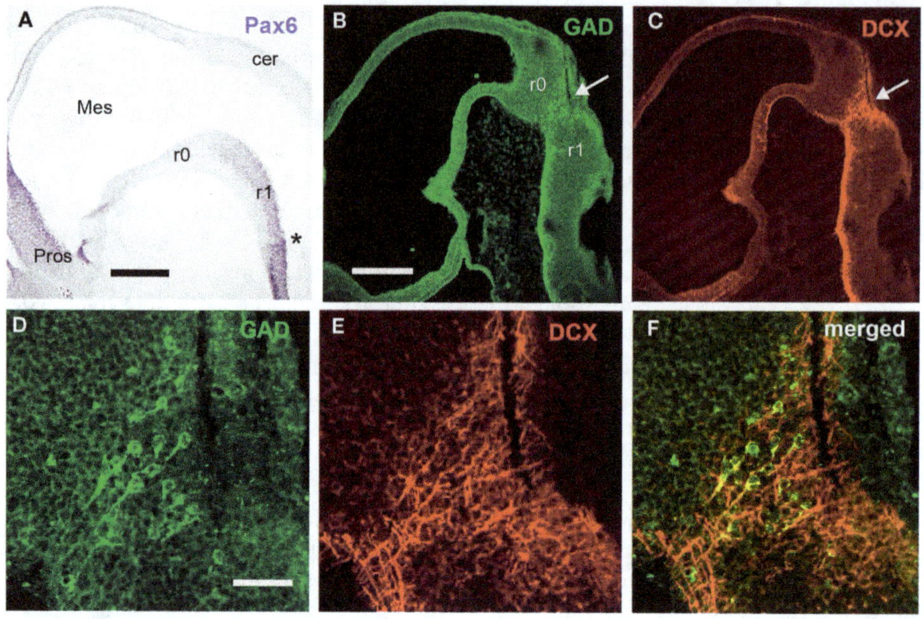

FIGURE 3 | The distribution of Pax6, GAD, and DCX cells reveals the r0/r1 boundary. (A–C) Panoramic views of sagittal sections of embryos at stage 26 to show the distribution of Pax6 **(A)**, GAD **(B)**, and DCX **(C)** in the rostral rhombencephalon. Note the absence of Pax6 cells in r0 and the dorsoventral band of GAD and DCX cells caudally to r0 (white arrow in **B,C**). **(D,E)** Detail of this cell band to show colocalization of both substances in some cells (yellow in **F**). Asterisk in A indicates the rostralmost intrarhombomeric boundary at r1. For abbreviations, see list. Scale bars: 500 μm **(A)**; 300 μm **(B,C)**; 50 μm **(D–F)**.

and Horigome, 2000). According this hypothesis, the late caudal location of the V nerve root is originated by a caudal shift of the trigeminal neural crest that arises initially from r2 (Neal, 1898; Kuratani and Horigome, 2000). However, since both the established nerve roots and the interrhombomeric boundaries are held to be fixed structural entities, incapable of active movement, this hypothesis of a caudally shifting root does not seem convincing. The massiveness of the V nerve root discards the possibility of a substitution of a new r3 trigeminal root for a disappearing r2 root (as conjectured above for the very slender glossopharyngeal and vagal roots). Our observations at later stages reveal that there is a root-less part of the hindbrain wall intercalated between the V and VII–VIII roots (**Figures 1C,E,H**; see also **Figure 4C**), which represents a possibly compressed r3. In any case the V root would actually lie in r2. Our results also suggest that, in dogfishes, an intrarhombomeric ventricular ridge develops rostral to the r1/r2 limit between early and late pharyngula stages, possibly due to large growth of this region. As noted above in relation to the HoxA2 results, there is a conspicuous ventricular ridge into r1 (asterisks in **Figures 1A–D**) that appears to subdivide this large rhombomere in a caudal region with an appearance of rhombomere and a more rostral one showing a different appearance (note in **Figure 1H** the maintaining of correspondence of proposed rhombomeres r2 and r4 with branchial arches). The r1 territory is noticeably larger than a normal rhombomere in all vertebrates, and Vaage (1969, 1973) already suggested that it may contain a cryptic subdivision into rostral and caudal parts in some vertebrates. The formation in *S. canicula* of an additional boundary rostral to the normal r1/r2 limit actually may explain the surprising "displacement" of the V nerve root exit claimed by some authors (Neal, 1898; Kuratani and Horigome, 2000). The solely use of morphology to assign rhombomeres based on von Kupffer (1906), which defined rhombomere 1 as the anterior region of the hindbrain between the meso-rhombencephalic border and the first distinct hindbrain interneuromeric border, would result in r2 to be counted as r3 in previous studies (and r3 + r4 to be identified as r4).

The identification of the caudal rhombomeres and the limit between the rhombencephalon and the spinal cord in *S. canicula* are unclear. Caudally to the conspicuous r5/r6 boundary there is a subtle ventricular ridge that could correspond to the r6/r7 boundary but there are not more evidences of intraventricular ridges, which preclude identification of r7 and r8 on the basis of such interrhombomeric limits. The position of the abducens (VI), glossopharyngeal (IX), and vagal (X) nerve roots may help to identify the caudal rhombomeres. In early embryos of *S. canicula* (S26) the root of the abducens nerve was located in r6 (**Figures 2 and 4E**), in agreement with the location of abducens motoneurons reported in adults of this species by ChAT immunohistochemistry (Anadón et al., 2000), and by tract-tracing methods in *Squalus* embryos (Gilland and Baker, 1992). The IX and X nerve roots emerge from the non-segmented region caudal to r6 that supposedly consists of r7 and r8 but, without specific molecular markers, their position in relation to rhombomeres could not be assessed. Even so, the IX nerve root emerges close to the r6–r7 border and the first X nerve root emerges somewhat caudally (**Figure 2**). In late pharyngula stages of the sharks *Squalus acanthias* (Scammon stages 24–26; Gilland and Baker, 1992, 1993, 2005) and *S. torazame* (stage V; Kuratani and Horigome, 2000) the emergence of IX and X roots has been established in r7 and r8, respectively (Gilland and Baker, 1992, 1993, 2005; Kuratani

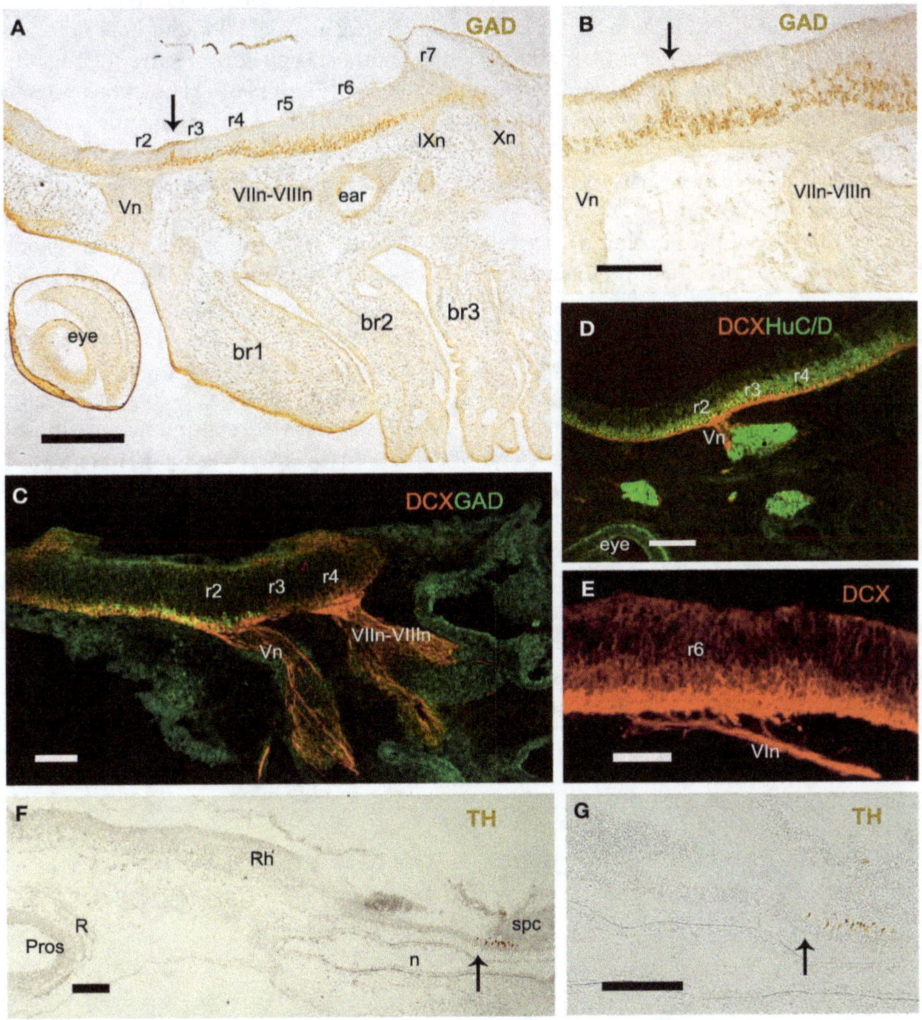

FIGURE 4 | Sagittal sections of embryos at stage 26 to show the position of nerve roots in relation to rhombomeres (A–E) and the caudal limit of the rhombencephalon (F,G). (A,B) Panoramic view and detail to show the roots of several branchiomeric nerves and the distribution of GAD-ir cells at the r2–r3 interrhombomeric boundary (arrows). **(C–E)** DCX labeled processes at the roots of V **(C,D)**, VII–VIII **(C)**, and VI **(E)** nerves. **(F,G)** Panoramic view and detail showing the rostral extension of the spinal TH-ir CSF-contacting neurons. Arrows indicate the possible rhombencephalon–spinal cord boundary. For abbreviations, see list. Scale bars: 200 μm **(A,C,D,F,G)**; 100 μm **(B,E)**.

and Horigome, 2000), although observations of Kuratani and Horigome (2000) in earlier pharyngula stages of *S. torazame* (Stage II) suggested that the initial entrance of the IX nerve root occurred in r6. The apparent caudal shift of the postotic branchiomeric nerve roots (or substitution of nerve roots) in dogfishes has been related to the growth of the otocyst (Kuratani and Horigome, 2000). The reported differences in segmental organization of the caudal rhombencephalon in elasmobranchs have been related to the possible caudal migration of IX neurons born in r6 and r7 to settle in rostral r8 (Gilland and Baker, 2005). As noted previously for the trigeminal, the differences in the rhombomere numeration caused by the existence of an additional visible boundary rostral to the r1/r2 limit may also explain the apparent displacement of the IX and X roots claimed in sharks by some authors (Gilland and Baker, 1992, 1993, 2005; Kuratani and Horigome, 2000). These nerves exit from r6 and r7 in other vertebrates, including zebrafish in which a caudal migration of VII, IX, and X motoneurons has been reported (Chandrasekhar et al., 1997). The use of molecular markers appears necessary to decipher unequivocally the segmental organization of the caudal rhombencephalon in *S. canicula*.

The spinal floor plate in *S. canicula* shows characteristic GABAergic and catecholaminergic cerebrospinal fluid (CSF)-contacting cells, which by contrast are absent from the rhombencephalic floor plate (Sueiro et al., 2003, 2004). A re-analysis of these results reveals that the rostral most CSF-contacting cell populations of the floor plate are located at a level just caudal to the last X nerve root. We suggest to use this level as reference for the rhombencephalon–spinal cord boundary (**Figures 4F,G**). However, in chicken this limit was traced at the middle level of the 5th somite owing the existence of additional rhombomere-like regions (pseudorhombomeres; Cambronero and Puelles, 2000; Marín et al., 2008), which is more caudal than that proposed for *S. canicula*. Whether pseudorhombomeres also exist in dogfish need be investigated.

Longitudinal columns

Here we also explored the longitudinal organization in the early rhombencephalon of *S. canicula*. At the earlier stages of *S. canicula* studied, longitudinal ventricular *sulci* are not evident and specific molecular markers for the alar–basal boundary have not been tested. However, the existence of rhombencephalic longitudinal zones, and the boundary between alar and basal plates can be roughly identified on the basis of the columnar distribution of Pax6- and GAD-positive cells.

At early stages, Pax6-labeled cells formed a column continuous with that of the spinal cord. They occupied the majority of the rhombencephalic lateral wall excepting the floor plate and the adjacent region of the basal plate, as inferred from the comparison with parallel sections immunostained for sonic hedgehog (Shh), a well known hindbrain floor plate marker in other vertebrates (**Figures 5A–I**). However, differences in the intensity of Pax6 expression allowed us to distinguish between a ventrolateral column that contained the most intensely labeled Pax6 cells and coincided in part with the extent of the basal plate (excepting the negative region adjacent to the floor plate), and a dorsolateral alar column containing weakly labeled Pax6 cells. At the level of VII-VIII nerve roots (r4), this dorsolateral column extended dorsally up to the developing roof plate choroid plexus, thus probably corresponding with the full extent of the alar plate. Rostrally, the dorsal rhombencephalic region that gives rise to the cerebellar primordium (cerebellar plate) did not contain Pax6 cells (**Figure 1H**).

At stage 26, the GAD-immunoreactive (ir) populations appeared clearly organized in longitudinal columns extending all along the rhombencephalon (**Figure 6**). Sagittal (**Figures 6B–D**) and transverse (**Figures 6E–H**) sections revealed two main bands of GAD-ir cells located in the mantle layer; one was dorsolateral (in the alar plate; open arrow in **Figures 6B–H**) and the other was ventrolateral (in the basal plate; solid arrow in **Figures 6B–H**), and they were separated by a band of GAD-negative cells (asterisks in **Figures 6C–H**). Ventral commissural axons that mainly emerged from cells of the ventrolateral group were observed throughout the rhombencephalon. From the level of the "acoustic-facial" (VII–VIII) nerve roots (r4) down to caudal rhombencephalic levels, the dorsolateral and ventrolateral columns each appeared subdivided into dorsal and ventral sub-columns (**Figures 6F–H**). The ventrolateral columns were continuous with those observed in the rostral spinal cord (Sueiro et al., 2004). In contrast with what was observed in the spinal cord (Sueiro et al., 2004), no CSF-contacting GAD-ir cells were present in the hindbrain floor plate.

REGIONALIZATION OF THE HINDBRAIN IN INTERMEDIATE EMBRYOS (SECOND PERIOD)

Longitudinal columns

In intermediate embryo stages, the Pax6-ir cells also formed longitudinal columns in the dorsal, laterodorsal (alar plate) and lateroventral (basal plate) rhombencephalic walls. Pax6 expression in

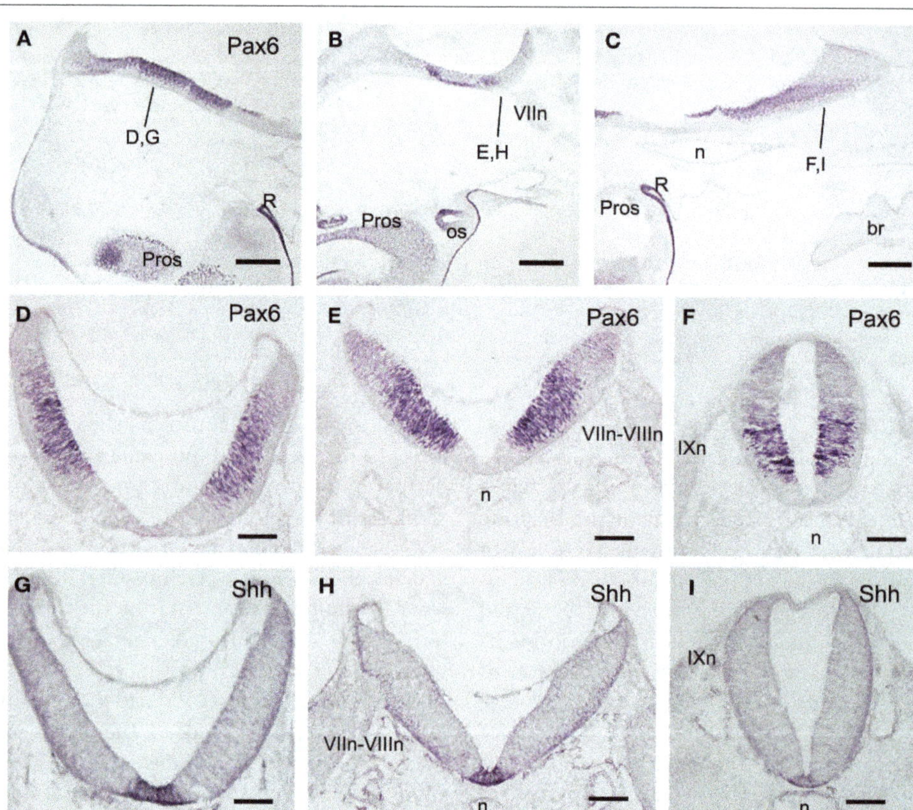

FIGURE 5 | Sagittal (A–C) and transverse (D–I) sections of embryos at stage 25 to show the distribution of Pax6- (A–F) and Sonic hedgehog-immunoreactive cells (G–I). The levels of **(D–I)** are indicated in **(A–C)** and in **Figure 2**. Scale bars: 500 μm **(A–C)**; 200 μm **(D–I)**.

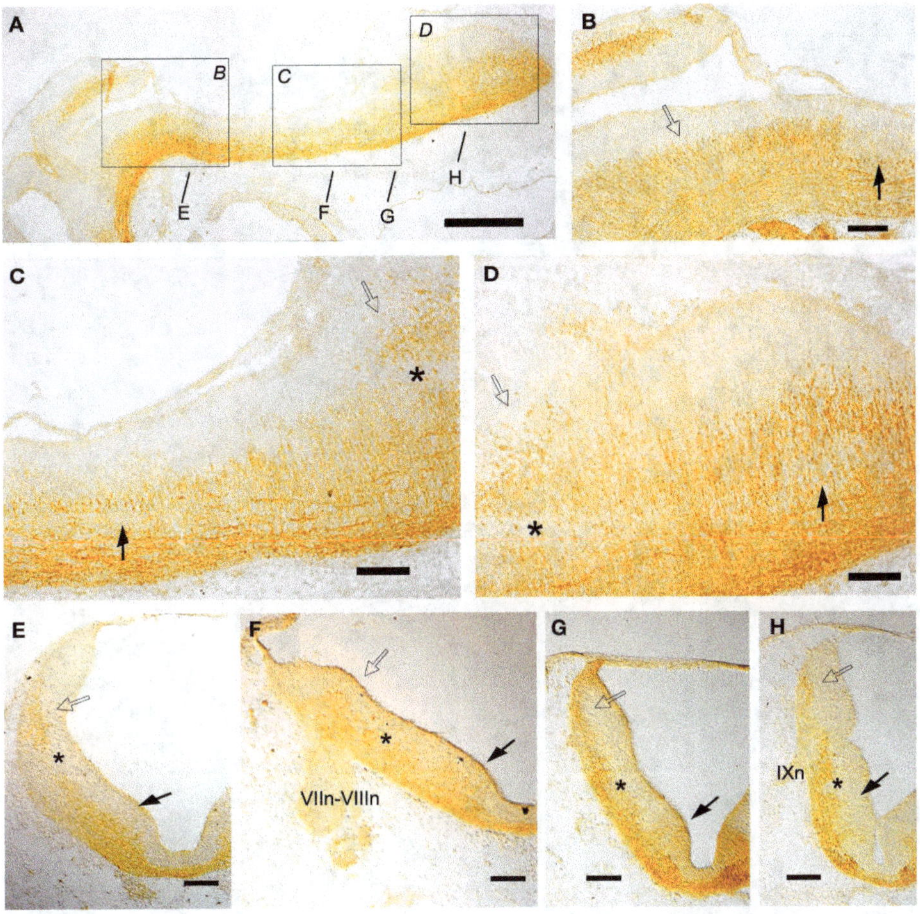

FIGURE 6 | Sagittal (A–D) and transverse (E–H) sections of embryos at stage 26 showing the columnar distribution of GAD-ir populations. The levels of (E–I) are indicated in **(A)** and in **Figure 2**. Dorsolateral and ventrolateral columns are continuous along the rhombencephalon from rostral to caudal levels **(A–H)** but from r4 these columns appeared subdivided into dorsal and ventral subgroups **(F–H)**. Scale bars: 500 μm **(A)**; 100 μm **(B–H)**.

the ventricular zone decreased, being reduced to the dorsal portion of the alar and basal plates, i.e., the dorsal and lateroventral wall sectors (**Figures 7A–D**), although rostrally the decrease in immunoreactivity of dorsal cells was less evident.

With regard to GAD-ir longitudinal cell columns, they were more evident than in the previously studied stage, and four longitudinal columns were clearly distinguished along most of the rhombencephalon. These four longitudinal GABAergic columns were located respectively in the four classic functional columns: somatosensory, viscerosensory, visceromotor, and somatomotor (**Figures 7F–H**). However, at rostral levels (r1–r2) only two main columns were noted (**Figure 7E**).

There was no obvious overlap between Pax6-ir and GABAergic cell columns, which were located in the ventricular and mantle zones, respectively. However, double labeling revealed a correlation between the sharp limit separating the intensely and weakly Pax6-ir ventricular cells, and the limit between the dorsolateral and ventrolateral GAD columns (**Figures 7I–O**). This limit may represent the alar–basal boundary.

No CR-ir cells were observed in *S. canicula* embryos at early stages, but from the intermediate stage (S29) onward, CR-ir populations were noticed in different brain areas (**Figure 8**). At stage 29, CR-ir cells were observed in all brain vesicles but were more abundant in the posterior brain (**Figure 8**). These cells were scarce at alar prosencephalic (subpallium and thalamus) and mesencephalic (optic tectum) levels and moderately abundant in the basal diencephalon (posterior tubercle and basal synencephalon, where formed the primordium of the nucleus of the medial longitudinal fascicle). In contrast, the rhombencephalon contained abundant CR-ir cells along the whole extension of alar and basal regions. To identify all the rhombencephalic CR-ir cell groups exceeds the aims of this study, as they develop on later stages. However, the apparent columnar organization of rhombencephalic CR-ir populations in an intermediate stage (S29) makes CR a very suitable marker to analyze the longitudinal columnar organization both in alar and basal territories (**Figure 9**).

In the basal rhombencephalon, CR-ir cells formed an almost continuous column from isthmic to spinal levels (**Figures 9A–J**). Most of them form part of the reticular formation, which contains raphe (midline) populations organized as a continuous field in the superior reticular formation (r1–r4) and more lateral reticular populations that extended down to caudal rhombencephalic levels (**Figures 9B–I**). Other basal CR-ir populations identified at this intermediate stage were the visceromotor nuclei (**Figures 9D,E,I,J**).

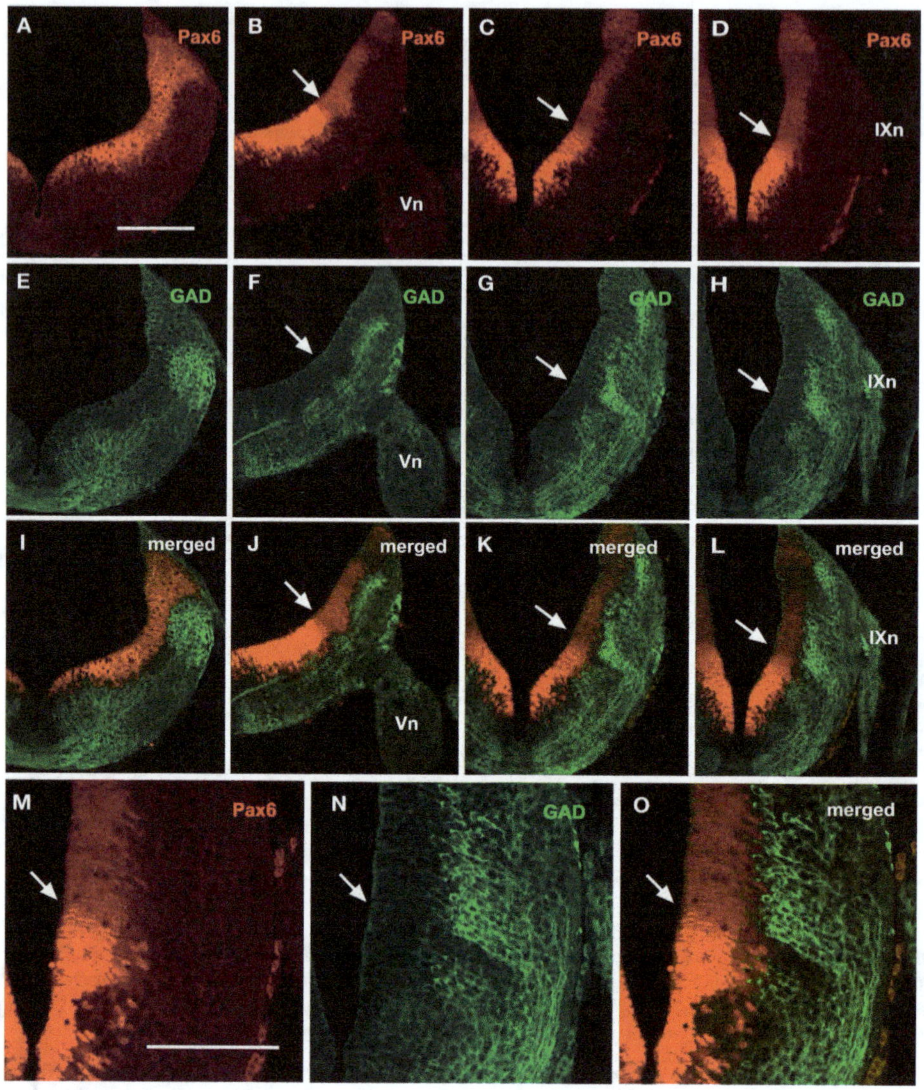

FIGURE 7 | Transverse sections from rostral (A,E,I) to caudal (D,H,L) rhombencephalic levels of embryos at stage 29 showing the comparative distribution of Pax6 (A–D) and GAD (E–H) cells. Double labeling **(I–L)** reveals a band of GAD-negative cells coinciding with the interface between intense and weak Pax6 cells that may corresponds to the alar–basal boundary (white arrows). **(M–O)** Detail of this boundary. Scale bar: 200 μm **(A–L)**; 100 μm **(M–O)**.

At isthmic levels, some small CR-ir cells were located medially, probably forming part of the primordial interpeduncular nucleus (not shown). At caudal rhombencephalic levels (at the level of entrance of the X nerve roots), some weakly CR-ir cells were found ventrally to the medial longitudinal fascicle, which at these levels contained moderately labeled fibers. This caudal CR-ir population of the basal rhombencephalon probably corresponds to the inferior olive primordium (**Figures 8 and 9E,J**).

In the rhombencephalic alar plate, no CR-ir cells were observed at the intermediate stage (S29) in the cerebellar plate (**Figure 9A**) but later in development, abundant cells were found in the molecular layer of the cerebellar body and related cerebellar-like structures (Rodríguez-Moldes et al., 2008; Anadón et al., 2009). Moreover, CR-ir cells were observed along the alar dorsolateral column from rostral to caudal rhombencephalic levels. Along its extent, different subgroups could be distinguished. A dorsolateral population containing large CR-ir cells intermingled with smaller elements extended from r2 to r6, and probably represents primordial nuclei of the octavolateral area (**Figures 9G,H**). Another subgroup of the dorsolateral column contained few small weakly labeled CR-ir cells that occupied the ventricular protrusion that extended from 4 to 8 and represents cells of the primordial viscerosensory lobe (**Figures 9G–J**).

Transverse segmental regions

At the intermediate stage (S29), the interrhombomeric boundaries become blurred and are no longer detectable morphologically. In spite of this, the transversal organization in rhombomeres 1 to 8 of the *S. canicula* rhombencephalon may be inferred on the basis of the position of (a) the nerve roots, as their relationship with rhombomeres does not change with respect to earlier stages and (b) the reticular cells, motoneurons and other

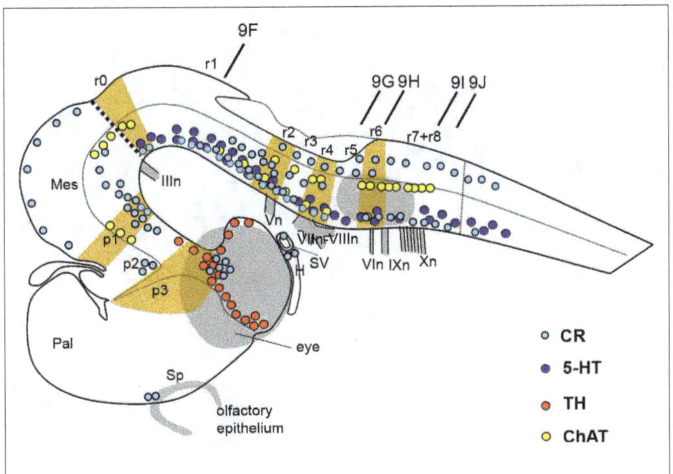

FIGURE 8 | Schematic representation of the embryonic brain at stage 29 showing the distribution of CR- (bright blue dots), 5-HT- (dark blue dots), TH- (red dots), and ChAT-ir (yellow dots) immunoreactive cells and the relation to transverse segments. The dotted line indicates the alar–basal boundary. The vertical bars indicate the approximate levels of sections of **Figure 9**. For abbreviations, see list.

rhombencephalic populations which are distributed following a segmental organization. A segmental organization can also be revealed by using antibodies raised against TH, 5-HT, and ChAT, which label catecholaminergic, serotoninergic, and cholinergic populations, respectively, and against CR. Accordingly, we studied the possible extent of rhombomeres in the hindbrain of *S. canicula* S29 embryos by identifying conspicuous chemoarchitectonic boundaries (**Figure 8**).

A previous work has reported the development of catecholaminergic (TH-ir) populations in the embryonic brain of *S. canicula* (Carrera et al., 2005). Although TH-ir cells were already present in the hypothalamus and diencephalon by stage 29 (**Figure 8**), in the rhombencephalon TH-ir cells started to appear at stages 30–31 (Carrera et al., 2005). Here, we briefly re-examined the rhombencephalic catecholaminergic populations in the context of the rhombomere organization raised by analysis of *HoxA2* and *Wnt8* genes (see above). From stage 30 onward, the rostral rhombencephalic TH-ir groups, i.e., the locus coeruleus (rostral) and subcoeruleus (caudal) were recognized as located at r1 and r2, respectively (not shown in **Figure 8**, as it represents the stage 29). They occupied dorsal territories of the basal region since the first time in which became detectable by TH immunohistochemistry (although in chick and mouse they originate from the alar plate; Aroca et al., 2006). Caudal rhombencephalic TH-ir cell groups were related to alar (viscerosensory column) and basal (visceromotor column and reticular cells) regions. Populations of the viscerosensory and visceromotor columns extended from a level caudal to the entrance of the VII–VIII nerves down to the obex, i.e., from r5 to r8, while the ventrolateral reticular TH-ir cells extended from levels of the VI motor nucleus to the obex, occupying therefore r6–r8.

The development of serotoninergic populations in *S. canicula* has been previously described (Carrera et al., 2008). All serotoninergic (5-HT-ir) cell groups of the adult rhombencephalon were already differentiated at stage 29 but not those of more rostral brain levels (Carrera et al., 2008), which is in sharp contrast to that happens with catecholaminergic populations (**Figure 8**). In the rhombencephalon, serotoninergic cells occupied basal reticular territories and formed midline (raphe) and lateral (reticular) populations, both arising from cells adjacent to the floor plate (Carrera et al., 2008). The reticular 5-HT-ir cell groups exhibited a clear segmental pattern, which allowed to correlate them with rhombomeres. In the study of Carrera et al. (2008), the description of hindbrain populations followed the rhombomere numeration proposed by Neal (1898) and others (Gilland and Baker, 1993, 2005; Kuratani and Horigome, 2000). After re-examining the results of Carrera et al. (2008) at the light of the present rhombomeric numeration, we confirm that the mid/hindbrain boundary coincides approximately with the rostral end of three 5-HT-ir nuclei (raphe linearis, raphe dorsalis anterioris, and reticular B9 cell group) but disagree with our previous interpretation in the r1/r2 and r2/r3 location. Under the present view, the r1/r2 boundary actually coincides with the caudal end of three reticular 5-HT-ir nuclei (subcoeruleus, raphe pontis oralis medialis, and lateralis) and the rostral end of the raphe dorsalis, while the r2/r3 boundary corresponds to the raphe dorsalis caudal end. There were no 5-HT-ir neurons between levels caudal to the V motor nucleus and rostral to the facial nerve root, which may correspond at some extent to r3 levels. This rhombomere also marks the separation between the superior and inferior sets of 5-HT-ir nuclei.

The segmental organization of the motor nuclei has been reported in adult *S. canicula* by using ChAT as a marker for cholinergic neurons (Anadón et al., 2000). The same marker is used in the present study to identify motor nuclei in the rhombencephalon of S29 embryos (**Figures 8 and 10**). The rhombomere distribution of some motor nuclei of S29 embryos varied in relation to what was described in adults although, owing the change in numeration of rhombomeres. The ChAT-ir trochlear cells were located in the basal region of the isthmus (r0), separated by a clear-cut gap from the ChAT-ir oculomotor cells, which were located just rostrally in the mesencephalic tegmentum (**Figures 10A,B**). The ChAT-ir cells located at the level of the V nerve root probably correspond to the V motor nucleus, which is located in r2, and not in r3 as previously described (Anadón et al., 2000). The rostral end of this motor nucleus roughly coincides with the r1/r2 boundary (**Figures 10A,C**). The large ChAT-ir cell aggregate at the level of the VII–VIII nerve roots corresponds to the magnocellular octaval nucleus, which extended in r4 and the caudal part of r3 (**Figures 10A,D,E**). In r6, the group of labeled cells located at ventral levels probably corresponds to the VI nucleus. The cholinergic neurons of the visceromotor column were distinguished more dorsally, forming a column that extended along r6 and r7 (**Figures 10E,F**). The presence of some rostrocaudal discontinuities revealed the existence of three ChAT-ir cell clusters; the rostralmost probably represents the facial motor nucleus (located just rostral to the level of entrance of the IX nerve), while the groups that correspond to IX and X nuclei were located more caudally, just ventral to the viscerosensory lobe, where the roots of IX and X nerves were clearly discerned (**Figure 10E,F**). This observation reveals that in *S. canicula* intermediate embryos the facial motor nucleus is located in the same segment as in the adult (Anadón et al., 2000). Studies in embryos with earlier markers

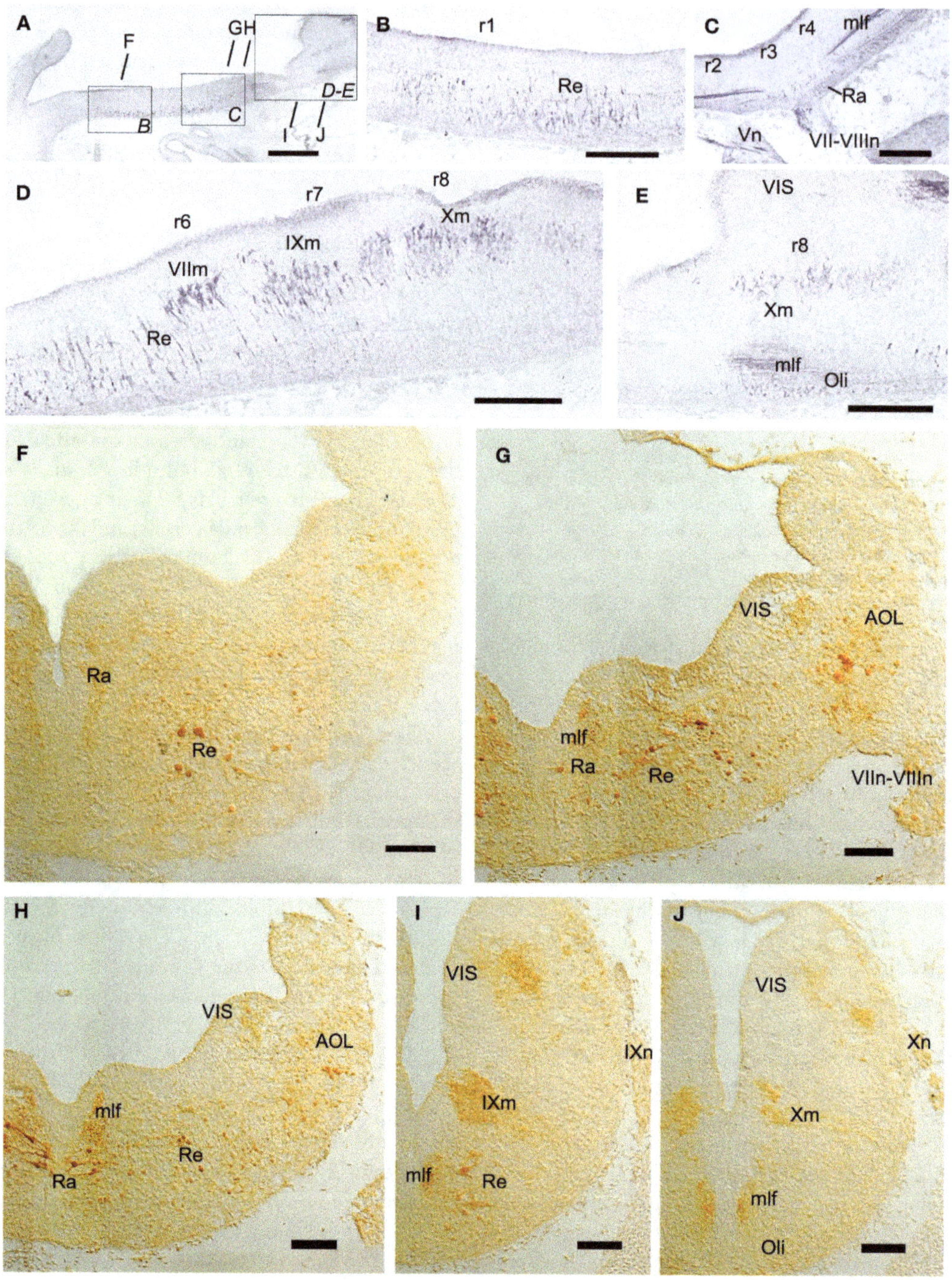

FIGURE 9 | Sagittal (A–E) and transverse (F–J) sections of embryos at stage 29 showing the columnar distribution of CR-ir populations. The levels of **(F–J)** are indicated in **(A)** and in **Figure 8.** Note that CR-ir cells are more abundant in the basal than in the alar rhombencephalon and form midline (Ra) and lateral (Re) populations of the reticular formation. Scale bars: 500 μm **(A)**; 200 μm **(B–E)**; 100 μm **(F–I)**.

of these motor populations are necessary in order to know if these cells originate from this rhombomere or from more rostral rhombomeres (r4–r5) and then migrate caudally, as it has been described in *Squalus* (Gilland and Baker, 1992) and in zebrafish (Chandrasekhar et al., 1997).

The columns of CR-ir cells along the alar and basal plates present some discontinuities that revealed the existence of clusters roughly related to rhombomeres. Raphe (midline) CR-ir cells formed two major groups; one extends along r1–r2 and contained small weakly labeled cells (**Figure 9F**) while the other occupies r3–r4 and contained large intensely labeled cells with their processes oriented mainly mediolaterally, some of them crossing the midline (**Figures 9C,G,H**). Reticular (lateral) cells were scarce in the rostral part of r1, but more caudally they formed a relatively abundant population of large cells that extended from the caudal part of r1–r4 (**Figures 9B,C,F,G**). In r5 and r6, CR-ir reticular cells

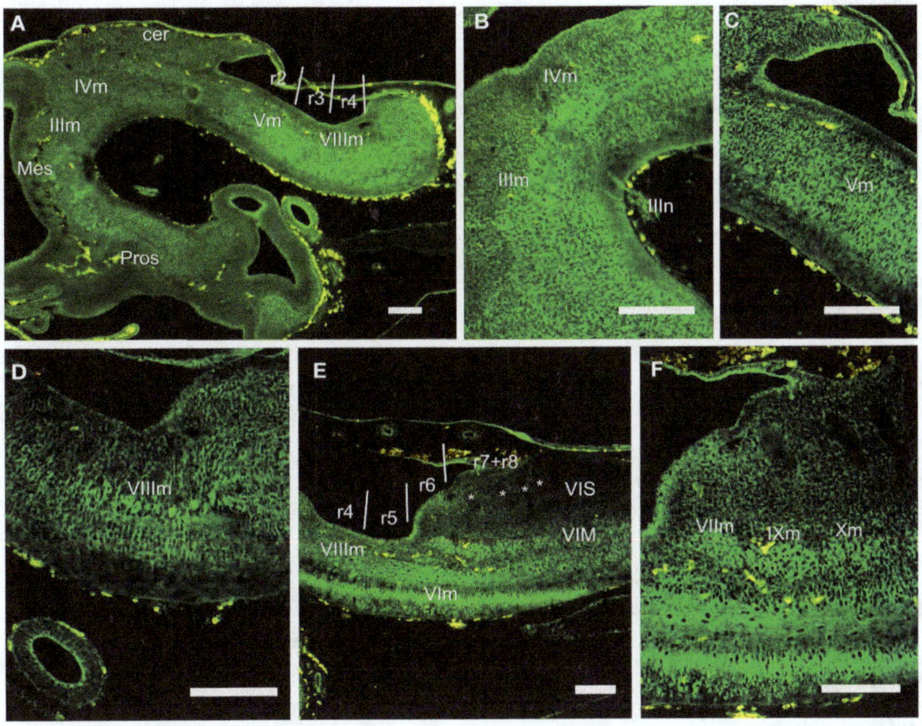

FIGURE 10 | Sagittal sections showing the distribution of ChAT-ir cell groups in the rhombencephalon at the stage 29. (A–D) Panoramic view **(A)** and details **(B–D)** of ChAT-ir cells of the oculomotor and trochlear nucleus **(B)**, trigeminal motor nucleus **(C)**, and magnocellular octaval nucleus **(D)**. **(E,F)** Panoramic view and detail of ChAT-ir cells in the visceromotor column. Asterisks label the negative roots of the glossopharyngeal and vagal nerves. For abbreviations, see list. Scale bars: 200 μm.

were small and scarce (**Figure 9D,H**), while large reticular CR-ir cells were present in the putative r7 (**Figure 9I**). More caudally the small weakly labeled cells of the inferior olive were observed (**Figures 9E,J**).

Although the molecular markers used in this study reveal some interesting features in the embryonic brain of the lesser spotted dogfish, further studies are necessary to give a more precise account of the rhombomeric limits and rhombomere identities, specially in the caudal rhombencephalon.

ACKNOWLEDGMENTS

The present study was supported by grants of Spanish Dirección General de Investigación-FEDER (BFU2007-61154, BFU2010-15816) and of Xunta de Galicia (PGIDIT07PXIB200102PR; 10PXIB200051PR; INCITE09ENA200048ES). Authors also acknowledge the support of the European Community – Research Infrastructure Action under the FP7 "Capacities" Specific Programme (ASSEMBLE grant agreement no. 227799). The EST sequencing project was taken in charge by Génoscope, Evry, France.

REFERENCES

Alexander, T., Nolte, C., and Krumlauf, R. (2009). Hox genes and segmentation of the hindbrain and axial skeleton. *Annu. Rev. Cell Dev. Biol.* 25, 431–456.

Anadón, R., Ferreiro-Galve, S., Sueiro, C., Graña, P., Carrera, I., Yañez, J., and Rodríguez-Moldes, I. (2009). Calretinin-immunoreactive systems in the cerebellum and cerebellum-related lateral-line medullary nuclei of an elasmobranch, *Scyliorhinus canicula*. *J. Chem. Neuroanat.* 37, 46–54.

Anadón, R., Molist, P., Rodríguez-Moldes, I., López, J. M., Quintela, I., Cerviño, M. C., Barja, P., and González, A. (2000). Distribution of choline acetyltransferase immunoreactivity in the brain of an elasmobranch, the lesser spotted dogfish (*Scyliorhinus canicula*). *J. Comp. Neurol.* 420, 139–170.

Aroca, P., Lorente-Cánovas, B., Mateos, F. R., and Puelles, L. (2006). Locus coeruleus neurons originate in alar rhombomere 1 and migrate into the basal plate: studies in chick and mouse embryos. *J. Comp. Neurol.* 496, 802–818.

Aroca, P., and Puelles, L. (2005). Postulated boundaries and differential fate in the developing rostral hindbrain. *Brain Res. Rev.* 49, 179–190.

Ballard, W. W., Mellinger, J., and Lechenault, H. (1993). A series on normal stages for development of *Scyliorhinus canicula*, the lesser spotted dogfish (Chondrichthyes: Scyliorhinidae). *J. Exp. Zool.* 267, 318–336.

Bouillet, P., Oulad-Abdelghani, M., Ward, S. J., Bronner, S., Chambon, P., and Dollé, P. (1996). A new mouse member of the Wnt gene family, mWnt-8, is expressed during early embryogenesis and is ectopically induced by retinoic acid. *Mech. Dev.* 58, 141–152.

Briscoe, J., Pierani, A., Jessell, T. M., and Ericson, J. (2000). A homeodomain protein code specifies progenitor cell identity and neuronal fate in the ventral neural tube. *Cell* 101, 435–445.

Cambronero, F., and Puelles, L. (2000). Rostrocaudal nuclear relationships in the avian medulla oblongata: a fate map with quail chick chimeras. *J. Comp. Neurol.* 427, 522–545.

Carrera, I., Molist, P., Anadón, R., and Rodríguez-Moldes, I. (2008). Development of the serotoninergic system in the central nervous system of a shark, the lesser spotted dogfish *Scyliorhinus canicula*. *J. Comp. Neurol.* 511, 804–831.

Carrera, I., Sueiro, C., Molist, P., Ferreiro, S., Adrio, F., Rodríguez, M. A., Anadón, R., and Rodríguez-Moldes, I. (2005). Temporal and spatial organization of tyrosine hydroxylase-immunoreactive cell groups in the embryonic brain of an elasmobranch, the lesser-spotted dogfish *Scyliorhinus canicula*. *Brain Res. Bull.* 66, 541–545.

Castro, A., Becerra, M., Manso, M. J., and Anadón, R. (2006). Calretinin immunoreactivity in the brain of the zebrafish, *Danio rerio*: distribution and comparison with some neuropeptides and neurotransmitter-synthesizing enzymes. II. Midbrain, hindbrain, and rostral spinal cord. *J. Comp. Neurol.* 494, 792–814.

Chandrasekhar, A., Moens, C. B., Warren, J. T. Jr., Kimmel, C. B., and Kuwada, J. Y. (1997). Development of branchiomotor neurons in zebrafish. *Development* 124, 2633–2644.

Coolen, M., Menuet, A., Chassoux, D., Compagnucci, C., Henry, S., Lévèque, L., Da Silva, C., Gavory, F., Samain, S., Wincker, P., Thermes, C., D'Aubenton-Carafa, Y., Rodríguez-Moldes, I., Naylor, G., Depew, M., Sourdaine, P., and Mazan, S. (2009). "The dogfish *Scyliorhinus canicula*, a reference in jawed vertebrates," in *Emerging Model Organisms. A Laboratory Manual*, Vol. 1, eds R. R. Behringer, A. D. Johnson, and R. E Krumlauf (New York: Cold Spring Harbor Laboratory Press), 431–446.

Coolen, M., Sauka-Spengler, T., Nicolle, D., Le-Mentec, C., Lallemand, Y., Da Silva, C., Plouhinec J.-L., Robert, B., Wincker, P., Shi, D.-L., and Mazan, S. (2007). Evolution of axis specification mechanisms in jawed vertebrates: insights from a chondrichthyan. *PLoS ONE* 2, e374. doi: 10.1371/journal.pone.0000374

Derobert, Y., Baratte, B., Lepage, M., and Mazan, S. (2002). Pax6 expression patterns in *Lampetra fluviatilis* and *Scyliorhinus canicula* embryos suggest highly conserved roles in the early regionalization of the vertebrate brain. *Brain Res. Bull.* 57, 277–280.

Díaz-Regueira, S., and Anadón, R. (2000). Calretinin expression in specific neuronal systems in the brain of an advanced teleost, the grey mullet (*Chelon labrosus*). *J. Comp. Neurol.* 426, 81–105.

Ferreiro-Galve, S., Rodríguez-Moldes, I., and Candal, E. (2010). Calretinin immunoreactivity in the developing retina of sharks: comparison with cell proliferation and GABAergic system markers. *Exp. Eye Res.* 91, 378–386.

Freitas, R., and Cohn, M. J. (2004). Analysis of EphA4 in the lesser spotted catshark identifies a primitive gnathostome expression pattern and reveals co-option during evolution of shark-specific morphology. *Dev. Genes Evol.* 214, 466–472.

Gaskell, W. (1886). On the structure, distribution and function of the nerves which innervate the visceral and vascular systems. *J. Physiol.* 7, 1–81.

Gaskell, W. (1889). On the relation between the structure, function, distribution and origin of the cranial nerves; together with an theory of the origin of the nervous system of vertebrata. *J. Physiol.* 10, 153–211.

Gilland, E., and Baker, R. (1992). Longitudinal and tangential migration of cranial nerve efferent neurons in the developing hindbrain of *Squalus acanthias. Biol. Bull.* 183, 356–358.

Gilland, E., and Baker, R. (1993). Conservation of neuroepithelial and mesodermal segments in the embryonic vertebrate head. *Acta Anat. (Basel)* 148, 110–123.

Gilland, E., and Baker, R. (2005). Evolutionary patterns of cranial nerve efferent nuclei in vertebrates. *Brain Behav. Evol.* 66, 234–254.

Glover, J. C. (2001). Correlated patterns of neuron differentiation and Hox gene expression in the hindbrain: a comparative analysis. *Brain Res. Bull.* 55, 683–693.

Hamburger, V., and Hamilton, H. L. (1951). A series of normal stages in the development of the chick embryo. *J. Morphol.* 88, 49–92.

Herrick, C. J. (1918). *An Introduction to Neurology*, 2nd Edn. Philadelphia: W.B. Saunders Company.

Heyman, I., Kent, A., and Lumsden, A. (1993). Cellular morphology and extracellular space at rhombomere boundaries in the chick embryo hindbrain. *Dev. Dyn.* 198, 241–253.

Ju, M. J., Aroca, P., Luo, J., Puelles, L., and Redies, C. (2004). Molecular profiling indicates avian branchiomotor nuclei invade the hindbrain alar plate. *Neuroscience* 128, 785–796.

Kuratani, S., and Horigome, N. (2000). Developmental morphology of branchiomeric nerves in a cat shark, *Scyliorhinus torazame*, with special reference to rhombomeres, cephalic mesoderm, and distribution patterns of cephalic crest cells. *Zool. Sci.* 17, 893–909.

Marín, F., Aroca, P., and Puelles, L. (2008). Hox gene colinear expression in the avian medulla oblongata is correlated with pseudorhombomeric domains. *Dev. Biol.* 323, 230–247.

Marín, F., and Puelles, L. (1995). Morphological fate of rhombomeres in quail/chick chimeras: a segmental analysis of hindbrain nuclei. *Eur. J. Neurosci.* 7, 1714–1738.

Morona, R., and González, A. (2009). Immunohistochemical localization of calbindin-D28k and calretinin in the brainstem of anuran and urodele amphibians. *J. Comp. Neurol.* 515, 503–537.

Murakami, Y., Ogasawara, M., Sugahara, F., Hirano, S., Satoh, N., and Kuratani, S. (2001). Identification and expression of the lamprey Pax6 gene: evolutionary origin of the segmented brain of vertebrates. *Development* 128, 3521–3531.

Neal, H. V. (1898). The segmentation of the nervous system in *Squalus acanthias. Bull. Mus. Comp. Zool. Harvard* 31, 147–294.

O'Neill, P., McCole, R. B., and Baker, C. V. (2007). A molecular analysis of neurogenic placode and cranial sensory ganglion development in the shark, *Scyliorhinus canicula. Dev. Biol.* 304, 156–181.

Oulion, S., Debiais-Thibaud, M., d'Aubenton-Carafa, Y., Thermes, C., Da Silva, C., Bernard-Samain, S., Gavory, F., Wincker, P., Mazan, S., and Casane, D. (2010). Evolution of Hox gene clusters in gnathostomes: insights from a survey of a shark (*Scyliorhinus canicula*) transcriptome. *Mol. Biol. Evol.* 27, 2829–2838

Prince, V. E., Moens, C. B., Kimmel, C. B., and Ho, R. K. (1998). Zebrafish hox genes: expression in the hindbrain region of wild-type and mutants of the segmentation gene, valentino. *Development* 125, 393–406.

Pritz, M. B. (1999). Rhombomere development in a reptilian embryo. *J. Comp. Neurol.* 411, 317–326.

Puelles, L. (2001). Brain segmentation and forebrain development in amniotes. *Brain Res. Bull.* 55, 695–710.

Rodríguez-Moldes, I., Ferreiro-Galve, S., Carrera, I., Sueiro, C., Candal, E., Mazan, S., and Anadón, R. (2008). Development of the cerebellar body in sharks: spatiotemporal relations of Pax6 expression, cell proliferation and differentiation. *Neurosci. Lett.* 432, 105–110.

Sieber, M. A., Storm, R., Martinez-de-la-Torre, M., Müller, T., Wende, H., Reuter, K., Vasyutina, E., and Birchmeier, C. (2007). Lbx1 acts as a selector gene in the fate determination of somatosensory and viscerosensory relay neurons in the hindbrain. *J. Neurosci.* 27, 4902–4909.

Straka, H., Baker, R., and Gilland, E. (2002). The frog as a unique vertebrate model for studying the rhombomeric organization of functionally identified hindbrain neurons. *Brain Res. Bull.* 57, 301–305.

Sueiro, C., Carrera, I., Molist, P., Rodríguez-Moldes, I., and Anadón, R. (2004). Development and distribution of glutamic acid decarboxylase (GAD)-immunoreactive systems in the spinal cord of the dogfish *Scyliorhinus canicula* (elasmobranchs). *J. Comp. Neurol.* 478, 189–206.

Sueiro, C., Carrera, I., Rodríguez-Moldes, I., Molist, P., and Anadón, R. (2003). Development of catecholaminergic systems in the spinal cord of the dogfish *Scyliorhinus canicula* (elasmobranchs). *Dev. Brain Res.* 142, 141–150.

Tümpel, S., Cambronero, F., Sims, C., Krumlauf, R., and Wiedemann, L. M. (2008). A regulatory module embedded in the coding region of HoxA2 controls expression in rhombomere 2. *Proc. Natl. Acad. Sci. U.S.A.* 105, 20077–20082.

Vaage, S. (1969). The segmentation of the primitive neural tube in chick embryos (*Gallus domesticus*). A morphological, histochemical and autoradiographical investigation. *Ergeb. Anat. Entwicklungsgesch.* 41, 3–87.

Vaage, S. (1973). The histogenesis of the isthmic nuclei in chick embryos (*Gallus domesticus*): I. A morphological study. *Z. Anat. Entwicklungsgesch.* 142, 283–314.

von Kupffer, C. (1906). "Die Morphogenie des Zentralnervensystems," in *Handbuch der vergleichenden und experimentellen Entwicklungslehre der Wirbeltiere*, Vol. 2, Part 3, ed. O. Hertwig (Jena: Fischer), 1–272.

Conflict of Interest Statement: The authors declare that the research was conducted in the absence of any commercial or financial relationships that could be construed as a potential conflict of interest.

13

Cladistic analysis of olfactory and vomeronasal systems

Isabel Ubeda-Bañon[1], Palma Pro-Sistiaga[2], Alicia Mohedano-Moriano[3], Daniel Saiz-Sanchez[1], Carlos de la Rosa-Prieto[1], Nicolás Gutierrez-Castellanos[4], Enrique Lanuza[4], Fernando Martinez-Garcia[4] and Alino Martinez-Marcos[1]*

[1] *Laboratorio de Neuroplasticidad y Neurodegeneración, Departamento de Ciencias Médicas, Centro Regional de Investigaciones Biomédicas, Facultad de Medicina de Ciudad Real, Universidad de Castilla-la Mancha, Ciudad Real, Spain*

[2] *GIP Cyceron, Campus Jules Horowiz, Caen, France*

[3] *Laboratorio de Neuroanatomía Humana, Departamento de Ciencias Médicas, Centro Regional de Investigaciones Biomédicas, Facultad de Medicina de Albacete, Universidad de Castilla-La Mancha, Albacete, Spain*

[4] *Laboratori de Neuroanatomia Funcional i Comparada, Departaments de Biologia Cel·lular i Biologia Funcional, Facultat de Ciències Biològiques, Universitat de Valencia, València, Spain*

Edited by:
Agustín González, Universida Complutense de Madrid, Spain

Reviewed by:
Jorge A. Larriva-Sahd, Universidad Nacional Autónoma de México, Mexico
Carla Mucignat, Università degli Studi di Padova, Italy

****Correspondence:***
Alino Martinez-Marcos, Facultad de Medicina de Ciudad Real, Universidad de Castilla-La Mancha, Avda. de Moledores S/N, 13071 Ciudad Real, Spain.
e-mail: alino.martinez@uclm.es

Most tetrapods possess two nasal organs for detecting chemicals in their environment, which are the sensory detectors of the olfactory and vomeronasal systems. The seventies' view that the olfactory system was only devoted to sense volatiles, whereas the vomeronasal system was exclusively specialized for pheromone detection was challenged by accumulating data showing deep anatomical and functional interrelationships between both systems. In addition, the assumption that the vomeronasal system appeared as an adaptation to terrestrial life is being questioned as well. The aim of the present work is to use a comparative strategy to gain insight in our understanding of the evolution of chemical "cortex." We have analyzed the organization of the olfactory and vomeronasal cortices of reptiles, marsupials, and placental mammals and we have compared our findings with data from other taxa in order to better understand the evolutionary history of the nasal sensory systems in vertebrates. The olfactory and vomeronsasal cortices have been re-investigated in garter snakes (*Thamnophis sirtalis*), short-tailed opossums (*Monodelphis domestica*), and rats (*Rattus norvegicus*) by tracing the efferents of the main and accessory olfactory bulbs using injections of neuroanatomical anterograde tracers (dextran-amines). In snakes, the medial olfactory tract is quite evident, whereas the main vomeronasal-recipient structure, the nucleus sphaericus is a folded cortical-like structure, located at the caudal edge of the amygdala. In marsupials, which are acallosal mammals, the rhinal fissure is relatively dorsal and the olfactory and vomeronasal cortices relatively expanded. Placental mammals, like marsupials, show partially overlapping olfactory and vomeronasal projections in the rostral basal telencephalon. These data raise the interesting question of how the telencephalon has been re-organized in different groups according to the biological relevance of chemical senses.

Keywords: amygdala, cortex, evolution, olfaction, olfactory bulb, vomeronasal

INTRODUCTION

Odor perception is initiated by interactions between odorants (*sensu lato*) and a diverse repertoire of receptors in sensory neurons (Ache and Young, 2005; Bargmann, 2006; Kaupp, 2010). Classical neuroanatomical studies have investigated the olfactory system in a number of species of different taxa including fishes (s.l.; Hara, 1975; Laberge and Hara, 2001; Hamdani el and Doving, 2007), amphibians (Duchamp-Viret and Duchamp, 1997), reptiles (Lohman and Smeets, 1993), birds (Rieke and Wenzel, 1978), and mammals (Shepherd, 1972). These reports have allowed the characterization of the olfactory "cortex" in most vertebrates. Also, neuroanatomical investigations lead to the identification of the vomeronasal "cortex" in mammals (Winans and Scalia, 1970; Raisman, 1972; Scalia and Winans, 1975). The main conclusions of all these reports were that chemosensory cortex lacks odotopy and that olfactory and vomeronasal projections reached adjacent, non-overlapping zones in the telencephalon.

During the last two decades, the cloning of different olfactory (Buck and Axel, 1991; Liberles and Buck, 2006) and vomeronasal (Dulac and Axel, 1995; Bargmann, 1997, 1999; Herrada and Dulac, 1997; Matsunami and Buck, 1997; Ryba and Tirindelli, 1997) receptors has allowed considerable progress in tracing olfactory and vomeronasal perception from receptors to the activity of sensory

Abbreviations: ac, anterior commissure; ACo, anterior cortical amygdaloid area; ADVR, anterior dorsal ventricular ridge; AOB, accessory olfactory bulb; aot: accessory olfactory tract; BAOT, bed nucleus accessory olfactory tract; BNST, bed nucleus stria terminalis; CA, cornu ammonis areas; CA1-3, fields CA1-3 of cornu ammonis; CxA, cortex–amygdala-transition zone; DC, dorsal cortex; DG, dentate gyrus; DLA, dorsolateral amygdaloid nucleus; dlo, dorsal lateral olfactory tract; dmRF, dorsomedial retrobulbar formation; GL, glomerular layer; GrL, granular cell layer; IC, islands of calleja; iot, intermediate olfactory tract; LC, lateral cortex; LE, lateral entorhinal cortex; lfb, lateral forebrain bundle; lot, lateral olfactory tract; MC, medial cortex; Me, median eminence; MeAD, medial amygdaloid nucleus, anterodorsal; MeAV, medial amygdaloid nucleus, anteroventral part; meot, medial olfactory tract; MePD, medial amygdaloid nucleus, posterodorsal part; MePV, medial amygdaloid nucleus, posteroventral part; NS, nucleus sphaericus; MOB, main olfactory bulb; mot, medial olfactory tract; OG, olfactory gray; OT, olfactory tubercle; ot, optic tract; PDVR, posterior dorsal ventricular ridge; Pir, piriform cortex; PMCo, posteromedial cortical amygdaloid area; PMLo, posterolateral cortical amygdaloid area; S, septum; sm, stria medullaris; ST, striatum; Tu, olfactory tubercle; TT, taenia tecta; VPA, ventral posterior amygdala.

neurons to higher processing centers and, ultimately, to behavior (Buck, 1995, 1996, 2000, 2004; Mombaerts, 1996, 1999a,b, 2004; Mombaerts et al., 1996; Dulac, 1997, 2000; Dulac and Torello, 2003; Brennan and Keverne, 2004; Brennan and Zufall, 2006; Dulac and Wagner, 2006; Cleland, 2010). Interactions and synergic activation of both systems, however, occurs in early stages of neural processing (Xu et al., 2005; Slotnick et al., 2010).

The genetic and molecular approaches to the study of the organization of chemosensory systems have allowed a step forward to understand the organization of chemosensory systems. Genetic tracing of given receptors constitutes a valuable tool for this aim. The present review tries to provide a global panorama on the organization and evolution of olfactory and vomeronasal cortices with emphasis on recent advances including tract-tracing as well as genetic and molecular approaches. Own data of reptiles, marsupials and placental mammals are re-analyzed in the context of current knowledge of main taxa of vertebrates.

TAXONOMIC OVERVIEW OF VERTEBRATES

Although a complete description of the taxonomic classification of vertebrates is out of the scope of the present manuscript, a brief outline of the main vertebrate taxa will be useful not only for the comparative strategy herein used but also to help non-familiarized readers to understand such organization. For the sake of clarity, the main taxonomic categories have been maintained but simplified. This hierarchical organization is explained below and has been adapted from Hickman and collaborators (Hickman et al., 2007).

The Phylum Chordata is defined by the presence of notochord. In its basic plan these animals are bilateral, coelomed, metameric, and cephalized. This Phylum includes the Groups Prochordata (with the Subphyla Urochordata–tunicates–and Cephalochordata–amphioxus) and Craniata (with the Subphylum Vertebrata). Within Subphylum Vertebrata are included the Superclasses Agnata (jawless, with the Classes Mixinoidea –mixins – and Cephalaspidomorpha –lampreys) and Gnathostomata (jawed, with the Classes Chondrichthyes – cartilaginous fishes – Osteichthyes –bony fishes – Amphibia, Reptilia, Aves, and Mammalia. The Class Mammalia includes the Subclasses Prototheria –monotremas – and Theria. The Subclasse Theria comprises the Infraclasses Metatheria – marsupials – and Eutheria with several Orders in which highlights the Order Primate. Finally, within the Order Primate consist of the Superfamilies Platyrrhini –new world monkeys – Catarrhini – old world monkeys – and Hominidae in which we are included.

AGNATA, JAWLESS

Among superclass Agnata most data in the literature regarding the organization of the olfactory system have been obtained in lampreys. Reports on the lamprey olfactory system has been devoted to the organization of the olfactory mucosa (Thornhill, 1967; Suzuki, 1984; VanDenbossche et al., 1995; Laframboise et al., 2007), olfactory bulbs (Iwahori et al., 1987a; Melendez-Ferro et al., 2001; Pombal et al., 2002), and telencephalon (Chiba, 1999; Pombal et al., 2002; Perez-Costas et al., 2004). The projections from the olfactory bulb identified medial and lateral olfactory tracts (LOT) reaching dorsal, lateral, and probably medial pallium as well as the posterior diencephalon as well as reciprocal, centrifugal projections to the bulb (Northcutt and Puzdrowski, 1988; Polenova and Vesselkin, 1993). On the other hand, the origin of the vomeronasal system is uncertain. It was classically considered that the vomeronasal system was developed by tetrapods and it was hypothesized to be an adaptation to terrestrial life (Eisthen, 1997). It has been demonstrated that lampreys detect pheromones (Fine and Sorensen, 2008) and display some genetic components of the vomeronasal system (Grus and Zhang, 2009). Also, an accessory olfactory organ has been shown to send separated projections from those of the main olfactory epithelium to the medial portion of the bulb (Ren et al., 2009). No further differential projections from this medial portion of the bulb to the pallium have been investigated. Therefore, data in the literature suggests that primordial elements of the vomeronasal system could be already present in jawless vertebrates.

CHONDRICHTHYES, CARTILAGINOUS FISHES

The olfactory system, including the olfactory epithelium (Ferrando et al., 2006, 2007, 2009; Zaccone et al., 2010) and the secondary connections from the olfactory bulbs have been investigated in sharks and rays (Smeets, 1983). Secondary olfactory centers have been neurochemically characterized as well (Yuen et al., 2005). Like lampreys, cartilaginous fishes display some genetic components of the vomeronasal system (Grus and Zhang, 2009). The distribution of G proteins suggests incipient segregated primary olfactory projections (Ferrando et al., 2009).

OSTEICHTHYES, BONY FISHES

The teleosts olfactory system has been investigated including the olfactory organs (Wilson and Westerman, 1967; Westerman and Wilson, 1968; Goel, 1978; Jain and Sahai, 1991), olfactory bulbs (Kosaka and Hama, 1982; Alonso et al., 1989; Satou, 1990), and olfactory-recipient areas (Singru et al., 2003; Gaikwad et al., 2004). The olfactory projections from the olfactory bulbs have been investigated in teleosts, with studies including early anatomical reports (Scalia and Ebbesson, 1971; Finger, 1975; Murakami et al., 1983). These projections have been re-investigated using modern genetic approaches (Miyasaka et al., 2009). In teleost fishes, whose telencephalon is everted (Butler, 2000; Mueller and Wullimann, 2009), the secondary olfactory projections terminate in non-cortical areas of the telencephalon (Folgueira et al., 2004). Interestingly, three pathways from different receptors to different areas in the olfactory bulb and to different areas in the telencephalon have been characterized in teleost fishes devoted to detect social cues, sex pheromones, and food odors (Hamdani el and Doving, 2007). In fact, not only vomeronasal receptors have been described in several species (Pfister et al., 2007), but, in lungfishes, it has been recently reported a complete vomeronasal system (Gonzalez et al., 2010).

AMPHIBIA

Studies on the amphibian olfactory system include reports focused in the olfactory epithelium (Getchell et al., 1989; Daston et al., 1990; Crowe and Pixley, 1992; Krishna et al., 1992), olfactory bulb (Scalia et al., 1991b), and olfactory-recipient areas (Gonzalez and Smeets, 1991; Petko and Santa, 1992; Marin et al., 1997; Brox et al., 2004). The differential projections from the olfactory and vomeronasal epithelia to the main and accessory olfactory bulbs (AOB) were reported in several species (Taniguchi et al., 2008). The amphibian AOB has been investigated as well (Saito et al., 2006).

Secondary olfactory projections were early addressed in amphibians (Northcutt and Royce, 1975). The differential projections from the main and AOBs were reported later on reaching cortical and non-cortical areas of the telencephalon, respectively (Scalia, 1972; Scalia et al., 1991a). The vomeronasal system was fully described more recently including not only hodology, but neurochemical and gene expression characterization (Moreno et al., 2005; Moreno and Gonzalez, 2007). Interestingly, heterogeneous expression of G proteins have been reported in the amphibian olfactory and vomeronasal epithelia (Jungblut et al., 2009). Vomeronasal receptor genes have been reported to be also expressed in the main olfactory epithelium indicating that some pheromone-like triggered behaviors (Woodley, 2010) are mediated via the olfactory system in some amphibians species (Date-Ito et al., 2008).

REPTILIA

Research on the reptilian olfactory system includes reports focused to olfactory receptors (Steiger et al., 2009), olfactory and vomeronasal epithelia (Wang and Halpern, 1982a,b, 1988; Iwahori et al., 1987b; Kondoh et al., 2010), olfactory bulbs (Iwahori et al., 1989a,b; Kosaka et al., 1991), and olfactory-recipient telencephalic areas (Smeets et al., 1986, 1987; Smeets, 1988; Smeets and Steinbusch, 1990). In reptiles, the main and AOBs projections were investigated in a number of species, mainly lizards and snakes (Gamble, 1952, 1956; Halpern, 1976; Lohman et al., 1988; Martinez-Garcia et al., 1991; Lanuza and Halpern, 1998). These projections have also reviewed (Lohman and Smeets, 1993). Both projections are reciprocated by backwards centrifugal projections (Martinez-Garcia et al., 1991; Lanuza and Halpern, 1998). The projections from the main olfactory bulb (MOB) are characterized by lateral, intermediate, and medial olfactory tracts (MOT; **Figure 1**). The lateral projection is the most robust projection and ends in the superficial layer of the reptilian lateral cortex (**Figure 1**). The projection from the AOB courses through the accessory olfactory tract (AOT) to reach the vomeronasal amygdala, within the reptilian amygdaloid complex (Martinez-Garcia et al., 1993; Martinez-Marcos et al., 1999). The vomeronasal amygdala is mainly composed by the nucleus sphericus, a folded, cortical-like structure. The vomeronasal projection ends in the inner layer of this nucleus (**Figure 2**). The projections from the main and AOBs in reptiles are summarized in **Figure 3**.

AVES

The avian olfactory system has been investigated from olfactory receptors (Nef et al., 1996) to olfactory epithelium (Slaby, 1987), olfactory bulb (Cobb, 1960; Ioale and Papi, 1989), and olfactory-recipient areas (Dietl and Palacios, 1988). The olfactory bulb projections in Aves were studied with Fink–Heimer technique demonstrating a bilateral non-symmetrical terminal field (Rieke and Wenzel, 1978). Using autoradiographic techniques, the avian olfactory bulb projections were compared to those of turtles. The main conclusions were that both projections were similar regarding "olfactory cortex," but they do differ significantly regarding projections to the amygdaloid region, being this latter reduced to the nucleus taeniae in the case of birds (Reiner and Karten, 1985). These projections have been characterized using neural tracers as well (Ebinger et al., 1992). Avian olfaction have been largely related to navigation (Gagliardo et al., 2009). In fact, the olfactory forebrain is quite specialized in migratory birds like anseriforms (Ebinger et al., 1992). New techniques based on the combinatorial expression patterns of neural markers and developmental regulatory genes have allowed to identify zones in the olfatorecipient area of the ventral pallium comparable to piriform, entorhinal, amygdalopiriform, and amygdaloid cortices of mammals (Martinez-Garcia et al., 2002; Abellan et al., 2009). Finally, analysis of olfactory receptor gene repertoires show that in all species studied, amplified olfactory receptor sequences were predicted to be from potentially functional genes thus suggesting that olfaction in birds may be a more important sense than generally believed (Steiger et al., 2008; Balthazart and Taziaux, 2009). The issue of avian pheromones is still far from been resolved (Caro and Balthazart, 2010).

METATHERIA, MARSUPIALS

Marsupials lack corpus callosum and consequently the telencephalon shows a different organization as compared to placental mammals. The rhinal fissure is located more dorsal in marsupials than in placental mammals and their anterior commissure is hypertrophied to communicate both hemispheres (Gloor, 1997). The olfactory epithelium (Kratzing, 1982) and olfactory bulbs are organized in a particular way in marsupials (Switzer and Johnson, 1977; Jia and Halpern, 2004). Olfactory projections were already investigated in the middle of twentieth century (Adey, 1953). The projections from the main and AOBs were described in opossums using the Fink–Heimer method (Scalia and Winans, 1975; Meyer, 1981; Shammah-Lagnado and Negrao, 1981). The olfactory-recipient and vomeronasal-recipient cortices occupied adjacent non-overlapping areas. Using neural tracers, the projections from the opossum main (Martinez-Marcos and Halpern, 2006) and accessory (Martinez-Marcos and Halpern, 1999b) olfactory bulbs were later re-investigated using modern neural tracers. The projections from the MOB course mainly via the LOT to reach the anterior olfactory nucleus, olfactory tubercle, nucleus of the LOT, anterior and posterolateral cortical amygdaloid nuclei and the piriform, and lateral entorhinal cortices (**Figure 4**). The projections from the AOB course through the AOT to reach the medial amgydaloid complex and the posteromedial cortical amygdaloid nucleus (**Figure 5**). Both projections converge at rostral levels such as the medial amygdala, whereas are non-overlapping at caudal levels (**Figure 6**). The differential expression of G proteins in the vomeronasal system (Halpern et al., 1995) and the cloning of the two families of vomeronasal receptors (Dulac and Axel, 1995; Herrada and Dulac, 1997; Matsunami and Buck, 1997; Ryba and Tirindelli, 1997) allowed to identify the differential projections to the anterior and posterior portions of the AOB (Jia and Halpern, 1996; Belluscio et al., 1999; Rodriguez et al., 1999). Both portions send convergent but also differential projections to the vomeronasal amygdala in opossums (Martinez-Marcos and Halpern, 1999b), which are also reciprocated by differential centrifugal projections to the anterior and posterior divisions of the AOB (Martinez-Marcos and Halpern, 1999a).

EUTHERIA, PLACENTAL MAMMALS

In placental mammals, the projections from the olfactory epithelium to the MOB (Clark, 1951) and from the bulb to the cortex (Clark and Meyer, 1947) were already addressed in the middle of

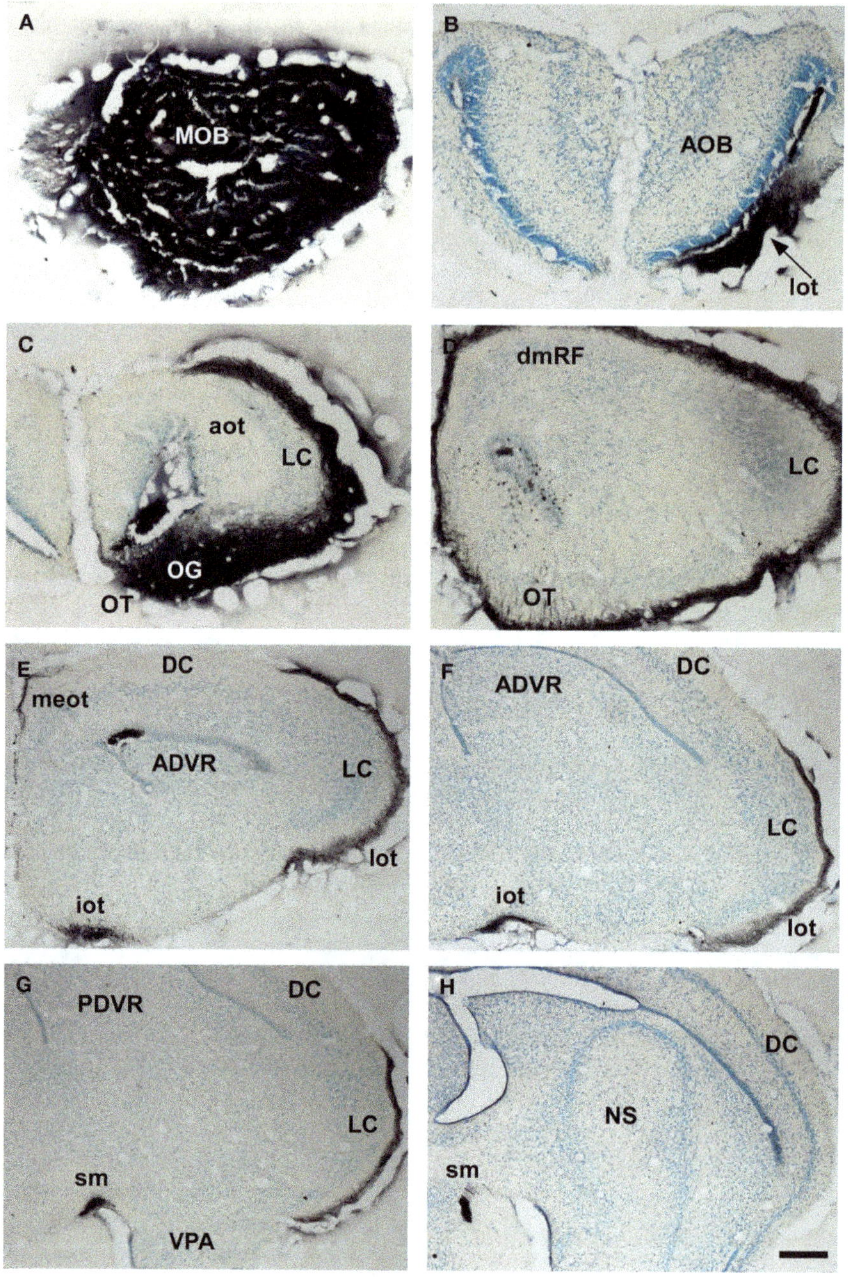

FIGURE 1 | Bright field microscopic images from rostral to caudal of coronal sections of one brain hemisphere showing biotinylated dextran-amine labeling Nissl-counterstained in the snake (*Thamnophis sirtalis*) olfactory cortices after one injection in the main olfactory bulb (MOB). (**A**) injection site in the MOB. (**B–H**) labeling in olfactory-recipient areas of the telencephalon. Scale bar **A–D** = 267; **E–H** = 400 μm.

the twentieth century. The characterization of projections from the main and AOBs were reported later on (Heimer, 1968; Winans and Scalia, 1970; Raisman, 1972; Price, 1973; Scalia and Winans, 1975; Devor, 1976; Skeen and Hall, 1977; Kosel et al., 1981; Schoenfeld and Macrides, 1984; Shipley and Adamek, 1984; De Carlos et al., 1989) including the centrifugal projections (Davis et al., 1978; de Olmos et al., 1978; Davis and Macrides, 1981; Shipley and Adamek, 1984; Coolen and Wood, 1998). As in marsupials, the projections from the MOB form a minor projection through the MOT and a major projection through the LOT to reach the anterior olfactory nucleus, taenia tecta, olfactory tubercle, the nucleus of the LOT, rostral levels of the medial amgydaloid complex and the anterior and posterolateral cortical amygdaloid nuclei as well as the piriform and lateral entorhinal cortices (**Figure 7**). The projections from the AOB (Larriva-Sahd, 2008) travel through the AOT to reach the cortex–amygdala-transition zone and the medial amgydaloid complex and posteromedial amygdaloid nucleus. Also, fibers course through the stria terminalis to reach the bed nucleus of the stria terminalis (**Figure 8**). Olfactory and vomeronasal projections converge at rostral levels of the basal telencephalon (Pro-Sistiaga et al., 2007) but not at

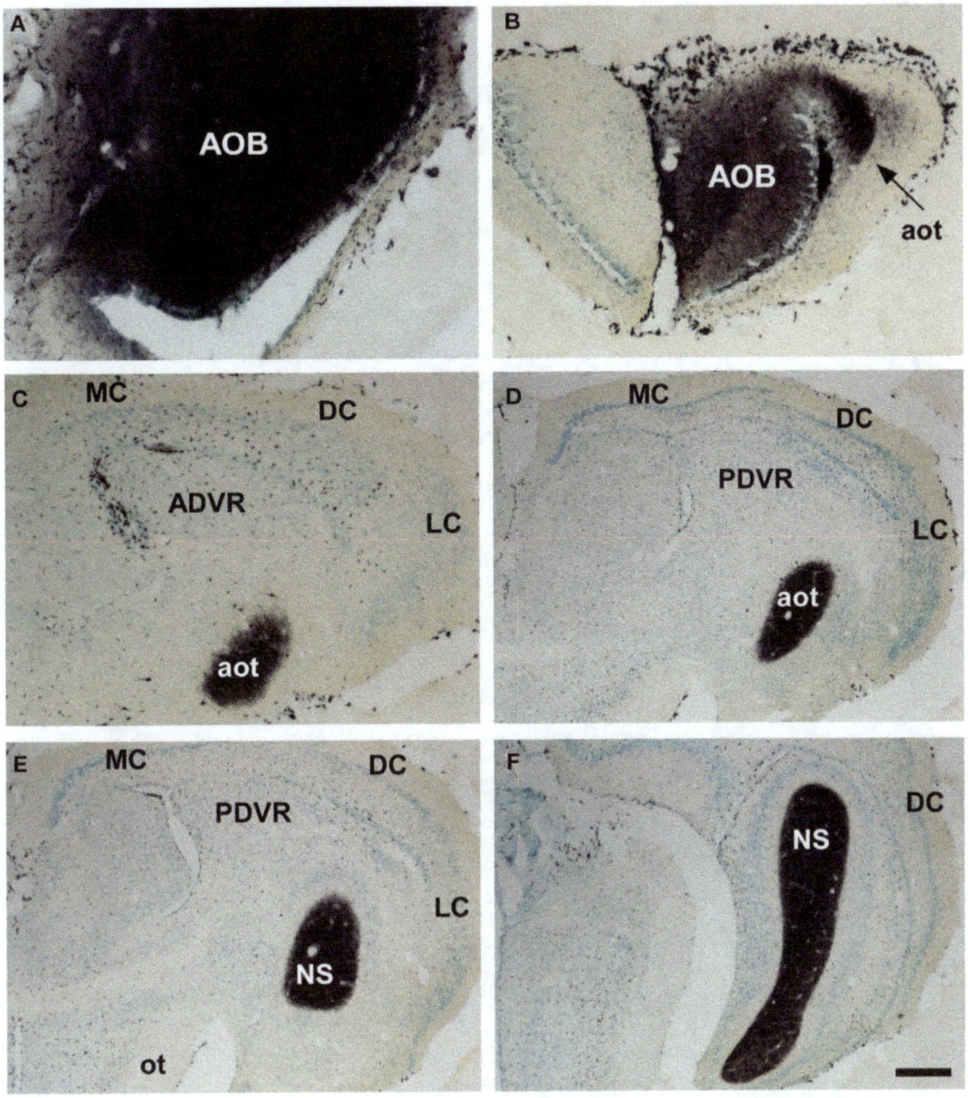

FIGURE 2 | Bright field microscopic images from rostral to caudal of coronal sections of one brain hemisphere showing biotinylated dextran-amine labeling Nissl-counterstained in the snake (*Thamnophis sirtalis*) vomeronasal amygdala after an injection in the accessory olfactory bulb (AOB). (**A**) injection site. (**B–F**) labeling in vomeronasal-recipient areas. Scale bar **A** = 160; **B–C** = 267; **D–E** = 400; **F** = 533 μm.

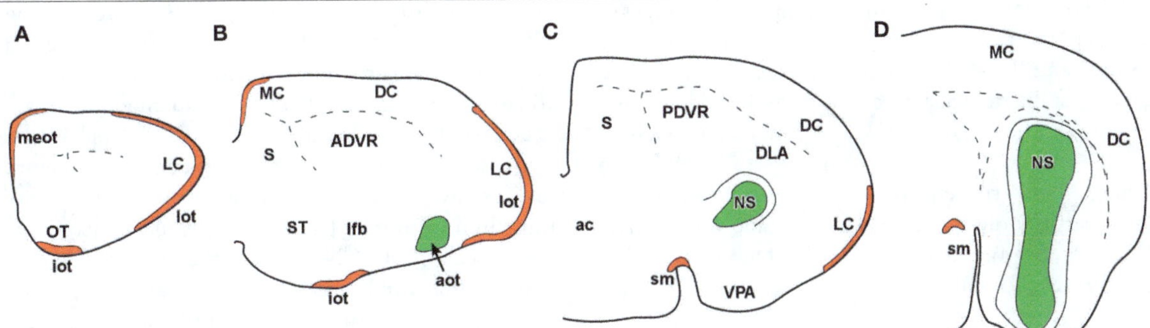

FIGURE 3 | Schematic representation of main (red) and accessory (green) projections from rostral to caudal (A-D) areas in the snake (*Thamnophis sirtalis*) olfactory – and vomeronasal-recipient areas.

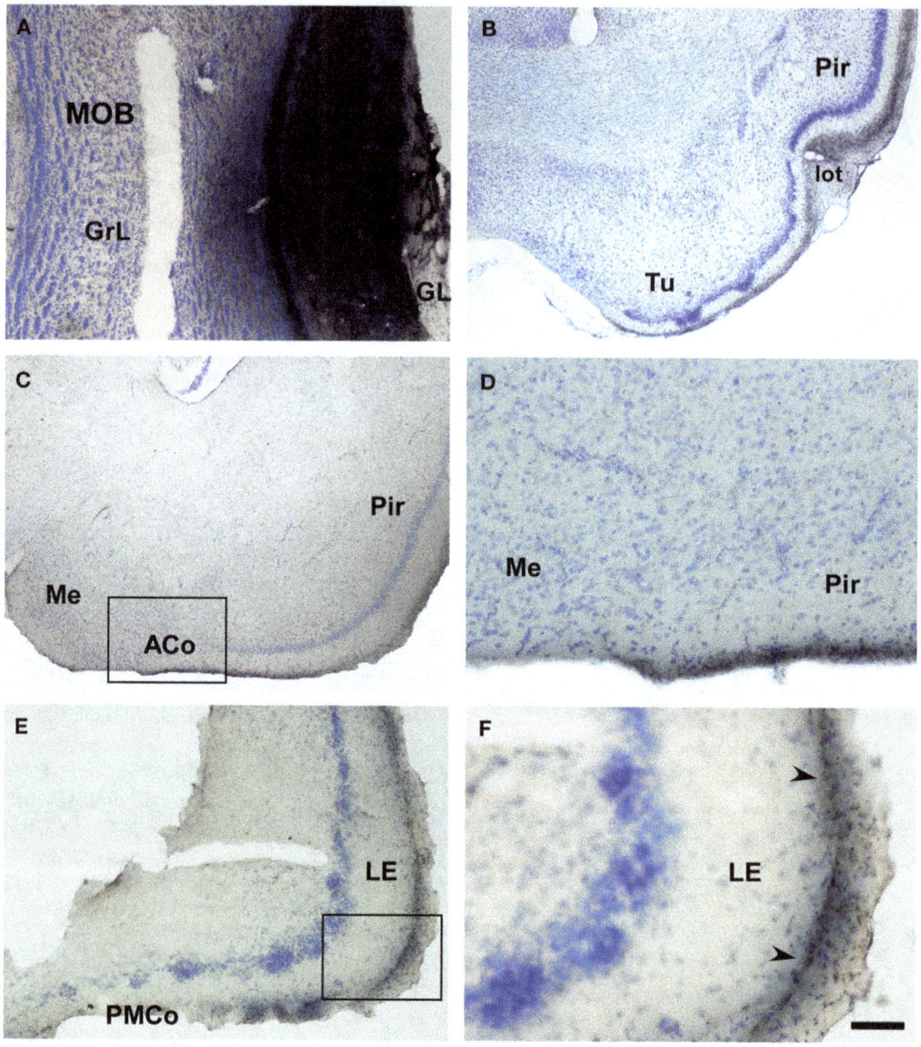

FIGURE 4 | Bright field microscopic images from rostral to caudal of coronal sections of one brain hemisphere showing biotinylated dextran-amine labeling Nissl-counterstained in the opossum (*Monodelphis domestica*) olfactory cortices after an injection in the main olfactory bulb (MOB). (**A**) injection site. (**B–F**) labeling in olfactory-recipient areas. Scale bar **A, D,** and **F** = 160; **B, C,** and **E** = 800 μm.

caudal ones (**Figure 9**; Martinez-Marcos, 2009; Gutierrez-Castellanos et al., 2010). The differential expression of G proteins in the vomeronasal system (Halpern et al., 1995) and the cloning of two families of vomeronasal receptors (Dulac and Axel, 1995; Herrada and Dulac, 1997; Matsunami and Buck, 1997; Ryba and Tirindelli, 1997) led to the description of differential projections from the vomeronasal epithelium to the anterior and posterior divisions of the AOB (Jia and Halpern, 1996; Belluscio et al., 1999; Rodriguez et al., 1999). Both divisions of the AOB show convergent (Von Campenhause and Mori, 2000), but also partially divergent projections in the vomeronasal amygdala (Mohedano-Moriano et al., 2007) that are preserved in the hypothalamus (Mohedano-Moriano et al., 2008).

PLATYRRHINI, NEW WORLD MONKEYS

The MOB connections were recently characterized in the marmoset (Liebetanz et al., 2002). Injections of anterograde tracers revealed the medial and LOTs as well as the olfactory-recipient structures including the anterior olfactory nucleus, piriform cortex, tenia tecta, periamygdaloid cortex, and rostral entorhinal cortex. Centrifugal projections were also revealed originating in olfactory-recipient areas by using retrograde tracers. The vomeronasal system exists, but it is poorly developed in New World monkeys. In marmoset, that possess an intact vomeronasal organ, sequences of vomeronasal receptors (V1R) appear to correspond to pseudogenes (Giorgi and Rouquier, 2002). Neuron-specific markers have been reported to be expressed in the vomeronasal epithelium of different species of primates including marmoset (Dennis et al., 2004). Neurons in the AOB express markers typical of mitral/tufted cells (Nakajima et al., 2003). Marmoset, like other mammals and in contrast to rodents and opossums, display a homogeneous vomeronasal system where only V1R and Gi proteins are expressed (Takigami et al., 2004). To our knowledge, the secondary vomeronasal projections from the AOB have not been traced in marmosets.

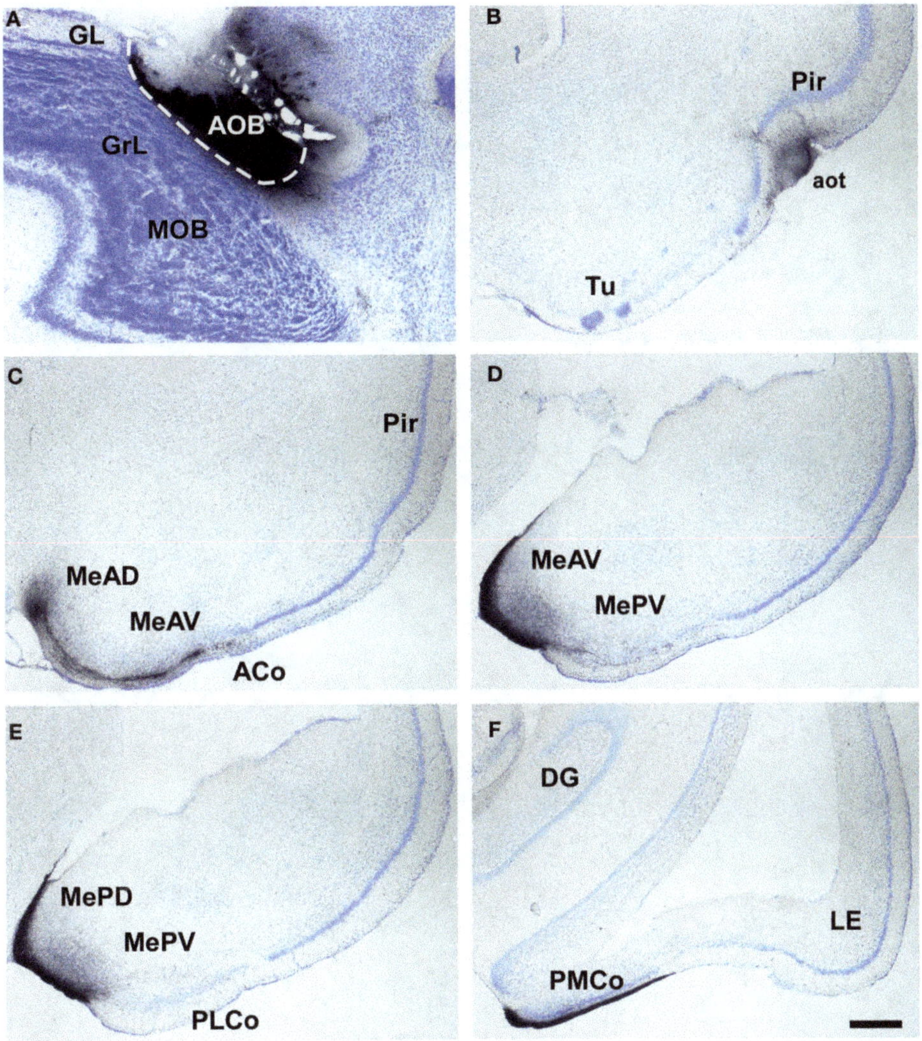

FIGURE 5 | Bright field microscope images from rostral to caudal of coronal (A is sagittal) sections of one brain hemisphere showing biotinylated dextran-amine labeling Nissl-counterstained in the opossum (*Monodelphis domestica*) vomeronasal cortices after an injection in the accessory olfactory bulb (AOB). (**A**) injection site. (**B**) labeling in vomeronasal-recipient areas. Scale bar **A** = 400; **B–F** = 800 μm.

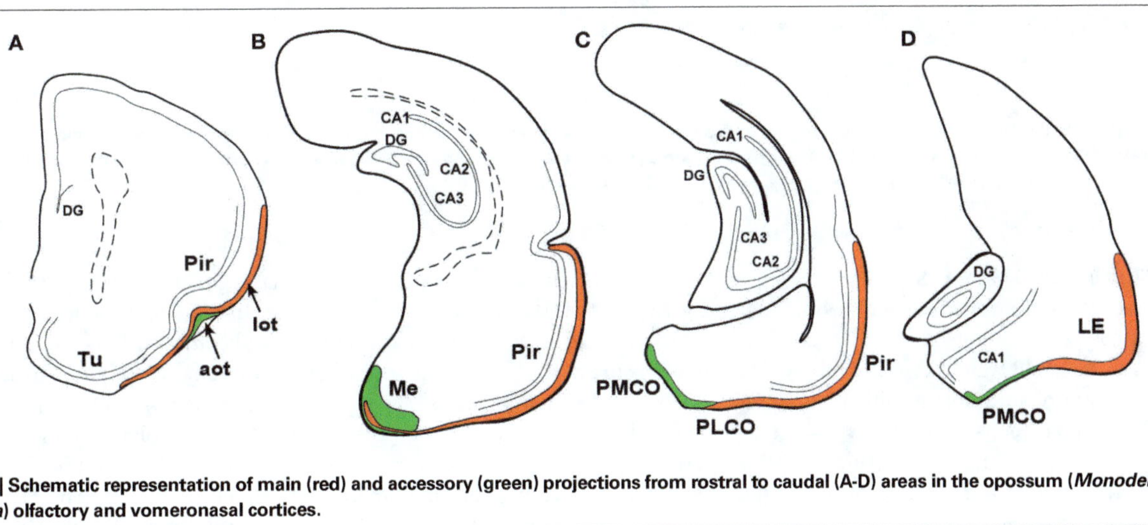

FIGURE 6 | Schematic representation of main (red) and accessory (green) projections from rostral to caudal (A-D) areas in the opossum (*Monodelphis domestica*) olfactory and vomeronasal cortices.

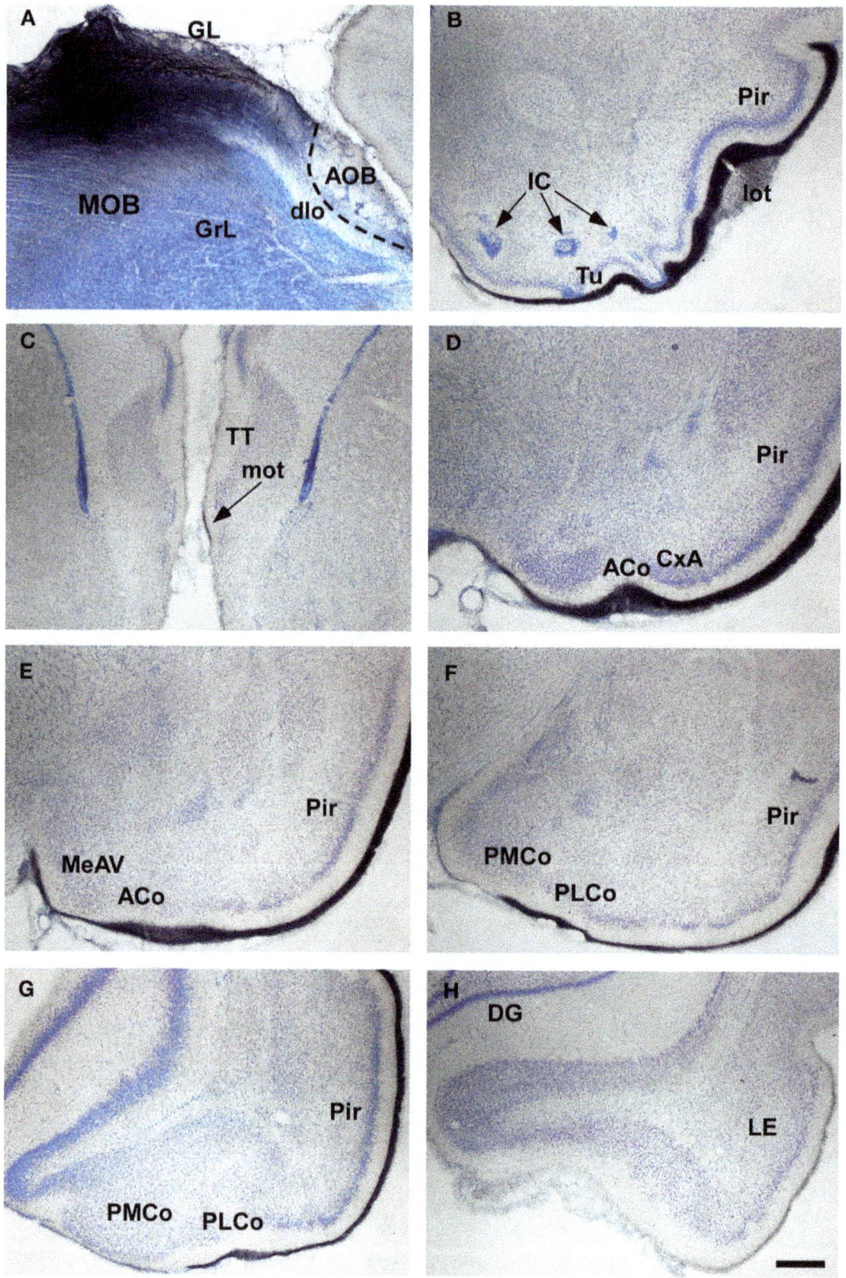

FIGURE 7 | Bright field microscopic images from rostral to caudal of coronal (A is sagittal) sections of one brain hemisphere showing biotinylated dextran-amine labeling Nissl-counterstained in the rat (*Rattus norvegicus*) olfactory cortices after an injection in the main olfactory bulb (MOB). **(A)** injection site. **(B–H)** labeling in olfactory-recipient areas. Scale bar **A–B** and **D–H** = 800; **C** = 400 μm.

CATARRHINI, OLD WORLD MONKEYS

Olfactory receptors are quite reduced in humans and great apes including a 40% of pseudogenes (Sharon et al., 1999). The projections from the MOB were traced in Old World monkeys using lesion–degeneration, autoradiographic (Turner et al., 1978), and neural tracing (Carmichael et al., 1994; Mohedano-Moriano et al., 2005) techniques. Among structures identified as olfactory-recipient were included the anterior olfactory nucleus, piriform cortex, ventral tenia tecta, olfactory tubercle, anterior cortical nucleus of the amygdala, periamygdaloid cortex, and olfactory division of the entorhinal cortex. Interestingly, olfactory fibers reach layer I of the medial amygdaloid complex. This structure has been traditionally described as a vomeronasal-recipient area, but recent data (Pro-Sistiaga et al., 2007; Kang et al., 2009) indicate that it is a mixed chemosensory structure receiving olfactory and vomeronasal inputs. Therefore, it could be hypothesized that this structure has changed from vomeronasal- to olfactory-recipient. Further investigations are needed to confirm this point (**Figure 10**).

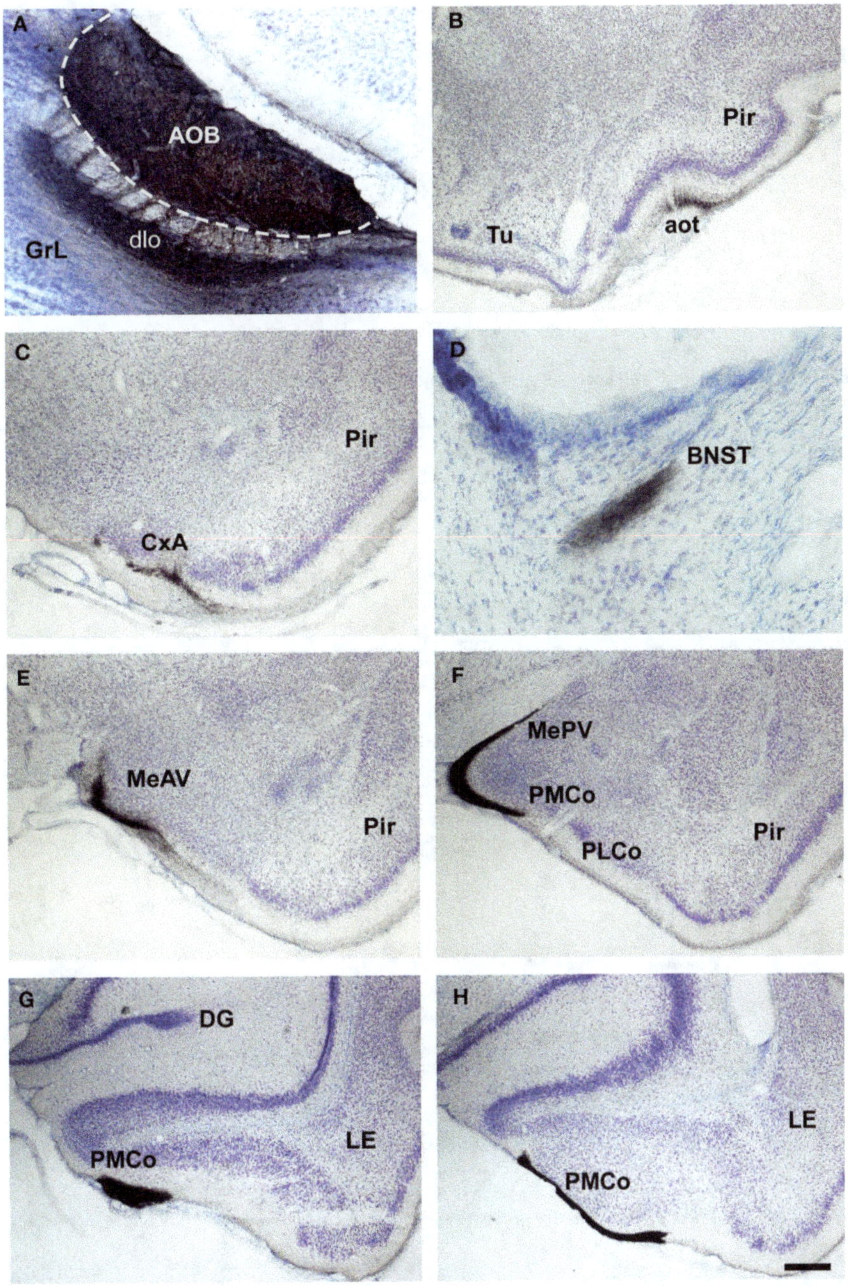

FIGURE 8 | Bright field microscopic images from rostral to caudal of coronal (A is sagittal) sections of one brain hemisphere showing biotinylated dextran-amine labeling Nissl-counterstained in the rat (*Rattus norvegicus*) vomeronasal cortices after an injection in the accessory olfactory bulb (AOB). **(A)** injection site. **(B–H)** labeling in vomeronasal-recipient areas. Scale bar **A** = 400; **B–C** and **E–H** = 800; **D** = 160 μm.

HOMINIDAE, HUMAN BEINGS

Olfactory receptor genes have been identified in humans (Ben-Arie et al., 1994; Glusman et al., 1996, 2000; Buettner et al., 1998; Rouquier et al., 1998), although up to 40% appear to correspond to pseudogenes (Sharon et al., 1999). In fact, evolutionary pressures have led to the loss of part of the olfactory receptor repertoire (Young et al., 2002; Gilad et al., 2003; Niimura and Nei, 2003). The characterizations of olfactory projections in human have been only addressed by indirect methods such as comparative approaches with other primates (Insausti, 1993; Insausti et al., 2002). Putative olfactory areas include the same structures identified in other primates such as anterior olfactory nucleus, piriform cortex, ventral tenia tecta, olfactory tubercle, anterior cortical nucleus of the amygdala, periamygdaloid cortex, and olfactory division of the entorhinal cortex. In humans, the vomeronasal system is vestigial. The vomeronasal organ is apparently only present during embryonic development and its presence is quite controversial in adult humans (Stensaas et al., 1991; Smith et al., 1998, 2001; Smith and Bhatnagar, 2000; Trotier et al., 2000; Abolmaali et al.,

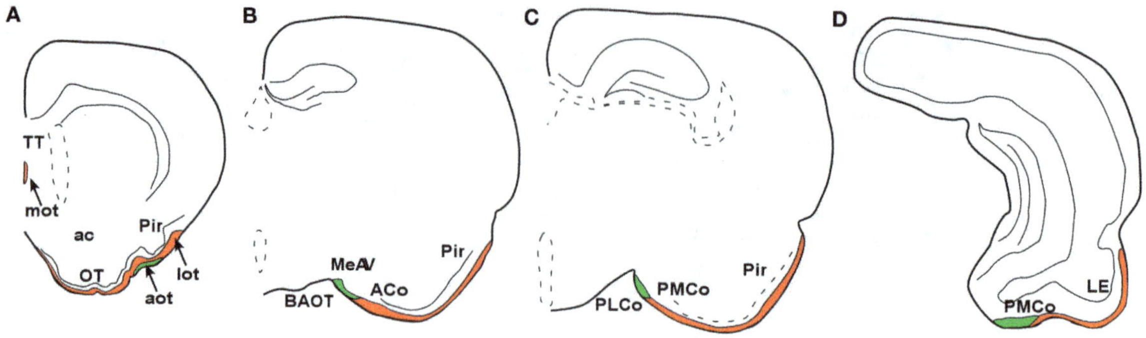

FIGURE 9 | Schematic representation of main (red) and accessory (green) projections from rostral to caudal (A-D) areas in the rat (*Rattus norvegicus*) olfactory and vomeronasal cortices.

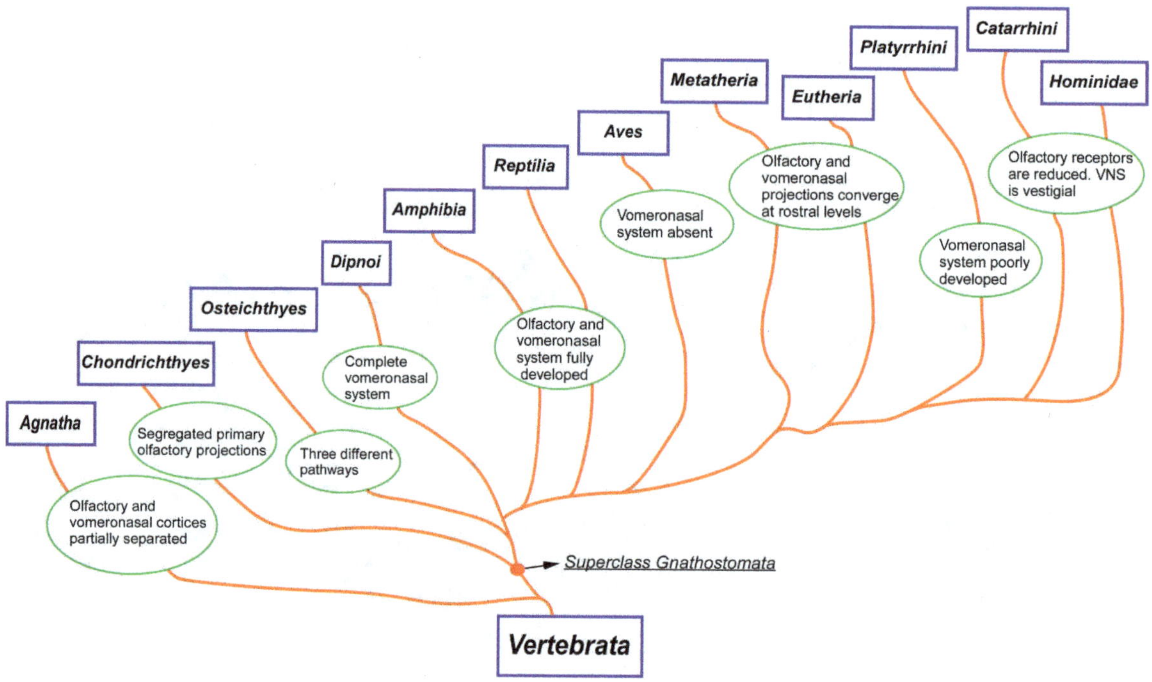

FIGURE 10 | Cladogram illustrating the main taxa analyzed in the present report and the main changes in the olfactory and vomeronasal systems occurred during evolution.

2001; Bhatnagar and Smith, 2001; Knecht et al., 2001, 2003; Meredith, 2001; Witt et al., 2002; Besli et al., 2004; Witt and Hummel, 2006; Witt and Wozniak, 2006). Putative pheromone receptors have been identified in human olfactory mucosa (Rodriguez et al., 2000; Rodriguez and Mombaerts, 2002). Further, to our knowledge, the human AOB has not been described. Therefore, the human "pheromonal-like" behaviors are probably mediated through the olfactory system (Mast and Samuelsen, 2009; Savic et al., 2009).

CONCLUSION

Olfaction plays a main role in most vertebrate taxa. Cladistic analysis of different vertebrates indicates that during evolution an early anatomical and functional subdivision of nasal chemical systems occurred – mainly olfactory and vomeronasal systems – including different receptors, and primary and secondary projection areas. The different chemical systems have suffered differential involution in given taxa due to evolutionary pressures.

ACKNOWLEDGMENTS

This work has been funded by the Spanish Ministry of Education and Science-FEDER (BFU2007-67912-CO2-01/BFI to Fernando Martinez-Garcia and BFU2007-62290/BFI to Alino Martinez-Marcos) and the Autonomous Government of Castilla-La Mancha (PCC08-0064 to Alino Martinez-Marcos and Enrique Lanuza).

REFERENCES

Abellan, A., Legaz, I., Vernier, B., Retaux, S., and Medina, L. (2009). Olfactory and amygdalar structures of the chicken ventral pallium based on the combinatorial expression patterns of LIM and other developmental regulatory genes. *Comp. J. Neurol.* 516, 166–186.

Abolmaali, N. D., Kuhnau, D., Knecht, M., Kohler, K., Huttenbrink, K. B., and Hummel, T. (2001). Imaging of the human vomeronasal duct. *Chem. Senses* 26, 35–39.

Ache, B. W., and Young, J. M. (2005). Olfaction: diverse species, conserved principles. *Neuron* 48, 417–430.

Adey, W. R. (1953). An experimental study of the central olfactory connexions in a marsupial (*Trichosurus Vulpecula*). *Brain* 76, 311–330.

Alonso, J. R., Covenas, R., Lara, J., Arevalo, R., de Leon, M., and Aijon, J. (1989). Tyrosine hydroxylase immunoreactivity in a subpopulation of granule cells in the olfactory bulb of teleost fish. *Brain Behav. Evol.* 34, 318–324.

Balthazart, J., and Taziaux, M. (2009). The underestimated role of olfaction in avian reproduction? *Behav. Brain Res.* 200, 248–259.

Bargmann, C. I. (1997). Olfactory receptors, vomeronasal receptors, and the organization of olfactory information. *Cell* 90, 585–587.

Bargmann, C. I. (1999). A complex sensory map for pheromones. *Neuron* 22, 640–642.

Bargmann, C. I. (2006). Comparative chemosensation from receptors to ecology. *Nature* 444, 295–301.

Belluscio, L., Koentges, G., Axel, R., and Dulac, C. (1999). A map of pheromone receptor activation in the mammalian brain. *Cell* 97, 209–220.

Ben-Arie, N., Lancet, D., Taylor, C., Khen, M., Walker, N., Ledbetter, D. H., Carrozzo, R., Patel, K., Sheer, D., Lehrach, H., and North, M. (1994). Olfactory receptor gene cluster on human chromosome 17: possible duplication of an ancestral receptor repertoire. *Hum. Mol. Genet.* 3, 229–235.

Besli, R., Saylam, C., Veral, A., Karl, B., and Ozek, C. (2004). The existence of the vomeronasal organ in human beings. *J. Craniofac. Surg.* 15, 730–735.

Bhatnagar, K. P., and Smith, T. D. (2001). The human vomeronasal organ. III. Postnatal development from infancy to the ninth decade. *J. Anat.* 199, 289–302.

Brennan, P. A., and Keverne, E. B. (2004). Something in the air? New insights into mammalian pheromones. *Curr. Biol.* 14, R81–R89.

Brennan, P. A., and Zufall, F. (2006). Pheromonal communication in vertebrates. *Nature* 444, 308–315.

Brox, A., Puelles, L., Ferreiro, B., and Medina, L. (2004). Expression of the genes Emx1, Tbr1, and Eomes (Tbr2) in the telencephalon of *Xenopus laevis* confirms the existence of a ventral pallial division in all tetrapods. *J. Comp. Neurol.* 474, 562–577.

Buck, L., and Axel, R. (1991). A novel multigene family may encode odorant receptors: a molecular basis for odor recognition. *Cell* 65, 175–187.

Buck, L. B. (1995). Unraveling chemosensory diversity. *Cell* 83, 349–352.

Buck, L. B. (1996). Information coding in the vertebrate olfactory system. *Annu. Rev. Neurosci.* 19, 517–544.

Buck, L. B. (2000). The molecular architecture of odor and pheromone sensing in mammals. *Cell* 100, 611–618.

Buck, L. B. (2004). Olfactory receptors and odor coding in mammals. *Nutr. Rev.* 62, S184–S188; discussion S141–S224.

Buettner, J. A., Glusman, G., Ben-Arie, N., Ramos, P., Lancet, D., and Evans, G. A. (1998). Organization and evolution of olfactory receptor genes on human chromosome 11. *Genomics* 53, 56–68.

Butler, A. B. (2000). Topography and topology of the teleost telencephalon: a paradox resolved. *Neurosci. Lett.* 293, 95–98.

Carmichael, S. T., Clugnet, M. C., and Price, J. L. (1994). Central olfactory connections in the macaque monkey. *J. Comp. Neurol.* 346, 403–434.

Caro, S. P., and Balthazart, J. (2010). Pheromones in birds: myth or reality? *J. Comp. Physiol.* 196, 751–766.

Chiba, A. (1999). Immunohistochemical distribution of neuropeptide Y-related substance in the brain and hypophysis of the arctic lamprey, *Lethenteron japonica*. *Brain Behav. Evol.* 53, 102–109.

Clark, W. E. (1951). The projection of the olfactory epithelium on the olfactory bulb in the rabbit. *J. Neurol. Neurosurg. Psychiatry* 14, 1–10.

Clark, W. E., and Meyer, M. (1947). The terminal connexions of the olfactory tract in the rabbit. *Brain* 70, 304–328.

Cleland, T. A. (2010). Early transformations in odor representation. *Trends Neurosci.* 33, 130–139.

Cobb, S. (1960). A note on the size of the avian olfactory bulb. *Epilepsia* 1, 394–402.

Coolen, L. M., and Wood, R. I. (1998). Bidirectional connections of the medial amygdaloid nucleus in the Syrian hamster brain: simultaneous anterograde and retrograde tract tracing. *J. Comp. Neurol.* 399, 189–209.

Crowe, M. J., and Pixley, S. K. (1992). Species differences in amphibian olfactory neuron reactivity to a monoclonal antibody. *Brain Res. Bull.* 28, 785–788.

Daston, M. M., Adamek, G. D., and Gesteland, R. C. (1990). Ultrastructural organization of receptor cell axons in frog olfactory nerve. *Brain Res.* 537, 69–75.

Date-Ito, A., Ohara, H., Ichikawa, M., Mori, Y., and Hagino-Yamagishi, K. (2008). Xenopus V1R vomeronasal receptor family is expressed in the main olfactory system. *Chem. Senses* 33, 339–346.

Davis, B. J., and Macrides, F. (1981). The organization of centrifugal projections from the anterior olfactory nucleus, ventral hippocampal rudiment, and piriform cortex to the main olfactory bulb in the hamster: an autoradiographic study. *J. Comp. Neurol.* 203, 475–493.

Davis, B. J., Macrides, F., Youngs, W. M., Schneider, S. P., and Rosene, D. L. (1978). Efferents and centrifugal afferents of the main and accessory olfactory bulbs in the hamster. *Brain Res. Bull.* 3, 59–72.

De Carlos, J. A., Lopez-Mascaraque, L., and Valverde, F. (1989). Connections of the olfactory bulb and nucleus olfactorius anterior in the hedgehog (*Erinaceus europaeus*): fluorescent tracers and HRP study. *J. Comp. Neurol.* 279, 601–618.

de Olmos, J., Hardy, H., and Heimer, L. (1978). The afferent connections of the main and the accessory olfactory bulb formations in the rat: an experimental HRP-study. *J. Comp. Neurol.* 181, 213–244.

Dennis, J. C., Smith, T. D., Bhatnagar, K. P., Bonar, C. J., Burrows, A. M., and Morrison, E. E. (2004). Expression of neuron-specific markers by the vomeronasal neuroepithelium in six species of primates. *Anat. Rec.* 281, 1190–1200.

Devor, M. (1976). Fiber trajectories of olfactory bulb efferents in the hamster. *J. Comp. Neurol.* 166, 31–47.

Dietl, M. M., and Palacios, J. M. (1988). Neurotransmitter receptors in the avian brain. I. Dopamine receptors. *Brain Res.* 439, 354–359.

Duchamp-Viret, P., and Duchamp, A. (1997). Odor processing in the frog olfactory system. *Prog. Neurobiol.* 53, 561–602.

Dulac, C. (1997). Molecular biology of pheromone perception in mammals. *Semin. Cell Dev. Biol.* 8, 197–205.

Dulac, C. (2000). Sensory coding of pheromone signals in mammals. *Curr. Opin. Neurobiol.* 10, 511–518.

Dulac, C., and Axel, R. (1995). A novel family of genes encoding putative pheromone receptors in mammals. *Cell* 83, 195–206.

Dulac, C., and Torello, A. T. (2003). Molecular detection of pheromone signals in mammals: from genes to behaviour. *Nat. Rev. Neurosci.* 4, 551–562.

Dulac, C., and Wagner, S. (2006). Genetic analysis of brain circuits underlying pheromone signaling. *Annu. Rev. Genet.* 40, 449–467.

Ebinger, P., Rehkamper, G., and Schroder, H. (1992). Forebrain specialization and the olfactory system in anseriform birds. An architectonic and tracing study. *Cell Tissue Res.* 268, 81–90.

Eisthen, H. L. (1997). Evolution of vertebrate olfactory systems. *Brain Behav. Evol.* 50, 222–233.

Ferrando, S., Bottaro, M., Gallus, L., Girosi, L., Vacchi, M., and Tagliafierro, G. (2006). Observations of crypt neuron-like cells in the olfactory epithelium of a cartilaginous fish. *Neurosci. Lett.* 403, 280–282.

Ferrando, S., Bottaro, M., Gallus, L., Girosi, L., Vacchi, M., and Tagliafierro, G. (2007). First detection of olfactory marker protein (OMP) immunoreactivity in the olfactory epithelium of a cartilaginous fish. *Neurosci. Lett.* 413, 173–176.

Ferrando, S., Gambardella, C., Ravera, S., Bottero, S., Ferrando, T., Gallus, L., Manno, V., Salati, A. P., Ramoino, P., and Tagliafierro, G. (2009). Immunolocalization of G-protein alpha subunits in the olfactory system of the cartilaginous fish Scyliorhinus canicula. *Anat. Rec. (Hoboken)* 292, 1771–1779.

Fine, J. M., and Sorensen, P. W. (2008). Isolation and biological activity of the multi-component sea lamprey migratory pheromone. *J. Chem. Ecol.* 34, 1259–1267.

Finger, T. E. (1975). The distribution of the olfactory tracts in the bullhead catfish, *Ictalurus nebulosus*. *J. Comp. Neurol.* 161, 125–141.

Folgueira, M., Anadon, R., and Yanez, J. (2004). An experimental study of the connections of the telencephalon in the rainbow trout (*Oncorhynchus mykiss*). I: olfactory bulb and ventral area. *J. Comp. Neurol.* 480, 180–203.

Gagliardo, A., Ioale, P., Savini, M., and Wild, J. M. (2009). Olfactory navigation in homing pigeons: the last challenge. *Ann. N.Y. Acad. Sci.* 1170, 434–437.

Gaikwad, A., Biju, K. C., Saha, S. G., and Subhedar, N. (2004). Neuropeptide Y in the olfactory system, forebrain and pituitary of the teleost, *Clarias batrachus*. *J. Chem. Neuroanat.* 27, 55–70.

Gamble, H. J. (1952). An experimental study of the secondary olfactory connexions in *Lacerta viridis*. *J. Anat.* 86, 180–196.

Gamble, H. J. (1956). An experimental study of the secondary olfactory connexions in *Testudo graeca*. *J. Anat.* 90, 15–29.

Getchell, M. L., Bouvet, J. F., Finger, T. E., Holley, A., and Getchell, T. V. (1989). Peptidergic regulation of secretory activity in amphibian olfactory mucosa: immunohistochemistry, neural stimulation, and pharmacology. *Cell Tissue Res.* 256, 381–389.

Gilad, Y., Man, O., Paabo, S., and Lancet, D. (2003). Human specific loss of olfactory receptor genes. *Proc. Natl. Acad. Sci. U.S.A.* 100, 3324–3327.

Giorgi, D., and Rouquier, S. (2002). Identification of V1R-like putative pheromone receptor sequences in non-human primates. Characterization of V1R pseudogenes in marmoset, a primate species that possesses an intact vomeronasal organ. *Chem. Senses* 27, 529–537.

Gloor, P. (1997). *The Temporal Lobe and Limbic System*. New York: Oxford University Press.

Glusman, G., Clifton, S., Roe, B., and Lancet, D. (1996). Sequence analysis in the olfactory receptor gene cluster on human chromosome 17: recombinatorial events affecting receptor diversity. *Genomics* 37, 147–160.

Glusman, G., Sosinsky, A., Ben-Asher, E., Avidan, N., Sonkin, D., Bahar, A., Rosenthal, A., Clifton, S., Roe, B., Ferraz, C., Demaille, J., and Lancet, D. (2000). Sequence, structure, and evolution of a complete human olfactory receptor gene cluster. *Genomics* 63, 227–245.

Goel, H. R. (1978). The structure and functions of the olfactory organs in the fresh water teleost Notopterus notopterus (HAM). *Folia Morphol.* 26, 392–396.

Gonzalez, A., Morona, R., Lopez, M. J., Moreno, N., and Northcutt, R. G. (2010). Lungfishes, like tetrapods, possess a vomeronasal system. *Front. Neuroanat.* 4:130. doi: 10.3389/fnana.2010.00130

Gonzalez, A., and Smeets, W. J. (1991). Comparative analysis of dopamine and tyrosine hydroxylase immunoreactivities in the brain of two amphibians, the anuran Rana ridibunda and the urodele *Pleurodeles waltlii*. *J. Comp. Neurol.* 303, 457–477.

Grus, W. E., and Zhang, J. (2009). Origin of the genetic components of the vomeronasal system in the common ancestor of all extant vertebrates. *Mol. Biol. Evol.* 26, 407–419.

Gutierrez-Castellanos, N., Martinez-Marcos, A., Martinez-Garcia, F., and Lanuza, E. (2010). Chemosensory function of the amygdala. *Vitam. Horm.* 83, 165–196.

Halpern, M. (1976). The efferent connections of the olfactory bulb and accessory olfactory bulb in the snakes, *Thamnophis sirtalis* and Thamnophis radix. *J. Morphol.* 150, 553–578.

Halpern, M., Shapiro, L. S., and Jia, C. (1995). Differential localization of G proteins in the opossum vomeronasal system. *Brain Res.* 677, 157–161.

Hamdani el, H., and Doving, K. B. (2007). The functional organization of the fish olfactory system. *Prog. Neurobiol.* 82, 80–86.

Hara, T. J. (1975). Olfaction in fish. *Prog. Neurobiol.* 5, 271–335.

Heimer, L. (1968). Synaptic distribution of centripetal and centrifugal nerve fibres in the olfactory system of the rat. An experimental anatomical study. *J. Anat.* 103, 413–432.

Herrada, G., and Dulac, C. (1997). A novel family of putative pheromone receptors in mammals with a topographically organized and sexually dimorphic distribution. *Cell* 90, 763–773.

Hickman, C. P., Roberts, L. S., and Larson, A. (2007). *Integrated Principles of Zoololgy*. New York: McGraw-Hill.

Insausti, R. (1993). Comparative anatomy of the entorhinal cortex and hippocampus in mammals. *Hippocampus* 3, 19–26.

Insausti, R., Marcos, P., Arroyo-Jimenez, M. M., Blaizot, X., and Martinez-Marcos, A. (2002). Comparative aspects of the olfactory portion of the entorhinal cortex and its projection to the hippocampus in rodents, nonhuman primates, and the human brain. *Brain Res. Bull.* 57, 557–560.

Ioale, P., and Papi, F. (1989). Olfactory bulb size, odor discrimination and magnetic insensitivity in hummingbirds. *Physiol. Behav.* 45, 995–999.

Iwahori, N., Kiyota, E., and Nakamura, K. (1987a). A Golgi study on the olfactory bulb in the lamprey, *Lampetra japonica*. *Neurosci. Res.* 5, 126–139.

Iwahori, N., Kiyota, E., and Nakamura, K. (1987b). Olfactory and respiratory epithelia in the snake, *Elaphe quadrivirgata*. *Okajimas Folia Anat. Jpn.* 64, 183–191.

Iwahori, N., Nakamura, K., and Mameya, C. (1989a). A Golgi study on the accessory olfactory bulb in the snake, *Elaphe quadrivirgata*. *Neurosci. Res.* 7, 55–70.

Iwahori, N., Nakamura, K., and Mameya, C. (1989b). A Golgi study on the main olfactory bulb in the snake *Elaphe quadrivirgata*. *Neurosci. Res.* 6, 411–425.

Jain, V. K., and Sahai, S. (1991). Anatomical and histochemical studies of the olfactory apparatus of three teleost fishes and its significance in their behaviour. *Funct. Dev. Morphol.* 1, 21–26.

Jia, C., and Halpern, M. (1996). Subclasses of vomeronasal receptor neurons: differential expression of G proteins (Gi alpha 2 and G(o alpha)) and segregated projections to the accessory olfactory bulb. *Brain Res.* 719, 117–128.

Jia, C., and Halpern, M. (2004). Calbindin D28k, parvalbumin, and calretinin immunoreactivity in the main and accessory olfactory bulbs of the gray short-tailed opossum, Monodelphis domestica. *J. Morphol.* 259, 271–280.

Jungblut, L. D., Paz, D. A., Lopez-Costa, J. J., and Pozzi, A. G. (2009). Heterogeneous distribution of G protein alpha subunits in the main olfactory and vomeronasal systems of Rhinella (Bufo) arenarum tadpoles. *Zool. Sci.* 26, 722–728.

Kang, N., Baum, M. J., and Cherry, J. A. (2009). A direct main olfactory bulb projection to the 'vomeronasal' amygdala in female mice selectively responds to volatile pheromones from males. *Eur. J. Neurosci.* 29, 624–634.

Kaupp, U. B. (2010). Olfactory signalling in vertebrates and insects: differences and commonalities. *Nat. Rev. Neurosci.* 11, 188–200.

Knecht, M., Kuhnau, D., Huttenbrink, B. K., Witt, M., and Hummel, T. (2001). Frequency and localization of the putative vomeronasal organ in humans in relation to age and gender. *Laryngoscope* 111, 448–452.

Knecht, M., Lundstrom, J. N., Witt, M., Huttenbrink, K. B., Heilmann, S., and Hummel, T. (2003). Assessment of olfactory function and androstenone odor thresholds in humans with or without functional occlusion of the vomeronasal duct. *Behav. Neurosci.* 117, 1135–1141.

Kondoh, D., Yamamoto, Y., Nakamuta, N., and Taniguchi, K. (2010). Lectin histochemical studies on the olfactory epithelium and vomeronasal organ in the Japanese striped snake, *Elaphe quadrivirgata*. *J. Morphol.* 271, 1197–1203.

Kosaka, T., and Hama, K. (1982). Synaptic organization in the teleost olfactory bulb. *J. Physiol.* 78, 707–719.

Kosaka, T., Kosaka, K., and Nagatsu, I. (1991). Tyrosine hydroxylase-like immunoreactive neurons in the olfactory bulb of the snake, *Elaphe quadrivirgata*, with special reference to the colocalization of tyrosine hydroxylase- and GABA-like immunoreactivities. *Exp. Brain Res.* 87, 353–362.

Kosel, K. C., Van Hoesen, G. W., and West, J. R. (1981). Olfactory bulb projections to the parahippocampal area of the rat. *J. Comp. Neurol.* 198, 467–482.

Kratzing, J. E. (1982). Regional variation in respiratory epithelium of the nasal cavity of the bandicoot (*Isoodon macrourus*). *J. Anat.* 134, 1–9.

Krishna, N. S., Getchell, T. V., Margolis, F. L., and Getchell, M. L. (1992). Amphibian olfactory receptor neurons express olfactory marker protein. *Brain Res.* 593, 295–298.

Laberge, F., and Hara, T. J. (2001). Neurobiology of fish olfaction: a review. *Brain Res. Rev.* 36, 46–59.

Laframboise, A. J., Ren, X., Chang, S., Dubuc, R., and Zielinski, B. S. (2007). Olfactory sensory neurons in the sea lamprey display polymorphisms. *Neurosci. Lett.* 414, 277–281.

Lanuza, E., and Halpern, M. (1998). Efferents and centrifugal afferents of the main and accessory olfactory bulbs in the snake *Thamnophis sirtalis*. *Brain Behav. Evol.* 51, 1–22.

Larriva-Sahd, J. (2008). The accessory olfactory bulb in the adult rat: a cytological study of its cell types, neuropil, neuronal modules, and interactions with the main olfactory system. *J. Comp. Neurol.* 510, 309–350.

Liberles, S. D., and Buck, L. B. (2006). A second class of chemosensory receptors in the olfactory epithelium. *Nature* 442, 645–650.

Liebetanz, D., Nitsche, M. A., Fromm, C., and Reyher, C. K. (2002). Central olfactory connections in the microsmatic marmoset monkey (*Callithrix jacchus*). *Cells Tissues Organs* 172, 53–69.

Lohman, A. H., Hoogland, P. V., and Witjes, R. J. G. M. (1988). "Projections from the main and accessory olfactory bulbs to the amygdaloid complex in the lizard gekko gecko," in *The Forebrain or Reptiles*, eds W. K. Schwerdtfeger and J. W. Smeets (Basel: Karger), 41–49.

Lohman, A. H., and Smeets, W. J. (1993). Overview of the main and accessory olfactory bulb projections in reptiles. *Brain Behav. Evol.* 41, 147–155.

Marin, O., Smeets, W. J., and Gonzalez, A. (1997). Distribution of choline acetyltransferase immunoreactivity in the brain of anuran (*Rana perezi*, *Xenopus laevis*) and urodele (*Pleurodeles waltl*) amphibians. *J. Comp. Neurol.* 382, 499–534.

Martinez-Garcia, F., Martinez-Marcos, A., and Lanuza, E. (2002). The pallial amygdala of amniote vertebrates: evolution of the concept, evolution of the structure. *Brain Res. Bull.* 57, 463–469.

Martinez-Garcia, F., Olucha, F. E., Teruel, V., and Lorente, M. J. (1993). Fiber connections of the amygdaloid formation of the lizard Podarcis hispanica. *Brain Behav. Evol.* 41, 156–162.

Martinez-Garcia, F., Olucha, F. E., Teruel, V., Lorente, M. J., and Schwerdtfeger, W. K. (1991). Afferent and efferent connections of the olfactory bulbs in the lizard Podarcis hispanica. *J. Comp. Neurol.* 305, 337–347.

Martinez-Marcos, A. (2009). On the organization of olfactory and vomeronasal cortices. *Prog. Neurobiol.* 87, 21–30.

Martinez-Marcos, A., and Halpern, M. (1999a). Differential centrifugal afferents to the anterior and posterior accessory olfactory bulb. *Neuroreport* 10, 2011–2015.

Martinez-Marcos, A., and Halpern, M. (1999b). Differential projections from the anterior and posterior divisions of the accessory olfactory bulb to the medial amygdala in the opossum, *Monodelphis domestica*. *Eur. J. Neurosci.* 11, 3789–3799.

Martinez-Marcos, A., and Halpern, M. (2006). Efferent connections of the main olfactory bulb in the opossum (*Monodelphis domestica*): a characterization of the olfactory entorhinal cortex in a marsupial. *Neurosci. Lett.* 395, 51–56.

Martinez-Marcos, A., Lanuza, E., and Halpern, M. (1999). Organization of the ophidian amygdala: chemosensory pathways to the hypothalamus. *J. Comp. Neurol.* 412, 51–68.

Mast, T. G., and Samuelsen, C. L. (2009). Human pheromone detection by the vomeronasal organ: unnecessary for mate selection? *Chem. Senses* 34, 529–531.

Matsunami, H., and Buck, L. B. (1997). A multigene family encoding a diverse array of putative pheromone receptors in mammals. *Cell* 90, 775–784.

Melendez-Ferro, M., Perez-Costas, E., Rodriguez-Munoz, R., Gomez-Lopez, M. P., Anadon, R., and Rodicio, M. C. (2001). GABA immunoreactivity in the olfactory bulbs of the adult sea lamprey *Petromyzon marinus* L. *Brain Res.* 893, 253–260.

Meredith, M. (2001). Human vomeronasal organ function: a critical review of best and worst cases. *Chem. Senses* 26, 433–445.

Meyer, R. P. (1981). Central connections of the olfactory bulb in the American opossum (*Didelphys virginiana*): a light microscopic degeneration study. *Anat. Rec.* 201, 141–156.

Miyasaka, N., Morimoto, K., Tsubokawa, T., Higashijima, S., Okamoto, H., and Yoshihara, Y. (2009). From the olfactory bulb to higher brain centers: genetic visualization of secondary olfactory pathways in zebrafish. *J. Neurosci.* 29, 4756–4767.

Mohedano-Moriano, A., Martinez-Marcos, A., Munoz, M., Arroyo-Jimenez, M. M., Marcos, P., Artacho-Perula, E., Blaizot, X., and Insausti, R. (2005). Reciprocal connections between olfactory structures and the cortex of the rostral superior temporal sulcus in the *Macaca fascicularis* monkey. *Eur. J. Neurosci.* 22, 2503–2518.

Mohedano-Moriano, A., Pro-Sistiaga, P., Ubeda-Banon, I., Crespo, C., Insausti, R., and Martinez-Marcos, A. (2007). Segregated pathways to the vomeronasal amygdala: differential projections from the anterior and posterior divisions of the accessory olfactory bulb. *Eur. J. Neurosci.* 25, 2065–2080.

Mohedano-Moriano, A., Pro-Sistiaga, P., Ubeda-Banon, I., de la Rosa-Prieto, C., Saiz-Sanchez, D., and Martinez-Marcos, A. (2008). V1R and V2R segregated vomeronasal pathways to the hypothalamus. *Neuroreport* 19, 1623–1626.

Mombaerts, P. (1996). Targeting olfaction. *Curr. Opin. Neurobiol.* 6, 481–486.

Mombaerts, P. (1999a). Molecular biology of odorant receptors in vertebrates. *Ann. Rev. Neurosci.* 22, 487–509.

Mombaerts, P. (1999b). Seven-transmembrane proteins as odorant and chemosensory receptors. *Science* 286, 707–711.

Mombaerts, P. (2004). Genes and ligands for odorant, vomeronasal and taste receptors. *Nat. Rev. Neurosci.* 5, 263–278.

Mombaerts, P., Wang, F., Dulac, C., Chao, S. K., Nemes, A., Mendelsohn, M., Edmondson, J., and Axel, R. (1996). Visualizing an olfactory sensory map. *Cell* 87, 675–686.

Moreno, N., and Gonzalez, A. (2007). Development of the vomeronasal amygdala in anuran amphibians: hodological, neurochemical, and gene expression characterization. *J. Comp. Neurol.* 503, 815–831.

Moreno, N., Morona, R., Lopez, J. M., Munoz, M., and Gonzalez, A. (2005). Lateral and medial amygdala of anuran amphibians and their relation to olfactory and vomeronasal information. *Brain Res. Bull.* 66, 332–336.

Mueller, T., and Wullimann, M. F. (2009). An evolutionary interpretation of teleostean forebrain anatomy. *Brain Behav. Evol.* 74, 30–42.

Murakami, T., Morita, Y., and Ito, H. (1983). Extrinsic and intrinsic fiber connections of the telencephalon in a teleost, *Sebastiscus marmoratus*. *J. Comp. Neurol.* 216, 115–131.

Nakajima, T., Tanioka, Y., and Taniguchi, K. (2003). Distribution of protein gene product 9.5-immunopositive and NADPH-diaphorase-positive neurons in the common marmoset (*Callithrix jacchus*) accessory olfactory bulb. *J. Vet. Med. Sci.* 65, 1307–1311.

Nef, S., Allaman, I., Fiumelli, H., De Castro, E., and Nef, P. (1996). Olfaction in birds: differential embryonic expression of nine putative odorant receptor genes in the avian olfactory system. *Mech. Dev.* 55, 65–77.

Niimura, Y., and Nei, M. (2003). Evolution of olfactory receptor genes in the human genome. *PNAS* 100, 12235–12240.

Northcutt, R. G., and Puzdrowski, R. L. (1988). Projections of the olfactory bulb and nervus terminalis in the silver lamprey. *Brain Behav. Evol.* 32, 96–107.

Northcutt, R. G., and Royce, G. J. (1975). Olfactory bulb projections in the bullfrog *Rana catesbeiana*. *J. Morphol.* 145, 251–267.

Perez-Costas, E., Melendez-Ferro, M., Perez-Garcia, C. G., Caruncho, H. J., and Rodicio, M. C. (2004). Reelin immunoreactivity in the adult sea lamprey brain. *J. Chem. Neuroanat.* 27, 7–21.

Petko, M., and Santa, A. (1992). Distribution of calcitonin gene-related peptide immunoreactivity in the central nervous system of the frog, *Rana esculenta*. *Cell Tissue Res.* 269, 525–534.

Pfister, P., Randall, J., Montoya-Burgos, J. I., and Rodriguez, I. (2007). Divergent evolution among teleost V1r receptor genes. *PLoS One* 2, e379. doi: 10.1371/journal.pone.0000379

Polenova, O. A., and Vesselkin, N. P. (1993). Olfactory and nonolfactory projections in the river lamprey (*Lampetra fluviatilis*) telencephalon. *J. Hirnforsch.* 34, 261–279.

Pombal, M. A., de Arriba, M. C., Sampedro, C., Alvarez, R., and Megias, M. (2002). Immunocytochemical localization of calretinin in the olfactory system of the adult lamprey, *Lampetra fluviatilis*. *Brain Res. Bull.* 57, 281–283.

Price, J. L. (1973). An autoradiographic study of complementary laminar patterns of termination of afferent fibers to the olfactory cortex. *J. Comp. Neurol.* 150, 87–108.

Pro-Sistiaga, P., Mohedano-Moriano, A., Ubeda-Banon, I., Del Mar Arroyo-Jimenez, M., Marcos, P., Artacho-Perula, E., Crespo, C., Insausti, R., and Martinez-Marcos, A. (2007). Convergence of olfactory and vomeronasal projections in the rat basal telencephalon. *J. Comp. Neurol.* 504, 346–362.

Raisman, G. (1972). An experimental study of the projection of the amygdala to the accessory olfactory bulb and its relationship to the concept of a dual olfactory system. *Exp. Brain Res.* 14, 395–408.

Reiner, A., and Karten, H. J. (1985). Comparison of olfactory bulb projections in pigeons and turtles. *Brain Behav. Evol.* 27, 11–27.

Ren, X., Chang, S., Laframboise, A., Green, W., Dubuc, R., and Zielinski, B. (2009). Projections from the accessory olfactory organ into the medial region of the olfactory bulb in the sea lamprey (*Petromyzon marinus*): a novel vertebrate sensory structure? *J. Comp. Neurol.* 516, 105–116.

Rieke, G. K., and Wenzel, B. M. (1978). Forebrain projections of the pigeon olfactory bulb. *J. Morphol.* 158, 41–55.

Rodriguez, I., Feinstein, P., and Mombaerts, P. (1999). Variable patterns of axonal projections of sensory neurons in the mouse vomeronasal system. *Cell* 97, 199–208.

Rodriguez, I., Greer, C. A., Mok, M. Y., and Mombaerts, P. (2000). A putative pheromone receptor gene expressed in human olfactory mucosa. *Nat. Genet.* 26, 18–19.

Rodriguez, I., and Mombaerts, P. (2002). Novel human vomeronasal receptor-like genes reveal species-specific families. *Curr. Biol.* 12, R409–R411.

Rouquier, S., Taviaux, S., Trask, B. J., Brand-Arpon, V., van den Engh, G., Demaille, J., and Giorgi, D. (1998). Distribution of olfactory receptor genes in the human genome. *Nat. Genet.* 18, 243–250.

Ryba, N. J., and Tirindelli, R. (1997). A new multigene family of putative pheromone receptors. *Neuron* 19, 371–379.

Saito, S., Kobayashi, N., and Atoji, Y. (2006). Subdivision of the accessory olfactory bulb in the Japanese common toad, *Bufo japonicus*, revealed by lectin histochemical analysis. *Anat. Embryol.* 211, 395–402.

Satou, M. (1990). Synaptic organization, local neuronal circuitry, and functional segregation of the teleost olfactory bulb. *Prog. Neurobiol.* 34, 115–142.

Savic, I., Heden-Blomqvist, E., and Berglund, H. (2009). Pheromone signal transduction in humans: what can be learned from olfactory loss. *Hum. Brain Mapp.* 30, 3057–3065.

Scalia, F. (1972). The projection of the accessory olfactory bulb in the frog. *Brain Res.* 36, 409–411.

Scalia, F., and Ebbesson, S. O. (1971). The central projections of the olfactory bulb in a teleost (*Gymnothorax funebris*). *Brain Behav. Evol.* 4, 376–399.

Scalia, F., Gallousis, G., and Roca, S. (1991a). Differential projections of the main and accessory olfactory bulb in the frog. *J. Comp. Neurol.* 305, 443–461.

Scalia, F., Gallousis, G., and Roca, S. (1991b). A note on the organization of the amphibian olfactory bulb. *J. Comp. Neurol.* 305, 435–442.

Scalia, F., and Winans, S. S. (1975). The differential projections of the olfactory bulb and accessory olfactory bulb in mammals. *J. Comp. Neurol.* 161, 31–55.

Schoenfeld, T. A., and Macrides, F. (1984). Topographic organization of connections between the main olfactory bulb and pars externa of the anterior olfactory nucleus in the hamster. *J. Comp. Neurol.* 227, 121–135.

Shammah-Lagnado, S. J., and Negrao, N. (1981). Efferent connections of the olfactory bulb in the opossum (*Didelphis marsupialis aurita*): a Fink-Heimer study. *J. Comp. Neurol.* 201, 51–63.

Sharon, D., Glusman, G., Pilpel, Y., Khen, M., Gruetzner, F., Haaf, T., and Lancet, D. (1999). Primate evolution of an olfactory receptor cluster: diversification by gene conversion and recent emergence of pseudogenes. *Genomics* 61, 24–36.

Shepherd, G. M. (1972). Synaptic organization of the mammalian olfactory bulb. *Physiol. Rev.* 52, 864–917.

Shipley, M. T., and Adamek, G. D. (1984). The connections of the mouse olfactory bulb: a study using orthograde and retrograde transport of wheat germ agglutinin conjugated to horseradish peroxidase. *Brain Res. Bull.* 12, 669–688.

Singru, P. S., Sakharkar, J. A., and Subhedar, N. (2003). Neuronal nitric oxide synthase in the olfactory system of an adult teleost fish *Oreochromis mossambicus*. *Brain Res.* 977, 157–168.

Skeen, L. C., and Hall, W. C. (1977). Efferent projections of the main and the accessory olfactory bulb in the tree shrew (*Tupaia glis*). *J. Comp. Neurol.* 172, 1–35.

Slaby, O. (1987). Morphological differences between the structure of the nasal apparatus of the swift (*Apus apus* L.) and the common "avian typus" during morphogenesis. Morphogenesis of the nasal capsule, the epithelial nasal tube and the organ of Jacobson in sauropsida. XVIII. *Folia Morphol.* 35, 436–440.

Slotnick, B., Restrepo, D., Schellinck, H., Archbold, G., Price, S., and Lin, W. (2010). Accessory olfactory bulb function is modulated by input from the main olfactory epithelium. *Eur. J. Neurosci.* 31, 1108–1116.

Smeets, W. J. (1983). The secondary olfactory connections in two chondrichthians, the shark Scyliorhinus canicula and the ray *Raja clavata*. *J. Comp. Neurol.* 218, 334–344.

Smeets, W. J. (1988). Distribution of dopamine immunoreactivity in the forebrain and midbrain of the snake Python regius: a study with antibodies against dopamine. *J. Comp. Neurol.* 271, 115–129.

Smeets, W. J., Hoogland, V. P., and Voorn, P. (1986). The distribution of dopamine immunoreactivity in the forebrain and midbrain of the lizard Gekko gecko: an immunohistochemical study with antibodies against dopamine. *J. Comp. Neurol.* 253, 46–60.

Smeets, W. J., Jonker, A. J., and Hoogland, P. V. (1987). Distribution of dopamine in the forebrain and midbrain of the red-eared turtle, Pseudemys scripta elegans, reinvestigated using antibodies against dopamine. *Brain Behav. Evol.* 30, 121–142.

Smeets, W. J., and Steinbusch, H. W. (1990). New insights into the reptilian catecholaminergic systems as revealed by antibodies against the neurotransmitters and their synthetic enzymes. *J. Chem. Neuroanat.* 3, 25–43.

Smith, T. D., and Bhatnagar, K. P. (2000). The human vomeronasal organ. Part II: prenatal development. *J. Anat.* 197(Pt 3), 421–436.

Smith, T. D., Buttery, T. A., Bhatnagar, K. P., Burrows, A. M., Mooney, M. P., and Siegel, M. I. (2001). Anatomical position of the vomeronasal organ in postnatal humans. *Ann. Anat.* 183, 475–479.

Smith, T. D., Siegel, M. I., Burrows, A. M., Mooney, M. P., Burdi, A. R., Fabrizio, P. A., and Clemente, F. R. (1998). Searching for the vomeronasal organ of adult humans: preliminary findings on location, structure, and size. *Microsc. Res. Tech.* 41, 483–491.

Steiger, S. S., Fidler, A. E., Valcu, M., and Kempenaers, B. (2008). Avian olfactory receptor gene repertoires: evidence for a well-developed sense of smell in birds? *Proc. Biol. Sci.* 275, 2309–2317.

Steiger, S. S., Kuryshev, V. Y., Stensmyr, M. C., Kempenaers, B., and Mueller, J. C. (2009). A comparison of reptilian and avian olfactory receptor gene repertoires: species-specific expansion of group gamma genes in birds. *BMC Genomics* 10, 446. doi: 10.1186/1471-2164-10-446

Stensaas, L. J., Lavker, R. M., Monti-Bloch, L., Grosser, B. I., and Berliner, D. L. (1991). Ultrastructure of the human vomeronasal organ. *J. Steroid Biochem. Mol. Biol.* 39, 553–560.

Suzuki, N. (1984). Anterograde fluorescent labeling of olfactory receptor neurons by Procion and Lucifer dyes. *Brain Res.* 311, 181–185.

Switzer, R. C. 3rd, and Johnson, J. I. Jr. (1977). Absence of mitral cells in monolayer in monotremes. Variations in vertebrate olfactory bulbs. *Acta Anat.* 99, 36–42.

Takigami, S., Mori, Y., Tanioka, Y., and Ichikawa, M. (2004). Morphological evidence for two types of mammalian vomeronasal system. *Chem. Senses* 29, 301–310.

Taniguchi, K., Saito, S., and Oikawa, T. (2008). Phylogenic aspects of the amphibian dual olfactory system. *J. Vet. Med. Sci.* 70, 1–9.

Thornhill, R. A. (1967). The ultrastructure of the olfactory epithelium of the lamprey *Lampetra fluviatilis*. *J. Cell Sci.* 2, 591–602.

Trotier, D., Eloit, C., Wassef, M., Talmain, G., Bensimon, J. L., Doving, K. B., and Ferrand, J. (2000). The vomeronasal cavity in adult humans. *Chem. Senses* 25, 369–380.

Turner, B. H., Gupta, K. C., and Mishkin, M. (1978). The locus and cytoarchitecture of the projection areas of the olfactory bulb in *Macaca mulatta*. *J. Comp. Neurol.* 177, 381–396.

VanDenbossche, J., Seelye, J. G., and Zielinski, B. S. (1995). The morphology of the olfactory epithelium in larval, juvenile and upstream migrant stages of the sea lamprey, *Petromyzon marinus*. *Brain Behav. Evol.* 45, 19–24.

Von Campenhause, H., and Mori, K. (2000). Convergence of segregated pheromonal pathways from the accesory olfactory bulb to the cortex in the mouse. *Eur. J. Neurosci.* 12, 33–46.

Wang, R. T., and Halpern, M. (1982a). Neurogenesis in the vomeronasal epithelium of adult garter snakes. 1. Degeneration of bipolar neurons and proliferation of undifferentiated cells following experimental vomeronasal axotomy. *Brain Res.* 237, 23–39.

Wang, R. T., and Halpern, M. (1982b). Neurogenesis in the vomeronasal epithelium of adult garter snakes. 2. Reconstitution of the bipolar neuron layer following experimental vomeronasal axotomy. *Brain Res.* 237, 41–59.

Wang, R. T., and Halpern, M. (1988). Neurogenesis in the vomeronasal epithelium of adult garter snakes: 3. Use of H3-thymidine autoradiography to trace the genesis and migration of bipolar neurons. *Am. J. Anat.* 183, 178–185.

Westerman, R. A., and Wilson, J. A. (1968). The fine structure of the olfactory tract in the teleost *Carassius carassius* L. *Z Zellforsch Mikrosk Anat.* 91, 186–199.

Wilson, J. A., and Westerman, R. A. (1967). The fine structure of the olfactory mucosa and nerver in the teleost *Carassius carassius* L. *Z Zellforsch Mikrosk Anat.* 83, 196–206.

Winans, S. S., and Scalia, F. (1970). Amygdaloid nucleus: new afferent input from the vomeronasal organ. *Science* 170, 330–332.

Witt, M., Georgiewa, B., Knecht, M., and Hummel, T. (2002). On the chemosensory nature of the vomeronasal epithelium in adult humans. *Histochem. Cell Biol.* 117, 493–509.

Witt, M., and Hummel, T. (2006). Vomeronasal versus olfactory epithelium: is there a cellular basis for human vomeronasal perception? *Int. Rev. Cytol.* 248, 209–259.

Witt, M., and Wozniak, W. (2006). Structure and function of the vomeronasal organ. *Adv. Otorhinolaryngol.* 63, 70–83.

Woodley, S. K. (2010). Pheromonal communication in amphibians. *J. Comp. Physiol. A. Neuroethol. Sens. Neural Behav. Physiol.* 196, 713–727.

Xu, F., Schaefer, M., Kida, I., Schafer, J., Liu, N., Rothman, D. L., Hyder, F., Restrepo, D., and Shepherd, G. M. (2005). Simultaneous activation of mouse main and accessory olfactory bulbs by odors or pheromones. *J. Comp. Neurol.* 489, 491–500.

Young, J. M., Friedman, C., Williams, E. M., Ross, J. A., Tonnes-Priddy, L., and Trask, B. J. (2002). Different evolutionary processes shaped the mouse and human olfactory receptor gene families. *Hum. Mol. Genet.* 11, 535–546.

Yuen, A. P., Fan, Y. W., Fung, C. F., and Hung, K. N. (2005). Endoscopic-assisted cranionasal resection of olfactory neuroblastoma. *Head Neck* 27, 488–493.

Zaccone, D., Cascio, P. L., Lauriano, R., Pergolizzi, S., Sfacteria, A., and Marino, F. (2010). Occurrence of neuropeptides and tyrosine hydroxylase in the olfactory epithelium of the lesser-spotted catshark (*Scyliorhinus canicula* Linnaeus, 1758). *Acta Histochem.* doi:10.1016/j.acthis.2010.09.010

Conflict of Interest Statement: The authors declare that the research was conducted in the absence of any commercial or financial relationships that could be construed as a potential conflict of interest.

14

The microcircuit concept applied to cortical evolution: from three-layer to six-layer cortex

Gordon M. Shepherd*

Department of Neurobiology, Yale University School of Medicine, New Haven, CT, USA

Edited by:
Fernando Martinez-Garcia, Universidad de Valencia, Spain

Reviewed by:
Bartlett W. Mel, University of Southern California, USA
Arnold Kriegstein, University of California San Francisco, USA

****Correspondence:***
Gordon M. Shepherd, Department of Neurobiology, Yale University School of Medicine, 333 Cedar Street, New Haven, CT 06510, USA.
e-mail: gordon.shepherd@yale.edu

Understanding the principles of organization of the cerebral cortex requires insight into its evolutionary history. This has traditionally been the province of anatomists, but evidence regarding the microcircuit organization of different cortical areas is providing new approaches to this problem. Here we use the microcircuit concept to focus first on the principles of microcircuit organization of three-layer cortex in the olfactory cortex, hippocampus, and turtle general cortex, and compare it with six-layer neocortex. From this perspective it is possible to identify basic circuit elements for recurrent excitation and lateral inhibition that are common across all the cortical regions. Special properties of the apical dendrites of pyramidal cells are reviewed that reflect the specific adaptations that characterize the functional operations in the different regions. These principles of microcircuit function provide a new approach to understanding the expanded functional capabilities elaborated by the evolution of the neocortex.

Keywords: olfactory cortex, dorsal general cortex, hippocampus, neocortex, pyramidal neuron, recurrent excitation, recurrent inhibition, apical dendrite

Recent evidence is allowing the patterns of synaptic organization in different brain regions to come more clearly into focus. These patterns have been characterized by various terms, including organization by contact (Ramon y Cajal, 1911), synaptic organization, basic circuit (Shepherd, 1974), local circuit (Rakic, 1976), canonical circuit (Douglas et al., 1989), and microcircuit (Byrne et al., 1978; Shepherd, 1978, 1994; Grillner et al., 2005; Graybiel and Grillner, 2006; Shepherd and Grillner, 2010). Whatever the terms used, the concepts are proving increasingly important in helping to guide experimental analysis of a system and construct computational simulations that aid the experimental analysis.

A brain microcircuit has been defined as the organization of nerve cells into specific patterns that carry out the information processing characteristic of a given brain region. This concept has been used to test whether it can provide the basis for comparing the principles of organization across different brain systems, in order to identify common principles as well as the special adaptations for each region. An early example was common principles across phyla in comparing mammalian and insect olfactory systems (Hildebrand and Shepherd, 1997). Microcircuits for over 50 brain regions, in both vertebrates and invertebrates, have been recently published (Shepherd and Grillner, 2010).

If this approach has merit in comparing different brain systems, it should be of further value in comparing systems for insights into evolution. Here we apply this approach to the evolution of the cerebral cortex. The key problem is well recognized. The cerebral cortex of fish, amphibians and reptiles is characterized by three layers, whereas mammals have developed a new type of "neocortex" with six layers (reviewed in Striedter, 2005). One of the most challenging problems in vertebrate evolution is understanding how this happened. (Solving this problem is not helped by the confusing terminology for the different parts of the cortex: see Swanson, 2000 for a discussion of this question.)

The problem is usually addressed looking backward from the neocortex. An alternative is a prospective view, beginning with three-layer cortex. This started with early work on olfactory cortex, perhaps the region of the cerebral cortex least changed through vertebrate evolution, hippocampus, and reptilian dorsal cortex. In the mammal, three-layer cortex persists in the olfactory cortex and the hippocampus. Early work (Shepherd, 1974, 1988; Smith et al., 1980; and Kriegstein and Connors, 1986) provided evidence for the hypothesis that these regions of three-layer cortex contain the basic microcircuit core that has been elaborated in six-layer neocortex.

This review will update that hypothesis, drawing together earlier and more recent work on cortical microcircuits to provide new evidence for how this might have occurred. A broad synthesis such as this is needed not only for fresh approaches to the problem of neocortical evolution, but also for providing a framework for integrating parallel approaches using molecular and genetic approaches. This framework should also contribute eventually to a better understanding of the new functions enabled by a neocortical architecture. I apologize that space does not permit citing of all the relevant literature.

CORTICAL MICROCIRCUITS: THE BASIC HYPOTHESIS

The traditional method for analyzing brain evolution has been neuroanatomy, with a focus on comparing such features as size and number of brain areas, patterns of cell lamination, and the connections between areas. However, a new approach at the cellular and microcircuit level became possible in the 1970s with the new studies revealing patterns of synaptic organization. This provided the first evidence for basic patterns of organization that are similar across different regions. This included the three main regions of the mammalian cerebral cortex: olfactory cortex, hippocampus, and neocortex. On this basis:

> It is suggested that the study of synaptic organization provides a basis for distinguishing certain characteristics of local organization that may be termed cortical.... It implies that certain modes of information processing are possible with a cortical type of organization that are not possible with other, noncortical, types.
>
> ...the study of synaptic organization [is] the necessary basis for understanding the particular contribution of the cortex to mammalian and human behavior. (Shepherd, 1974)

One of the first basic cortical circuits to be identified was of mammalian olfactory cortex. **Figure 1** (top) provides a reminder that olfactory cortex is defined as the main region that receives direct input through the lateral olfactory tract (LOT) from the output cells (mitral and tufted) of the olfactory bulb. We focus here on the region occupying the piriform cortex beneath and adjacent to the LOT. The hippocampus is located in the medial temporal area, and neocortex in the dorsal part, as we discuss below.

We begin by noting several features of the anatomy of the cells. First, the principal neurons have apical dendrites with radial parallel orientations; second, the principal neurons are situated within a framework of a non-repeating sequence of layers; and third, the principal neurons are graded in their size and morphology in the different layers. We will see these properties repeated in all the cortices of the forebrain.

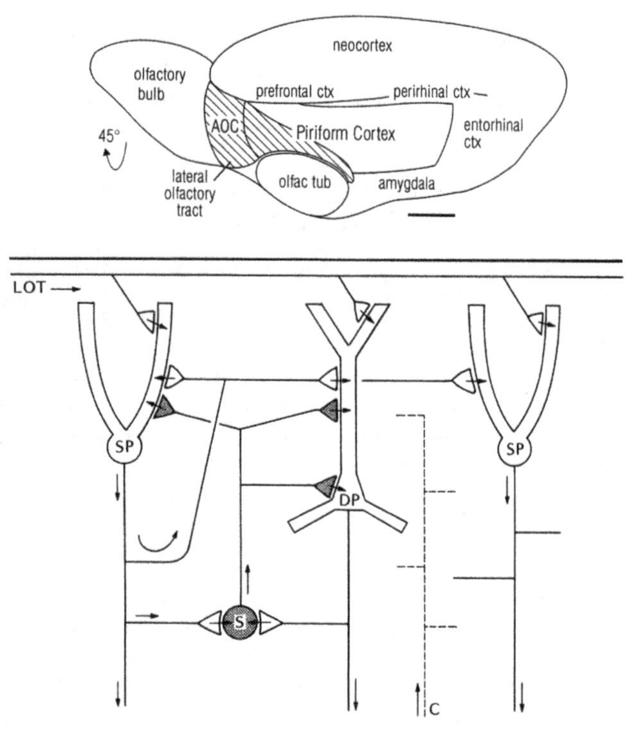

FIGURE 1 | Top: Olfactory cortical areas on the ventrolateral surface of the cerebrum of the rat. Abbreviations: AOC, anterior olfactory cortex; ctx, cortex; olfac tub, olfactory tubercle. From Neville and Haberly (2004). Bottom: Basic circuit of the mammalian piriform (olfactory) cortex. Abbreviations: LOT, lateral olfactory tract; SP, superficial pyramidal cell; DP, deep pyramidal cell; S, stellate cell; C, centrifugal fiber. Arrows indicate direction of flow of activity. Open profiles: excitatory synaptic action; filled profiles: inhibitory synaptic action. From Shepherd (1974).

Single cell recordings from the cat, and from a primitive mammal, the opossum, revealed the basic EPSP–IPSP responses of pyramidal cells to single shocks in the LOT, and the responses of interneurons (Biedenbach and Stevens, 1969; Haberly, 1973a,b). This provided a local circuit for excitation of the pyramidal cells through their distal apical dendrites, and recurrent feedback inhibition through their axon collaterals onto interneurons. A key further finding, using current source density analysis, was of pyramidal cell recurrent excitatory collaterals back onto pyramidal cell apical dendrites (Haberly and Shepherd, 1973).

To summarize these results, a basic circuit was composed, consisting of distal dendritic excitatory input to the pyramidal cells, which then generate recurrent excitation (RE) and recurrent inhibition (Haberly and Shepherd, 1973; see **Figure 1** bottom). These three synaptic operations were proposed to be key features of cerebral cortex in general (Shepherd, 1974).

The first place to test this hypothesis was the other main type of three-layer cortex in the mammal, the hippocampus. The basic anatomical connections within the hippocampus had been laid out by Ramon y Cajal (1911). The electrophysiology of the hippocampal pyramidal cell began with Andersen (1960) and Kandel et al. (1961), and the functional organization of the hippocampal circuits began to be revealed by the new work in the hippocampal slice (Andersen et al., 1971; Skrede and Westgaard, 1971). This gave rise to the classical three-synapse model (**Figure 2**).

At first glance the hippocampal circuit seems different from the olfactory cortex, with the special relay through the dentate gyrus, and the sequence of activation of CA3 followed by CA1. However, there are similarities: the excitatory inputs to the apical dendrites of CA3 and CA1 pyramidal cells, the recurrent excitatory axon collaterals of CA3 pyramidal cells onto CA3 and CA1 pyramidal cells, and the activation of local inhibitory feedback, could be seen as adaptations of the simpler architecture of the olfactory cortex.

Compared with these early successes, studies of the basic connectivity within the mammalian neocortex had barely begun. Nonetheless, evidence was obtained for thalamocortical activation of pyramidal cells, and the two types of actions through their axon collaterals: direct RE, and recurrent inhibition through inhibitory interneurons (see Phillips, 1959). There was an additional circuit element, thalamocortical activation through stellate cells onto the pyramidal cells, which could be viewed as analogous to the situation in the dentate and hippocampus, as an additional internal relay in the input pathway. An early version of the basic circuit for neocortex is shown in **Figure 3**.

In comparing these three early basic circuits, the common elements are evident: activation through apical dendrites, RE, and recurrent and lateral inhibition, both playing back onto different levels of the apical dendrites. That these basic features of the three-layer cortices should be embedded in the neocortex carried the seeds of a new way of thinking about cortical evolution.

TURTLE DORSAL CORTEX

This new way of thinking was stimulated by studies in reptilian forebrain of dorsal cortex, also called general cortex. This receives input from the thalamus, and is of special interest as occupying a position which can be regarded as a precursor of neocortex, based

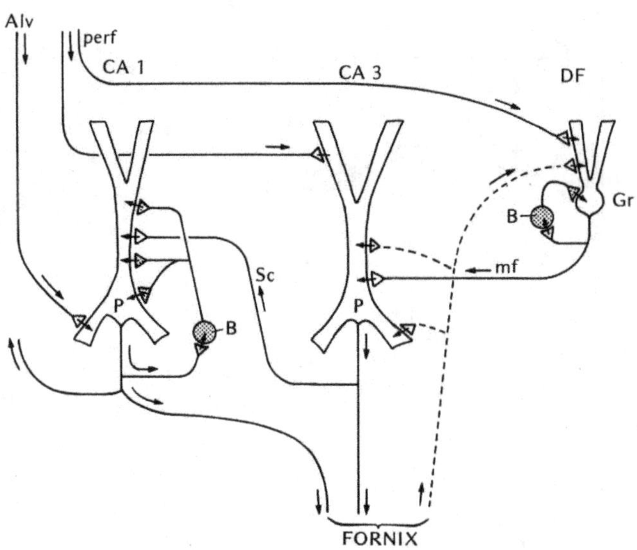

FIGURE 2 | Basic circuit of the mammalian hippocampus and dentate fascia. Abbreviations: Alv, alveus; perf, perforant pathway; CA1, CA3: regions of the hippocampus; DF, dentate fascia; P, pyramidal cell; B, basket cell; Gr, granule cell; mf, mossy fiber; Sc, Schaffer collateral. Arrows indicate direction of flow of activity. Open profiles: excitatory synaptic action; filled profiles: inhibitory synaptic action. From Shepherd (1974).

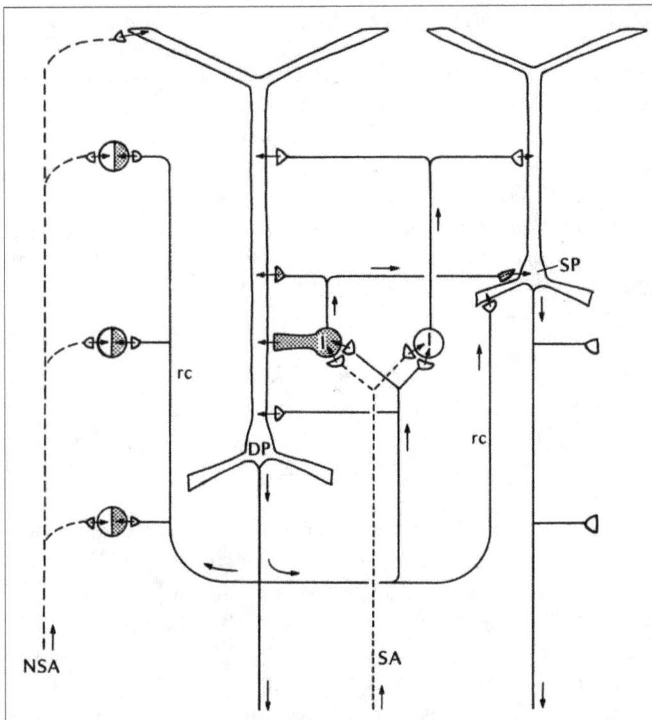

FIGURE 3 | Basic circuit of the mammalian neocortex. Abbreviations: SA, specific sensory afferents; NSA, non-specific sensory afferents; DP, deep pyramidal cell; SP, superficial pyramidal cell; I, intrinsic neurons (excitatory stellate cells and inhibitory interneurons are lumped together); rc, recurrent collateral. Arrows indicate direction of flow of activity. Open profiles: excitatory synaptic action; filled profiles: inhibitory synaptic action. From Shepherd (1974).

on its position, shown in **Figure 4** (left), on the dorsal surface of the forebrain, flanked on either side by the olfactory cortex and hippocampus. The strategy of exploring this cortex was explicit in a pioneering study by Smith et al. (1980):

> We have been studying cortical organization in the adult turtle because this neural system is simple enough for quantitative analysis, yet similar enough in its extrinsic connections to provide a model for some features of mammalian neocortex.

Building on previous studies in mammals using electronmicroscopy to observe degenerating axon terminals following unilateral ablation of the thalamus, they found synaptic connections onto spines of pyramidal cells and smooth dendrites of stellate interneurons. This suggested a pattern of organization in which there are feedforward as well as feedback inhibitory connections from stellate cells onto pyramidal cells (see **Figure 4**).

Stimulated by this anatomical study and the previous physiological studies of cortical organization, Connors and Kriegstein (1986; also Kriegstein and Connors, 1986) then undertook a landmark study to characterize the electrophysiological properties of these cells in a slice preparation of the turtle dorsal cortex. Using a combination of cell labeling, focal electrical stimulation, and responses to single volleys, they characterized the synaptic connections and physiological properties of both the pyramidal and stellate cells. Consistent with Smith et al. (1980), they found that thalamic afferents excite both pyramidal cell distal dendrites and stellate cells. They also obtained evidence that the stellate cells provide for both feedforward and feedback inhibition of the pyramidal cells. Finally, they also showed feedback excitation from the pyramidal cells back onto pyramidal cells.

They integrated their results by building on the circuit diagram of Smith et al. (1980). As shown in **Figure 5**, they also took into account the previous basic circuit diagrams for the other types of cortices in order to make comparisons with them. They summarized their conclusions as follows (Kriegstein and Connors, 1986):

> The general synaptic organization of turtle general cortex shows striking similarities with those of other cerebral cortical structures, including the pyriform cortex, hippocampus, and neocortex of several well-studied mammalian species (Shepherd, 1979). Each cortex has a principal cell type (or group of subtypes) that features prominent, spinous apical dendrites, and one or more types of sparsely spinous, GABA-utilizing interneuron. Similarities exist for both the general plan of local circuitry and the physiology of the synapses themselves. The uniqueness of each cortex is, of course, specified by many differences of organization. A comparison of these properties between and within species may yield clues about the principles of cortical function and its evolution.

The work of Smith et al. (1980) and of Kriegstein and Connors (1986) thus combined the previous work in the other cortical regions to suggest a new approach to understanding cortical evolution, focused on analysis of intrinsic circuit organization in different regions with detailed comparisons between them of specific circuits for basic functional operations.

SUMMARY OF THE EARLY CONCEPTS

These early studies were summarized in a review (Shepherd, 1988) whose aim was to test the original proposal that "there is a set of basic principles that governs the organization of intrinsic circuits

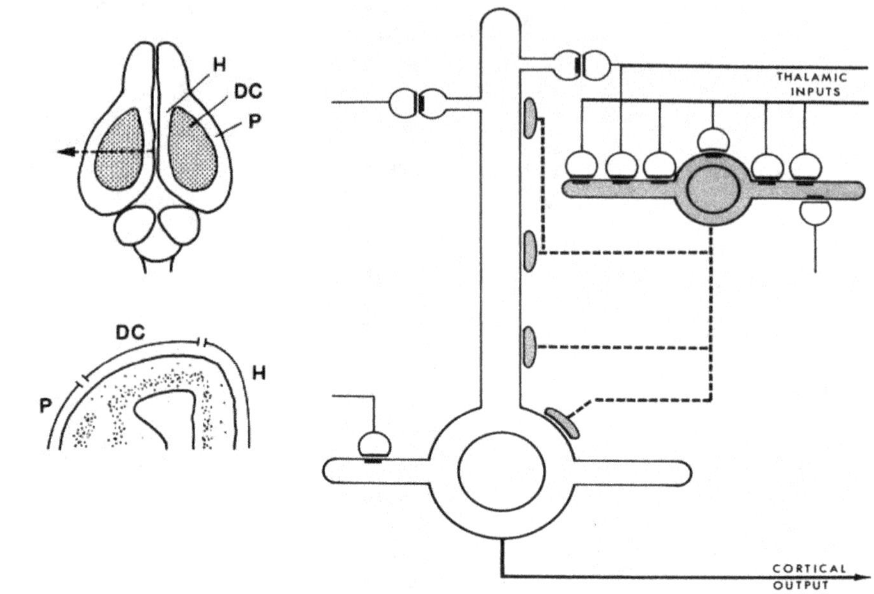

FIGURE 4 | Left, above: Dorsal view of the turtle brain. Abbreviations: DC, dorsal cortex; H, hippocampus; P, piriform (olfactory) cortex. Below, cross section of forebrain at level of arrow in top diagram. From Connors and Kriegstein (1986). Right: Model of circuit in turtle dorsal cortex based on degeneration studies of connectivity from the thalamus and resulting calculations. The circuit is dominated by massive thalamic input to inhibitory interneurons, which provide massive feedforward inhibition to the pyramidal neurons. Both pyramidal cells and interneurons also receive excitatory input from unspecified sources. Open profiles: excitatory synaptic action; filled profiles: inhibitory synaptic action. From Smith et al. (1980).

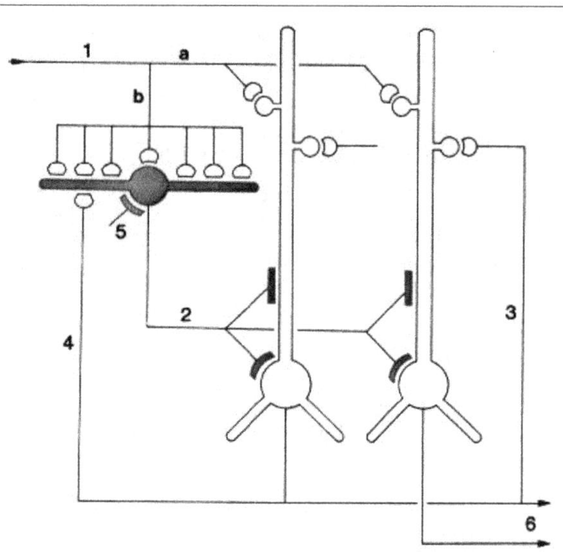

FIGURE 5 | "Schematic diagram of the principal intracortical connections of the turtle visual cortex based on neuroanatomical data (Smith et al., 1980) and the physiological observations reported here. Thalamocortical afferent volleys (1) provide direct excitation of pyramidal cell dendrites (a) and also powerfully excite inhibitory stellate cells (b). Feedforward inhibition is mediated by stellate cell-pyramidal cell contact (2). Local pathways also mediate reciprocal excitation between pyramidal cells (3) as well as feedback inhibition through pyramidal cell-stellate cell conact (4). There is also physiological support for inhibition of stellate interneurons (5), presumably arising from stellate cell-stellate cell contact. The pyramidal cells provide output from the cortex (6) by way of axons coursing primarily in the subcellular zone." Kriegstein and Connors (1986). Open profiles: excitatory synaptic action; filled profiles: inhibitory synaptic action.

Table 1 | Summary of elements common to cortical circuits (Shepherd, 1988).

Pyramidal cells with apical and basal dendrites;
Excitatory inputs to distal dendritic spines of pyramidal cells;
Feedforward inhibition through inhibitory interneurons;
Feedback and lateral inhibition through pyramidal cell axon collaterals;
Feedback excitation through pyramidal cell axon collaterals;
Modulation of pyramidal cell activity through layered inputs to apical dendrite and soma.

in the main types of cerebral cortex." A detailed consideration of the anatomy and physiology of the cells and intrinsic circuits in the three regions of three-layer cortex, and in six-layer neocortex, supported the proposal. At this stage, those key specific circuits could be summarized in **Table 1**.

It was emphasized that this common set of circuit elements was analogous to the common set of bones constituting the basic vertebrate skeleton. Just as the hand has been adapted from forelimb digits by evolutionary pressures, so have the circuit elements of the basic cortical microcircuit become adapted during neocortical evolution. It was suggested that these adaptations included addition of new neurons, new types of output neurons, new types of interneurons, and new types of intracortical connections and connection patterns. It was further suggested that novel physiological properties may have appeared, such as deployment of active properties in the dendrites, and the elaboration of second messengers and other biochemical mechanisms. In this way the basic circuit provides the substrate for evolving new functions during evolution. Specifically,

> ... there is an underlying logic to the construction of cortical local circuits and microcircuits that provides a common modular framework that is adapted to generate the special properties of the neocortex.

Among the circuit elements that may be critical for cortical processing, the dendritic spines are of special interest. It was noted that the large number on distal dendrites moves the site of synaptic inputs away from having a direct effect on spike generation at the soma, and makes the effects of those inputs "contingent on specific combinations of inputs and cascades of non-linear interactions between the spine." (Shepherd, 1988).

This period in the 1980s also saw the introduction of neural networks based on parallel processing for the purpose of simulating brain function (Rumelhart and McClelland, 1986). These were based on representations of neurons as single summing nodes, in contrast with the complex dendritic branching patterns and spatio-temporal integration in real neurons. The networks are characterized by all-to-all connectivity, in contrast to the specific connectivity of most neurons. An aim of the review was to clarify the limitations of this network architecture by showing the elements of the local circuits – particularly including the properties of dendrites and dendritic spines, and the specificity of excitatory and inhibitory interactions – that should be built into neural network models in order to simulate more accurately human cognitive functions, a goal that unfortunately still is far from realized (see also Shepherd, 1990).

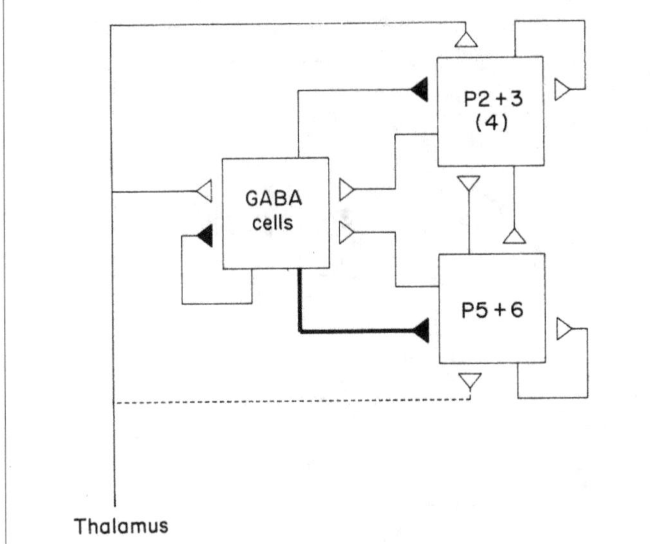

FIGURE 6 | A canonical microcircuit for mammalian visual cortex. P2 + 3 represent pyramidal cells of the superficial 2 and 3 layers of visual cortex. Also included are the stellate cells of layer 4, indicated by (4), whose properties resemble those of the superficial pyramidal cells. P5 + 6 represent pyramidal cells of the deep five and six layers. GABA cells represent inhibitory interneurons of all types. Strength of functional connection is indicated by thickness of line. The thalamic input is relatively limited in terms of numbers of synapses, but is amplified by the strong recurrent excitatory connections. From Douglas et al. (1989).

A CANONICAL NEOCORTICAL CIRCUIT

The emerging concept of a basic circuit for the neocortex was expressed in a distinct form in the "canonical cortical microcircuit" of Douglas et al. (1989). This was based on experimental studies in visual cortex of interactions between two populations of pyramidal neurons, superficial and deep, and a population of interneurons (**Figure 6**; stellate cells, being spiny, were grouped with the pyramidal cells). The pyramidal (and stellate) neurons are glutamatergic and excitatory, the interneurons GABAergic and inhibitory. Each pyramidal neuron population has intracortical connections onto three targets: itself (feedback excitation through its own axon collaterals); similarly on the other set of pyramidal neurons; and the population of inhibitory interneurons (giving rise to feed back inhibition onto its own population and onto the other population of pyramidal neurons). The inhibitory interneurons accordingly are excited by each population of pyramidal neurons and inhibit each population, as well as inhibiting themselves. Different weights of excitation and inhibition are indicated by the thickness of the arrows. The thalamic input is shown activating mainly the stellate cells of layer 4, which, being spiny and excitatory, are regarded as having properties similar to those of the spiny superficial pyramidal cells.

This scheme enabled Douglas et al. (2004) to summarize several important features of cortical connectivity and dynamics from their own and previous work. The preponderance of connections is between the excitatory pyramidal cells, including re-excitation. Because thalamic synapses account for only some 10% of the connections in the cortex, the excitatory and re-excitatory connections may be important in selectively amplifying the thalamic inputs. However, re-excitation is potentially dangerous in leading to hyperexcitability and seizures. Inhibition is therefore needed to oppose or modulate this potentially strong excitation. Cortical circuits can thus be seen to be poised on the knife edge of excitation restrained by inhibition, one of the risks of the computational power of the cortical microcircuit (see also below).

The canonical circuit of **Figure 6** can be seen to depict in flow-chart form the essential connectivity of the basic cortical circuit shown in **Figure 3**. It has been useful for testing for basic elements in neocortical microcircuits, as described further below.

FROM THREE LAYERS TO SIX LAYERS

In support of the hypothesis of Smith et al. (1980) and Kriegstein and Connors (1986), the intrinsic organization of three-layer cortical areas as a basis for the evolution of six-layer neocortex was made explicit in a hypothesis in 1994, which stated:

> These facts suggest that the basic circuit for olfactory–hippocampal–general cortex may represent a framework that has been elaborated into the neocortex in the course of mammalian evolution.

The hypothesis is illustrated in the diagrams of **Figure 7**. The basic circuit common to three-layer cortices is shown in A. The common elements of primary afferents, intrinsic circuits for feed-forward inhibition (FI) and lateral inhibition (LI), and RE, are indicated by the labels.

The possible evolutionary relation to six-layer neocortex is indicated by the arrow. The direct input from thalamus to pyramidal cells, characteristic of three-layer cortex, is indicated by the dashed lines. In addition, six-layer cortex has a new class of stellate cells, which also receive thalamocortical input, and relay it to

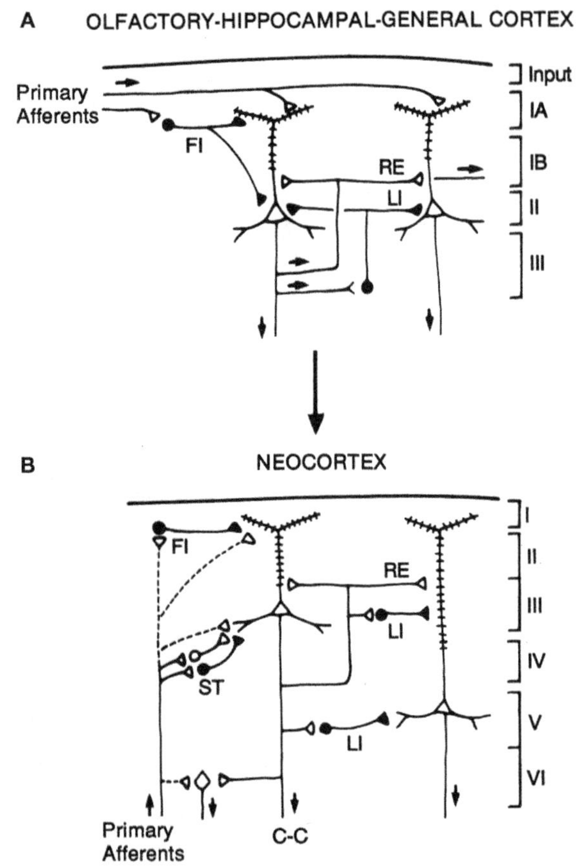

FIGURE 7 | Hypothesized relations between canonical microcircuits for three-layer simple cortex and six-layer neocortex. (A) Simplified representation of the three main types of three-layer microcircuits: olfactory (piriform) cortex, hippocampus; general (dorsal) reptilian cortex. Abbreviations: FI, feedforward inhibition; LI, lateral inhibition; RE, recurrent excitation. For the hippocampus, primary afferents represent the perforant pathway; RE represent the Schaffer collaterals, and LI represent local inhibitory feedback. Pyramidal cells and inhibitory interneurons as in **Figure 3**. Cortical layers shown on right. **(B)** Canonical microcircuit for neocortex. Abbreviations: same as A; C-C, cortico-cortical fibers; ST, stellate cell cortical layers shown on right. Arrows indicate direction of flow of activity. Open profiles: excitatory synaptic action; filled profiles: inhibitory synaptic action. From Shepherd (1994).

the pyramidal cells. In granular cortex such as the primary visual area, the stellate cells are concentrated in layer 4; in agranular cortex such as motor areas, the stellate cells are distributed in several layers. The stellate cells can be seen to constitute a kind of internal forward relay interposed between the afferents and the pyramidal cells, serving as a staging "preprocessing" site for transforming the thalamic input into its cortical form. This may be necessary because the thalamic input constitutes scarcely 10% of the synaptic connections in its layers of termination (Douglas and Martin, 2010); the vast majority come from intrinsic and cortico-cortical connections.

Apart from this difference in the input, the other main difference from three-layer cortex is the division into a superficial cortex (layers 1–3) and a deep cortex (layers 4–5), characterized by superficial and deep pyramidal cells, as indicated in the diagram. However, the diagram reiterates the original basic circuit of **Figure 1**, in showing that the pyramidal cells have their intrinsic circuits for LI and RE (not all possible combinations are shown for simplicity).

With this approach it was possible to begin to identify properties that are special about the basic circuit of the neocortex. First, it is accessible to every major sensory input, either directly from olfactory cortex or indirectly through the thalamus. Similarly, it provides a wide variety of motor outputs, that reach all levels of the neuraxis, from the cortex itself through the basal ganglia and brainstem to the spinal cord. Second, it expands the single layer of pyramidal cells in dorsal cortex to the superficial (layers 2–3) and deep (layers 5,6) layers of neocortex. This greatly expands the combinatorial possibilities for intracortical processing. Third, in contrast to dorsal cortex where the afferents come in at the top, the afferents ascend from the depths and efferents descend through the same layers. This means that both input and output have potential access to all the cells in every layer. When the intrinsic circuits through the axon collaterals and interneurons are added, the result is that "the potential ways by which information can be integrated, stored, and recombined becomes enormous" (Shepherd, 1994). Fourth, whereas in most regions there are one or two types of output neuron, in the cortex each layer is the potential source of output, either locally between layers (cells in layer 1 and 4) or distantly (cells in layers 2,3 and 5,6). This means that each layer can function as a semi-independent input-output unit, defined by its own unique combination of inputs, intrinsic connections, interactions with other layers, and output targets.

The final advantage of six-layer "neocortex" is that it arose in a favorable position from dorsal "general" cortex. On the flanks of dorsal cortex were olfactory cortex on the ventral lateral side and hippocampus on the medial side, both hemmed in by their locations. By contrast, dorsal cortex had the opportunity to expand, but on one condition: that the brain case could expand to give it room. This occurred throughout mammalian evolution, enabling neocortex to enlarge individual areas such as the major sensory receiving cortices or motor areas, or adding new areas such as for speech, "in order to combine information from new combinations of inputs or control different combinations of output targets." (Shepherd, 1994). An expanded summary of these properties common to three-layer cortex and elaborated in six-layer cortex is provided in **Table 2**.

TESTING THE HYPOTHESIS: RECENT STUDIES OF CORTICAL MICROCIRCUITS

This microcircuit approach provides a framework within which to assess studies of cortical properties at the neuron and circuit level. We consider recent and current work from this perspective. This work has focused on the two main types of neuron: pyramidal neuron and interneuron, and the two main types of connections between them: recurrent excitatory and inhibitory pathways through the pyramidal cell axon collaterals. Within the pyramidal neurons, the information processing that occurs in their dendrites is of key importance. We consider each of these features in turn, beginning with the axon collateral pathways for RE and inhibition.

OLFACTORY CORTEX AS A CONTENT-ADDRESSABLE MEMORY

We are accustomed to thinking of the inputs to the hippocampus and to visual cortex in terms of spatial patterns, but what about olfactory cortex? Work in the olfactory bulb (Sharp et al., 1975;

Table 2 | Current summary of the elements characterizing the microcircuit organization of three-layer and six-layer forebrain cortex.

1. Both three-layer and six-layer cortex are built on pyramidal cells with apical and basal dendritic trees.
2. Strong excitatory afferents are received in the spines of the branches of the apical and basal dendrites.
3. The spines and local branches create local sites with varying degrees of local information processing properties.
4. The spines, local branches, and main stems contain different combinations of Na, K, and Ca ionic channels, which create local sites of integration and boosting of input signals to reach the sites of action potential output in the cell body and axon hillock.
5. The pyramidal cells have well developed recurrent axon collaterals
6. The axon collaterals give rise to two main types of intrinsic circuit.
7. One type is direct feedback and lateral recurrent excitation.
8. This excitatory recurrent system has long lateral extensions, which enable widespread recombination of intrinsic excitation with the excitatory afferent input
9. The other type is feedback and lateral inhibition through inhibitory interneurons
10. Inhibitory interneurons are subdivided into multiple types which target different sites and levels of the soma-dendritic extent of the pyramidal cells.
11. Cortical information processing therefore involves a continual balance between excitatory and inhibitory circuits.
12. In three-layer cortex, these intrinsic circuits are organized around a single layer of pyramidal and pyramidal like neurons.
13. Five- and six-layer neocortex appears an expansion of the three-layer microcircuit into closely integrated superficial and deep layers.
14. Cortico-cortical afferents make synapses at different levels of the pyramidal cell soma-dendritic axis to excite, inhibit, or modulate the transfer of synaptic inputs and extent of backpropagating action potentials in the dendritic trees.
15. Brainstem systems provide differential modulation in different layers.

Stewart et al., 1979) using the 2-deoxyglucose activity mapping method showed that odor stimulation gives rise to spatial patterns of activity in the glomerular layer. Different odors produced different patterns, providing strong evidence that odor molecules are represented in the olfactory system by different spatial activity patterns, and that these are further processed by circuits in the olfactory bulb and olfactory cortex as the basis for odor perception and discrimination. This functional evidence for spatial patterns was strongly supported by the subsequent evidence for spatial organization of the projections of the olfactory receptor cells (Vassar et al., 1994; Ressler et al., 1994).

While the 2DG studies showed clear activity patterns in the olfactory bulb, they showed only diffuse uptake in the olfactory cortex (Sharp et al., 1977). This and other evidence indicated that the diffuse projections to the olfactory cortex, together with the internal system of long association fibers, provide for widespread processing of a given odor there. Based on these properties, Haberly (1985) suggested in a key paper that the olfactory cortex acts as a "content-addressable memory" system in which each site in the system contains information about the entire input. This fundamental insight has been the main organizing principle for understanding information processing in the olfactory cortex. Beginning with Wilson and Bower (1988) and Lynch and Baudry (1988) it has been incorporated into subsequent experimental studies, as well as computational models of olfactory cortex.

The olfactory patterns in the olfactory bulb have been termed "odor images" (see Xu et al., 2000). In the processing of these images, the olfactory bulb has been compared with visual area V1, and olfactory cortex with visual association cortex (Neville and Haberly, 2004). An analogy was drawn in this regard by Haberly (1985) with the visual association cortical area for processing information about faces. Thus, olfactory cortex, hippocampus, and dorsal cortex are all involved in processing information encoded as complex spatial patterns (see especially the review by Wilson and Stevenson, 2006).

Thanks to the pioneering studies of Lewis Haberly and more recently many others, much basic information is available on the mammalian olfactory pyramidal neurons and the olfactory cortical microcircuit. The afferent fibers in the LOT make excitatory glutamatergic synapses on the spines of distal apical dendrites of the pyramidal cells, acting on both AMPA and NMDA receptors. Synapses with similar properties are made by the axon collaterals that activate GABAergic inhibitory interneurons and also form the long re-excitatory association fibers. An addition to the classical microcircuit of **Figure 1** is the feedforward inhibitory interneuron in the superficial layer of the cortex. This work has been summarized in Neville and Haberly (2004) and Wilson and Stevenson (2006). It has enabled detailed dissection of the excitatory and inhibitory circuits within the olfactory cortex, as indicated in **Figure 8**.

COMPARISON OF OLFACTORY AND HIPPOCAMPAL MICROCIRCUITS

We have seen that a general similarity was early recognized between the microcircuit organization of olfactory cortex and hippocampus (**Figures 1 and 2**). This idea has been supported by subsequent work. **Figure 9** illustrates a close comparison by Neville and Haberly (2004) between the main excitatory circuits in the two systems. In the olfactory cortex, there is a sequence of input from the OB to the distal apical dendrites, an intrinsic long association feedforward recombining pathway from the anterior olfactory cortex, and the long recurrent association fibers directed mainly from the anterior cortex to the more posterior cortices. In the hippocampus, there is similarly a main afferent input to the distal apical dendrites, an intrinsic feedforward pathway through the dentate gyrus, and the recurrent association fibers directed from CA3 to CA1.

In this comparison, the main motif shared by these regions is the intrinsic sequential processing and recombination of input. It is known that both olfactory cortex and hippocampus are involved in processing spatial maps (olfactory cortex processes

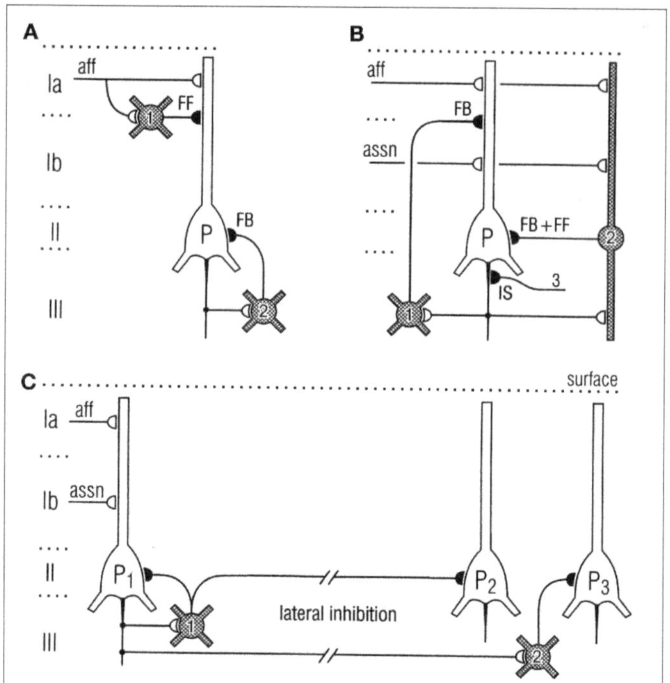

FIGURE 8 | Top: Circuits for excitatory input and different types of inhibition of pyramidal cells in the olfactory cortex. (A) Feedforward (FF) inhibitory (I) circuit from LOT afferents (aff) and feedback (FB) inhibitory circuit onto pyramidal cells (P). **(B)** Feedback and feedforward circuits from pyramidal cell axons, including inhibitory control of the initial segment (IS); assn, association fibers. **(C)** Pathways for lateral inhibition, through long axons of basket cell onto distant pyramidal cell, or long axon collateral of pyramidal cell onto distant basket cell. Open profiles: excitatory synaptic action; filled profiles: inhibitory synaptic action. From Neville and Haberly (2004).

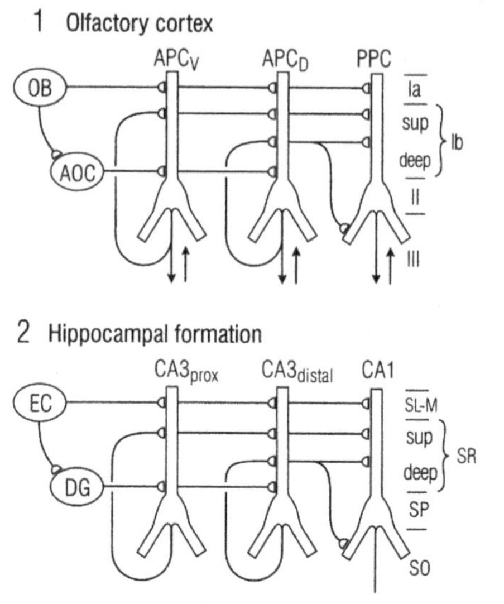

FIGURE 9 | Comparison between the microcircuit organization of olfactory cortex and hippocampus. "Note the parallels in both the horizontal dimension (connections between subdivisions) and the vertical dimension (laminar organization of fiber systems according to their areas of origin." Abbreviations: (1) OB, olfactory bulb; AOC, anterior olfactory cortex; APCV, ventral anterior piriform cortex; APCD, dorsal anterior piriform cortex; PPC, posterior piriform cortex; sup, superficial. (2) EC, entorhinal cortex; DG, dentate gyrus; prox, proximal; dist, distal; SL-M, stratum lacunosum-moleculare; SR, stratum radiatum; sup, superior; SP, stratum pyramidale; SO, stratum oriens. From Neville and Haberly (2004).

high-dimensional odor maps, as noted above, and hippocampus processes spatial cognitive maps – O'Keefe and Nadel, 1978; Moser et al., 2010). Neville and Haberly (2004) conclude that "These intriguing similarities in neuronal circuitry suggest that the two systems operate on similar functional principles."

In addition to the sequential processing within these regions, one of the output targets of olfactory cortex is the hippocampus through entorhinal cortex. The hippocampus is thus involved in higher level olfactory processing. The inclusion of hippocampus in the olfactory pathway was a part of the traditional neuroanatomical concept of the "rhinencephalon," but was denied or ignored during the upsurge of interest in the hippocampus in the 1950s and 1960s. However, sequential processing from olfactory cortex to hippocampus is now increasingly recognized (Yokota et al., 1970; Lynch and Baudry, 1988), so it is time to put the hippocampus back in the olfactory pathway.

RECENT STUDIES OF THE NEOCORTICAL CANONICAL MICROCIRCUIT

Douglas et al. (2004) have suggested that their canonical cortical microcircuit model can apply, with fine-tuning of the connectivity and physiological properties, across the cortex, from visual to motor areas, justifying calling it a "canonical" circuit. They argue that

> ... simplicity encourages the convergence of theory and biology through common models, and such convergence is imperative if we are to understand how the synaptic organization of the neocortex produces the complexity of cortical function

supporting the theme of this review.

The canonical model stimulated further work quantitating the proposed connectivity. Binzegger et al. (2009) carried out an analysis of synaptic connectivity within the cortex based on the location of axonal terminals of HRP injected cells. The results showed that the cortex is dominated by the large population of superficial pyramidal cells; that these cells have many re-excitatory connections; and that they have a large input to deep pyramidal cells. The deep pyramidal cells are dominated by this input; in contrast, they have few re-excitatory collaterals onto themselves, and few excitatory connections back on to the superficial pyramidal cells. Computational network simulations showed how stability arises from the connectivity, membrane properties, and inhibitory connections. The thalamic input is amplified through the dynamic re-excitatory network as earlier predicted. A parallel study of reconstructions of dendritic and axonal arbors provided evidence of strong connectivity within a column from excitatory pyramidal cells to inhibitory interneurons, with weaker connectivity in the reverse direction (Stepanyants et al., 2008).

Another approach to analyzing cortical microcircuits has been through experiments with laser scanning photostimulation of caged glutamate release. These have revealed strong excitatory flow from upper to lower layer neurons in both sensory and motor cortex (e.g., Weiler et al., 2008), suggesting that motor output is controlled by a top-down "pre-amplifier-like network" of upper-layer neurons. Here we see again the advantages of six-layer cortex in multiplying the combinatorial possibilities of interlaminar connectivity.

In summary, the microcircuit approach continues to focus studies on essential subsystems for intrinsic excitation and re-excitation together with recurrent/lateral inhibition. As we have seen (**Figure 7**), the parallels include similarities – the retention of basic excitatory and inhibitory subsystems – and differences – expansion to two main layers, and the addition of the stellate cell subsystem.

RECENT STUDIES OF INFORMATION PROCESSING IN PYRAMIDAL CELL DENDRITES

The pyramidal cell occupies a central place in the microcircuit organization of all the forebrain cortical regions. Attention therefore focuses on comparisons between the information capacities of the pyramidal cell dendrites. We consider several recent studies which address this issue.

APICAL DENDRITES OF OLFACTORY CORTICAL PYRAMIDAL CELLS

A recent study that has tested the olfactory cortex microcircuit has looked closely at the integrative properties of the apical dendrite of the pyramidal cell (Bathellier et al., 2009). These authors were intrigued by the finding (Poo and Isaacson, 2007) that olfactory bulb inputs vary widely in their potency in eliciting a pyramidal cell response. They wished to know whether this reflects numbers of input axons or strength of suprathreshold dendritic activity due to clustered inputs to a given dendrite. The methods used dual patch recordings in brain slices from pyramidal neurons activated by injected current or LOT fibers. Labeled cells had multiple apical branches 300–400 μm long. Dual patches on soma and distal dendrite showed that the dendrites were electrotonically relatively compact; for inputs in a distal dendrite, there was a maximum of 50% current loss at the soma. The dendrites were only weakly active. They were able to support backpropagating action potentials, as in neocortical and hippocampal pyramidal neurons, but could generate only small local Na+ spikes that had little effect at the soma. Also, unlike neocortex, they showed no dendritic Ca2+ or NMDA spikes, although Ca2+ entry occurred with backpropagating action potentials.

With regard to integrative activity in the apical dendrite, synaptic inputs following activation of axons in the LOT appeared to be uniformly distributed over distal dendrites. Bathellier et al. (2009) argue that this minimizes sublinear summation effects (no clustering). They conclude that many single fibers have contacts distributed widely over the dendritic tree, an arrangement that provides for efficient transmission of distributed co-active inputs. As a consequence, stimulus feature extraction must be based on linear summation at the soma of many inputs over many dendrites rather than clustered processing in targeted dendrites. They suggest that such clustering could be a neocortical pyramidal cell innovation.

Backpropagation of action potentials is shared with other cortical pyramidal cells, but is more variable in olfactory pyramidal cells as well as in turtle dorsal cortex (see below). This may be correlated with lack of reliability of plasticity of the input synapses (Poo and Isaacson, 2007). It is also correlated with the fact that in both olfactory and dorsal cortex the pyramidal cell dendrites are only weakly active. This points to active properties as possibly a specialization required for more complex processing in the hippocampus and neocortex.

LOGIC OPERATIONS IN APICAL DENDRITES OF HIPPOCAMPAL PYRAMIDAL NEURONS

Before the advent of dual patch recordings by Stuart et al. (1993), computational approaches provided the first insights into the information processing capabilities of active dendrites. Although the processing is universally regarded as integrative, what exactly is the nature of this integration, and what is the nature of the information that is processed?

This question was addressed with a computational study to test whether dendrites might be capable of generating logic operations. In a classic study, McCulloch and Pitts (1943) had shown that excitatory and inhibitory interconnections between nerve cells could generate basic logic operations of AND, OR, and AND–NOT; these three operations are sufficient for building a digital computer. This same paradigm transferred to equivalent interactions between dendritic spines within an apical dendritic tree of a pyramidal neuron such as in CA1 or CA3 of the hippocampus was tested by Shepherd and Brayton (1987). The results showed that in the presence of a thresholding mechanism in the spines, the basic logic operations emerged naturally from simple combinations of synaptic responses, all of them present in dendritic responses. AND operations are related to summation and coincidence detection; OR operations to simple responses of individual synapses; AND–NOT operations to inhibitory control, either at the site of an excited spine by an inhibitory input on an excited spine, or modulation of the output of the spine by a distant inhibitory input on the dendritic branch. The thresholding mechanisms can be the all-or-nothing response of a single spine to a single vesicle released at an active zone, or voltage gated Na+ or Ca2+ channels in subjacent dendritic branch (Shepherd et al., 1989).

These operations appear inherent in a system of dendritic branches or dendritic spines containing one or more of these thresholding properties (see **Figure 10**). They confer upon the apical (and possibly basal) dendritic system the ability to carry out information processing at a distance from the cell body. In this way the global input–output functions of the cell become conditional on the summated effects of multiple semi-independent compartments carrying out sub-threshold information processing.

This model was tested by Poirazi et al. (2003), who provide a good summary of the possible significance of active dendritic properties in pyramidal neurons:

"There is general agreement that pyramidal cell dendrites contain a large number and variety of voltage-dependent channels distributed non-uniformly throughout the dendritic tree, which heavily influence the cell's integrative behavior. Recent evidence also suggests that elemental synaptic conductances may vary systematically as a function of dendritic location (Magee and Cook, 2000). However, there remain quite different views as to the functional role that these dendritic and synaptic channels may play. One view is that voltage-dependent dendritic currents and scaling of synaptic conductances exist to transform the complex and physically sprawling cell into a virtual "point neuron." According to this view, dendritic non-linearities may exist to (1)

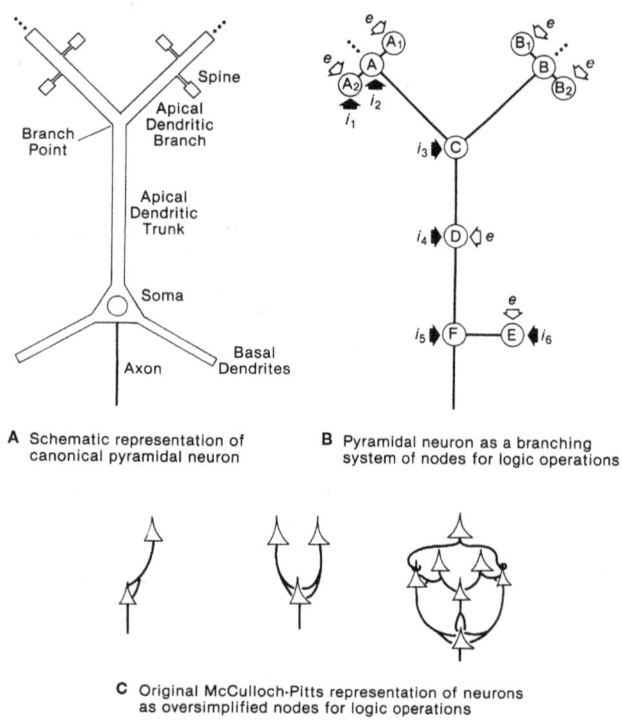

FIGURE 10 | Dendritic spines allow the pyramidal neuron to function as a complex multiunit processing system. (A): representation of a pyramidal neuron with multiple spine units. **(B)**: representation of the pyramidal neuron with multiple sites for coincidence detection (A, B) in its spines and distal dendritic branches, with spread to summation points by passive or active mechanisms (C), further spread boosted by active membrane and synaptic inputs) (D), similar mechanisms in the basal dendrites (E), and final summation at the ell body and axon hillock (F). Modulation occurs through excitation or inhibition at successive stages by layer-targeted inputs. Excitatory synapses indicated by open arrows; inhibitory synapses by filled arrows. **(C)**: Examples of interconnections between point neurons that could implement OR (left), AND (middle), or more complex logic operations (right), as represented by McCulloch and Pitts (1943). From Shepherd (1994).

make the cell more linear, by counteracting the classical synaptic non-linearity that arises from the summation of conductances (Bernander et al., 1994; Cash and Yuste, 1999), and in conjunction with synaptic scaling, they could (2) make the cell more functionally compact, by counteracting the distance-dependent attenuation of synaptic responses that arise from the cable properties of dendrites (Cauller and Connors, 1992; De Schutter and Bower, 1994; Magee and Cook, 2000). Both ideas emphasize the coupling of individual synapses to the cell body and the uniformity and linearity thereof.

A second view holds that the dendrites exist to create a number of independent functional compartments within which various kinds of non-linear computations can be carried out (Koch et al., 1983; Rall and Segev, 1987; Shepherd and Brayton, 1987; Mel, 1992a,b). Our results here support a particular version of this hypothesis in which the long, thin, unbranched, synapse-rich terminal dendrites may themselves act like classical neuron-like summing units, each with its own quasi-independent subunit non-linearity. The cell body for its part, fed either directly by the basal dendrites or by the main trunk which acts as a high-efficiency conduit from the apical dendrites, sums together the dendritic subunit outflows to determine the cell's overall response. We have previously explored some of the functional implications of such a model (Mel et al., 1998; Mel, 1999; Archie and Mel, 2000; Poirazi and Mel, 2001)".

It may be seen that many of the themes in the exploration of dendritic properties of pyramidal neurons are brought together in this summary.

Poirazi et al. (2003) implemented the experimental findings in a neuron with simulations that provided evidence that these local active interactions endow the cortical pyramidal neuron with the ability to function as a "two-layer neural network" (**Figure 11**). This model has received repeated experimental support (Antic, 2003; Losonczy and Magee, 2006; Polsky et al., 2008).

We have seen that the apical dendrite of the olfactory pyramidal neuron has a relatively low density of Na+ channels and is less able to generate local thresholding of responses to its distal synaptic inputs. It appears that this ability may have become more developed in the apical dendrites of hippocampal pyramidal neurons. We will see that this applies also to the apical dendrites of neocortical pyramidal neurons. Mammalian hippocampal pyramidal cell dendrites may thus have evolved toward some of the properties of neocortical pyramidal cells.

APICAL DENDRITES OF TURTLE DORSAL CORTICAL PYRAMIDAL NEURONS

After Kriegstein and Connors (1986) there was unfortunately little interest in the synaptic organization of turtle dorsal cortex. However, one hopes this situation will change with the recent study by William Ross and his colleagues (Larkum et al., 2008) of the physiological properties of turtle pyramidal cells. They have built on the work and concepts of Kriegstein and Connors (1986), citing them that turtle dorsal cortex "presents a logical foundation for studying the more elaborate six-layered cortex," and that "There is a broad range of evidence establishing that the more elaborate six-layered neocortex was derived from the pallium (e.g., Mulligan and Ulinski, 1990; Reiner, 2000)." These statements indicate that the

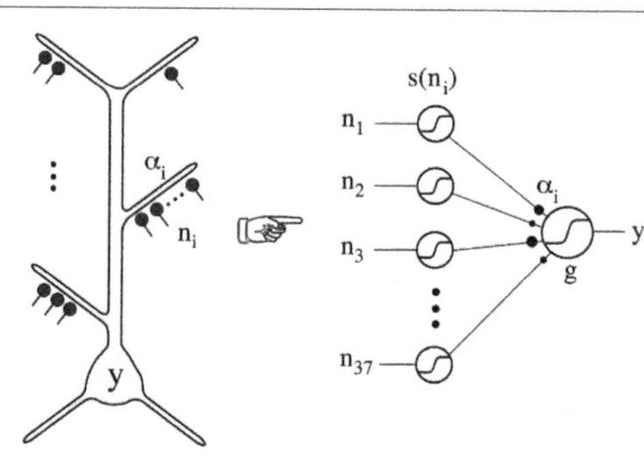

FIGURE 11 | Thin oblique and terminal dendritic branches allow the pyramidal neuron to function as a two-layered neural network. The thin oblique and apical terminal dendritic branches constitute semi-independent local integrating subunits. Their interactions through the intervening dendritic tree can be regarded as constituting a second layer of neural network, in addition to the first layer formed by their interacting cell bodies and their axons. From Poirazi et al. (2003).

foundation laid by the work discussed above is gaining acceptance for application to cortical evolution, at least among those working at the level of synaptic organization and brain microcircuits.

In revisiting and updating the work of Kriegstein and Connors (1986), Larkum et al. (2008) were particularly interested in the dendritic properties of the pyramidal neurons. The combination of dual patch recordings and cell imaging techniques has transformed this key area of research, and the authors used both approaches in their study. Their basic findings can be summarized as follows.

First, the basic findings of Kriegstein and Connors (1986) were confirmed. Most turtle "pyramidal cells" are characterized by multiple apical dendrites and usually no basal dendrites. It may be noted that the pyramidal cells in mammalian olfactory cortex come in two varieties: one also has multiple apical dendrites and no basal dendrites, and is called a "semilunar cell"; the other has the more conventional apical and basal dendritic trees (see Neville and Haberly, 2004). Mammalian pyramidal cells, especially those in layer 2, can often have multiple apical dendrites (E. G. Jones, personal communication).

Despite this morphological difference, many basic electrophysiological properties of turtle pyramidal neurons were found to resemble those of mammalian neocortical pyramidal neurons. For example, intracellular current injection elicits repetitive spikes, which initiate preferentially near the soma; dendritic spike initiation occurs with stronger dendritic depolarization, and Na+-spike backpropagation is accompanied by Ca2+ influx. Among differences, the authors found that there was a lack of the broad Ca2+ spikes characteristic of the distal dendrites of hippocampal and neocortical pyramidal cells. This, together with the lack of an apical tuft, suggests that an apical tuft able to generate broad Ca2+ spikes may be "a more recent specialization of mammalian neocortical and hippocampal pyramidal neurons." The lack of dendritic Ca2+ spikes in the turtle is associated with the inability of a dendritic input to change the firing pattern in the soma from regular spiking to bursting. In neocortical pyramidal neurons this ability is believed to be necessary "to associate feedback inputs arriving in the tuft with feed forward inputs in the basal regions" (Larkum et al., 2008). Bursting may be a key property allowing a neuron to have a more potent effect on a target, which could be important for inducing plastic changes underlying learning and memory.

The results indicate that backpropagating action potentials and dendritic calcium influx are fundamental properties of cortical pyramidal cells. In mammalian pyramidal cells these properties have been especially implicated in mechanisms of synaptic plasticity. The fact that they are present in dorsal cortical pyramidal cells provides a fresh perspective, because it indicates that they were present in the basic three-layer cortical microcircuit. This indicates that mechanisms of plasticity that we ascribe to neocortical neurons and microcircuits in fact were already present in the three-layer precursors of those neurons and microcircuits. As the authors conclude:

> ...these findings encourage continued use of the turtle cortical slice preparation in seeking the characteristics that define the fundamental functional properties of cortical cells and circuits across a wide range of vertebrates.

APICAL DENDRITES OF NEOCORTICAL PYRAMIDAL NEURONS

Recent studies have revealed what appear to be some special properties of neocortical pyramidal cell dendrites. Of particular interest are the most distal dendritic branches of the apical dendrite that form a tuft within layer 1. Using multiple patches (see **Figure 12**, left), Larkum et al. (2009) showed that these branches can generate NMDA spikes, which in turn can generate Ca2+ spikes at the Ca2+ spike initiation zone where the branches converge onto the apical dendritic trunk, from which spikes can propagate to the soma (**Figure 12**, middle column). Previous studies have demonstrated NMDA spikes in the basal dendrites which can spread to initiate Na+ spikes at the soma. This has suggested a unifying principle for the functional organization of the dendrites of the neocortical pyramidal neuron, in which the distal branches of the apical and basal dendrites generate NMDA spikes, which sum at their respective Ca2+ and Na+ spike initiation sites, leading to the final summation at the axon hillock to generate the axonal action potential output (see **Figure 12**, right).

This new model represents a further refining of the concept of semi-independent compartments within the dendritic trees, to which the rules for summation of responses to generate basic logic operations still apply. It gives further support to the evidence that the single cell is a multi-compartment functional system, that cannot be represented by a single summing node as in neural network formulations. The neocortical microcircuit thus needs to be expanded to include the special properties of the apical and basal dendrites.

CORTICAL INTERNEURONS AND CORTICAL COLUMNS

Pyramidal cells appear to dominate the neuronal population of the cerebral cortex, with 70–80% of the total, with interneurons comprising less 20–30% (as low as 10% in some estimates). However, the interneurons are attracting increasing interest because of their diversification into many subtypes. This is limited in olfactory cortex to the two main subtypes noted already: one deep type involved in feedback and LI onto the pyramidal cell somata, the other in superficial FI onto the pyramidal cell apical dendrites. In dorsal cortex the studies of Smith et al. (1980) showed a tremendous convergence of both input fibers and pyramidal cell axon collaterals onto one main type, suggesting that it played a key role in the inhibitory control of the pyramidal cells. Further studies are needed to test for subtypes within this population.

Diversification of subtypes reached its highest degree in hippocampus and neocortex. In the hippocampus, there are estimated to be at least 21 GABAergic interneuron subtypes, differentiated on the basis of multiple criteria: location of cell body, structure of dendritic trees, branching of axon, laminar and cellular synaptic targets, and molecular and physiological properties. As summarized by Somogyi (2010),

> Interneurons provide multiple modulatory operations, such as changing threshold, synchronization, gain control, input scaling, and so on, and assist the network in the selection of pyramidal cells for cell assemblies.

In the neocortex, diversification is even more profligate. According to Markram (2010), there are 13 major anatomical types of interneuron. "Each anatomical type of neuron can express up to 8 of 15 major types of electrical behaviors, giving rise to as many as 200 morpho-electrical types of interneurons in a neocortical

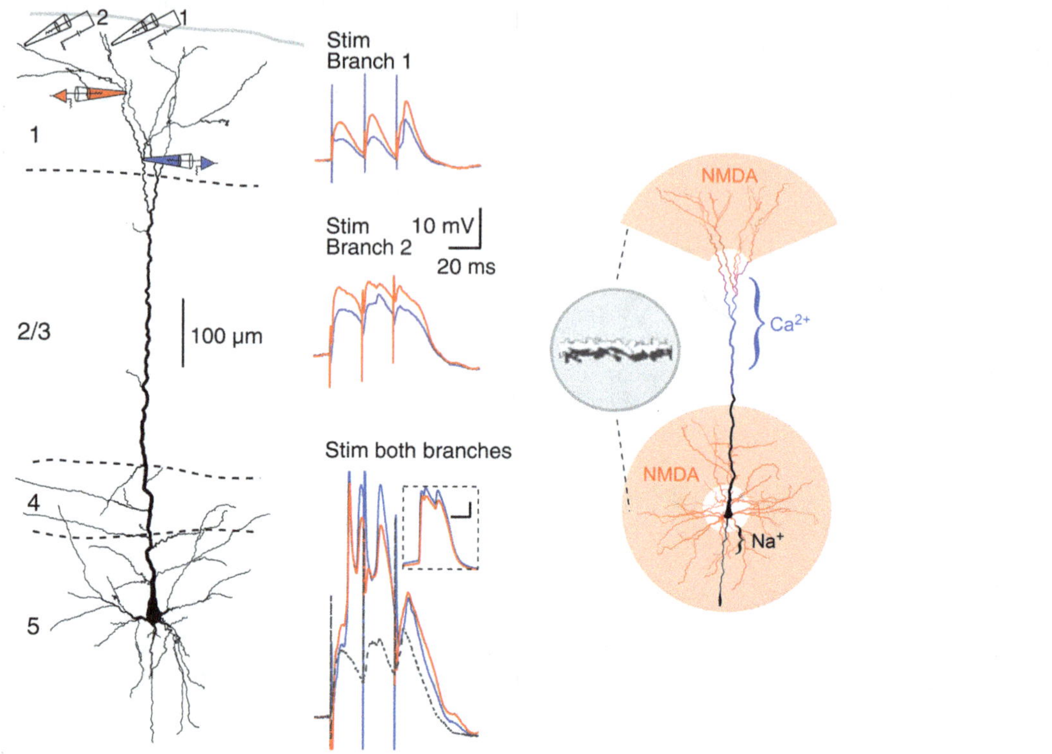

FIGURE 12 | Compartmentalization of the distal apical tuft of a neocortical pyramidal cell. Left column: Two different distal branches were stimulated (electrodes 1 and 2) while recordings were made from two more proximal sites (black electrodes 1 and 2). Stimulation at site 1 evoked a series of EPSPs (middle column, top), while stimulation at site 2 evoked NMDA spikes (middle column, middle). Simultaneous stimulation gave supralinear summation to produce a Ca^{2+} spike at the Ca^{2+} spike initiation zone in the apical dendrite (middle column, bottom). Right column: summary diagram of relation between NMDA spike generating distal branches and Ca^{2+} and Na^{2+} spike generating proximal sites. From Larkum et al. (2009).

column...." There is evidence that the morpho-electrical type of identified pyramidal cell and interneuronal subtype is predictive of the type of interactions between the two, giving rise to a large number of combinatorial possibilities. These studies in rodents may not map adequately onto the variety of interneurons in primate and human neocortex (E. G. Jones, personal communication).

These local interactions in the neocortex are widely regarded to be organized within radial columns. This has been a tremendously fertile idea in thinking about microcircuit organization in the cortex over the past half century (Mountcastle, 1957; Hubel and Wiesel, 1962). Barrels in somatosensory cortex of certain animals are another example of modular organization in the neocortex. It is attractive to consider the cortical column as a neocortical invention. However, olfactory glomeruli, the nervous system's most distinctive anatomical and molecular module, may serve a similar function in the olfactory bulb in organizing the input to olfactory cortex (see Willhite et al., 2006), as may cell clusters in entorhinal cortex for its input to the hippocampus.

ONE CORTICAL MICROCIRCUIT OR MANY? A BIOINFORMATICS APPROACH

The diversity of neuron properties, interneurons, and intra and interlaminar connectivity being revealed by current studies appears to be a hallmark of neocortex. In the face of this diversity it may be asked whether the concept of a basic microcircuit for cerebral cortex is viable. As Nelson (2002) put it in a review of a meeting on mammalian cerebral cortex: is there "a single canonical microcircuit: a kind of basic wiring diagram which, although embellished, remains fundamentally unaltered from mouse to man and across all cortical regions"? Is there a single canonical microcircuit or are there many? Should we be lumpers or splitters?

The approach taken in this review in dealing with this question is built on how bioinformatics deals with gene and protein diversity. Taking G-protein coupled receptors (GPCRs) as an example, there is a motif of seven transmembrane domain receptors coupled to G-protein effectors, which constitutes a family. Within this family are subfamilies of receptors activated by different transmitter molecules, and subfamilies which activate different types of G-proteins. These different combinations sort themselves out into classes and subclasses (see the IUPHAR nomenclature website of the International Union of Basic and Clinical Pharmcology: http://www.iuphar-db.org/index.jsp). This approach has been critical to the rise of molecular biology.

Applying this approach to cortical microcircuits, the basic elements we have identified, of pyramidal cells with apical and basal dendrites, giving rise to internal excitatory feedback and inhibitory feedback through interneurons, would describe the cerebral cortex family. The three- and six-layer cortical microcircuits would constitute subfamilies. Classes could be identified based on pyramidal cell properties and types of interneurons, as we have seen. Further diversification in relation to different cortical areas of different species might constitute subclasses. These suggestions indicate the need to have a conceptual framework such as the cortical microcircuit within which diversity can be prioritized. This framework in turn provides the basis for assessing the relative significance of each element of the diversity in the evolution of the cortex. It may be predicted that this hierarchical approach of bioinformatics can also be effective in promoting understanding of cortical microcircuit organization.

CONCLUDING DISCUSSION

The principles of organization at the microcircuit level underlying the evolution from three-layer to six-layer cortex may be summarized briefly in the following manner. The basic cortical microcircuit family consists of pyramidal cells interacting through recurrent excitatory and inhibitory intrinsic circuits, expanded from a single layer of pyramidal cell bodies in the subfamily represented by reptilian dorsal cortex, olfactory cortex, and hippocampus, to the multiple layers of pyramidal cell bodies of the mammalian neocortex subfamily. Within the neocortical subfamily, variations (classes and subclasses) at the molecular, cellular, and circuit level occur that are specific for each species.

A more complete inventory of the elements upon which the principles of cortical microcircuit organization are built is summarized in **Table 2**.

These properties taken together define the microcircuit organization of the cerebral cortex throughout most of vertebrate evolution. It may be proposed that this constitutes a unique set of properties found nowhere else in the vertebrate nervous system, uniquely adapted to the demands of providing the highest level of information processing in controlling and elaborating the behavior of any given vertebrate species. There are of course many variations on this theme in the basic cortical circuits suggested by a number of investigators (neocortex: DeFelipe and Jones, 2010; Markram, 2010; Georgopoulos and Stefanis, 2010; Svoboda et al., 2010; Wang, 2010; hippocampus: Buzsaki, 2006; Somogyi, 2010; entorhinal cortex: Moser et al., 2010; and olfactory cortex: Wilson and Barkai, 2010), but they all recognize at least the main features.

These shared properties are only the starting points for addressing the really interesting questions that will lead to identifying the unique subset of properties that characterizes neocortex. Although this goes beyond the focus of the present review, some promising directions may be indicated.

First (and foremost), what are the gene mechanisms that generate the expansion of the layers of microcircuits, to produce the quantal leap from three to six layers? Current studies of cortical development in rodents and in primates are providing critical insights into these processes (Cheung et al., 2007; Rakic, 2009; Montiel et al., this volume). A possible mechanism may be found in the fact that genesis of cortical layers occurs by the migration of new neurons along radial glia to their final layer in an inside-out sequence. New layers could have been added by mutations in the stop signals for the migrating neurons (P. Rakic, personal communication). A new initiative to map the entire human transcriptome, with focus on the cortex, is likely to give a new perspective on this question (Johnson et al., 2009).

How is the microcircuit concept related to the tremendous expansion of the neocortex that occurred during mammalian evolution, especially among certain species such as cetacea and primates, and especially humans? It is evidence that the neocortical microcircuit can be easily extended laterally to expand the cortex and differentiate into new regions. A leading hypothesis is that this cortical expansion occurred through elaboration from "protomaps" (Rakic, 2009). It may be hypothesized that each protomap contains a "protomicrocircuit" fine-tuned for its emerging cell properties and potential connectivity.

The physiological properties of the cortical cells require much more study. Building on the classical differentiation of cortical neurons into thick and thin spikes and regular and burst firing (McCormick et al., 1985), physiologists are identifying increasingly complex subtypes, especially of interneurons. The functions of the interneurons in synchronizing and desynchronizing cortical microcircuits through chemical and electrical synapses is a rapidly growing field in itself (Buzsaki, 2006; Mancilla et al., 2007). Cortical network activity is increasingly recognized as reflecting a balance between RE and inhibition (Haider et al., 2006). This balance is critical in all three types of mammalian cortex, as shown by the susceptibility of all of them to seizure activity from an excess of RE or reduction in recurrent inhibition.

Are there unique physiological properties of pyramidal cell dendrites in the pyramidal cells of humans compared with subhuman primates and other species that make their own critical contribution to human cognitive capabilities? Studies of human cortical cells are now possible from surgery for relief of epilepsy, which is providing valuable material for species-specific human properties at the biochemical and electrophysiological (Chen et al., 1996) level. And cells specific for humans open another angle on specific human properties (Allman et al., 2010).

How does this approach reconcile with other approaches to cortical evolution? A comprehensive review of cortical evolution (Striedter, 2005) has supported the basic focus here on reptilian dorsal cortex as the nearest approximation to the postulated precursor of mammalian neocortex. Reconciliation between current theories involving evolutionary routes through the dorsal ventricular ridge and the avian brain (Jarvis et al., 2005) is beyond the scope of this review. It can however be proposed that the concept of the microcircuit as an organizing principle, beginning with three-layer cortex, needs to be central to that discussion.

ACKNOWLEDGMENTS

This review is based on work generously supported by the National Institute for Deafness and other Communicative Disorders. I am grateful to Donald Wilson, Edward Jones, Zoltan Molnar, Ford Ebner, Pasko Rakic, and Gordon M. G. Shepherd for valuable comments on the manuscript. I dedicate this article to Lewis B. Haberly, student, colleague, friend, for his pioneering experiments and conceptual insights in constructing the microcircuit of the olfactory cortex and extending it to principles of cortical organization.

REFERENCES

Allman, J. M., Tetreault, N. A., Hakeem, A. U., Manaye, K. F., Semendeferi, K., Erwin, J. M., Goubert, V., and Hof, P. R. (2010). The von Economo neurons in the frontoinsular and anterior cingulate cortex in great apes and humans. *Brain Struct. Funct.* 214, 495–517.

Andersen, P. (1960). Interhippocampal impulses. II. Apical dendritic activation of CAI neurons. *Acta Physiol. Scand.* 48, 178–208.

Andersen, P., Bliss, T. V. P., and Skrede, K. K. (1971). Lamellar organization of hippocampal excitatory pathways. *Exp. Brain Res.* 13, 222–238.

Antic, S. D. (2003). Action potentials in basal and oblique dendrites of rat neocortical pyramidal neurons. *J. Physiol.* 550, 35–50

Archie, K. A., and Mel, B. W. (2000). A model for intradendritic computation of binocular disparity. *Nat. Neurosci.* 3, 54–63.

Bathellier, B., Margrie, T. W., and Larkum, M. E. (2009). Properties of piriform cortex pyramidal cell dendrites: implications for olfactory circuit design. *J. Neurosci.* 29, 12641–12652.

Bernander, O., Koch, C., and Douglas, R. J. (1994). Amplification and linearization of distal synaptic input to cortical pyramidal cells. *J. Neurophysiol.* 72, 2743–2753.

Biedenbach, M. A., and Stevens, C. F. (1969). Synaptic organization of cat olfactory cortex as revealed by intracellular recording. *J. Neurophysiol.* 32, 204–214.

Binzegger, T., Douglas, R. J., and Martin, K. A. (2009). Topology and dynamics of the canonical circuit of cat V1. *Neural Netw.* 22, 1071–1078.

Buzsaki, G. (2006). *Rhythms of the Brain.* New York: Oxford University Press.

Byrne, J. H., Castellucci, V. F., and Kandel, E. R. (1978). Contribution of individual mechanoreceptor sensory neurons to defensive gill-withdrawal reflex in Aplysia. *J. Neurophysiol.* 41, 418–431.

Cash, S., and Yuste, R. (1999). Linear summation of excitatory inputs by CA1 pyramidal neurons. *Neuron* 22, 383–394.

Cauller, L. J., and Connors, B. W. (1992). "Functions of very distal dendrites: Experimental and computational studies of layer I synapses on neocortical pyramidal cells," in *Single Neuron Computation*, eds. T. McKenna, J. Davis, and S. Zornetzer (Boston: Academic Press), 199–229.

Chen, W. R., Lee, S., Kato, K., Spencer, D. D., Shepherd, G. M., and Williamson, A. (1996). Long-term modifications of synaptic efficacy in the human inferior and middle temporal cortex. *Proc. Natl. Acad. Sci. U.S.A.* 93, 8011–8015.

Cheung, A. F., Pollen, A. A., Tavare, A., DeProto, J., and Molnar, Z. (2007). Comparative aspects of cortical neurogenesis in vertebrates. *J. Anat.* 211, 164–176.

Connors, B. W., and Kriegstein, A. R. (1986). Cellular physiology of the turtle visual cortex: distinctive properties of pyramidal and stellate neurons. *J. Neurosci.* 6, 164–177.

De Schutter, E., and Bower, J. M. (1994). Simulated responses of cerebellar Purkinje cells are independent of the dendritic location of granule cell synaptic inputs. *Proc. Natl. Acad. Sci. U.S.A.* 91, 4736–4740.

DeFelipe, J., and Jones, E. G. (2010). "Neocortical microcircuits," in *Handbook of Brain Microcircuits*, eds G. M. Shepherd and S. Grillner (New York: Oxford University Press), 5–14.

Douglas, R. J., Markram, H., and Martin, K. (2004). "Neocortex," in *The Synaptic Organization of the Brain*, ed. G. M. Shepherd (New York: Oxford University Press), 499–558.

Douglas, R. J., and Martin, K. A. C. (2010). "Canonical cortical circuits," in *Handbook of Brain Microcircuits*, eds G. M. Shepherd and S. Grillner (New York: Oxford University Press), 15–21.

Douglas, R. J., Martin, K. A. C., and Whitteridge, D. (1989). A canonical microcircuit for neocortex. *Neural Comput.* 1, 480–488.

Georgopoulos, A. P., and Stefanis, C. N. (2010). "The motor cortical circuit," in *Handbook of Brain Microcircuits*, eds G. M. Shepherd and S. Grillner (New York: Oxford University Press), 39–45.

Graybiel, A.M., and Grillner, S. (2006). *Microcircuits: The Interface between Neurons and Global Brain Function.* Cambridge, MA: MIT Press.

Grillner, S., Markram, H., De Schutter, E., Silberberg, G., and LeBeau, F. E. (2005). Microcircuits in action – from CPGs to neocortex. *Trends Neurosci.* 28, 525–533.

Haberly, L. B. (1973a). Summed potentials evoked in opossum prepyriform cortex. *J. Neurophysiol.* 36, 775–788.

Haberly, L. B. (1973b). Unitary analysis of opossum prepyriform cortex. *J. Neurophysiol.* 36, 762–774.

Haberly, L. B. (1985). Neuronal circuity in olfactory cortex. Anatomy and functional implications. *Chem. Senses* 10, 219–238.

Haberly, L. B., and Shepherd, G. M. (1973). Current-density analysis of summed evoked potentials in opossum prepyriform cortex. *J. Neurophysiol.* 36, 789–802.

Haider, G., Duque, A., Hasenstaub, A. R., and McCormick, D. A. (2006). Neocortical network activity in vivo is generated through a dynamic balance of excitation and inhibition. *J. Neurosci.* 26, 4535–4545.

Hildebrand, J. G., and Shepherd, G. M. (1997). Mechanisms of olfactory discrimination: converging evidence for common principles across phyla. *Annu. Rev. Neurosci.* 20, 595–631.

Hubel, D. H., and Wiesel, T. N. (1962). Receptive fields, binocular interaction and functional architecture in the cat's visual cortex. *J. Physiol.* 160, 106–154.

Jarvis, E. D., Güntürkün, O., Bruce, L., Csillag, A., Karten, H., Kuenzel, W., Medina, L., Paxinos, G., Perkel, D.J., Shimizu, T., Striedter, G., Wild J.M., Ball, G.F., Dugas-Ford, J., Durand, S.E., Hough, G.E, Husband, S., Kubikova, L., Lee, D.W., Mello, C.V., Powers, A., Siang, C., Smulders, T.V., Wada, K., White, S.A., Yamamoto, K., Yu, J., Reiner, A., Butler, A.B., Avian Brain Nomenclature Consortium. (2005). Avian brains and a new understanding of vertebrate brain evolution. *Nat. Rev. Neurosci.* 6, 151–159.

Johnson, M. B., Kawasawa, Y. I., Mason, C. E., Kranik, Z., Coppola, G., Bogdanović, D., Geschwind, D. H., Mane, S. M., State, M.W., and Sestan, N. (2009). Functional and evolutionary insights into human brain development through global transcriptome analysis. *Neuron* 62, 494–509.

Kandel, E. R., Spencer, W. A., and Brinley, F. J. Jr. (1961). Electrophysiology of hippocampal neurons. I. Sequential invasion and synaptic organization. *J. Neurophysiol.* 24, 225–242.

Koch, C., Poggio, T., and Torre, V. (1983). Nonlinear interactions in a dendritic tree: localization, timing, and role in information processing. *Proc. Natl. Acad. Sci. U.S.A.* 80, 2799–2802.

Kriegstein, A. R., and Connors, B. W. (1986). Cellular physiology of the turtle visual cortex: synaptic properties and intrinsic circuitry. *J. Neurosci.* 6, 178–191.

Larkum, M. E., Nevian, T., Sandler, M., Polsky, A., and Schiller, J. (2009). Synaptic integration in tuft dendrites of layer 5 pyramidal neurons: a new unifying principle. *Science* 325, 756–760.

Larkum, M. E., Watanabe, S., Lasser-Ross, N., Rhodes, P., and Ross, W. N. (2008). Dendritic properties of turtle pyramidal neurons. *J. Neurophysiol.* 99, 683–694.

Losonczy, A., and Magee, J. C. (2006). Integrative properties of radial oblique dendrites in hippocampal CA1 pyramidal cell neurons. *Neuron* 50, 291-307

Lynch, G., and Baudry, M. (1988). "Structure-function relationships in the organization of memory," in *Pespectives in Memory Research*, ed. M. S. Gazzaniga (Cambridge, MA: MIT Press), 23–91.

Magee, J. C., and Cook, E. P. (2000). Somatic EPSP amplitude is independent of synapse location in hippocampal pyramidal neurons. *Nat. Neurosci.* 3, 895–903.

Mancilla, J. G., Lewis, T. J., Pinto, D. J., Rinzel, J., and Connors, B. W. (2007). Synchronization of electrically coupled pairs of inhibitory interneurons in neocortex. *J. Neurosci.* 27, 205802973.

Markram, H. (2010). "Microcircuitry of the neocortex," in *Handbook of Brain Microcircuits*, eds G. M. Shepherd and S. Grillner (New York: Oxford University Press), 22–30.

McCormick, D. A., Connors, B. W., Lighthall, J. S., and Prince, D. A. (1985). Comparative electrophysiology of pyramidal and sparsely spiny stellate neurons of the neocortex. *J. Neurophysiol.* 54, 782–806.

McCulloch, W. W., and Pitts, W. H. (1943). A logical calculus of ideas immanent in nervous activity. *Bull. Math. Biophys.* 5, 115–133.

Mel, B. W. (1999). Computational neuroscience. Think positive to find parts. *Nature* 401, 759–760.

Mel, B. W. (1992a). "The clusteron: toward a simple abstraction for a complex neuron," in *Advances in Neural Information Processing*, Vol. 4, eds. J. Moody, S. Hanson, and R. Lippmann (San Mateo, CA: Morgan Kaufmann), 3542.

Mel, B. W. (1992b). NMDA-based pattern discrimination in a modeled cortical neuron. *Neural. Comput.* 4, 502–516.

Mel, B. W., Rudelman, D. L., and Archie, K. A. (1998). Translation invariant orientation tuning in visual complex cells could derive from intradendritic computations. *J. Neurosci.* 17, 4325–4334.

Moser, E. I., Witteer, P. M., and Moser, M.-B. (2010). "Entorhinal cortex," in *Handbook of Brain Microcircuits*, eds G. M. Shepherd and S. Grillner (New York: Oxford University Press), 175–189.

Mountcastle, V. B. (1957). Modality and topographic properties of single neurons of cat's somatic sensory cortex. *J. Neurophysiol.* 20, 408–434.

Mulligan, K. A., and Ulinski, P. S. (1990). Organization of geniculocortical projections in turtles: isoazimuth lamellae in the visual cortex. *J. Comp. Neurol.* 296, 531–547.

Nelson, S. B. (2002). Cortical microcircuits: diverse or canonical? *Neuron* 36, 19–27.

Neville, K. R., and Haberly, L. B. (2004). "Olfactory cortex," in *The Synaptic Organization of the Brain*, ed. G. M. Shepherd (New York: Oxford University Press), 415–454.

O'Keefe, J., and Nadel, L. (1978). *The Hippocampus as a Cognitive Map.* New York: Oxford University Press.

Phillips, C. G. (1959). Actions of antidromic pyramidal volleys ob single Betz cells in the cat. *Quart. J. Exp. Physiol.* 44, 1–25.

Poirazi, P., Brannon, T., and Mel, B. W. (2003). Pyramidal neuron as a two-layer neural network. *Neuron* 37, 989–999.

Poirazi, P., and Mel, B. W. (2001). Impact of active dendrites and structural plasticity on the memory capacity of neural tissue. *Neuron* 29, 779–796.

Polsky, A., Mel, B. W., and Schiller, J. (2008). Computational subunits in thin dendrites of pyramidal cells. *Nat. Neurosci.* 7, 621–627.

Poo, C., and Isaacson, J. S. (2007). An early critical period for long-term plasticity and structural modification of sensory synapses in olfactory cortex. *J. Neurosci.* 27, 7553–7558.

Rakic, P. (ed.). (1976). *Local Circuit Neurons.* Cambridge MA: MIT Press.

Rakic, P. (2009). Evolution of the neocortex: a perspective from developmental biology. *Nat. Rev. Neurosci.* 10, 724–735.

Rall, W., and Segev, I. (1987). "Functional possibilities for synapses on dendrites and on dendritic spines," in *Synaptic Function*, eds G. M. Edelman, W. Gall, and W. M. Cowan (New York: John Wiley and Sojs), 605–636.

Ramon y Cajal, S. (1911). *Histologie du système nerveux de l'homme et des vertébrés.* Transl. L. Azoulay. Paris: Maloine. English translation by Swanson, N., and Swanson, L.W. (1995) Histology of the Nervous System. New York: Oxford University Press.

Reiner, A. J. (2000). A hypothesis as to the organization of cerebral cortex in the common amniote ancestor of modern reptiles and mammals. *Novartis Found. Symp.* 228, 83–102.

Ressler, K. J., Sullivan, S. L., and Buck, L. B. (1994). Information coding in the olfactory system: evidence for a stereotyped and highly organized epitope map in the olfactory bulb. *Cell* 79, 1245–1255.

Rumelhart, D. E., and McClelland, J. L. (eds). (1986). *Parallel Distributed Processsing. Explorations in the Microstructure of Cognition.* Cambridge, MA: MIT Press.

Sharp, F. R., Kauer, J. S., and Shepherd, G. M. (1975). Local sites of activity-related glucose metabolism in rat olfactory bulb during olfactory stimulation. *Brain Res.* 98, 596–600.

Sharp, F. R., Kauer, J. S., and Shepherd, G. M. (1977). Laminar analysis of 2-deoxyglucose uptake in olfactory bulb and olfactory cortex of rabbit and rat. *J. Neurophysiol.* 40, 800–813.

Shepherd, G. M. (1974). *The Synaptic Organization of the Brain.* New York: Oxford University Press.

Shepherd, G. M. (1978). Microcircuits in the nervous system. *Sci. Am.* 238, 93–103.

Shepherd, G. M. (1979). *The Synaptic Organization of the Brain*, 2nd Edn. New York: Oxford University Press.

Shepherd, G. M. (1988). "A basic circuit of cortical organization," in *Perspectives in Memory Research*, ed. M. S. Gazzaniga (Cambridge, MA: MIT Press), 93–134.

Shepherd, G. M. (1990). "The significance of real neuron architectures for neural network simulations," in *Computational Neuroscience*, ed. E. Schwartz (Cambridge, MA: MIT Press), 82–96.

Shepherd, G. M. (1994). *Neurobiology*, 3rd Edn. New York: Oxford University Press.

Shepherd, G. M., and Brayton, R. K. (1987). Logic operations are properties of computer-simulated interactions between excitable dendritic spines. *Neuroscience* 21, 151–165.

Shepherd, G. M., and Grillner, S. (eds). (2010). *Handbook of Brain Microcircuits.* New York: Oxford University Press.

Shepherd, G. M., Woolf, T. B., and Carnevale, N. T. (1989). Comparisons between active properties of distal dendritic branches and spines: implications for neuronal computations. *J. Cogn. Neurosci.* 1, 273–286.

Skrede, K. K., and Westgaard, R. H. (1971). The transverse hippocampal slice: a well-defined cortical structure maintained in vitro. *Brain Res.* 35, 589–593.

Smith, L. M., Ebner, F. F., and Colonnier, M. (1980). The thalamocortical projection in Pseudemys turtles: a quantitative electron microscopic study. *J. Comp. Neurol.* 190, 445–461.

Somogyi, P. (2010). "Hippocampus: intrinsic organization," in *Handbook of Brain Microcircuits*, eds. G. M. Shepherd and S. Grillner (New York: Oxford University Press), 148–164.

Stepanyants, A., Hirsch, J. A., Martinez, I. M., Kisvarday, A. F., Ferecsko, A. S., and Chklovskii, D. B. (2008). Local potential connectivity in cat primary visual cortex. *Cereb. Cortex* 18, 13–28.

Stewart, W. B., Kauer, J. S., and Shepherd, G. M. (1979). Functional organization of rat olfactory bulb analysed by the 2-deoxyglucose method. *J. Comp. Neurol.* 185, 715–734.

Striedter, G. (2005). *Principles of Brain Evolution.* Sunderland, MA: Sinauer.

Stuart, G. J., Dodt, H. U., and Sakmann, B. (1993). Patch-clamp recordings from the soma and dendrites of neurons in brain slices using infrared video microscopy. *Pflugers Arch.* 423, 511–518.

Svoboda, K., Hooks, B. M., and Shepherd, G. M. G. (2010). "Barrel cortex," in *Handbook of Brain Microcircuits*, eds G. M. Shepherd and S. Grillner (New York: Oxford University Press), 31–38.

Swanson, L. W. (2000). What is the brain? *Trends Neurosci.* 23, 519–527.

Vassar, R., Chao, S. K., Sitcheran, R., Nunez, J. M., Vosshall, L. B., and Axel, R. (1994). Topographic organization of sensory projections to the olfactory bulb. *Cell* 79, 981–991.

Wang, X.-J. (2010). "Prefrontal cortex," in *Handbook of Brain Microcircuits*, eds G. M. Shepherd and S. Grillner (New York: Oxford University Press), 46–56.

Weiler, N., Wood, L., Yu, J., Solla, S. A., and Shepherd, G. M. G. (2008). Top-down laminar organization of the excitatory network in motor cortex. *Nat. Neurosci.* 11, 360–366.

Willhite, D. C., Nguyen, K.T., Masurkar, A.V., Greer, C. A., Shepherd, G. M., and Chen, W. R.(2006). Viral tracing identified distributed columnar organization in the olfactory bulb. *Proc. Natl. Acad. Sci. U.S.A.* 103, 12592–12597.

Wilson, D. A., and Barkai, E. (2010). "Olfactory cortex," in *Handbook of Brain Microcircuits*, eds G. M. Shepherd and S. Grillner (New York: Oxford University Press), 263–276.

Wilson, M. A., and Bower, J. M. (1988). "A computer simulation of olfactory cortex with functional implications for storage and retrieval of olfactory information," in *Neural Information Processing Systems*, ed. D. Z. Andersen (New York: American Institute of Physics), 114–126.

Wilson, D. A., and Stevenson, R. J. (2006). *Learning to Smell. Olfactory Perception from Neurobiology to Behavior.* Baltimore, MD: Johns Hopkins.

Xu, F., Greer, C. A., and Shepherd, G. M. (2000). Odor maps in the olfactory bulb. *J. Comp. Neurol.* 422, 489–495.

Yokota, T., Reeves, A. G., and MacLean, P. D. (1970). Differential effects of septal and olfactory volleys on intracellular responses of hippocampal neurons in awake, sitting monkeys. *J. Neurophysiol.* 33, 96–107.

Conflict of Interest Statement: The authors declare that the research was conducted in the absence of any commercial or financial relationships that could be construed as a potential conflict of interest.

15

Comparison of pretectal genoarchitectonic pattern between quail and chicken embryos

Paloma Merchán[1], Sylvia M. Bardet[2], Luis Puelles[1] and José L. Ferran[1]*

[1] Department of Human Anatomy and Psychobiology, Centre for Biomedical Research on Rare Diseases (CIBERER 736), School of Medicine, University of Murcia, Murcia, Spain

[2] Unité de Génétique Moléculaire Animale, INRA UMR 1061, University of Limoges, Limoges, France

Edited by:
Fernando Martinez-Garcia, University of Valencia, Spain

Reviewed by:
Frank Schubert, University of Portsmouth, UK
Ruth Morona, Complutense University, Spain
Salvador Martinez, University Miguel Hernandez, Spain

***Correspondence:**
José L. Ferran, Department of Human Anatomy and Psychobiology, School of Medicine, University of Murcia, Campus Espinardo E30071, Murcia, Spain.
e-mail: jlferran@um.es

Regionalization of the central nervous system is controlled by local networks of transcription factors that establish and maintain the identities of neuroepithelial progenitor areas and their neuronal derivatives. The conserved cerebral Bauplan of vertebrates must result essentially from conserved patterns of developmentally expressed transcription factors. We have previously produced detailed molecular maps for the alar plate of prosomere 1 (the *pretectal region*) in chicken (Ferran et al., 2007, 2008, 2009). Here we compare the early molecular signature of the pretectum of two closely related avian species of the family Phasianidae, *Coturnix japonica* (Japanese quail) and *Gallus gallus* (chicken), aiming to test conservation of the described pattern at a microevolutionary level. We studied the developmental pretectal expression of *Bhlhb4*, *Dbx1*, *Ebf1*, *Gata3*, *Gbx2*, *Lim1*, *Meis1*, *Meis2*, *Pax3*, *Pax6*, *Six3*, *Tal2*, and *Tcf7l2* (*Tcf4*) mRNA, using *in situ* hybridization, and PAX7 immunohistochemistry. The genoarchitectonic profile of individual pretectal domains and strata was produced, using comparable section planes. Remarkable conservation of the combinatorial genoarchitectonic code was observed, fundamented in a tripartite anteroposterior subdivision. However, we found that at corresponding developmental stages the pretectal region of *G. gallus* was approximately 30% larger than that of *C. japonica*, but seemed relatively less mature. Altogether, our results on a conserved genoarchitectonic pattern highlight the importance of early developmental gene networks that causally underlie the production of homologous derivatives in these two evolutionarily closely related species. The shared patterns probably apply to sauropsids in general, as well as to more distantly related vertebrate species.

Keywords: prosomere 1, precommissural pretectum, juxtacommissural pretectum, commissural pretectum, Galliformes, Phasianidae, forebrain, diencephalon

INTRODUCTION

Starting from early induction processes taking place at the neural plate stages, the partitions of the central nervous system are established sequentially by positional information created by morphogens secreted from various organizers. Prior to neural tube closure the major brain subdivisions – forebrain, midbrain, and hindbrain – are molecularly delimited one from another. Each of these partitions becomes regionalized subsequently by expressing specific combinations of genes, including transcription factors and cell-signaling, cell-cycle-regulating, and cell-adhesion molecules, which work in a networked way to generate different position-dependent molecular identities, specific neuronal, and glial populations and the resulting differential histogenesis of each molecularly individualized sector of the neural wall. Among the different types of genes, those coding for transcription factors (which represent collectively the core of the developmental network) play a key role in this process, since they specify, modifying, or stabilizing, the molecular codes active during the developmental process of any given brain region. The diffusible morphogens released from the secondary organizers establish gradiental concentration fields of signals whose interpretation by competent cells can change the primary molecular identity of the local histogenetic area (the neural progenitor cells) by up/down-regulation of downstream transcription factors (Puelles, 1995, 2001; Echevarria et al., 2003; Puelles et al., 2004; Kiecker and Lumsden, 2004; Davidson, 2006; Davidson and Erwin, 2006, 2009; Guillemot, 2007; Sánchez-Arrones et al., 2009). Supporting the idea that specific genetic codes identify each neural partition (and establish the respective boundaries), several comparative studies of gene expression patterns have revealed that homologous neural regions largely share a common molecular code at early stages of development across vertebrates (Fernandez et al., 1998; Hauptmann and Gerster, 2000; Puelles et al., 2000; Bachy et al., 2001; Murakami et al., 2001; Hauptmann et al., 2002; Puelles and Rubenstein, 2003; Ferran et al., 2007, 2008;

Abbreviations: AAB, alar–basal boundary; CNS, central nervous system; CoP, commissural pretectum; Di, deep intermediate zone; DMB, di-mesencephalic boundary; Hab, habenula; Hyp, hypothalamus; i, intermediate zone; JcP, juxtacommissural pretectum; MCPC, magnocellular nucleus of the posterior commissure; mes, mesencephalon; mi, middle intermediate; oi, outer-intermediate zone; OT, optic tectum; p1, prosomere 1; p2, prosomere 2; p3, prosomere 3; p1MT, p1 medial terminal nucleus; PcP, precommissural pretectum; pe, periventricular zone; PG, pineal gland; rh, rhombencephalon; RP, roof plate; Tel, telencephalon; TG, tectal gray; Th, thalamus; TPB, thalamo-pretectal boundary; tt, tecto-thalamic tract; su, superficial zone; v, ventricular zone.

García-López et al., 2008; Abellán and Medina, 2009; Bardet et al., 2010; Morona et al., 2010). A shared molecular pattern underpinning conserved morphogenesis may be held to represent the topological and molecularly conserved Bauplan of the neural tube, common to all vertebrates (Puelles and Rubenstein, 1993, 2003; Puelles, 1995, 2001; Puelles et al., 2004, 2007). Within this paradigm, combined gene expression patterns *properly correlated to their topological position* are highly relevant for dissecting the molecular code of each region, domain, layer, or nucleus. This is a scientific endeavor recently defined as the study of cerebral genoarchitecture (Ferran et al., 2009; Puelles, this volume). It is proving to be extremely useful for identifying homologous regions and derivatives between different vertebrates (Puelles and Medina, 2002; Puelles and Rubenstein, 2003; Ferran et al., 2007, 2008, 2009).

The pretectal region is the alar plate of prosomere 1 (p1), placed between the thalamus and the midbrain (Puelles et al., 2007). Building upon the pioneering studies on the chicken pretectum done by Rendahl (1924) and Kuhlenbeck (1939), several recent contributions have improved our knowledge of the anatomy of this region, both in terms of its subdivision into histogenetic domains and the characterization of its various derivatives (Redies et al., 1997, 2000; De Castro et al., 1998; Yoon et al., 2000; Ferran et al., 2007, 2008, 2009; Puelles et al., 2007). We defined a number of molecular characteristics of the pretectal identity codes from stage HH13 to posthatched chicken (Ferran et al., 2007, 2009). Specific molecular markers identify the rostral or precto-thalamic boundary (*Pax3*, *Meis1*) and the caudal or pretecto-mesencephalic boundary (*Pax6*, *Meis2*). In addition, the pretectal region was subdivided molecularly into three anteroposterior domains described as *precommissural pretectum* (PcP; *Bhlb4*, *Ebf1*), *juxtacommissural pretectum* (JcP; *Six3*, *Tal2*, *Lim1*), and *commissural pretectum* (CoP, *Pax7*, *Tal2*, *Lim1*). Several molecularly distinct dorsoventral subdomains of the three primary AP domains were detected as well (Ferran et al., 2007, 2009). Importantly, these molecular partitions were largely consistent with the fate map studies of García-López et al. (2004). The same tripartite molecular subdivision was found in the pretectum of the mouse (Ferran et al., 2008) and the *Xenopus laevis* frog (Morona et al., 2010).

Our present aim was to analyze the degree of conservation of pretectal genoarchitecture at a microevolutionary scale. For this purpose, we studied two closely related avian species (*Coturnix japonica* and *Gallus gallus*) that belong to the family Phasianidae, from the order Galliformes (Kimball et al., 1999; Crowe et al., 2006; Kan et al., 2010a,b; Shen et al., 2010). We chose to perform our study at the intermediate stages Q26/HH26 and Q28/HH28 (Q = Ainsworth et al., 2010 quail stages; HH = Hamburger and Hamilton, 1951 chicken stages). These stages represent in the chick the transition between early neurogenesis (HH20–HH27) and incipient mantle layer transformation into pronuclei (HH28–HH32; Crossland and Uchwat, 1982; Martínez, 1987; Puelles et al., 1987; Ferran et al., 2009). These embryos are still far from the period when definitive nuclei start to be distinguished (HH33–HH36). These important "hinge stages" have not been analyzed in depth previously. Therefore, we obtained a molecular map of selected markers for these developmental stages in both avian species, studying the previously defined molecular codes for each anteroposterior pretectal domain, as well as the relative pattern in which the incipient mantle strata became segregated molecularly. We included detailed studies of expression patterns for some genes that were not previously analyzed, or had been only superficially explored at these stages (*Ebf1*, *Gata3*, *Meis1*, *Meis2*, *Pax3*, and *Tcf712* [*Tcf4*]). We found in both species remarkable conservation at the studied stages of the combinatorial genoarchitectonic codes across the tripartite anteroposterior subdivision, and virtually the same combinatorial code with regard to radial stratification.

MATERIALS AND METHODS

The present research conforms to the stipulations of the European Community (86/609/EEC) and the Spanish Government (Royal Decree 223/1998) on care and use of laboratory animals.

ANIMALS

Fertilized quail (*Coturnix coturnix japonica*) and chicken eggs (*Gallus gallus domesticus*) from a local farm were incubated at 37°C in a forced-air incubator until the desired embryonic stage (Q26/HH26 to Q28/HH28). Around 60 embryos were staged according to Ainsworth et al. (2010) for quails and Hamburger and Hamilton (1951) for chickens. The embryos were fixed overnight by immersion in 4% paraformaldehyde in phosphate-buffered saline (PBS, pH7.4) at 4°C. Some embryos used for *in situ* hybridization (with or without immunochemical counterstain) were processed as wholemounts (or as brain halves, each half serving for 1–2 contrasting markers). The rest of the embryo heads were fixed overnight, washed 24 h in cold PBS, cryoprotected overnight in 20% sucrose in PBS, and finally embedded in 15% gelatin and 20% sucrose in PBS. The blocks were cryostat-sectioned 18 µm-thick in topologically true horizontal and transversal section planes relative to the length axis of p1 (pretectum). The sections were adhered onto SuperFrost-Plus slides (Menzel-Gläser, Braunschweig, Germany), separated into four or five parallel series. Each series was processed subsequently for *in situ* hybridization with a different mRNA probe. Some series were immunoreacted after the *in situ* hybridization reaction.

RT-PCR

RNA was extracted from fresh dissected brains of *G. gallus* embryos at stages HH24, HH30, or HH33 and *C. japonica* at stage Q26 using Trizol reagent (10296-028, Invitrogen). The RNA was treated with DNAse I (18068-015, Invitrogen) during 15 min at room temperature, and then the enzyme was inactivated at 65°C. The RNA was reverse-transcribed into single-stranded cDNA with Superscript II reverse transcriptase and oligo dT anchored primers (11904-018, SuperScript First-Strand Synthesis System for RT-PCR; Invitrogen). The resulting first-strand cDNA (0.5 µl of the reverse transcription reaction) was used as a template for PCR, performed with Taq polymerase (M8305, Promega). Specific primers listed below were designed to clone gene fragments from *Bhlhb4*, *Ebf1*, *Gbx2*, *Pax3* from *G. gallus* sequences; and *Bhlhb4*, *Dbx1*, *Ebf1*, *Gata3*, *Lim1*, *Meis1*, *Meis2*, *Pax3*, *Pax6*, *Pax7*, *Six3*, *and Tcf7l2* from *C. japonica* sequences (*G. gallus* sequences were used for primer design).

CQ*Bhlhb4*F1: 5′-ATGGCCGAGCTCAAGTCGCT-3′;
CQ*Bhlhb4*F2: 5′-TGGGCAAGTCGGCAGAGAG-3′.
CQ*Bhlhb4*R: 5′-TCAAGGCTTGTCGCTGCAGT-3′.
CQ*Ebf1*F1: 5′-CAGTCAATGTTGATGGCCAT-3′;
CQ*Ebf1*F2: 5′-GCACAACAATTCCAAGCAT-3′;
CQ*Ebf1*R: 5′-AGGAGAAGTTTGCGGTCTCA-3′.

*C*Gbx2F: 5′-AGCGACCTCGACTACAGCTC-3′;
*C*Gbx2R: 5′-ATTCACAAGACGGGAGTTGG-3′.
*C*Pax3F: 5′-GCCGCCGCGATGACCACG-3′;
*C*Pax3R: 5′-GAGCGAGACCGGAAAATAACACCA-3′;
*Q*Dbx1F: 5′-GTCCCCGCTACACAAGGCAC-3′.
*Q*Dbx1R: 5′-CTTCCTGCTCCAGGTATTCG-3′.
*Q*Gata3F: 5′-TGGAACCTCAGCCCTTTTTCC-3′.
*Q*Gata3R: 5′-GTTAAAGGAGCTGCTCTTGG-3′.
*Q*Lim1F: 5′-GGAGCAAAGTGTTCCACTTG-3′.
*Q*Lim1R: 5′-CGGTTCTGGAACCACACCTGG-3′;
*Q*Meis1F: 5′-GTGTTCGCCAAACAGATCCG-3′;
*Q*Meis1R: 5′-CCTCCATGCCCATATTCATGC-3′.
*Q*Meis2F: 5′-ATGGCGCAAAGGTACGATGAG-3′;
*Q*Meis2R: 5′-TTGCGACTGATTTACAAGAT-3′.
*Q*Pax3F: 5′-TCGGCGGCAGCAAACCCAAG-3′.
*Q*Pax3R: 5′-GGCTCCTGCCTGCTTCCTCC-3′.
*Q*Pax6F: 5′-GCAGGTATTACGAAACTGGC-3′.
*Q*Pax6R: 5′-GGGTTGCATAGGCAGGTTGT-3′.
*Q*Pax7F: 5′-GATGTTCAGCTGGGAGATCC-3′.
*Q*Pax7R: 5′-ACAGGATTCATGTGGTTG-3′.
*Q*Six3F: 5′-GTGGCCAGCGTCTGCGAGAC-3′.
*Q*Six3R: 5′-GTTAAAGGAGCTGCTCTTGG-3′.
*Q*Tcf7l2F: 5′-CACCCGCACCATGTACACCC-3′.
*Q*Tcf7l2R: 5′-CCTTCACCTTGTATGTAGCG-3′.

PCR conditions were as follows: 5 min at 94°C, then 35 cycles (30 s at 94°C, plus 1 min at Tm temperature −57°C, and 1 min at 72°C), followed by 20 min at 72°C. The PCR products were cloned into pGEM-T Easy Vector (Promega) and sequenced (SAI, University of Murcia). *C. japonica* and *G. gallus* sequences were submitted to GenBank (accession numbers: HQ436513, *Bhlhb4 C. japonica*; HQ436514, *Dbx1 C. japonica*; HQ436515, *Ebf1 C. japonica*; HQ436512, *Ebf1 G. gallus;* JF297589, *Gata3 C. japonica;* HQ436511, *Gbx2 G. gallus*; JF719578, *Lim1 C. japonica;* JF304296, Meis1A.2 *C. japonica*; HQ436516, *Meis2A.1 C. japonica;* HQ436517, *Pax3 C. japonica;* HQ436518, *Pax6 C. japonica;* HQ436519, *Pax7 C. japonica;* JF297588, *Six3 C. japonica*; HQ436520, *Tcf7l2 C. japonica*).

IN SITU HYBRIDIZATION

Digoxygenin-11-UTP (Roche, Lewes, UK) was used for RNA probe synthesis. Plasmid information is provided in **Table 1**.

The whole-mount *in situ* hybridization protocol used was that of Shimamura et al. (1994), whereas the ISH reaction on cryostat-sectioned material followed the protocol of Hidalgo-Sánchez et al. (2005). After ISH, the sections were washed, and the hybridized product was detected immunocytochemically using anti-digoxigenin antiserum coupled to alkaline phosphatase (Roche Diagnostics, Mannheim, Germany). Nitroblue tetrazolium/bromochloroindolyl phosphate (NBT/BCIP) was used as chromogenic substrate for the final alkaline phosphatase reaction (Boehringer, Mannheim, Germany).

IMMUNOHISTOCHEMISTRY

After *in situ* hybridization, immunocytochemical reaction for PAX7 was performed in whole-mounts according to Ferran et al. (2007). Hybridized cryostat sections were processed for

Table 1 | List of gene markers used, sequence of the gene in the construct, and origin of the plasmid construction.

Gen	Species	NCBI number/ size/position	Laboratory/references
Bhlhb4	*G. gallus*	NM_204504.2 (663bp;77–739)	Present results
Bhlhb4	*C. japonica*	HQ436513 (666bp;1–666)	Present results
Dbx1	*G. gallus*	XR_026947.1 (1511bp; 1–1511)	Ferran et al. (2007)
Dbx1	*C. japonica*	HQ436514 (441bp;1–441)	Present results
Ebf1	*G. gallus*	HQ436512 (1055bp;1–1055)	Present results
Ebf1	*C. japonica*	HQ436515 (1004bp;1–1004)	Present results
Gbx2	*G. gallus*	HQ436511 (977bp, 1–977)	Present results
Gata3	*G. gallus*	NM_001008444.1 (779bp;758–1533)	EST clon: ChEST663o17; Boardman et al. (2002)
Gata3	*C. japonica*	JF297589 (844bp; 1–844)	Present results
Lim1	*G. gallus*	NM_205413.1 (1348bp; 105–1453)	Matsunaga et al. (2000)
Lim1	*C. japonica*	JF719578 (454bp; 1-454)	Present results
Tal2	*G. gallus*	XM_424886.2 (898bp; 17–915)	EST clon: ChEST45a19; Boardman et al. (2002)
Meis1A.2	*G. gallus*	FJ265709.1 (1230bp;1–1230)	Sánchez-Guardado et al. (2011)
Meis1A.2	*C. japonica*	JF304296 (787bp; 1–787)	Present results
Meis2A.1	*G. gallus*	HQ436521 (1231bp;1–1231)	Sánchez-Guardado et al. (2011)
Meis2A.1	*C. japonica*	HQ436516 (905bp;1–905)	Present results
Pax3	*G. gallus*	NM_204269.1 (1514bp; 12–1525)	Present results
Pax3	*C. japonica*	HQ436517 (344bp;1–344)	Present results
Pax6	*G. gallus*	NM_205066.1 (1327bp; 553–1880)	Ferran et al. (2007)
Pax6	*C. japonica*	HQ436518 (845bp;1–845)	Present results
Pax7	*C. japonica*	HQ436519 (744 bp;1–744)	Present results
Six3	*G. gallus*	NM_204364 (798bp; 406–1204)	Bovolenta et al. (1998)
Six3	*C. japonica*	JF297588 (647bp; 1–647)	Present results
Tcf712	*G. gallus*	AB040438.1 (2345bp; 1–2345)	Matsunaga et al. (2000)
Tcf7l2	*C. japonica*	HQ436520 (827bp;1–827)	Present results

immunocytochemistry in a similar way. After several washes in 0.1 M PBS with 0.75% Triton X-100 (PBT), sections were treated with 3% hydrogen peroxide in PBT for 15 min in the dark to inactivate endogenous peroxidase activity. After several rinses in PBT, they were blocked with 0.2% gelatin (PBTG) and 0.1 M lysine during 1–4 h. The anti-PAX7 primary antibody diluted in PBGT was incubated for 48 h at 4°C (1:20; Developmental Studies Hybridoma Bank, Iowa City, IA, USA). After washes in PBT and PBTG, the tissues were incubated with biotinylated goat anti-mouse IgG (1:200 in PBT, 1.5 h; Vector Laboratories, Burlingame, CA, USA), passing thereafter to streptavidin/horseradish peroxidase complex (Vectastain-ABC kit; Vector Laboratories; 1:350, 1 h). The brown peroxidase reaction was performed with a 15-min soak in 3,3-diaminobenzidine [Sigma, St. Louis, MO, USA; 50 mg/100 ml in 0.05 M Tris–HCl buffer (pH 7.6)], plus 5–10 min with added 0.03% hydrogen peroxide. The reaction was stopped with 0.05 M Tris buffer. Sections were coverslipped with Eukitt.

IMAGING

Digital microphotographs of the whole-mounts were obtained with a Zeiss Axiocam camera (Carl Zeiss, Oberkochen, Germany), and a ScanScope digital scanner (Aperio, Technologies, Inc.; Vista, CA, USA) was used for the cryostat sections (exported as TIF files). The images were corrected for contrast and brightness in Photoshop 7.0. In order to compare different gene expression patterns, images were artificially pseudocolored (from blue to red or green) and superimposed using Photoshop 7.0. The plates were labeled using Adobe Photoshop IllustratorCS2 (Adobe Systems, San José, CA, USA). Representative sections from comparable chicken and quail embryos were measured using Image-ProPlus (Media Cibernetics Inc.). Image J software was used to delineate contours around areas to be compared quantitatively, obtaining the areas (in arbitrary units) of the whole pretectum at several sections levels, as well as the individual precommissural, juxtacommissural, and commissural domains. Considering volume proportional to sectioned surface, the promediated values of the individual domains were calculated as percentage of the total pretectal area, giving a rough estimate of relative proportions. No statistic was possible due to the small number of data.

RESULTS

PRELIMINARY REMARKS ON THE SELECTION OF SPECIES, GENES, AND DEVELOPMENTAL STAGES

The goal of the present work was to make a comparative study of the spatio-temporal distribution of key mRNAs in the pretectal region of two closely related species. Since a previous detailed study was made in *G. gallus* (Chicken; Ferran et al., 2007, 2009), we decided to use *C. japonica*, a member of the same avian family (Phasianidae). This species is commonly used as tissue-donor for quail–chicken grafting experiments (**Figure 1A**). Regarding the stages, we aimed to characterize early combinatorial molecular codes and test pattern profiles defining the general pretectal Bauplan during initial steps of pronuclear generation (after radial migration of postmitotic neurons into the mantle layer). Therefore, we decided to perform our study between stages Q26/HH26 and Q28/HH28, thus also expanding our previous chicken studies. Finally, the genes chosen as markers were selected according to our previous knowledge of their importance for delimiting boundaries or a specific domain, layer, or nuclear derivative (Ferran et al., 2007, 2009).

DIFFERENCES IN TRANSCRIPT SEQUENCES BETWEEN *C. japonica* AND *G. gallus*

Coturnix japonica and *G. gallus* underwent 40 million years of independent evolution as members of the Coturnicinae and Gallininae subfamilies, respectively (**Figure 1A**). Therefore, our first aim was to assess any differences at the nucleotide and aminoacidic level of the studied genes. For this purpose, we cloned the complete coding sequence of *Bhlhb4*, obtained partial coding sequences from *Ebf1*, *Gata3*, *Lim1*, *Meis1*, *Meis2*, *Pax3*, *Pax6*, *Pax7*, *Six3*, and *Tcf7l2*, we also studied the 3′UTR of *Dbx1* from *C. japonica*, comparing them to available *G. gallus* sequences. We found >93 and >96% (often ~99%) similarity at the nucleotide and protein levels, respectively, for all the analyzed *C. japonica* and *G. gallus* genes (**Figure 1B**). In addition, we compared the four published gene sequences from *C. coturnix* obtained from GenBank, finding a similar level of conservation in *G. gallus* and *C. japonica* (data not shown). These results indicate a high level of mRNA sequence conservation between *C. japonica* and *G. gallus*, which is likely to represent the general degree of divergence among the subfamilies of the family Phasianidae.

PRETECTAL BOUNDARIES AND DOMAINS ARE DEFINED BY THE SAME GENOARCHITECTONIC CODES IN *C. japonica* AND *G. gallus*

A major conclusion of our previous studies was that the combined expression patterns of three genes were enough to define the antero-posterior pretectal boundaries and its internal tripartition (Ferran et al., 2007, 2008). Here we corroborated that the same molecular code applies to *C. japonica*. In both species, pretectal expression of *Pax3* stops rostrally at the thalamo-pretectal boundary (TPB; p2/p1), whereas that of *Pax6* ends caudally at the pretecto-mesencephalic limit (p1/m1); these patterns jointly define the pretectal region (alar p1; **Figures 2A,C,D,E,H,I**). In addition, expression of *Six3* neatly distinguished in both cases the intermediate pretectal domain (JcP; **Figures 2B,F,G**). Therefore, the combination of markers *Six3/Pax3/Pax6* also identifies the rostral and caudal pretectal domains (PcP and commissural pretectum, or CoP, respectively). As previously found in the chicken, the quail CoP domain showed extensive PAX7 immunoreaction (**Figures 2E,I**).

Next, we analyzed *Gbx2*, *Meis1*, and *Pax3* expression patterns in cryostat sections in order to define more precisely the molecular TPB. In both species, *Gbx2* is strongly expressed in the thalamic mantle zone, stopping caudally at the TPB; *Gbx2* is absent at the overlying habenular region (**Figures 2J,O,O′,Y and 3M–P,AE,AF**). In addition, we observed a periventricular patch expressing *Gbx2* in the rostral pretectum (see below; asterisk in **Figures 2O and 3N,P,AF**). *Pax3* expression is largely restricted to the pretectal ventricular zone, though its signal appears as well in the mantle of the CoP domain (see below). *Pax3* transcripts generally stop rostrally at the TPB (**Figures 2A,D,E,K, O′,P,Y and 3I–L**). However, at the dorsal-most levels, *Pax3* expression expands into the habenular dorsal p2 domain, and is accordingly not useful as a p2/p1 limit marker at that specific position (blue arrowhead; **Figures 2A,D,E**). *Meis1* appears expressed in the pretectum but not in the thalamus. Its domain stops precisely at the rostral pretectal boundary,

A

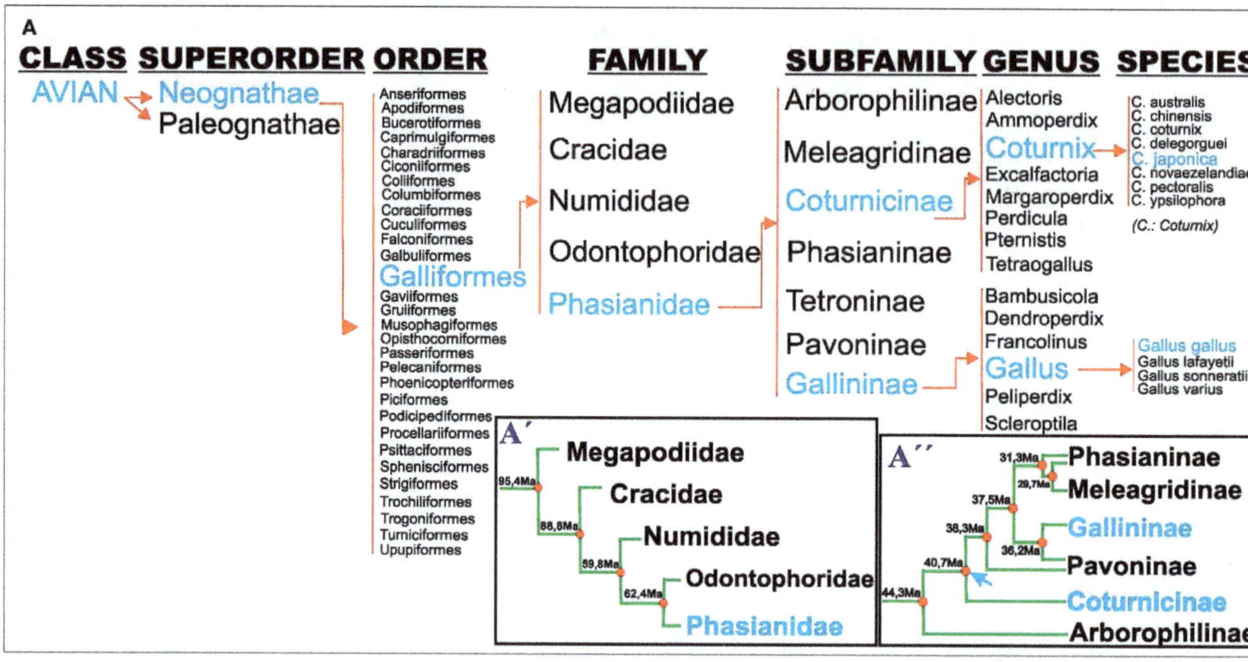

B

Gene	*C. japonica* NCBI Acc. number	*G. gallus* NCBI Acc. number	Nucleotide sequence length	% of similarity *C. japonica*/ *G. gallus*	Protein sequence length	% of similarity *C. japonica*/ *G. gallus*
Bhlhb4	HQ436513	NM_20450402.2	666	94%	221	96%
Ebf1	HQ436515	HQ436512	1004	99 %	334	99 %
Gata3	JF297589	NM_001008444.1	844	99 %	281	99 %
Lim1	JF719578	NM_205413.1	454	99 %	150	99 %
Meis1A.2	JF304296	FJ265709.1	787	98%	262	99%
Meis2A.1	HQ436516	HQ436521	905	99%	292	99%
Pax3	HQ436517	NM_204269.1	344	98%	114	99%
Pax6	HQ436518	NM_205066.1	845	97%	281	98%
Pax7	HQ436519	NM_205065.1	744	99%	247	100%
Six3	JF297588	NM_204364	647	99%	215	99%
Tcf7l2	HQ436520	XM_421760.2	788	99%	262	99%
Dbx1	HQ436514	XR_026947.1	447	93%	3′UTR	3′UTR

FIGURE 1 | (A) Taxonomic classification of Galliformes according to Crowe et al. (2006). **(A′)** Postulated phylogenetic relationships between families of the order *galliformes*. The timetree represents the mean times of independent evolution, estimated from several studies, according to Pereira and Baker (2009). **(A″)** Phylogenetic relationships among members of the family Phasianidae according to Kan et al. (2010a,b). *Blue arrow:* time point of Gallininae and Coturnicinae split. **(B)** Comparison of the codifying and protein sequences of the listed genes between *G. gallus* and *C. japonica*.

including its dorsal-most part, showing no expansion into p2, in contrast to *Pax3*. Moreover, *Meis1* shows strong expression in the ventricular and mantle zones of the PcP domain in both species (see below; **Figures 2L,Q,Y and 3A–D**). Altogether, these genes allow the precise identification not only of the early TPB, but also of the different mantle derivatives abutting at this boundary from either side (*Meis1*, pretectum; *Gbx2*, thalamus; **Figure 2Y**).

Additionally, we compared markers that recognize the pretecto- or diencephalo-mesencephalic boundary (DMB). To this end, we studied *Pax6*, *Meis2*, *Tcf7l2* (previously named *Tcf4*), and PAX7 expression patterns. *Pax6* is consistently expressed in the ventricular and mantle zones of the caudal pretectum (CoP), with a clearcut caudal end at the DMB in both animal models (**Figures 2C,H,M,R,Y**). We found that *Meis2* expression, which appears extensively at the mesencephalic ventricular and mantle zones, stops rostrally at the mesencephalic side of the DMB boundary up to stage Q26/HH27. From Q27/HH28 onward, *Meis2* expression emerges in some periventricular and superficial cells of CoP (see below; green arrows **Figures 2S,T,W,Y**). *Tcf7l2* was previously reported to be expressed in the alar plate of the caudal diencephalon (thalamus and pretectum), stopping at the DMB up to stage HH24 (Ferran et al., 2007). From HH25 onward, we found that *Tcf7l2* transcripts expand progressively caudalward within the mesencephalic alar mantle. However, *Tcf7l2* signal remains restricted to the diencephalon at the level of the ventricular zone, stopping caudally at the DMB; therefore, this marker continues being useful for identifying this boundary (**Figures 2U,X,Y**). Finally, as previously described in chicken, PAX7 is widely expressed in the ventricular and mantle zones of the caudal

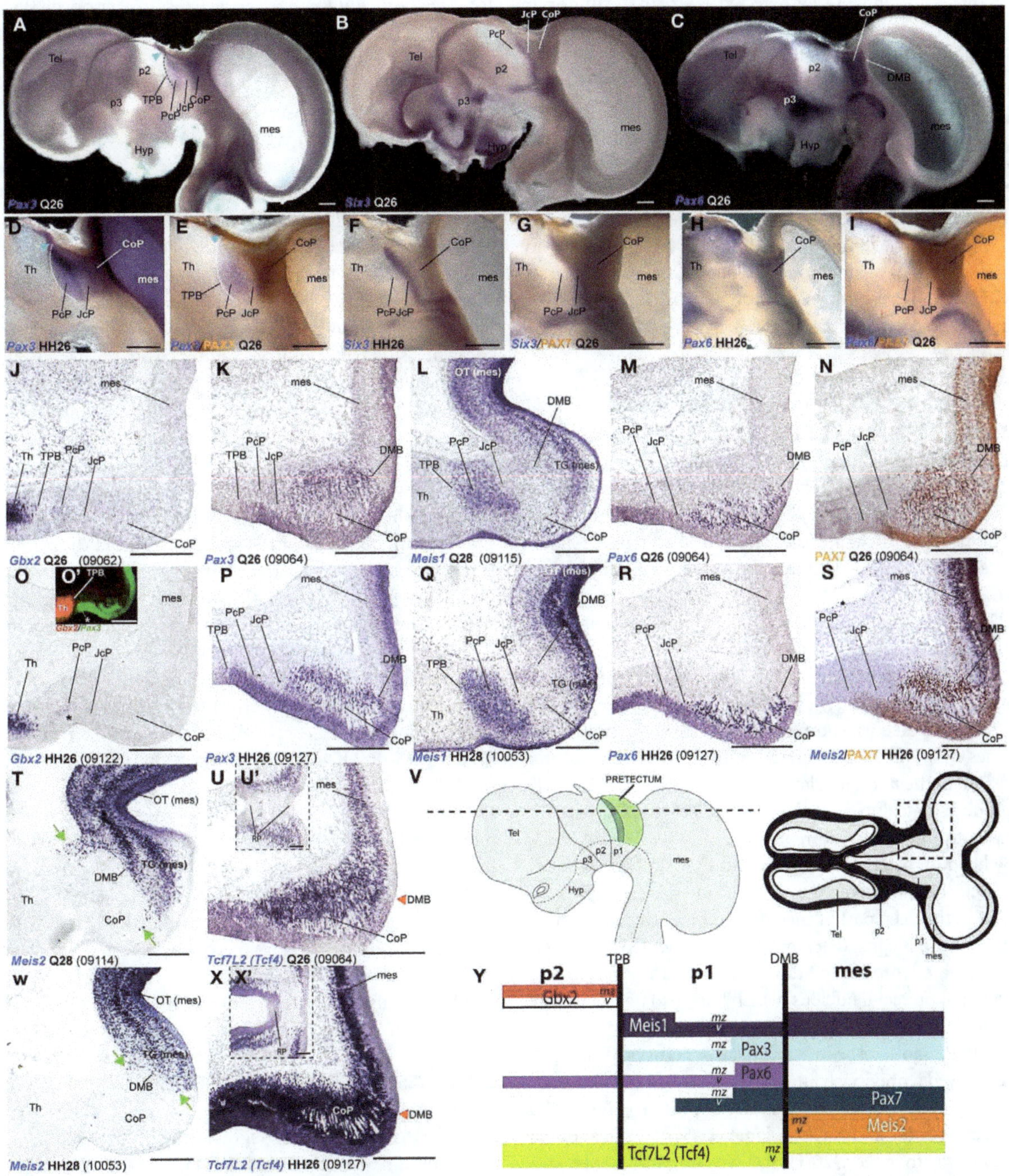

FIGURE 2 | Pairwise comparison of gene patterns in the developing pretectum of Q26 quail or HH26 chicken embryos (as identified at left bottom corner of each panel). The markers shown are *Pax3* **(A,D,E,K,P)**, *Six3* **(B,F,G)**, *Pax6* **(C,H,I,M,R)**, PAX7 **(E,I,N,S)**, *Gbx2* **(J,O,O′)**, *Meis1* **(L,Q)**, *Meis2* **(S,T,W)**, and *Tcf7l2* **(U,U′,X,X′)**. **(A–I)** Whole-mount *in situ* hybridization and immunoreaction processed material identify the main pretectal boundaries and define an anteroposterior tripartition. *Blue arrowhead* in **(A,D,E)**: *Pax3* expression extends continuously from the pretectum into the thalamic habenular region. **(J–X)** Horizontal sections at corresponding levels in both species illustrating distribution along the radial dimension of the studied markers. The pairwise comparable panels are organized one on top of the other **(J,O,K,P, …)**. The numbers between brackets at the bottom of each panel give the code identifying the specimen in our collection (data from the same specimen may appear in different panels or plates). Inset **(O′)** compares in pseudocolor the patterns of *Gbx2* and *Pax3*, demonstrating that the cell group marked with an asterisk **(O,O′)** lies caudal to the thalamo-pretectal boundary. Insets **(U′,X′)** show horizontal sections passing through the roof of the pretectum, where *Tcf7l2* is not expressed. *Green arrows* in **(T,W)**: *Meis2* positive cells at the CoP. The schemata in **(V)** represent a lateral view of the brain indicating the horizontal section plane used, and the position in such sections of the pretectal region that appears magnified in the panels (dashed box). **(Y)** Schema of gene combinations mapped in the midbrain (mes) and diencephalic prosomeres p1 and p2. Each gene is represented by a color-coded bar. The upper and lower halves of each bar represent gene expression in the mantle (mz) or ventricular zones (v) respectively. Scale bars = 300 μm.

pretectum (CoP). Although PAX7 is detected as well in the midbrain tectum, its expression is downregulated caudal to the DMB in a rostral alar midbrain territory intercalated between the pretectum and the optic tectum proper, the primordium of the tectal gray (TG; Ferran et al., 2007, 2009; see also García-Calero et al., 2002 and Puelles et al., 2007). Therefore, both species showed a sharp boundary at the DMB through the combination of PAX7 immunohistochemistry and *Meis2/Tcf712* mRNA *in situ* hybridization (**Figures 2I,N,S,Y**).

As regards the ventral boundary of the pretectum, marked in chicken by *Pax6* expression (neither *Pax3* or PAX7 reach ventrally the alar–basal boundary), it also was comparable in the quail (**Figures 2C,H and 8J**). In both cases, moreover Tcf712 expression reaches dorsally the roof–alar plate boundary (**Figures 2U′,X′ and 8K**).

CONSERVED MOLECULAR PROFILE OF THE PRECOMMISSURAL PRETECTUM DURING EARLY MANTLE HISTOGENESIS

Ventricular (*v*), periventricular (*pe*), intermediate (*i*), and superficial strata (*su*) can be distinguished in the PcP at the stages analyzed (Rendahl, 1924; Senn, 1970, 1979; Ferran et al., 2009). During the pronuclear period, the thick intermediate stratum becomes subdivided into *deep* (*di*), *middle* (mi), and *outer* (*oi*) intermediate layers (Ferran et al., 2009).

Bhlhb4, Dbx1, Ebf1, Meis1, and *Pax3* mRNA expression mark the PcP derivatives, therefore we compared these patterns with those of *Gbx2, Lim1*, and *Six3* in order to clearly identify the rostral and caudal boundaries of PcP (**Figure 3**). *Meis1* appears expressed at the PcP ventricular zone and all corresponding mantle layers in both avian species at stages Q26/HH26–Q27/HH27, but at Q28/HH28 its signal clearly decreased in the *pe* mantle layer (**Figures 3A–D, 4A–F,Y–AD, and 7**). A pioneering group of *Meis1*-positive PcP cells apparently moving incipiently into the JcP domain was clearly observed at HH26 (green arrowhead, or asterisk, in **Figures 3B,D,F,AK,AL**). At stages Q27/HH27–Q28/HH28 there is a population of cells expressing strongly *Meis1* in the deep part of the intermediate layer (*di*), which, when compared to *Six3* signal (a JcP marker), are revealed as PcP cells that have translocated into the JcP domain. This is the primordium of the dorsocaudal pretectal nucleus, which later also penetrates the CoP (Ferran et al., 2009). *Pax3* mRNA was only detected at the *v* and *pe* layer of the PcP mantle zone in both species (**Figures 3I–L, 5G,V, and 7**). We observed a previously undescribed stream of *Gbx2* positive cells localized in the periventricular layer of the PcP (**Figures 2O, 3N,N′,P,P′,AF,AF′, and 7**). This *Gbx2* signal was visualized at dorsal levels of the PcP from stage Q26/HH26 onward, and it increased progressively at later stages (asterisk in **Figures 2O′, 3N,P,AF**). *Bhlhb4* mRNA expression was strongly present at the PcP *pe* and *i* strata in both species. As described for *Meis1*, we observed a few *Bhlhb4* positive cells originated from the PcP *di* layer that apparently translocate into the JcP domain (green arrow, **Figures 3Q–T,AH,AI and 7**). *Dbx1* transcripts appear in the PcP *pe* layer and in a salt and pepper pattern at the *v* stratum, in both species. The expression of this gene does not stop at the thalamo-pretectal limit, but continues in p2 within the habenular region (**Figures 3U–X and 7**). *Ebf1* mRNA expression was observed throughout the PcP mantle layers, but not at the ventricular stratum. At dorsal PcP levels, *Ebf1* expression extends also into the habenular region of p2, but more ventrally it clearly stops at the boundary between thalamus and pretectum. As reported above for *Meis1*and *Bhlhb4*-positive cells, comparison of the expression patterns of *Ebf1* and *Lim1* (JcP marker) showed some *Ebf1*-positive cells from the PcP *di* layer entering the JcP domain (green arrow, or asterisk; **Figures 3Y–AD,AM and 7**). Finally, a cluster of *Gata3*-expressing cells was observed at the PcP *oi* and *su* strata from both species (**Figures 4S–V,AQ–AT**).

CONSERVED MOLECULAR PROFILE OF THE JUXTACOMMISSURAL PRETECTUM DURING EARLY MANTLE HISTOGENESIS

To analyze the JcP region, we studied the *Six3, Gata3, Lim1*, and *Tal2* gene expression patterns. We had previously demonstrated in chicken that *Six3* is a selective cell marker for the mantle zone of the JcP domain from HH17/18 onward (Ferran et al., 2007). Here we first compared the expression patterns of *Six3* and *Meis1* to double-check the rostral JcP boundary along the full radial dimension (**Figures 4A–L,Y–AJ**). Then, we compared *Six3* with the *Lim1, Gata3*, and *Tal2* markers – all expressed throughout the JcP and CoP domains – to identify the caudal JcP boundary within these patterns (**Figures 4G–X,AE–AV, 6E–L,Q–X, and 7**). Between Q26/HH26 and Q28/HH28 all JcP mantle layers show *Six3* expression (**Figures 4G–J,AE–AH and 7**), but the *i* stratum, in most of the sections, and the *su* stratum, at dorsal levels, already have started to downregulate *Six3* expression at Q27/HH27 (asterisk in **Figures 4I,J,AE–AH**). This change in the pattern seems correlated with the onset of *FoxP1* expression at the same loci (Data not shown; see Discussion). *Lim1* is strongly expressed in all JcP mantle derivatives of both species, with a particularly compact appearance of the *oi* layer from the *i* stratum, which mainly represents the primordium of the lateral spiriform nucleus (asterisk **Figures 4M–R,AK–AP**; Ferran et al., 2009). JcP expression of *Gata3* mRNA, which has not been described previously, is similar to that of *Lim1* in both species (**Figures 4S–V,AQ–AT**). Nevertheless, a relatively stronger *Gata3* signal at the JcP *pe* and *di* strata distinguishes them from the CoP ones (**Figures 4U–X,AS–AV and 7**). *Tal2* signal is strong at the JcP *pe* and *di*, but decreases slightly at the *oi* layer from the dorsal and lateral subdomains; this signal is absent at the ventral JcP and CoP subdomains of both species (**Figures 6E–H,Q–T and 7**). *Pax3* and *Pax6* are expressed in the JcP ventricular zone, and PAX7 only appears in overlap at the level of the most dorsal JcP subdomains (**Figures 5 and 7**).

CONSERVED MOLECULAR PROFILE OF THE COMMISSURAL PRETECTUM DURING MANTLE HISTOGENESIS

In order to study radial segregation of strata and layers in the CoP domain, we compared *Gata3, Lim1, Pax3, Pax6, Pax7*, and *Tal2* mRNA expression, adding occasional data from the *Bhblb4, Dbx1, Ebf1, Meis1, Meis2*, and *Six3* expression patterns. The genes of the PAX family are variously combined within CoP, generating by themselves a molecular code that identifies the four strata observed from the ventricle to the pial surface (*v, pe, i, su*). The *v* zone is characterized by the expression of *Pax3, Pax6*, and *Pax7*, though *Pax7* expression is absent at the most ventral alar plate levels (arrowhead; **Figures 5 and 7**). The *pe* stratum expresses strongly *Pax6* and *Pax7*, and shows a weak *Pax3* signal (**Figures 5 and 7**).

Starting at stages Q26 in quail and HH27 in chicken, the CoP *i* stratum started to be segregated in three parts, the deep, middle and outer intermediate layers (*di, mi, oi*). The thin *di* layer shows *Pax7*- and *Pax3*-positive cells (**Figures 5I,J,N,O**).

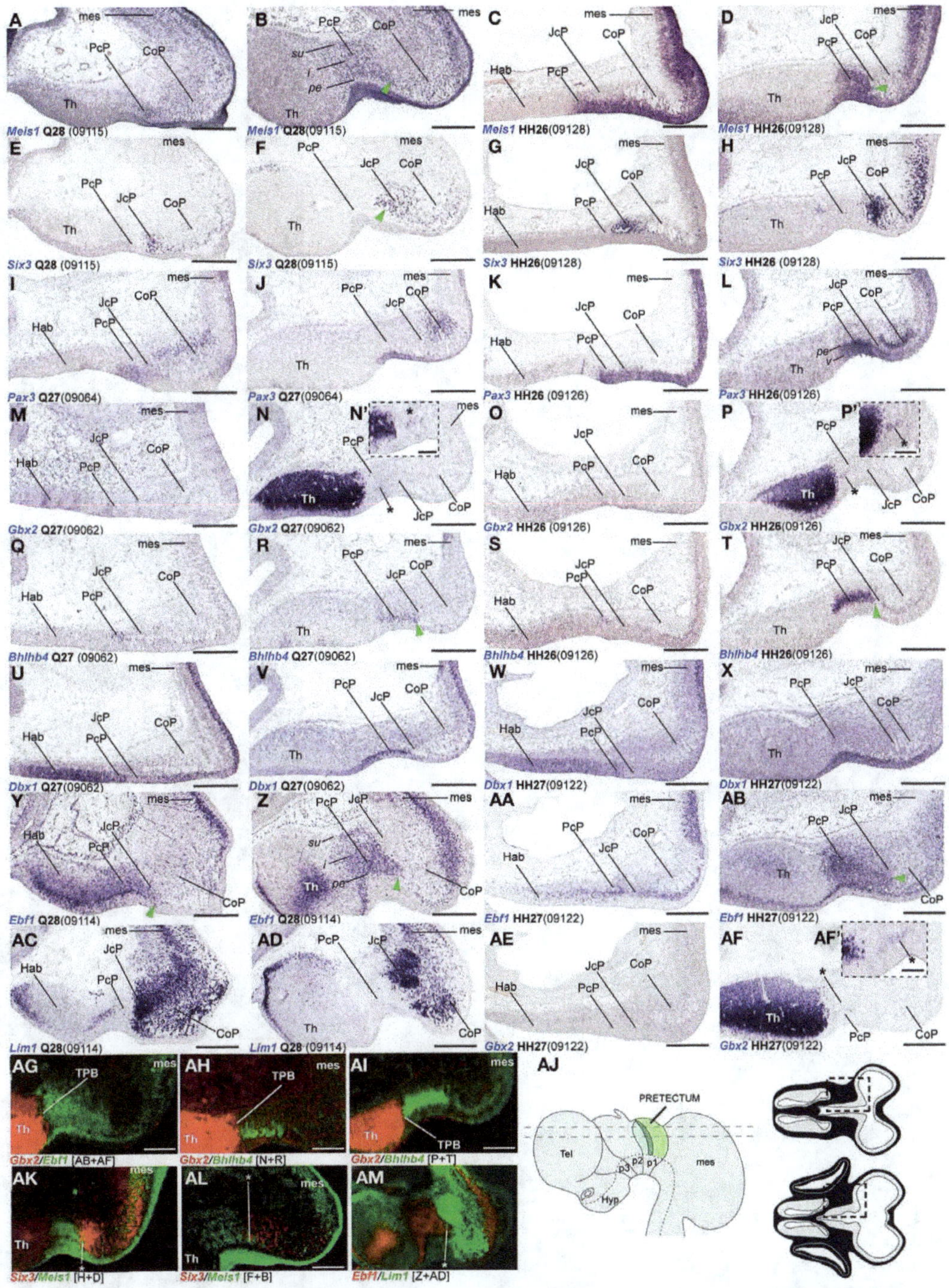

FIGURE 3 | (A–AM) Comparisons of *in situ* hybridization data for PcP markers at HH26/27-Q27/28 in horizontal cryostat sections. From top to bottom of the plate, each row of four panels generally contains data on one gene: *Meis1* **(A–D)**, *Six3* **(E–H)**, *Pax3* **(I–L)**, *Gbx2* **(M–P,AE,AF)**, *Bhlhb4* **(Q–T)**, *Dbx1* **(U–X)**, *Ebf1* **(Y–AB)**, *Lim1* **(AC–AD)**. Note that material from different specimens (identifying codes in brackets) was pooled into this plate. Each adjacent pair of panels from left to right corresponds to two different section levels in one species (in dorsoventral order), to be compared with the next two panels of corresponding section levels in the other species [e.g., for *Meis1*, **(A,B)** are two quail section levels to be compared with **(C,D)**, showing the same marker at equivalent levels in the chick]. Patterns comparable between quail and chicken are thus shown horizontally. The panels illustrating the other markers in successive rows represent corresponding section levels (though sometimes a different specimen is compared), so that different gene patterns are compared vertically. *Green arrowheads* in **(B,D,F,R,T,Y,Z,AB)** and *asterisks* in **(AK–AM)** indicate small groups of cells expressing a PcP marker that lie within the molecularly identified JcP domain, suggesting a tangential migratory displacement. *Asterisks* in **(N/N′,P/P′,AF/AF′)**: *Gbx2* positive cells within the PcP. **(AG–AI,AK–AM)** Pseudocolored superposition of the indicated pairs of marker domains from adjacent sections, to illustrate boundary relationships between them. **(AJ)** Schematic view of the brain indicating the two horizontal section planes illustrated in this plate, and the position in such sections of the pretectal region that appears magnified in the panels (dashed boxes). Scale bars = 300 μm for **(A–AM)** and 100 μm for **(N′,P′,AF′)**.

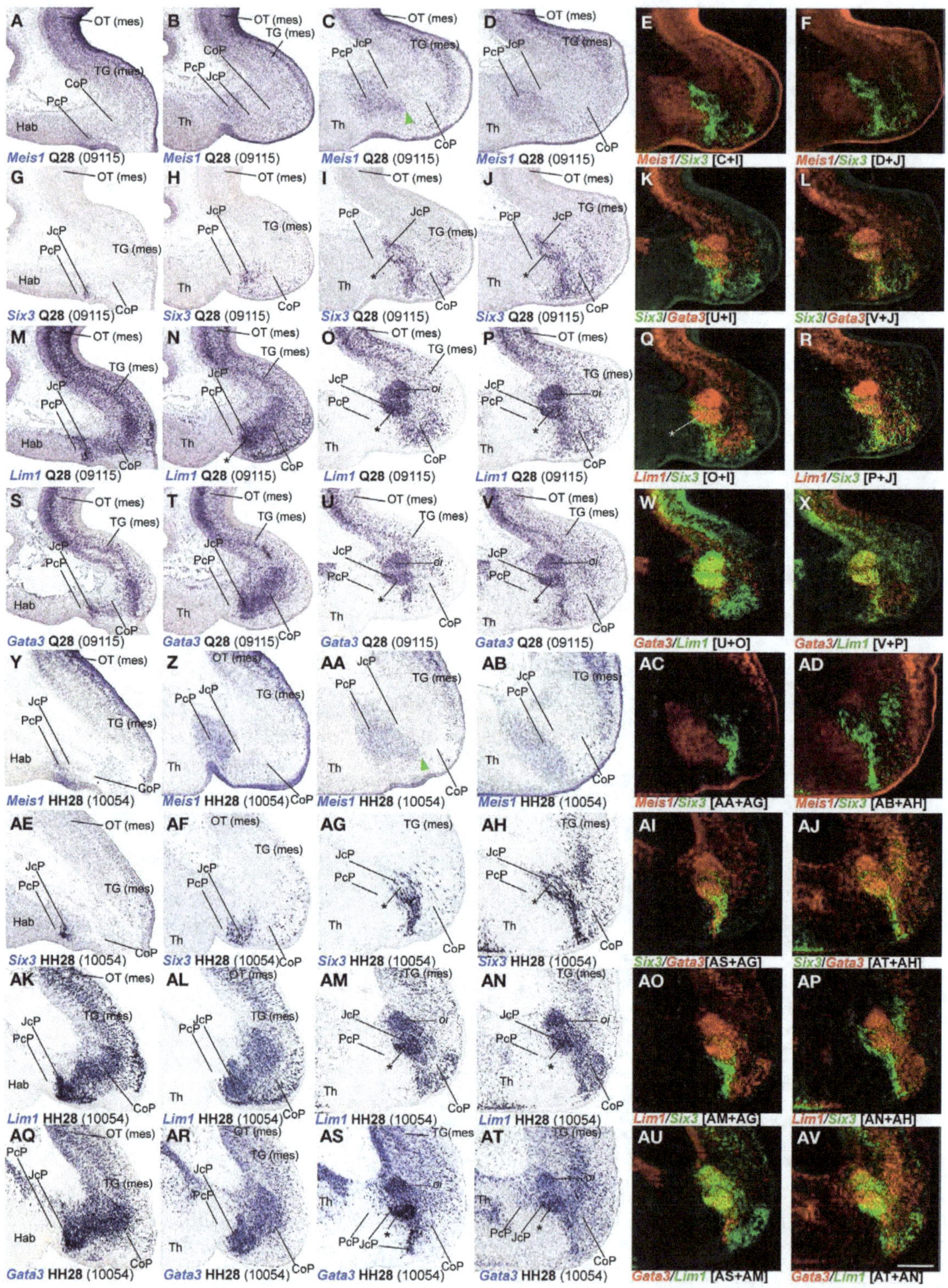

FIGURE 4 | (A-AV) Comparisons of *in situ* hybridization data for four JcP markers at Q28/HH28 in horizontal cryostat sections at four section levels (in each case a single specimen). The markers are identified at the bottom left corner of each panel. Each row of panels [e.g., **(A–F)**] shows from left to right four section levels (dorsal to ventral sequence) reacted for a particular marker, followed by two pseudocolored images comparing the same marker, but paired with another at the two ventral-most levels studied. The first four rows show different markers in the quail, and the last four rows contain comparable material for the chick, so that panels taken long the vertical columns represent essentially the same section level and are comparable across the species. *Green arrowheads* in **(C,AA)** mark cells expressing a PcP marker that are found inside the differentially specified JcP domain. *Asterisks* in **(I,J,O,P,U,V,AG,AH,AM,AN,AS,AT)** identify the developing lateral spiriform nucleus. Numbers between brackets: code of the specimen in our collection. Scale bar = 300 μm.

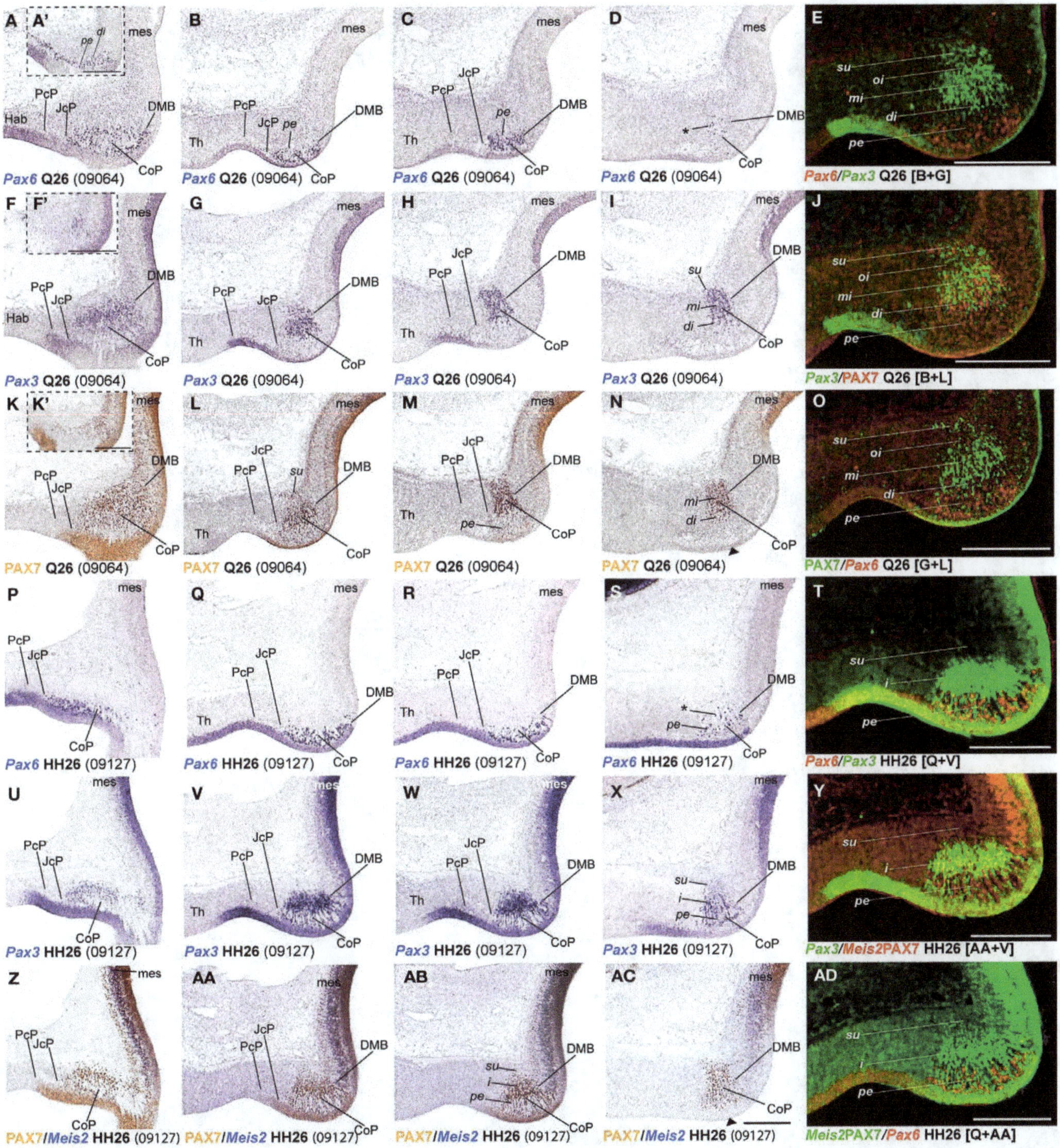

FIGURE 5 | (A–AD) Comparisons of *in situ* hybridization/immunochemical data for three CoP markers at Q26-HH26 in horizontal cryostat sections at four section levels (in each case a single specimen). The markers are identified at the bottom left corner of each panel. Each row of panels [e.g., **(A–E)**] shows from left to right four section levels (dorsal to ventral sequence) reacted for a particular marker, followed by a pseudocolored image comparing the same marker, but paired with another at the second level studied. The first three rows show different markers in the quail, and the last three rows contain comparable material for the chick, so that panels taken long the vertical columns represent essentially the same section level and are comparable across the species. Insets **(A',F',K')** show a more dorsal section level, illustrating details of expression of the corresponding marker. *Black arrowheads* in **(N,AC)** indicate ventral levels of CoP ventricular zone lacking PAX7 immunoreaction. *Asterisks* in **(D,S)** identify *Pax6* positive cells in the CoP deep intermediate layer. Numbers between brackets: code of the specimen in our collection. Scale bar in **(AC)** applies as well to **(A–D,F–I,K–N,P–S,U–X,Z–AB)**. Scale bars = 300 μm.

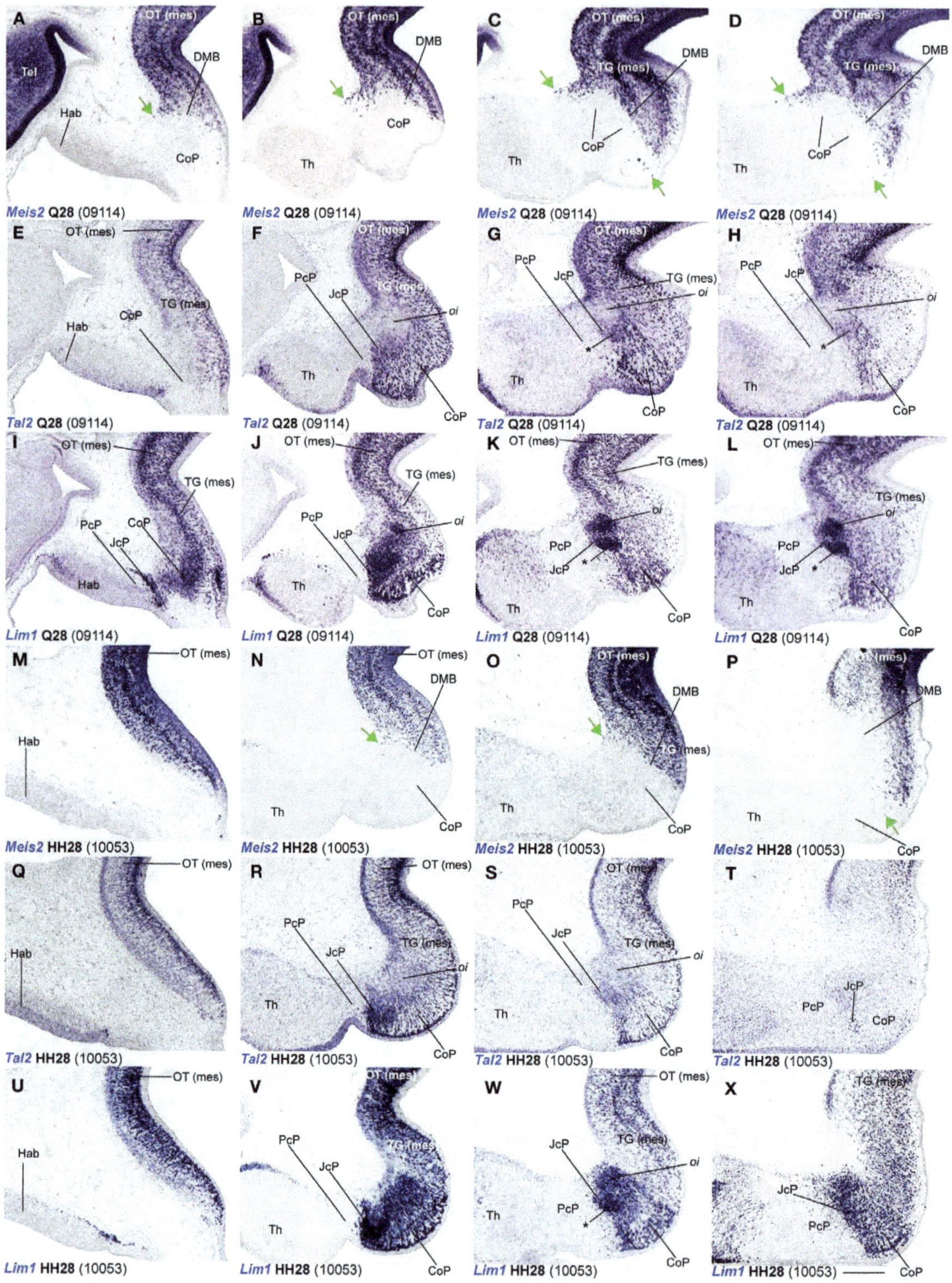

FIGURE 6 | (A–X) Comparisons of *in situ* hybridization data for three markers labeling JcP and CoP at Q28/HH28 in horizontal cryostat sections at four section levels (in each case a single specimen). The markers are identified at the bottom left corner of each panel. Each row of panels [e.g., **(A–D)**] shows from left to right four section levels (dorsal to ventral sequence) reacted for a particular marker. The first three rows show different markers in the quail, and the last three rows contain comparable material for the chick, so that panels taken long the vertical columns represent essentially the same section level and are comparable across the species. *Green arrows* in **(A–D,N–P)** indicate apparently ectopic cells expressing *Meis2* (midbrain marker) at the CoP *su* and *pe* strata. *Asterisks* in **(G,H,K,L,W)** identify the developing lateral spiriform nucleus, exhibiting high expression levels of *Lim1* and a low *Tal2* signal. Numbers between brackets: code of the specimen in our collection. Scale bar = 300 μm.

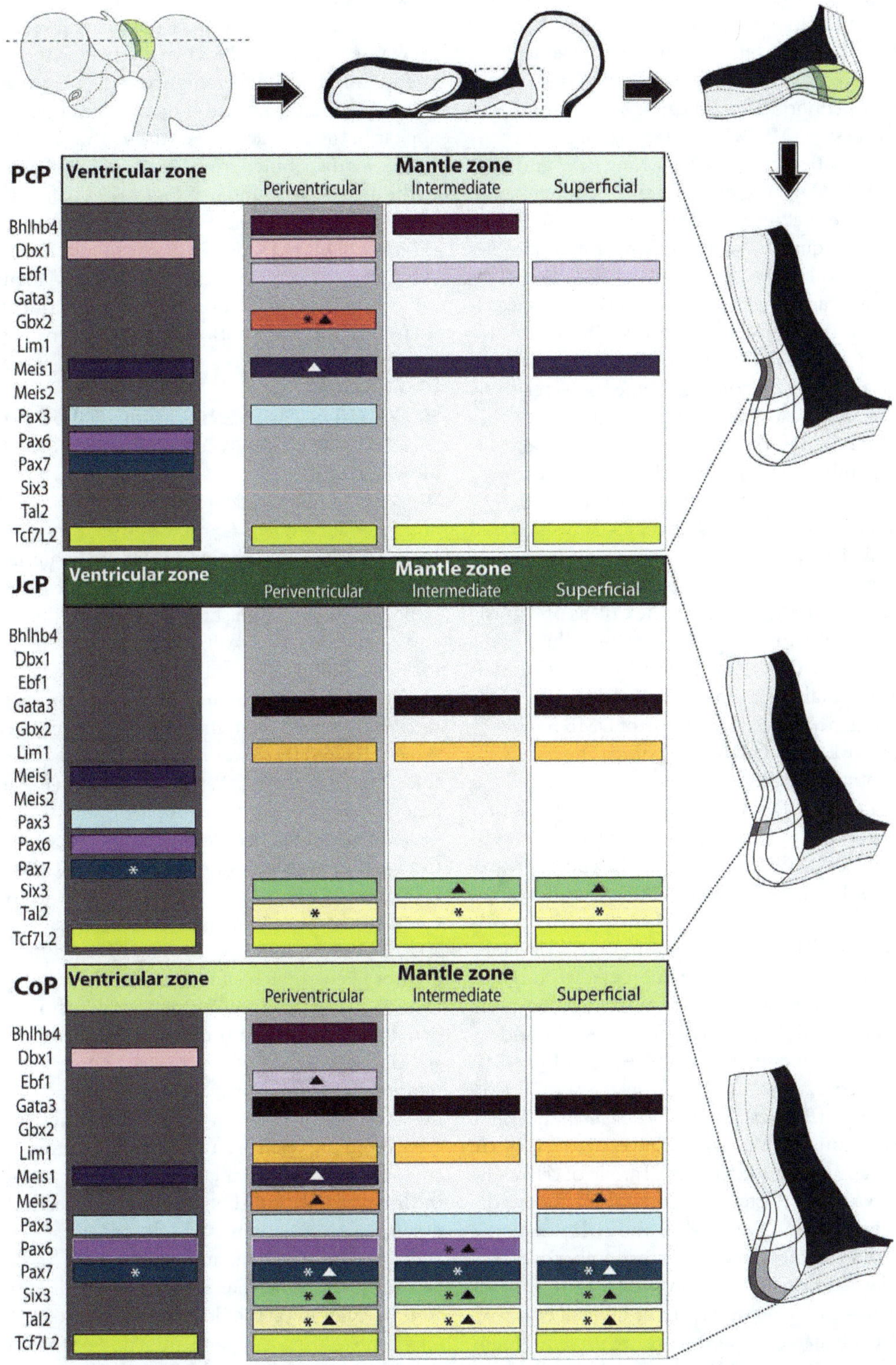

FIGURE 7 | Schematic synthesis of the shared molecular profile examined in avian pretectal domains. Schematics on top: a lateral view of the brain shows the section plane of a representative horizontal across the three pretectal domains (color coded); such a section is illustrated next, with the boxed pretectal region; finally the topography of the three pretectal domains is shown in detail. Schematics along the right side: Enlarged and rotated copies of the detail schema above, highlighting the basic strata in the pretectum and the specific domain whose molecular profile per strata is shown at left (*Dark gray*: ventricular zone; *light gray*: periventricular stratum). Schematics at the left side: Each block represents an entire domain (PcP, JcP, CoP), where the expression of the listed genes – represented by a colored bar – is attributed to the relevant strata. The asterisks imply that this gene is not expressed throughout the dorsoventral extent of the stratum. Solid triangles imply that some cells in the stratum downregulate this mRNA (see Results).

Additionally, at stage Q26/HH27 an incipient patch of *Pax6* expression was observed at the dorsal-most portion of the CoP *di* layer (**Figures 5A,A′**). At the ventral-most levels we detected a few cells of the same layer with strong *Pax6* expression, which possibly constitute the primordium of the magnocelular nucleus of the posterior commissure (MCPC; **Figures 5D,S**). The overlying *mi*, *oi*, and *su* CoP mantle layers showed strong *Pax7* and *Pax3* signal (**Figures 5F–O,U–AD**). Interestingly, the specimens used to study PAX family genes belonged precisely to the same stage, according to the respective quail and chicken developmental tables (Hamburger and Hamilton, 1951; Ainsworth et al., 2010). This allowed us to detect two variant aspects between the two species. First, the relative size of the pretectum and its CoP domain was larger in chicken than in quail (**Figures 9A,B**). Secondly, quail specimens at an equivalent stage in contrast seemed to be relatively slightly more advanced in development, since their layering process was more advanced than in the chicken (**Figure 9C**; and see Discussion). In quail embryos at Q26, we observed an incipient segregation of the intermediate stratum into *di*, *mi*, and *oi* layers, a structural pattern that was present only in chicken from HH27 onward (**Figures 5A,A′,I,J,N,O,P,X,Y,AC,AD**).

Leaving apart *Gata3*, which had not been studied previously in this region, *Lim1* and *Tal2* were expressed in the CoP as previously described (Ferran et al., 2007). To determine precisely the anteroposterior boundaries of the CoP, we combined these expression patterns with *Six3*, thus obtaining the anterior CoP boundary, and with *Meis2*, highlighting the caudal limit of CoP or DMB boundary (**Figures 4G–L,Q,R and 6E,F,K,L,Q,R,W,X**). Comparing *Lim1* with *Gata3* and *Tal2*, we noticed that *Lim1* and *Tal2* are both present at the CoP *pe* stratum (although *Tal2* signal disappears at the ventral subdomains). In addition, only a few *Gata3* cells were observed at the *pe* of the dorsal CoP levels, though their number increases ventralward (**Figures 4M–X,AK–AV and 6E–Q,X**). The *di*, *mi*, and *oi* layers of the *i* mantle stratum express *Lim1* and *Gata3*, but *Tal2* was virtually absent there. The compact group of cells developing at the *oi* layer (the prospective pretectal-subpretectal complex; Ferran et al., 2009) and at the su stratum (terminal nuclei) express strongly *Lim1* and *Gata3* mRNAs (**Figures 4M–X,AK–AV and 7**).

Dbx1 shows a salt and pepper pattern in the *v* zone of the CoP, and a stronger and wider expression domain in the ventral CoP subdomains in both species (**Figures 3U–X**). *Ebf1*, *Bhlhb4*, and *Meis1* are expressed in the *pe* stratum of the CoP (**Figures 2L, 3S,T,Y–AB, 4B–F,Z–AD, and 7**). *Meis2* is expressed in a small group of cells at the CoP *pe* stratum and in a major cluster at the *su* stratum close to the DMB (green arrow, **Figures 2T,W, 6A–D, M–P, and 7**). Interestingly, the latter *Meis2* expression was observed in a larger number of cells in the quail than in chicken of the same stage, possibly suggesting again a relatively more advanced developmental status of quail embryos. Finally, *Six3* – the main JcP marker – is also expressed in some groups of cells at the CoP *pe* layer, a pattern that best visible at the level of ventral subdomains (CoV). Moreover, the CoV *Six3* expression expands into the *i* mantle layers (**Figures 3E–H and 4F–J,AD–AH**).

SHARED MOLECULAR PROFILE IN THE DORSOVENTRAL SUBDOMAINS

Using horizontal and transversal (coronal) sections, we were able to make a first approach to examine conservation of genoarchitectonic pattern in pretectal dorsoventral subdomains. We found strikingly identical patterns in both species. *Pax6* signal at the level of the *vz* reaches the alar–basal boundary throughout the pretectum (Ferran et al., 2009). PAX7 expression is restricted to dorsal and lateral CoP subdomains (**Figures 2, 3, 5, 7, and 8A,J–L**). *Six3* signal is observed in all DV subdomains of JcP and its transcripts also appear in the mantle zone of the ventral CoP subdomains. *Tcf712 signal* was distributed from the most dorsal basal plate domains up to the alar–roof boundary (**Figures 2U,U′,X,X′, 4I–J,AG,AH, and 8C,G,K,N**). *Bhlhb4* and *Ebf1* were observed in all DV parts of PcP (**Figures 8D,E,H,I,O,P**). *Pax3* was found in nearly all pretectal DV subdomains, except the ventral-most ones (**Figures 8B,F,M**). *Meis1* DV expression stopped ventrally at the alar–basal boundary of all pretectal domains in both quail and chicken (**Figures 4A–F,Y–AD**).

DISCUSSION

EQUIVALENT DEVELOPMENTAL STAGES FROM *C. japonica* (QUAIL) AND *G. gallus* (CHICKEN) SHOW DIFFERENT PRETECTAL SIZE AND DEGREE OF DIFFERENTIATION

We staged embryos according to Ainsworth et al. (2010) for quail, and Hamburger and Hamilton (1951) for chicken. Both staging tables were generated based on standard criteria about useful external anatomical landmarks, and their stages are essentially comparable one-to-one, at least in the period examined here (Hamburger and Hamilton, 1951; Ainsworth et al., 2010). However, we found that identically staged embryos from chicken and quail are not fully equivalent as regards pretectal development (in fact, brain development in general). First, the pretectal region of chicken embryos at stages HH26–HH28 was significantly larger by roughly 30% than that of quail embryos at stages Q26–Q28 (**Figure 9A**). Differences among close species in the proportions of adult brain regions have been suggested to be caused by changes in cell-cycle rates and/or the timing of neurogenesis, as well as by alterations of brain patterning (Finlay and Darlington, 1995; Striedter, 2005; Menuet et al., 2007; Charvet and Striedter, 2008; Charvet et al., 2010; Sylvester et al., 2010). Our results strongly suggest that differences in patterning are not likely to be responsible for the observed variation in pretectum size. Therefore, further studies should address the effect of cell-cycle rates and timing of neurogenesis upon the observed size differences. It is of course well known that, under comparable temperature conditions, the incubation period up to hatching of quail is shorter by 84 h than the chicken one. However, comparative data about the relative length of neuroepithelial cell cycles in these two species are not available. Our results suggest that differences in brain proportions between these closely related species begin during early development, as described for mesencephalic differences between parrots and galliformes (McGowan et al., 2010). Secondly, we found that the molecularly identified quail pretectal strata developing at the CoP domain appeared slightly more mature – by representing a larger proportion of the total domain volume than the corresponding chicken counterparts at equivalent stages (**Figure 9C**). These differences reflect an unavoidable inaccuracy of current staging tables in predicting detailed microscopic traits heterochronic relative to macroscopic morphologic features. More complex and detailed distinctive molecular features of particular organs will be needed to upgrade the standard staging tables (e.g., as done for chicken primitive streak stages by López-Sánchez et al., 2005).

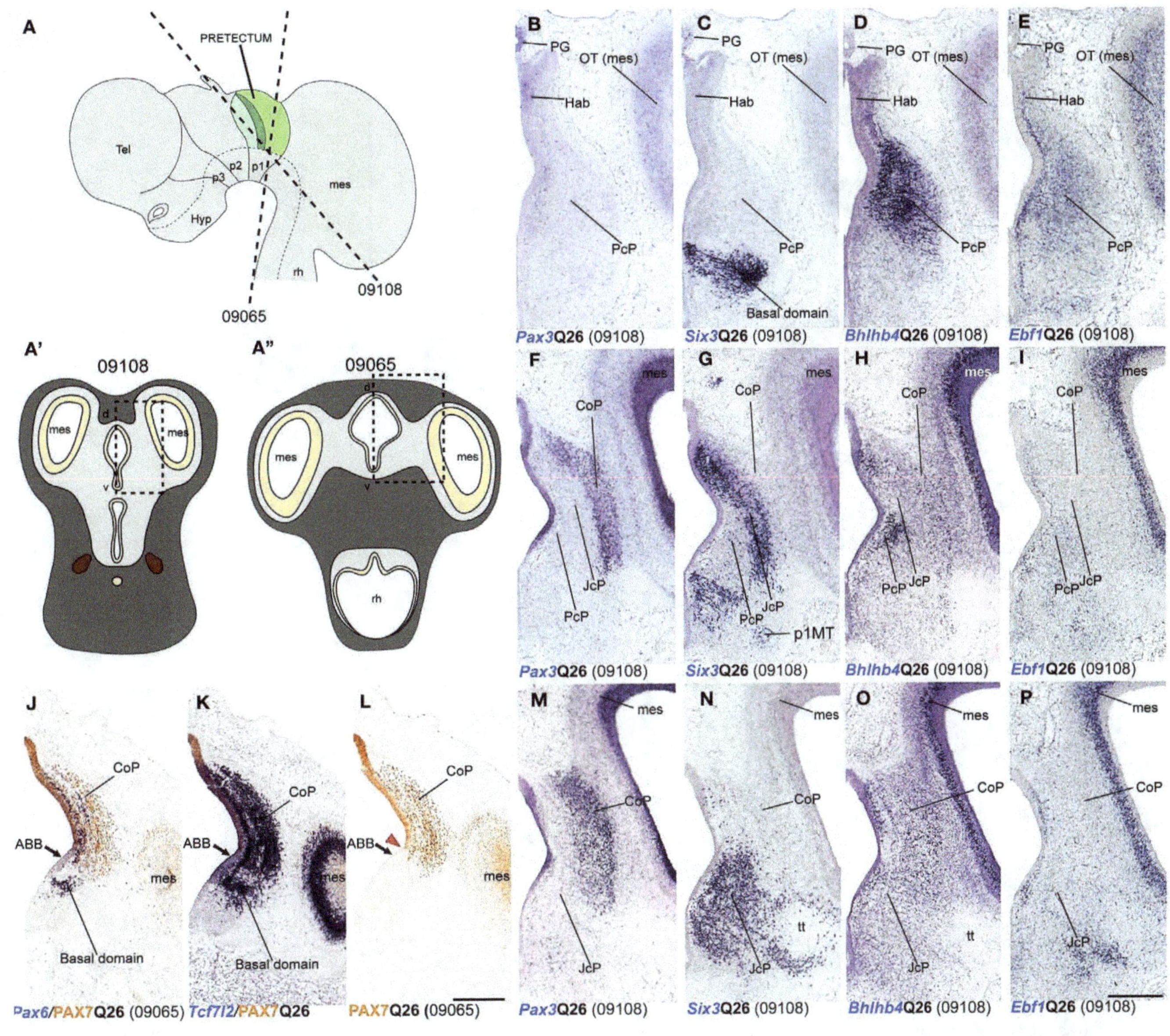

FIGURE 8 | Dorsoventral extent of seven pretectal markers in the quail, studied by *in situ* hybridization/immunoreaction in transversal cryostat sections at Q26 (two specimens). (A,A′,A″) Schemata showing a lateral view with two variant transversal section planes used (see specimen code in brackets) and the respective aspect of such transversal sections, in order to illustrate the brain region analyzed in both specimens. [Block comprising **(B–I,M–P)**] comparisons of four markers (*Pax3, Six3, Bhlhb4, Ebf1*) at three section levels from rostral to caudal from a single specimen (levels arranged top to bottom along the columns). **(J–L)** Three adjacent transversal sections at CoP level, allowing comparison of *Pax6*, PAX7, and *Tcf7l2* dorsoventral patterns in a different quail specimen. The *red arrowhead* in **(L)** shows the ventral-most limit of PAX7 expression, slightly above the alar–basal boundary(ABB; black arrow). Numbers between brackets: code of the specimen in our collection. Scale bar = 300 μm.

CONSERVED GENOARCHICTECTONIC PROFILE OF THE PRETECTAL DOMAIN IN PHASIANIDAE

We present a detailed comparative characterization of molecularly distinct pretectal progenitor areas from chicken (*G. gallus*) and quail (*C. japonica*) at early stages of mantle development (Q26/HH26–Q28/HH28). We found a strikingly conserved combinatorial genetic code that patterns this region in both species, strongly suggesting that this corresponds to the ancestral pretectal code for members of the family Phasianidae. We had previously defined the molecular code identifying each region, domain and subdomain (progenitor areas), as well as their respective mantle derivatives, in chicken embryos (Ferran et al., 2007, 2008, 2009). The present study adds information for new gene expression patterns and expands our previous knowledge for some domains, in some cases modifying previously established notions.

The rostral pretectal boundary (TPB) is identified by the rostral limit of expression of *Bhlbh4*, *Ebf1*, *Meis1*, and *Pax3* genes in both species (Ferran et al., 2007, 2008, 2009; present results). Here we confirmed that the thalamic expression of *Gbx2* is a complementary boundary marker for the TPB at the studied stages. Similar thalamic

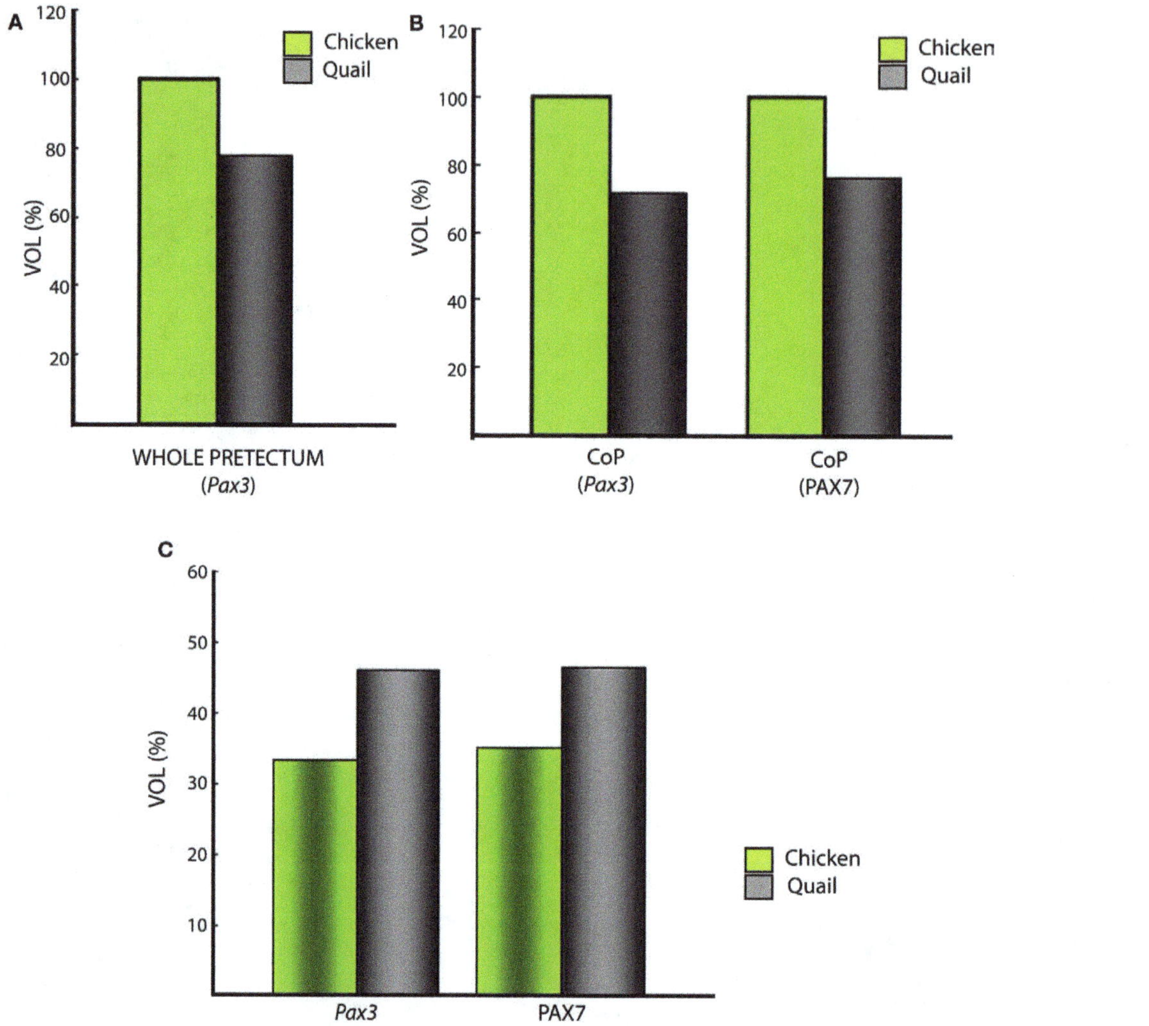

FIGURE 9 | Comparative analysis between quail and chicken of roughly estimated relative pretectal volumes, either of whole pretectum or of selected portions. (A) Total estimated volume of pretectum extrapolated from the domain expressing *Pax3*. The volume in the chicken was standardized as 100%. Note the quail pretectum is about 28% smaller. **(B)** The color-coded bars represent the estimated volumes of the quail/chicken CoP domain, separately extrapolated from ventricular and mantle expression of the genes *Pax3* and PAX7. The CoP volume of the chicken was standardized as 100%. Both calculations using *Pax3* or PAX7 suggest a similar smaller size of CoP in the quail. **(C)** The color-coded bars represent the estimated proportion of the intermediate CoP stratum of each species relative to the respective total volume of CoP, separately extrapolated from the expression of the genes *Pax3* and PAX7 (similar proportion in both cases).

Gbx2 expression was previously observed in mouse, chicken (older stages), zebrafish, and *Xenopus* (Bulfone et al., 1993; Niss and Leutz, 1998; Martínez-de-la-Torre et al., 2002; Kikuta et al., 2003); however, the strict complementarity of thalamic *Gbx2* with pretectal *Pax3* was demonstrated only recently in *Xenopus* (Morona et al., 2010). We nevertheless observed as well a patch of *Gbx2* signal within the rostral *pe* stratum of PcP. It can be speculated that this result is due to some thalamic cells migrating tangentially into the neighboring pretectum. This possibility acquires relevance because observations in a mutant mouse line in which the gene Gbx2 was deleted ($Gbx2^{CreER/-}$; R26R mutants) was thought to produce abnormally such a displacement of thalamic cells into the pretectum (Chen et al., 2009). Our present data suggest instead the possibility that such a movement may be constitutive in the wild type.

While *Meis1* delineates the TPB (the p2/p1 interprosomeric boundary) across the whole alar plate, up to the diencephalic roof, the *Dbx1*, *Ebf1*, and *Pax3* expression domains present in PcP extend across the pretecto-habenular limit into the habenular region of prosomere 2, as is also true of *Pax6* and PAX7, whose CoP domains similarly extend rostralward at this dorsal level (**Figures 2A,C,D,E,H,I, 3U,W,Y,AA, and 5A,P**; Ferran et al., 2007, 2008, 2009). We think that the primary pattern causing these shared properties of the habenular region and the cited dorsocaudal pretectal regions is probably *Pax6*. At earlier stages this gene is first expressed throughout the diencephalic alar plate. Subsequently it becomes progressively downregulated at both sides of the zona limitans intrathalamica (probably a SHH-mediated effect; Hashimoto-Torii et al., 2003; Kiecker and Lumsden, 2004; Vieira et al., 2005;

Vieira and Martínez, 2006; see Discussion in Ferran et al., 2007). The downregulated *Pax6* expression at the level of the alar domain caudal to the zona limitans involves the thalamus proper in p2 and the PcP and JcP domains in p1; so that *Pax6* expression persists at the habenula, in p2, as well as at dorsal parts of PcP and JcP, and at the entire CoP, in p1, that is, the sites farthest from the zona limitans intrathalamica. This *Pax6* pattern possibly stabilizes *Pax3* and *Pax7* in the same mixed area, with a corresponding distribution of genes such as *Dbx1*, *Ebf1* (*Pax6* transiently upstream of them before it becomes downregulated at PcP). The *Meis1* pattern thus importantly establishes the neuromeric limit at this dorsal level between the thalamic habenular region and the pretectum. The overlapping distribution of pretectal *Meis1* and *Pax3* was also observed for the mouse, and comparable *Pax3* data exist also for *Xenopus* (Toresson et al., 2000; Ferran et al., 2008; Morona et al., 2010). Interestingly, *Pax3* and *Meis* genes have been suggested to be part of a specific regulatory network involved in the development of the rhombencephalon in *Xenopus* (Elkouby et al., 2010; Gutkovich et al., 2010); further studies should address whether a similar relationship of these transcription factors exists in the patterning of the pretectal region of vertebrates.

The caudal pretectal boundary was marked by the expression domains of *Pax6* and *Tcf7l2* (*Tcf4*; rostral side) and *Meis2* (caudal side) during early chicken development. However, only *Pax6* has been studied extensively throughout development (Ferran et al., 2007, 2008, 2009). Here we found that *Tcf7l2* (*Tcf4*) is also expressed in the midbrain mantle from stage Q25/HH25 onwards, but its DMB boundary persists at the ventricular zone at the stages analyzed. The same early diencephalic pattern and added mesencephalic expression in the mantle at later stages was observed in the mouse (Ferran et al., in preparation) and *X. laevis* (Morona et al., 2010, and unpublished observations). In *Xenopus*, some authors have misinterpreted early diencephalic *Tcf7l2* expression as "rostral mesencephalon" (Kunz et al., 2004; Koenig et al., 2008, 2010); nonetheless, comparison with the *Pax6* expression pattern illustrated in the same studies, as well as by Schlosser and Ahrens, (2004), clearly indicates that *Tcf7l2* expression was only diencephalic (thalamus and pretectum) at those stages. According to the genoarchitectonic data from Schlosser and Ahrens, (2004), the distinction between p1, p2, p3, and midbrain in *Xenopus* is established at stages 24–27, whereas *Tcf7l2* (*Tcf4*) is clearly expressed only in the diencephalon until at least stages 33–34 (Figure 1 in Morona et al., 2010). *Meis2* expression in the alar mesencephalon, stopping rostrally at the DMB boundary, was described in chicken from stage HH9/10 onward (Ferran et al., 2007; Sánchez-Guardado et al., 2011). In the present study, we identified at Q27/HH28 some *Meis2*-positive cells in the *pe* and *su* strata from the CoP, which progressively increased in number. Those cells lying at the CoP *su* stratum will become part of the lateral and dorsal terminal nuclei of the accessory optic tract at later stages (data not shown), whereas the deep *pe* ones apparently are integrated in the pretectal periaqueductal gray. The progression of *Meis2* mRNA expression suggests that the positive cells at the CoP increased progressively in clear connection with a stream of *Meis2*-positive cells translocating from the mesencephalic TG; a radial migration of the *su* cells is inconsistent with the fact that such cells never are found within the *i* stratum. Our analysis therefore suggests that these cells may be migrating from the TG at the rostral mesencephalon, unless, alternatively, these cells are selectively upregulating *Meis2* expression independently. The few *Meis2*-positive cells observed in the *pe* stratum at all stages analyzed also show a pattern suggesting a periventricular mesencephalic TG origin. In contrast, various studies using quail/chicken chimeras or lineage analysis after infection with a recombinant retrovirus showed no quail-derived cells migrating from mesencephalon to diencephalon (Senut and Alvarado-Mallart, 1987; Gray et al., 1988; Gray and Sanes, 1991; Martínez et al., 1992; García-López et al., 2004; García-López, 2005). Nearly all of the cited quail/chicken chimera studies involved grafts of the rostral prospective optic tectum, which demonstrated a rostralward tangential migration of given tectal cell types restricted within the tectum itself, but never penetrating the TG, or crossing into diencephalic domains (Senut and Alvarado-Mallart, 1987; Figure 1 in Martínez et al., 1992; García-López et al., 2004; García-López, 2005). Similarly, the lineage studies labeled clones that were restricted to the optic tectum and confirmed strictly tectal radial and tangential migration patterns (Gray et al., 1988; Gray and Sanes, 1991; Ferran, 2002), but no rostral translocation into the diencephalon. Due either to the small size of the TG primordium, or to the traditional tendency to disregard it, no experiment so far has properly tested the fate of TG derivatives. However, alar mesencephalic quail tissue transplanted heterotopically into the chicken diencephalic alar plate produced a massive superficial dispersion of quail cells, which invaded selectively all primary retinorecipient nuclei of the chick diencephalon; it was not determined whether prospective TG tissue was included in these grafts (Martínez and Alvarado-Mallart, 1989). Notably, most of the *Meis2*-positive cells apparently entering the CoP from the TG occupy the superficial stratum. Further studies will be needed to test whether the TG is indeed a source of *Meis2*-positive cells for the pretectum or the observed pattern is a consequence of independent gene expression recruitment by pretectal cells.

At the level of the PcP domain, we similarly found *Gbx2* expression in the *pe* layer that might be related either to migration of thalamic cells (note the signal extending caudalward from the thalamus in **Figure 3P′**), or to gene expression recruitment. Among available lineage tracing and fate-mapping studies relevant to the TPB, the reports of Figdor and Stern (1993) and García-López et al. (2004) did not identify thalamic clones or derivatives crossing the p1–p2 boundary, whereas Larsen et al. (2001) did observe cell movement between thalamus and pretectum, concluding that this boundary is not clonally restricted. More studies are needed to resolve this controversy. *Pax6* expression starts to appear at the dorsal PcP *di* stratum at HH27, earlier than previously observed by us (shown at HH30/32 in Ferran et al., 2009; see asterisk in their Figures 4J,S). These cells will become part of the core of the medial pretectal nucleus (Figure 10F in Ferran et al., 2009).

The dorsocaudal nucleus (DCa), originally described by Rendahl (1924), and also known as the "medial or dorsomedial spiriform nucleus" (Edinger and Wallenberg, 1899; Kuhlenbeck, 1939; see Table 3 in Ferran et al., 2009) was found to be derived from the PcP domain on the basis of a characteristic genoarchitectonic code (expression of *Bhlhb4*, *Ebf1*, and *Nbea*; Figures 11–14 in Ferran et al., 2009). In our earlier study, we concluded that DCa cells migrate through the JcP domain at stage HH31 (Figures 14A,B in Ferran et al., 2009). In our present analysis, we compared in chicken and quail markers for PcP (*Meis1*, *Ebf1*, *Bhlhb4*) and JcP derivatives (*Six3*, *Lim1*, *Tal2*, *Gata3*), and corroborated this migration, finding in addition that the first cells that move into the JcP domain constitute a pioneering migratory group departing from the PcP *di* stratum at around Q27/HH27.

At the level of JcP, its characteristic marker *Six3* was previously shown to become secondarily downregulated at a middle locus of the intermediate mantle stratum starting at HH27, while *Lim1* and *Tal2* continue to be expressed in this cluster of cells that also begins to express selectively *FoxP1* and matures as the lateral spiriform nucleus (Ferran et al., 2007, 2009). Here we confirmed the whole pattern for these genes in both species, and added *Gata3* expression to the molecular code characteristic of the cells constituting the prospective lateral spiriform nucleus.

The intermediate mantle layer of CoP was previously described by us to be segregated into *di*, *mi*, and *oi* layers at least from HH30 onward (Figure 4 in Ferran et al., 2009). Here, we provide evidence (combining *Pax3*, *Pax7*, *Gata3*, *Lim1*, and *Tal2* expression patterns) that this segregation of the intermediate mantle stratum actually begins at Q26/HH27 (**Figures 5 and 7**).

MICROEVOLUTION OF CODING SEQUENCES AND PRETECTAL GENOARCHITECTURE IN THE PHASIANIDAE FAMILY

The two species analyzed here belong to the well known avian order Galliformes; however, the phylogenetic relationships within this order are not well resolved yet, primarily due to the low variability in anatomical, and osteological traits, as well as to inconclusive molecular studies (Kimball et al., 1999; Crowe et al., 2006; Kriegs et al., 2007; Mayr, 2008; Tavares and Baker, 2008; Kan et al., 2010a,b; Shen et al., 2010). Based on the combined evidence from different phylogenetic analyses, Crowe et al. (2006) put forward a tentative revised classification of the Galliformes. In this classification, the order Galliformes comprises five families (Megapodiidae, Cracidae, Numididae, Odontophoridae, and Phasianidae), and the family Phasianidae encompasses seven subfamilies (Arborophilinae, Coturnicinae, Pavoninae, Gallininae, Meleagridinae, Tetraoninae, and Phasianinae). The Coturnicinae and Gallininae subfamilies include the *C. japonica* and *G. gallus* species, respectively (**Figure 1A**). The order Galliformes apparently started to evolve 90 million years ago, whereas the split between the families Phasianidae and Odontophoridae occurred ~60 million years ago (**Figures 1A,A′**; Puelles and Medina, 2002). Analysis of mitochondrial genomes suggested that the subfamilies Phasianinae, Gallininae, and Coturnicinae evolved independently from ~40 million years (Kan et al., 2010b; blue arrow, **Figure 1A′**). Therefore, the species analyzed here, *C. japonica* and *G. gallus*, have undergone a combined time of divergent evolution of ~80 million years. We sequenced and compared the coding sequences of 12 genes, finding very low rates of genomic variation, consistent with the analyses of mitochondrial genomes. This high level of coding sequence conservation was associated with a striking degree of genoarchitectonic Bauplan conservation during early stages of nervous system development in both species. Since genoarchitectonic codes are expected to be controlled by *cis* regulatory elements, our data also suggest a high level of conservation of the underlying genomic regulatory sequences between both species (Davidson, 2006; Carroll, 2008).

PRETECTAL GENOARCHITECTURE IN VERTEBRATES: DEGREE OF PHENOTYPIC CONSERVATION THROUGHOUT ONTOGENY

Our previous studies on the genoarchitecture of the chicken pretectum have provided a starting point for comparing this region at an unprecedented level of detail among different vertebrates (Ferran et al., 2007, 2009). The present results have shown that chicken and quail pretectal genoarchitecture patterns are strikingly conserved, thus likely representing an ancestral pattern within the Phasianidae. Outgroup comparisons with other species, such as the avian superorder Neognathae (ostriches; **Figure 1A**), and archosaurian reptiles (e.g., a crocodile) or lepidosaurians (e.g., lizards), should corroborate whether the observed pretectal genoarchitectonic profile is plesiomorphic in all birds and reptiles. Furthermore, there is already evidence that the same molecular map and a structural anteroposterior tripartition exists in the pretectum of the mouse and *Xenopus* frog (Ferran et al., 2008; Morona et al., 2010), suggesting that the referred plesiomorphy may apply as well to tetrapods in general. A tripartite pretectum has been postulated as well for lamprey larvae (Pombal and Puelles, 1999; Pombal et al., 2009), which suggest we deal here with a fundamental aspect of forebrain structure in all vertebrates. Some elements of the studied pretectal molecular code were, in fact, used in *Xenopus* larvae to identify precisely the pretectal region, and its main subdivisions (Morona et al., 2010) working within the context of field homology in the brain (Puelles and Medina, 2002). The present results also reveal that the pattern of radial segregation of molecularly characterized mantle components (pronuclei) described for the chicken (Ferran et al., 2007, 2009) are most likely representative for all members of the family Phasianidae. This is independent of the different absolute sizes of the respective populations and domains in chicken and quail, or of the heterochronic aspects of maturation commented above. Although late stages of differentiation are commonly thought to present more phenotypic variations (Davidson, 2006), the nuclear anatomy of the adult pretectum shows little variation among studied adult birds (Karten and Hodos, 1967; Zweers, 1971; Kuenzel and Masson, 1988; Puelles et al., 2007). Our results nevertheless allow making very detailed molecular comparative analyses at the level of strata segregation or differentiation of distinct neuronal subpopulations among different bird species, or between birds and other vertebrates, thus exploring any significant variations. For example, our study in *Xenopus* disclosed that at early stages PAX7 was observed in the mantle zone of the JcP domain, an expression trait that we did not find in chicken or quail (Morona et al., 2010; Ferran et al., 2007, 2009; present results).

ACKNOWLEDGMENTS

We thank Manuel Irimia for helpful comments and discussion; Dr. J. Balthazart and Dr. S. Martínez for *C. japonica* embryos. This work was supported by MICINN grant BFU2008-04156 and SENECA Foundation contract 04548/GERM/06-10891 to L. Puelles. P. Merchán is a postdoctoral fellow of NIH grant 1-R01-MH070370-01A2 at the L.P. lab. EST clones from the UK Chick EST Project were provided by ARK-Genomics (www.ark-genomics.org). The PAX7 monoclonal antibody developed by A. Kawakami was obtained from the Developmental Studies Hybridoma Bank, developed under the auspices of the NICHD and maintained by the University of Iowa, Department of Biological Sciences, Iowa City, IA, USA.

REFERENCES

Abellán, A., and Medina, L. (2009). Subdivisions and derivatives of the chicken subpallium based on expression of *LIM* and other regulatory genes and markers of neuron subpopulations during development. *J. Comp. Neurol.* 515, 465–501.

Ainsworth, S. J., Stanley, R. L., and Evans, D. J. R. (2010). Developmental stages of the Japanese quail. *J. Anat.* 216, 3–15.

Bachy, I., Vernier, P., and Rétaux, S. (2001). The *LIM*-homeodomain gene family in the developing *Xenopus* brain: conservation and divergences with the mouse related to the evolution of the forebrain. *J. Neurosci.* 21, 7620–7629.

Bardet, S. M., Ferran, J. L., Sánchez-Arrones, L., and Puelles, L. (2010). Ontogenetic expression of Sonic hedgehog in the chicken supallium. *Front. Neuroanat.* 4:28. doi: 10.3389/fnana.2010.00028

Boardman, P. E., Sanz-Ezquerro, J., Overton, I. M., Burt, D. W., Bosch, E., Fong, W. T., Tickle, C., Brown, W. R., Wilson, S. A., and Hubbard, S. J. (2002). A comprehensive collection of chicken cDNAs. *Curr. Biol.* 19, 1965–1969.

Bovolenta, P., Mallamaci, A., Puelles, L., and Boncinelli, E. (1998). Expression pattern of cSix3, a member of the Six/sine oculis family of transcription factors. *Mech. Dev.* 70, 201–203.

Bulfone, A., Puelles, L., Porteus, M. H., Frohman, M. A., Martin, G. R., and Rubenstein, J. L. (1993). Spatially restricted expression of *Dlx-1*, *Dlx-2 (Tes-1)*, *Gbx-2*, and *Wnt- 3* in the embryonic day 12.5 mouse forebrain defines potential transverse and longitudinal segmental boundaries. *J. Neurosci.* 13, 3155–3172.

Carroll, S. B. (2008). Evo-devo and an expanding evolutionary synthesis: a genetic theory of morphological evolution. *Cell* 134, 25–36.

Charvet, C. J., Sandoval, A. L., and Striedter, G. F. (2010). Phylogenetic origins of early alterations in brain region proportions. *Brain Behav. Evol.* 75, 104–110.

Charvet, C. J., and Striedter, G. F. (2008). Developmental species differences in brain cell cycle rates between northern bobwhite quail and parakeets. *Brain Behav. Evol* 72, 295–306.

Chen, L., Guo, Q., and Li, J. Y. H. (2009). Transcription factor *Gbx2* acts cell-nonautonomously to regulate the formation of lineage-restriction boundaries of the thalamus. *Development* 136, 1317–1326.

Crossland, W. J., and Uchwat, C. J. (1982). Neurogenesis in the chick ventral lateral geniculate and ectomammillary nuclei: relationship of soma size to birthdate. *Brain Res.* 282, 33–46.

Crowe, T. M., Bowie, R. C. K., Bloomer, P., Mandiwana, T. G., Hedderson, T. A. J., Randi, E., Pereira, S. L., and Wakeling, J. (2006). Phylogenetics, biogeography and classification of, and character evolution in, gamebirds (Aves: Galliformes): effects of character exclusion, data partitioning and missing data. *Cladistics* 22, 495–532.

Davidson, E. (2006). *The Regulatory Genome: Gene Regulatory Networks in Development and Evolution*. San Diego: Academic Press, Elsevier.

Davidson, E. H., and Erwin, D. H. (2006). Gene regulatory networks and the evolution of animal body plans. *Science* 311, 796–800.

Davidson, E. H., and Erwin, D. H. (2009). Evolutionary innovation and stability in animal gene networks. *J. Exp. Zool. B Mol. Dev. Evol.* 314, 182–186.

De Castro, F., Cobos, I., Puelles, L., and Martínez, S. (1998). Calretinin in pretecto- and olivocerebellar projections in the chick: immunohistochemical and experimental study. *J. Comp. Neurol.* 397, 149–162.

Echevarria, D., Vieira, C., Gimeno, L., and Martínez, S. (2003). Neuroepithelial secondary organizers and cell fate specification in the developing brain. *Brain Res. Brain Res. Rev.* 43, 179–191.

Edinger, L., and Wallenberg, A. (1899). Untersuchungen uber das Gehirn derTauben. *Anat. Anz.* 15, 245–271.

Elkouby, Y. M., Elias, S., Casey, E. S., Blythe, S. A., Tsabar, N., Klein, P. S., Root, H., Liu, K. J., and Frank, D. (2010). Mesodermal *Wnt* signaling organizes the neural plate via Meis3. *Development* 137, 1531–1541.

Fernandez, A. S, Pieau, C., Repérant, J., Boncinelli, E., and Wassef, M. (1998). Expression of the *Emx-1* and *Dlx-1* homeobox genes define three molecularly distinct domains in the telencephalon of mouse, chick, turtle and frog embryos: implications for the evolution of telencephalic subdivisions in amniotes. *Development* 125, 2099–2111.

Ferran, J. L. (2002). *Desarrollo embrionario y plasticidad del sistema nervioso central. El tectum óptico como modelo*. Ph.D. dissertation, University of Buenos Aires, Argentina.

Ferran, J. L., de Oliveira, E. D., Merchán, P., Sandoval, J. E., Sánchez-Arrones, L., Martínez-de-la-Torre, M., and Puelles, L. (2009). Genoarchitectonic profile of developing nuclear groups in the chicken pretectum. *J. Comp. Neurol.* 517, 405–451.

Ferran, J. L., Sánchez-Arrones, L., Bardet, S. M., Sandoval, J. E., Martínez-de-la-Torre, M., and Puelles, L. (2008). Early pretectal gene expression pattern shows a conserved anteroposterior tripartition in mouse and chicken. *Brain Res. Bull.* 75, 295–298.

Ferran, J. L., Sánchez-Arrones, L., Sandoval, J. E., and Puelles, L. (2007). A model of early molecular regionalization in the chicken embryonic pretectum. *J. Comp. Neurol.* 505, 379–403.

Figdor, M. C., and Stern, C. D. (1993). Segmental organization of embryonic diencephalon. *Nature* 363, 630–634.

Finlay, B. L., and Darlington, R. B. (1995). Linked regularities in the development and evolution of mammalian brains. *Science* 268, 1578–1584.

García-Calero, E., Martínez-de-la-Torre, M., and Puelles, L. (2002). The avian griseum tectale: cytoarchitecture, NOS expression and neurogenesis. *Brain Res. Bull.* 57, 353–357.

García-López, M., Abellán, A., Legaz, I., Rubenstein, J. L., Puelles, L., and Medina, L. (2008). Histogenetic compartments of the mouse centromedial and extended amygdala based on gene expression patterns during development. *J. Comp. Neurol.* 506, 46–74.

García-López, R. (2005). *Estudio experimental de las regiones prospectivas y la migración celular en el diencéfalo de aves*. Ph.D. dissertation, Miguel Hernández University, Spain.

García-López, R., Vieira, C., Echevarria, D., and Martínez, S. (2004). Fate map of the diencephalon and the zona limitans at the 10-somites stage in chick embryos. *Dev. Biol.* 268, 514–530.

Gray, G. E., Glover, J. C., Majors, J., and Sanes, J. R. (1988). Radial arrangement of clonally related cells in the chicken optic tectum: lineage analysis with a recombinant retrovirus. *Proc. Natl. Acad. Sci. U.S.A.* 85, 7356–7360.

Gray, G. E., and Sanes, J. R. (1991). Migratory paths and phenotypic choices of clonally related cells in the avian optic tectum. *Neuron* 6, 211–225.

Guillemot, F. (2007). Spatial and temporal specification of neural fates by transcription factor codes. *Development* 134, 3771–3780.

Gutkovich, Y. E., Ofir, R., Elkouby, Y. M., Dibner, C., Gefen, A., Elias, S., and Frank, D. (2010). Xenopus Meis3 protein lies at a nexus downstream to *Zic1* and *Pax3* proteins, regulating multiple cell-fates during early nervous system development. *Dev. Biol.* 338, 50–62.

Hamburger, V., and Hamilton, H. L. (1951). A series of normal stages in the development of the chick embryo. *J. Morphol.* 88, 49–92.

Hashimoto-Torii, K., Motoyama, J., Hui, C. C., Kuroiwa, A., Nakafuku, M., and Shimamura, K. (2003). Differential activities of Sonic hedgehog mediated by *Gli* transcription factors define distinct neuronal subtypes in the dorsal thalamus. *Mech. Dev.* 120, 1097–1111.

Hauptmann, G., and Gerster, T. (2000). Regulatory gene expression patterns reveal transverse and longitudinal subdivisions of the embryonic zebrafish forebrain. *Mech. Dev.* 91, 105–118.

Hauptmann, G., Soll, I., and Gerster, T. (2002). The early embryonic zebrafish forebrain is subdivided into molecularly distinct transverse and longitudinal domains. *Brain Res. Bull.* 57, 371–375.

Hidalgo-Sánchez, M., Martínez-de-la-Torre, M., Alvarado-Mallart, R. M., and Puelles, L. (2005). Distinct preisthmic domain, defined by overlap of *Otx2* and *Pax2* expression domains in the chicken caudal midbrain. *J. Comp. Neurol.* 483, 17–29.

Kan, X. Z., Li, X. F., Lei, Z. P., Chen, L., Gao, H., Yang, Z. I., Yang, J. K., Guo, Z. C., Yu, L., Zhang, L. Q., and Qian, C. J. (2010a). Estimation of divergent times for major lineages of galliform birds: evidence from complete mitochondrial genome sequences. *Afr. J. Biotechnol.* 9, 3073–3078.

Kan, X. Z., Yang, J. K., Li, X. F., Chen, L., Lei, Z. P., Wang, M., Qian, C. J., Gao, H., and Yang, Z. I. (2010b). Phylogeny of major lineages of galliform birds (Aves: Galliformes) based on complete mitochondrial genomes. *Genet. Mol. Res.* 9, 1625–1633.

Karten, H. J., and Hodos, W. (1967). *A stereotaxic atlas of the brain of the pigeon (Columba livia)*. Baltimore, MD: The John Hopkins Press.

Kiecker, C., and Lumsden, A. (2004). Hedgehog signaling from the ZLI regulates diencephalic regional identity. *Nat. Neurosci.* 7, 1242–1249.

Kikuta, H., Kanai, M., Ito, Y., and Yamasu, K. (2003). *Gbx2* homeobox gene is required for the maintenance of the isthmic region in the zebrafish embryonic brain. *Dev. Dyn.* 228, 433–450.

Kimball, R. T., Braun, E. L., Zwartjes, P. W., Crowe, T. M., and Ligon, J. D. (1999). A molecular phylogeny of the Pheasants and Partridges suggests that these lineages are not monphyletic. *Mol. Phylogenet. Evol.* 11, 38–54.

Koenig, S. F., Brentle, S., Hamdi, K., Fichtner, D., Wedlich, D., and Gradl, D. (2010). *En2*, *Pax2/5* and *Tcf-4* transcription factors cooperate in patterning the *Xenopus* brain. *Dev. Biol.* 340, 318–328.

Koenig, S. F., Lattanzio, R., Mansperger, K., Rupp, R. A., Wedlich, D., and Gradl, D. (2008). Autoregulation of *XTcf-4* depends on a Lef/Tcf site on the *XTcf-4* promoter. *Genesis* 46, 81–86.

Kriegs, J. O., Matzke, A., Churakov, G., Kuritzin, A., Mayr, G., Brosius, J., and Schmitz, J. (2007). Waves of genomic hitchhikers shed light on the evolution of gamebirds (Aves: Galliformes). *BMC Evol. Biol.* 7, 190. doi: 10.1186/1471-2148-7-190

Kuenzel, W. J., and Masson, M. (1988). *A Stereotaxic Atlas of the Brain of the Chick (Gallus domesticus).* Baltimore, MD: Johns Hopkins University Press.

Kuhlenbeck, H. (1939). The development and structure of the pretectal cell masses in the chick. *J. Comp. Neurol.* 71, 361–386.

Kunz, M., Herrmann, M., Wedlich, D., and Gradl, D. (2004). Autoregulation of canonical Wnt signaling controls midbrain development. *Dev. Biol.* 273, 390–401.

Larsen, C. W., Zeltser, L. M., and Lumsden, A. (2001). Boundary formation and compartition in the avian diencephalon. *J. Neurosci.* 21, 4699–4711.

López-Sánchez, C., Puelles, L., García-MartínezMartínez, V., and Rodríguez-Gallardo, L. (2005). Morphological and molecular analysis of the early developing chick requires an expanded series of primitive streak stages. *J. Morphol.* 264, 105–116.

Martínez, S. (1987). *Estudio experimental de la conectividad tectal en relación con la región pretectal y la comisura posterior: aspectos estructurales, citoquímicos y ontogenéticos.* Ph.D. dissertation, University of Murcia, Spain.

Martínez, S., and Alvarado-Mallart, R. M. (1989). Transplanted mesencephalic quail cells colonize selectively all primary visual nuclei of chick diencephalon: a study using heterotopic transplants. *Brain Res. Dev. Brain. Res.* 47, 263–274.

Martínez, S., Puelles, L., and Alvarado-Mallart, R. M. (1992). Tangential neuronal migration in the avian tectum: cell type identification and mapping of regional differences with quail/chick homotopic transplants. *Brain Res. Dev. Brain Res.* 66, 153–163.

Martínez-de-la-Torre, M., Garda, A. L., Puelles, E., and Puelles, L. (2002). *Gbx2* expression in the late embryonic chick dorsal thalamus. *Brain Res. Bull.* 57, 435–438.

Matsunaga, E., Araki, I., and Nakamura, H. (2000). Pax6 defines the di-mesencephalic boundary by repressing En1 and Pax2. *Development* 127, 2357–2365.

Mayr, G. (2008). The fossil record of galliform birds: comments on Crowe et al. (2006). *Cladistics* 24, 74–76.

McGowan, L., Kuo, E., Martin, A., Monuki, E. S., and Striedter, G. (2010). Species differences in early patterning of the avian brain. *Evolution* 65, 907–911.

Menuet, A., Alunni, A., Joly, J. S., Jeffery, W. R., and Rétaux, S. (2007). Expanded expression of Sonic hedgehog in *Astyanax cavefish*: multiple consequences on forebrain development and evolution. *Development* 134, 845–855.

Morona, R., Ferran, J. L., Puelles, L., and González, A. (2010). Embryonic genoarchitecture of the pretectum in *Xenopus laevis*: a conserved pattern in tetrapods. *J. Comp. Neurol.* 519, 1024–1050.

Murakami, Y., Ogasawara, M., Sugahara, F., Hirano, S., Satoh, N., and Kuratani, S. (2001). Identification and expression of the lamprey *Pax6* gene: evolutionary origin of the segmented brain of vertebrates. *Development* 128, 3521–3531.

Niss, K., and Leutz, A. (1998). Expression of the homeobox gene *GBX2* during chicken development. *Mech. Dev.* 76, 151–155.

Pereira, S. L., and Baker, A. J. (2009). "Waterfowl and gamefowl (Galloanserae)," in *The Time Tree of Life*, eds B. S. Hedges and S. Kumar (New York: Oxford University Press), 415–418.

Pombal, M. A., Megías, M., Bardet, S. M., and Puelles, L. (2009). New and old thoughts on the segmental organization of the forebrain in lampreys. *Brain Behav. Evol.* 74, 7–19.

Pombal, M. A., and Puelles, L. (1999). Prosomeric map of the lamprey forebrain based on calretinin immunocytochemistry, Nissl stain, and ancillary markers. *J. Comp. Neurol.* 414, 391–422.

Puelles, L. (1995). A segmental morphological paradigm for understanding vertebrate forebrains. *Brain Behav. Evol.* 46, 319–337.

Puelles, L. (2001). Brain segmentation and forebrain development in amniotes. *Brain Res. Bull.* 55, 695–710.

Puelles, L., Amat, J. A., and Martínez-de-la-Torre, M. (1987). Segment-related, mosaic neurogenetic pattern in the forebrain and mesencephalon of early chick embryos: I. Topography of AChE-positive neuroblasts up to stage HH18. *J. Comp. Neurol.* 266, 247–268.

Puelles, L., Kuwana, E., Puelles, E., Bulfone, A., Shimamura, K., Keleher, J., Smiga, S., and Rubenstein, J. L. (2000). Pallial and subpallial derivatives in the embryonic chick and mouse telencephalon, traced by the expression of the genes *Dlx-2*, *Emx-1*, *Nkx- 2.1*, *Pax-6*, and *Tbr-1*. *J. Comp. Neurol.* 424, 409–438.

Puelles, L., Martínez, S., Martínez-de-la-Torre, M., and Rubenstein, J. L. (2004). "Gene maps and related histogenetic domains in the forebrain and midbrain," in *The Rat Nervous System*, ed. G. Paxinos (New York: Elsevier), 3–25.

Puelles, L., Martínez-de-la-Torre, M., Paxinos, G., Watson, C., and Martínez, S. (2007). *The Chick Brain in Stereotaxic Coordinates. An Atlas Featuring Neuromeric Subdivisions and Mammalian Homologies.* San Diego: Academic Press, Elsevier.

Puelles, L., and Medina, L. (2002). Field homology as a way to reconcile genetic and developmental variability with adult homology. *Brain Res. Bull.* 57, 243–255.

Puelles, L., and Rubenstein, J. L. (1993). Expression patterns of homeobox and other putative regulatory genes in the embryonic mouse forebrain suggest a neuromeric organization. *Trends Neurosci.* 16, 472–479.

Puelles, L., and Rubenstein, J. L. (2003). Forebrain gene expression domains and the evolving prosomeric model. *Trends Neurosci.* 26, 469–476.

Redies, C., Arndt, K., and Ast, M. (1997). Expression of the cell adhesion molecule axonin-1 in neuromeres of the chicken diencephalon. *J. Comp. Neurol.* 381, 230–252.

Redies, C., Ast, M., Nakagawa, S., Takeichi, M., Martínez-de-la-Torre, M., and Puelles, L. (2000). Morphologic fate of diencephalic prosomeres and their subdivisions revealed by mapping cadherin expression. *J. Comp. Neurol.* 421, 481–514.

Rendahl, H. (1924). Embryologische und morphologische Studien über das Zwischenhirn beim Huhn. *Acta Zool.* 5, 241–344.

Sánchez-Arrones, L., Ferran, J. L., Rodríguez-Gallardo, L., and Puelles, L. (2009). Incipient forebrain boundaries traced by differential gene expression and fate mapping in the chick neural plate. *Dev. Biol.* 335, 43–65.

Sánchez-Guardado, L. Ó., Irimia, M., Sánchez-Arrones, L., Burguera, D., Rodríguez-Gallardo, L., García-Fernández, J., Puelles, L., Ferran, J. L., and Hidalgo-Sánchez, M. (2011). Distinct and redundant expression and transcriptional diversity of *Meis* gene paralogs during chicken development. *Dev. Dyn.* doi:10.1002/dvdy.22621

Schlosser, G., and Ahrens, K., (2004). Molecular anatomy of placode development in *Xenopus laevis*. Dev. Biol. 271, 439–466.

Senn, D. G. (1970). The stratification in the reptilian central nervous system. *Acta Anat. (Basel)* 75, 521–552.

Senn, D. G. (1979). "Embryonic development of the central nervous system," in *Biology of the Reptilia, Chapter 4, Vol. 9, Neurology A (RG. Northcutt and PH. Ulinski)*, ed. C. Gans (London: Academic Press). 173–244.

Senut, M. C., and Alvarado-Mallart, R. M. (1987). Cytodifferentiation of quail tectal primordium transplanted homotopically into the chick embryo. *Brain Res.* 429, 187–205.

Shen, Y. Y., Liang, L., Sun, Y. B., Yue, B. S., Yang, X. J., Murphy, R. W., and Zhang, Y. P. (2010). A mitogenomic perspective on the ancient, rapid radiation in the Galliformes with an emphasis on the Phasianidae. *BMC Evol. Biol.* 10, 132. doi: 10.1186/1471-2148-10-132

Shimamura, K., Hirano, S., McMahon, A. P., and Takeichi, M. (1994). *Wnt-1*-dependent regulation of local E-cadherin and alpha N-catenin expression in the embryonic mouse brain. *Development* 120, 2225–2234.

Striedter, G. F. (2005). *Principles of Brain Evolution*. Sunderland, MA: Sinauer.

Sylvester, J. B., Rich, C. A., Loh, Y. H., van Staaden, M. J., Fraser, G. J., and Streelman, J. T. (2010). Brain diversity evolves via differences in patterning. *Proc. Natl. Acad. Sci. U.S.A.* 107, 9718–9723.

Tavares, E. S., and Baker, A. J. (2008). Single mitochondrial gene barcodes reliably identify sister-species in diverse clades of birds. *BMC Evol. Biol.* 8, 81. doi: 10.1186/1471-2148-8-81

Toresson, H., Parmar, M., and Campbell, K. (2000). Expression of *Meis* and *Pbx* genes and their protein products in the developing telencephalon: implications for regional differentiation. *Mech. Dev.* 94, 183–187.

Vieira, C., Garda, A. L., Shimamura, K., and Martínez, S. (2005). Thalamic development induced by *Shh* in the chick embryo. *Dev. Biol.* 284, 351–363.

Vieira, C., and Martínez, S. (2006). Sonic hedgehog from the basal plate and the zona limitans intrathalamica exhibits differential activity on diencephalic molecular regionalization and nuclear structure. *Neuroscience* 143, 129–140.

Yoon, M. S., Puelles, L., and Redies, C. (2000). Formation of cadherin-expressing brain nuclei in diencephalic alar plate divisions. *J. Comp. Neurol.* 421, 461–480.

Zweers, G. A. (1971). *A Stereotaxic Atlas of the Brainstem of the Mallard (Anas platyrhynchos L.).* Assen: Van Gorcum.

Conflict of Interest Statement: The authors declare that the research was conducted in the absence of any commercial or financial relationships that could be construed as a potential conflict of interest.

16

The long adventurous journey of rhombic lip cells in jawed vertebrates: a comparative developmental analysis

Mario F. Wullimann[1]*, Thomas Mueller[2], Martin Distel[3†], Andreas Babaryka[3], Benedikt Grothe[1] and Reinhard W. Köster[3†]

[1] Graduate School of Systemic Neurosciences and Department Biology II, Ludwig-Maximilians-Universität Munich, Planegg, Germany
[2] Department Developmental Biology, Institute of Biology I, University of Freiburg, Freiburg, Germany
[3] Institute of Developmental Genetics, Helmholtz Zentrum München, German Research Center for Environmental Health, Neuherberg, Germany

Edited by:
Agustín González, Universidad Complutense de Madrid, Spain

Reviewed by:
Susan Dymecki, Harvard University, USA
Rob Machold, New York University School of Medicine, USA
Pilar Aroca, University of Murcia, Spain

***Correspondence:**
Mario F. Wullimann, Graduate School of Systemic Neurosciences and Division of Neurobiology, Department Biology II, Ludwig-Maximilians-Universität Munich, Grosshadernerstr. 2, D-82152 Planegg, Bavaria, Germany.
e-mail: wullimann@bio.lmu.de

†Current address:
Martin Distel, Department of Cellular and Molecular Medicine, University of California San Diego, 9500 Gilman Drive, La Jolla, CA 92093-0380, USA;
Reinhard W. Köster, Cell Biology and Cell Physiology, Institute of Zoology, Technische Universität Braunschweig, Spielmannstr. 7, D-38106 Braunschweig, Germany.

This review summarizes vertebrate rhombic lip and early cerebellar development covering classic approaches up to modern developmental genetics which identifies the relevant differential gene expression domains and their progeny. Most of this information is derived from amniotes. However, progress in anamniotes, particularly in the zebrafish, has recently been made. The current picture suggests that rhombic lip and cerebellar development in jawed vertebrates (gnathostomes) share many characteristics. Regarding cerebellar development, these include a *ptf1a* expressing ventral cerebellar proliferation (VCP) giving rise to Purkinje cells and other inhibitory cerebellar cell types, and an *atoh1* expressing upper rhombic lip giving rise to an external granular layer (EGL, i.e., excitatory granule cells) and an early ventral migration into the anterior rhombencephalon (cholinergic nuclei). As for the lower rhombic lip (LRL), gnathostome commonalities likely include the formation of precerebellar nuclei (mossy fiber origins) and partially primary auditory nuclei (likely convergently evolved) from the *atoh1* expressing dorsal zone. The fate of the *ptf1a* expressing ventral LRL zone which gives rise to (excitatory cells of) the inferior olive (climbing fiber origin) and (inhibitory cells of) cochlear nuclei in amniotes, has not been determined in anamniotes. Special for the zebrafish in comparison to amniotes is the predominant origin of anamniote excitatory deep cerebellar nuclei homologs (i.e., eurydendroid cells) from *ptf1a* expressing VCP cells, the sequential activity of various *atoh1* paralogs and the incomplete coverage of the subpial cerebellar plate with proliferative EGL cells. Nevertheless, the conclusion that a rhombic lip and its major derivatives evolved with gnathostome vertebrates only and are thus not an ancestral craniate character complex is supported by the absence of a cerebellum (and likely absence of its afferent and efferent nuclei) in jawless fishes

Keywords: atoh1, cerebellum, cochlear nuclei, precerebellar systems, ptf1a, wnt1, zebrafish, rhombic lip

AMNIOTE RHOMBIC LIP AND CEREBELLAR DEVELOPMENT

GENERAL

The vertebrate hindbrain (rhombencephalon) consists of an anterior metencephalon (rhombomere 1), including the cerebellum and pons, and a posterior myelencephalon (remaining rhombomeres). The embryonic anterior rhombencephalon has a dorsal rhombic groove (rhombic fossa) because the dorsal part of the neural tube wall, the alar plates, are laterally extended and form a V-shaped medulla oblongata in transverse section (**Figures 1A,B**). In contrast, the alar plates of the posterior rhombencephalon and the spinal cord approach each other closely in the dorsal midline and are kept together by a thin roof plate, reminiscent of a closed embryonic neural tube (**Figure 1C**). However, the alar plates of the anterior rhombencephalon are also interconnected by the roof plate which is greatly mediolaterally extended (**Figure 1B**). This epithelial tela covers the rhombic fossa and will generate (together with mesodermal vascular tissue at its peripheral side) a convoluted chorioideal plexus that is involved in cerebrospinal fluid production (Redzic et al., 2005). Interestingly, the secreted factor Sonic Hedgehog plays a specific signaling role for both the proliferation of the neuroectodermal tela itself – by acting on its germinative domain at its lateral point of attachment at the alar plate – as well as for the mesodermal vascularization of the developing choroid plexus (Huang et al., 2009; Nielsen and Dymecki, 2010). During embryonic development, the laterally displaced alar plate edges in amniotes constitute the rhombic lip which have long been known to be highly proliferative and to give rise to various brain structures that are finally located remote from their rhombic lip origin. Here, we will first review major steps in the understanding of amniote rhombic lip (including cerebellar) development before discussing related progress in anamniotes, particularly in zebrafish. With regard to amniotes, the organization of the review aims to give a sketch of how the field progressed historically ("Lower rhombic lip," "Cerebellum/Upper rhombic lip") before going into modern molecular data in amniotes ("Molecular revolutions").

LOWER RHOMBIC LIP

Both proliferation in the rhombic lip (*Rautenlippe*) and cellular migration into the pontine and inferior olivary regions are visible in normal histological material and were first described beginning in the late nineteenth century by Wilhelm His followed by various contemporaries (see Nieuwenhuys, 1998 for a review) who

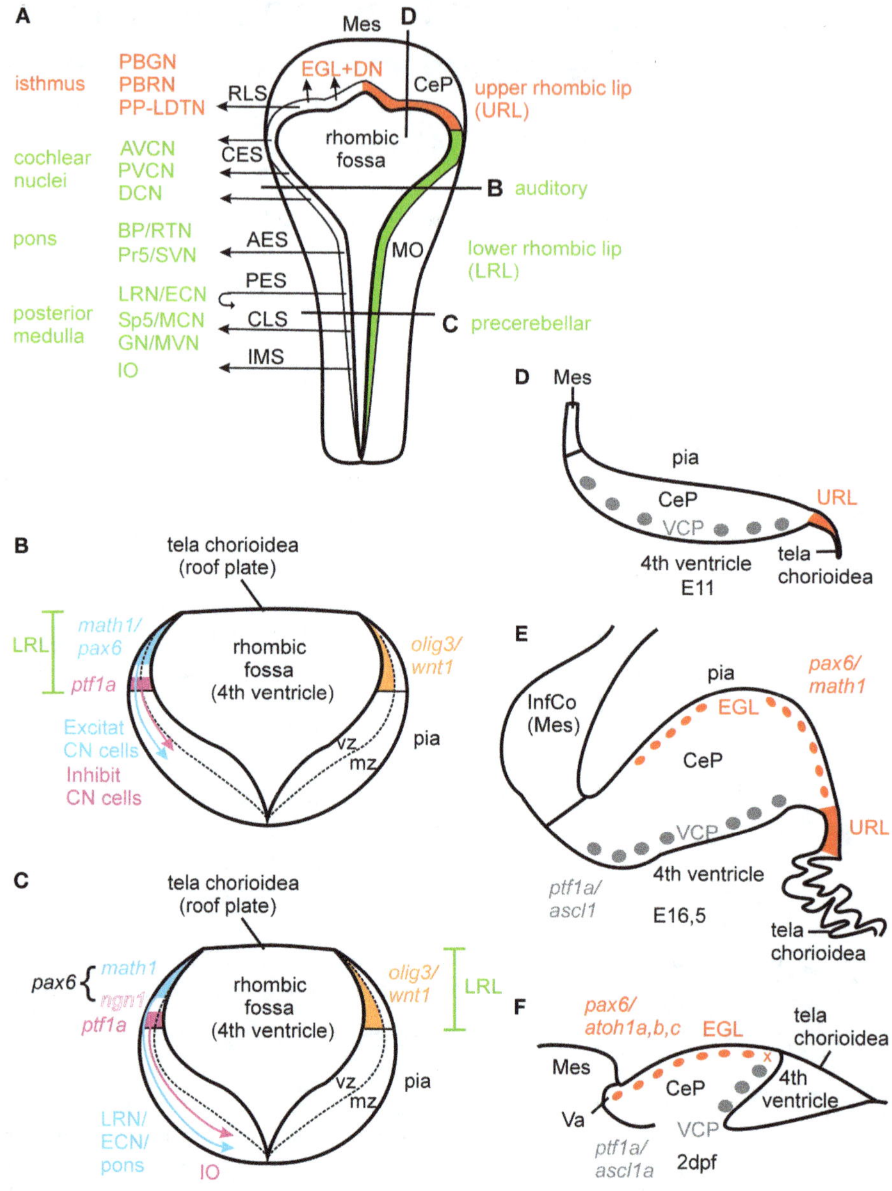

FIGURE 1 | (A–E) Amniote rhombic lip development. **(A)** Dorsal schematic view of embryonic amniote rhombencephalon showing rhombic lip and its derivatives. Many of these facts were first revealed by pre-genetic studies (see text for older citations) and later confirmed and detailed by molecular and genetic approaches. Anterior origin of primary auditory nuclei is indicated for mammals, in birds they originate along the entire lower rhombic lip (see text). **(B–C)** Schematic transverse section trough lower rhombic lip at two levels showing critical differential gene expression patterns. Compiled from Hoshino et al. (2005), Machold and Fishell (2005), Wang et al. (2005), Landsberg et al. (2005), Farago et al. (2006), Machold et al. (2007), Liu et al. (2008), Rose et al. (2009), Fujiyama et al. (2009), and Storm et al. (2009). Note that the *lmx1a/wnt1* positive generative zone for the choroid plexus in the most dorsal lower rhombic lip (Landsberg et al., 2005; Huang et al., 2009; Nielsen and Dymecki, 2010) is not shown. See text for some additional *math1* dependent medullary nuclei as shown in Rose et al. (2009). **(D–E)** Schematic view of sagittal sections of mouse cerebellum at E11 when EGL has not yet formed (after photo in Goldowitz and Hamre, 1998) and E16.5 when EGL has formed (after photo in Sillitoe and Joyner, 2007). Note that this difference between an anterior ventricular proliferative zone and URL emerges around E10 (DN cells formation) and that classical descriptions of the earlier upper rhombic lip include both (see text). **(F)** Sagittal section of zebrafish cerebellar plate at 2 dpf (redrawn after Kani et al., 2010). The x symbol indicates the hypothetical site of the ventricular origin of subpial *atoh1* positive cells and, thus, the structure corresponding to the amniote URL (see text). AES, anterior extramural stream; AVCN, anteroventral cochlear nucleus; BP, basal pons; CeP, cerebellar plate; CES, cochlear extramural stream; CLS, caudal rhombic lip stream (of Rose et al., 2009); CN, cochlear nucleus; DCN, dorsal cochlear nucleus; DN, deep cerebellar nuclei; ECN, external cuneate nucleus; EGL, external granular (or germinative) layer; GN, gracile nucleus; IMS, intramural stream; InfCo, inferior colliculus; IO, inferior olive; LRL, lower rhombic lip; LRN, lateral reticular nucleus; MCN, medial cuneate nucleus; Mes, mesencephalon; MO, medulla oblongata; MVN, medial vestibular nucleus; PBGN, parabigeminal nucleus; PBRN, parabrachial nucleus; PES, posterior extramural stream; PP-LDTN, pedunculopontine-laterodorsal tegmental nuclei; Pr5, principal sensory trigeminal nucleus; PVCN, posteroventral cochlear nucleus; RLS, rostral rhombic lip stream; RTN, reticulotegmental pontine nucleus; Sp5, spinal trigeminal nucleus; SVN, superior vestibular nucleus; URL, upper rhombic lip; VCP, ventral cerebellar proliferation (ventricular germinal matrix).

reported the situation for the human embryo. Later, Harkmark (1954) reported rhombic lip derived migration into inferior olive and pons in the chicken embryo describing how mitotic activity in the rhombic lip is followed by the appearance of ventrally directed streams of increasingly differentiating cells into inferior olive and pons. He additionally performed lesion experiments which – while not directly demonstrating the fate of lesioned rhombic lip cells – allowed a first hypothesis on the spatiotemporal origin of migrating rhombic lip cells. An important step forward in this field emerged with autoradiography (Taber-Pierce, 1966; Altman and Bayer, 1987a,b,c,d). These studies applied tritiated thymidine to embryonic rodents and used short and long term survival times to infer birth dates, migration routes and final destination of rhombic lip derived cells within the ventral medulla oblongata (**Figure 1**). During embryonic days 13–19, the rhombic lip of the rat brain produces – in the following order – neurons destined for the inferior olive (intramural stream, IMS), the lateral reticular and external cuneate nuclei (posterior extramural stream), the pontine reticulotegmental nucleus and the basal pontine gray (anterior extramural stream). The posterior extramural stream crosses the midline floor plate and, thus, the lateral reticular and external cuneate cells become to lie on the contralateral side. All these structures are called precerebellar, since they provide axonal input to the cerebellum (mossy fibers to granule cells, except for inferior olive: climbing fibers to Purkinje cells). Most of these afferent cerebellar projections occur in a contralateral manner. Even the adult ipsilaterally projecting lateral reticular and external cuneate nuclei have a developmental origin in the contralateral rhombic lip. Horseradish peroxidase injections at various relevant developmental time points confirmed that intramural (submarginal) and extramural (marginal) streams contribute inferior olivary and lateral reticular/external cuneate neurons, respectively (Bourrat and Sotelo, 1988, 1990). The latter studies in the embryonic rat brain also showed how leading neurites pioneer the migration path of lateral reticular/external cuneate and inferior olivary neurons and provided many details of this neuronal maturation. Similar migration events of precerebellar rhombic lip neurons were also described in the mouse by SEM/TEM studies (Ono and Kawamura, 1989, 1990) and in the chick by transfecting rhombic lip cells with enhanced green fluorescent protein (EGFP) expression vectors by electroporation (Ono et al., 2004). Also, the chick–quail transplantation system was used to show inferior olive/pons origins in rhombic lip (Tan and LeDouarin, 1991). Diffusible molecules (such as Netrin1 and Slit1/2 in the floor plate) and their receptors (Netrin1 receptors DCC and Unc5, Slit receptor Robo-2), as well as Ephrins and Eph receptors are involved in neurite guided migration (incl. its termination) of precerebellar neuronal somata in a complex manner. After settlement of these neurons, these factors also regulate topographically ordered axonal pathfinding toward their cerebellar projection targets (Chédotal et al., 1997; Bloch-Gallego et al., 1999; Wingate, 2001; Sotelo, 2004).

All of these studies document rare cases of central nervous system tangential migration of neural cells, which runs perpendicular to conventional radial migration (during the latter, cells move along radial glia fibers from ventricle toward pia). Tangential migrations also exist in other parts of the brain, for example the tangentially moving cell streams from the medial ganglionic eminence into the cortex or the dorsoventral neuronal migration in the spinal cord. Thus, rhombic lip derived migration involves a massive transgression of longitudinal zones, because these migrating alar plate cells eventually end up in the basal plate (inferior olive, pons, lateral reticular nucleus) or migrate at least through it before ending in the alar plate of the other brain side (external cuneate nucleus).

Much later – probably because of their less spectacular, shorter-distance migration – all three (dorsal, anteroventral, posteroventral) mammalian cochlear nuclei (DCN, AVCN, PVCN) were also described to derive at least partially from the rhombic lip (autoradiography: Taber-Pierce, 1967, HRP-labeling: Willard and Martin, 1986; cerebellar mutant studies: Berrebi et al., 1990, BrDU/DiI labeling: Ivanova and Yuasa, 1998). Finally, genetic studies showed in more detail that the mammalian cochlear nuclei develop from a portion of the rhombic lip that lies anterior to the region of the rhombic lip which gives rise to the extra- and intramural stream for precerebellar nuclei. For example, a sophisticated approach of intersectional and subtractive genetic mapping of *wingless* homolog *wnt1* (longitudinally expressed in the rhombic lip, see below) expressing cells in rhombomeres 3/5 (where the zinc-finger transcription factor gene *Krox20* is selectively expressed; Farago et al., 2006) or specific transgenic fate mapping of *Math5* expressing cells (*Atoh7*; Saul et al., 2008) revealed cochlear derivatives in detail. A rhombic lip origin was also reported for the chick primary auditory nuclei (Golgi stains and DiI labeling; Book and Morest, 1990). Interestingly however, the origin of chick primary auditory nuclei is not restricted to the anterior rhombic lip as in mammals, but extends throughout the medulla oblongata (Marín and Puelles, 1995; Cambronero and Puelles, 2000). This is strong evidence for an independent origin of archosaur and mammalian hearing, which is in line with the fossil record indicating an independent evolution of tympanic ears (Clack, 1997) and with parallel evolution of neuronal mechanisms, for instance for sound localization (Grothe, 2003; Grothe et al., 2004).

In summary, the longitudinally running amniote rhombic lip that flanks the rhombic fossa laterally, the so-called caudal or lower rhombic lip (LRL) gives rise to cochlear nuclei anteriorly in mammals (but all along the rhombic lip in birds) and precerebellar nuclei more posteriorly (**Figure 1**).

CEREBELLUM/UPPER RHOMBIC LIP

At their anterior pole, the longitudinally running rhombic lips fuse by forming a transverse bridge which will give rise to the primordium of the cerebellum (cerebellar plate), the deep cerebellar nuclei (DN), and the proliferative external granular layer (EGL, **Figure 1A**). To discriminate it from the caudal or lower rhombic lip, this anterior rhombic lip bridge has variedly been refered to as the rostral, cerebellar, or upper rhombic lip (URL). During embryonic development (around E10 in the mouse), it separates into two germinative zones: a fastly expanding anterior, ventricularly located ventral cerebellar proliferation (VCP, **Figure 1D**) and the so-called germinal trigone, which is the posterior rim of the initial cerebellar rhombic lip bridge (nicely depicted in Goldowitz and Hamre, 1998). While classical descriptions of the very early rhombic lip implicitly included both germinative zones, a consensus emerged meanwhile to refer only to the posterior proliferative zone (germinal trigone) as the URL and we follow this restricted definition of URL (**Figure 1A**). For our purpose here it is important to realize that both the VCP in the developing cerebellar plate and the URL are principally ventricularly located proliferative areas, unlike the later emerging and continued proliferative EGL which is subpially located.

In amniote cerebellar development, different classes of neuronal cells were described in classical histology to be generated in subsequent waves (for an excellent review see Sotelo, 2004; for adult cerebellar organization, see: Ito, 2006). In chick cerebellar development, the first wave of postmitotic neuronal cells destined to become the deep cerebellar nuclei (DN) originates at the ventricle of the early cerebellar plate, apparently in the VCP (work of Feirabend, discussed by Dubbeldam, 1998). After migrating somewhat toward the periphery, these future DN cells move laterally down to the base of the cerebellum to their adult location. A later wave of postmitotic neuronal cells leaves the chick VCP and moves toward the periphery to eventually become Purkinje (and probably Golgi) cells. A similar early embryonic origin of DN cells was seen in autoradiographic studies in rodents, followed by Purkinje (and maybe early Golgi) cells, while late Golgi cells and molecular layer cells (basket and stellate cells) originate postnatally (mouse: Miale and Sidman, 1961; Taber-Pierce, 1975; rat: Altman and Bayer, 1985, 1987e) from interstitial proliferative cells in the ventral white matter (Sotelo, 2004).

An even later embryonic wave of amniote cerebellar neuronal cells is generated in the URL (or germinal trigone), the ventricular epithelium posterior to the now already existing cerebellar plate and has been described in normal histological and autoradiographic studies to invade the uttermost periphery of the cerebellar plate in a tangential ventrolateral to dorsomedial (e.g., mouse; Miale and Sidman, 1961) or posterior to rostral (rat: Altman and Bayer, 1987e) direction. Since these neuronal progenitors will postnatally continue to proliferate and migrate ventrally to develop into (internal) cerebellar granule cells (as first seen around 1900 by Santiago Ramon y Cajal in embryonic human brains), this peripheral cell sheet is called *external granular* or *germinal layer* (EGL). Hanaway (1967) noted in the chick that the future EGL cells are produced in the entire mediolateral extent of the ventricular cerebellar plate (presumably the URL) and move radially out into the periphery instead of tangentially invading it. The EGL of the lateral cerebellar plate is formed first, preceding that of the medial one, which possibly explains the earlier observations of an apparent lateromedial tangential invasion. Later, the entire URL was described in amniotes to give rise to cells migrating tangentially (mostly in caudorostral direction) into a subpial EGL position (retrovirally labeled clones: Ryder and Cepko, 1994; chick–quail transplants, DiI labeling: Wingate and Hatten, 1999; Wingate, 2001; DiI: Gilthorpe et al., 2002). URL cells invading the subpial cerebellar plate use clues in the overlying meninges for organized migration and the resulting adult internal granular cell masses maintain the mediolateral topology of their rhombic lip origin (reviewed in Chédotal, 2010). Thus, the founder cells of the amniote subpial EGL arise in the (ventricular) proliferative zone of the URL (posterior part of the cerebellar plate) while the rostrally expanded VCP at the ventricular side of the cerebellar plate at this developmental time point may be considered a different ventricular zone. In contrast to the DN and Purkinje neurons formed by cell waves described above, the EGL cells remain mitotic during postnatal development and eventually give rise to an immense number of postmitotic neurons which migrate basally (e.g., Fujta, 1967; Alder et al., 1996; Zhang and Goldman, 1996; Komuro and Rakic, 1998a).

The proliferative activity of the EGL is regulated by differentiated Purkinje neurons via the Sonic Hedgehog signaling (SHH)-ligand, which acts on SHH receptors (Patched, Smoothened) and transcription factors (Gli) expressed by EGL cells (Traiffort et al., 1998, 1999; review: Martí and Bovolenta, 2002; Sillitoe and Joyner, 2007; Chédotal, 2010). Thus, this represents a case of transit amplification (Kriegstein and Alvarez-Buylla, 2009). After entering the Vitronectin-rich premigratory zone, EGL cells become postmitotic (reviewed in Sotelo, 2004). During further cerebellar cortex development in amniotes, granule cells migrate ventrally in a radial glia guided fashion and will eventually cross the Purkinje cell layer to generate the densely populated deep adult internal granular layer (IGL; for reviews on this issue, see: Hatten, 1990, 1999; Hatten and Mason, 1990; Rakic, 1990; Hatten and Heintz, 1995; Hatten et al., 1997; Curran and D'Arcangelo, 1998; D'Arcangelo and Curran, 1998; Komuro and Rakic, 1998b; Goldowitz and Hamre, 1998; Voogd and Glickstein, 1998; Sotelo, 2004; Chédotal, 2010).

More recently, using an EGFP-expressing transgenic rat strain as source for transplants into wild type rats, the ventricular VCP was shown to produce all inhibitory cerebellar cell types (GABA-/glycinergic) in the emerging cerebellar plate (Purkinje cells/Golgi and Lugaro cells of internal granule layer/basket and stellate cells of the molecular layer; Leto et al., 2006; recent review on adult cerebellar organization: Ito, 2006), as similarly found in mice (Weisheit et al., 2006). The VCP also generates the inhibitory fraction of deep cerebellar nuclei (DN; see more details below). In complement, the URL gives rise to an early stream of excitatory (glutamatergic) deep cerebellar nuclear cells (mouse: between E10–E12), which invade tangentially the subpial developing cerebellar plate (the so-called nuclear transition zone, a forerunner of the EGL) and then descend ventrolaterally to contribute to the DN shown with *in situ* hybridization (ISH) studies of transcription factor expressing genes *tbr1*, *tbr2*, and *pax6* (Fink et al., 2006). Subsequently, the URL forms the EGL on the peripheral (subpial) side of the cerebellar plate (mouse: between E13 and E 16) which will continue to proliferate during postnatal development (mouse: 2 weeks) and it will produce myriads of excitatory (internal) granule and unipolar brush cells (Englund et al., 2006; Leto et al., 2006, review: Sillitoe and Joyner, 2007).

MOLECULAR REVOLUTIONS

NEW TOOLS

At the turn of the millennium, sophisticated genetic studies extended rhombic lip and cerebellar development toward an improved understanding of the underlying genetic processes (mostly mouse, but see Wilson and Wingate, 2006 for chicken). The early active genetic network in the midbrain–hindbrain boundary (MHB) involving transcription factor-encoding genes *otx2* (midbrain), *gbx2* (hindbrain), *pax2/5* (MHB), and *fgf8* and *wnt1* (both encode for proteins that can act as secreted morphogens) eventually leads to the formation of the cerebellar anlage defined by the expression of the homeodomain encoding genes *engrailed 1/2* (Acampora et al., 2001; Liu and Joyner, 2001; Wang and Zoghbi, 2001; Wurst and Bally-Cuif, 2001; Sgaier et al., 2005). Genes with later continued expression in rhombic lip/cerebellar plate derivates may serve as "natural" markers to trace their fate (such as *tbr1* for glutamatergic DN cells; see above). Most importantly, site specific recombinase systems (Cre-*loxP* and Flp-*FTR*) were introduced (Branda and Dymecki, 2004) to demonstrate the fate of cells expressing developmentally relevant genes expressed in the early cerebellar plate and rhombic lip after embryonic downregulation of this informative gene expression. Also, detailed comparisons of gene expression and phenotype in wild type and mutant organisms helped to decipher developmental mechanisms. An example is the paired-box/homeobox gene *pax6*, whose diverse roles in eye, nose, and cortex development are complemented by critical functions in rhombic lip and cerebellar development (Engelkamp et al., 1999). In the mouse, *pax6* is strongly expressed between 12.5 and 13.5 days in the LRL and URL plus the latter's derivative, the EGL, but not in the remaining cells of the cerebellar plate. The *pax6* expressing LRL progeny can be followed in anterior (AES) and posterior extramural streams (PES) toward their destination, i.e., reticulotegmental and basal pontine nuclei, lateral reticular/external cuneate nuclei, respectively, but not in the intramural stream (IMS) and its destination, the inferior olive (**Figure 1A**). In the *pax6* homozygous loss of function mutant *small eye (sey)*, the formation of basal pons (but not reticulotegmental nucleus and inferior olive) and LNR/ECN is impaired. Since in the *sey* mutant, proliferation in the LRL is not affected (premigratory cells actually accumulate there), and the Netrin1 receptor DCC fails to be expressed in AES cells (in those few that migrate to form the reticulotegmental nucleus), *pax6* may be associated with a function in migration, not proliferation. Proliferation is also not affected in the EGL of *sey* mutants: postmitotic cells accumulate in the premigratory zone of the cerebellar plate, but fail to migrate. In cells destined for the reticulotegmental pontine nucleus, *pax6* function must be redundantly taken over by other gene(s).

GENES INVOLVED IN INHIBITORY VS EXCITATORY NEURON DEVELOPMENT

The basic Helix-Loop-Helix (bHLH)-factor-encoding gene *ptf1a* is expressed in the ventricular ventral cerebellar proliferation (VCP) and adult animals of its corresponding mouse mutant *cerebelless* have only a rudimentary cerebellum and show associated motor deficits (Hoshino et al., 2005; Hoshino, 2006). The adult cerebellar rudiment contains large glutamatergic (DN type) cells, but no GABAergic cells. However, during embryonic cerebellar plate development, the EGL does initially develop and glutamatergic markers (Calretinin) are expressed in its descendents (while GABAergic markers such as Calbindin remain absent). The EGL eventually disappears gradually during postnatal stages. Further, lineage tracing involving a Cre-recombinase-*lacZ* strain allowing for the visualization of *ptf1a* expressing cells and their progeny revealed that these cells only develop into cerebellar GABAergic and glial cells, but not glutamatergic cells (Hoshino et al., 2005). Thus, the primary effect in *cerebelless* mutants is that no GABAergic cells are formed from the ventricular cerebellar proliferation (VCP), while EGL formation and glutamatergic cell production from it is initially unaffected (large DN cells, see above). Later, presumably because of the missing mitogenic SHH signal from Purkinje cells (see above), the EGL disappears and granule cells and a functional cerebellum are not formed as a secondary consequence.

Interestingly, adult *cerebelless* mutants also lack (glutamatergic) inferior olive and pontine nuclei, which – although embryonically formed – disappear postnatally. This likely occurs as a secondary consequence because these precerebellar nuclei lack a cerebellar innervation target (see above). In the hindbrain, *ptf1a* is also expressed in the ventral part of the LRL (apparently not affected in *cerebelless*) and cells descending from this area develop into all types of inhibitory (GABAergic, glycinergic) cells of the cochlear nuclei (Fujiyama et al., 2009), while glutamatergic cochlear nuclear cell types develop from the dorsal part of the LRL where another bHLH factor, the *atonal* homolog *atoh1* or *math1* – and also *pax6* – are expressed. Surprisingly, inferior olivary neurons (although glutamatergic) develop mostly from the *ptf1a* expressing cells in the posterior part of the ventral LRL (see below; **Figures 1B,C**).

In-depth analyses of mouse LRL revealed that *wnt1* is expressed throughout the entire dorsoventral extent of the developing LRL, while *math1* and the bHLH gene *neurogenin1* (*ngn1*) are restricted to its dorsal and a ventrally adjacent part, respectively (Landsberg et al., 2005; see **Figure 1C**). Importantly, *wnt1* is expressed in a decreasing dorsoventral gradient in the LRL, likely extending ventrally beyond the *ngn1* domain (Landsberg et al., 2005; Ray and Dymecki, 2009). Using Cre and Flp based fate mapping studies, Rodriguez and Dymecki (2000) and Landsberg et al. (2005) showed that mossy fiber-type precerebellar nuclei (BP, RTN, LRN, ECN) derive from the strongly *wnt1* and *math1* expressing dorsal LRL domain, while the climbing fiber system (IO) derives from weakly *wnt1* and strongly *ngn1* expressing ventral LRL domain. This is consistent with the reported *ptfa1* expression domain origin of IO (Hoshino et al., 2005; Yamada et al., 2007), although the *ptf1a* domain may be even more ventral than that of *ngn1* in the posteroventral LRL (Ray and Dymecki, 2009), and thus, the IO cells might be molecularly parcellated (Landsberg et al., 2005; Ray and Dymecki, 2009). In any case, the anteroventral LRL has a *ptf1a* domain, but lacks *ngn1* expression – and gives rise to inhibitory cochlear nuclei cells (Fujiyama et al., 2009; see above). In *pax6* mutant *sey* mice, a dorsal expansion of *ngn1* expression and concurrent regression of *math1* expression is seen, accompanied by the disruption of extramural streams (mossy fiber cells) and an increase of migrating cells in the intramural stream (IMS) to the IO (Landsberg et al., 2005), consistent with an earlier report on the *pax6* mutant sey phenotype (Engelkamp et al., 1999). This indicates that PAX6 acts in rhombic lip development and rhombic lip derived migration by limiting *ngn1* expression.

The bHLH gene *olig3* has a similar graded expression in the LRL as *wnt1* does (**Figures 1B,C** covering dorsoventrally *math1*, *ngn1*, and *ptf1* domains, with the gradient tapering out more slowly ventrally than that of *wnt1* (Liu et al., 2008; Ray and Dymecki, 2009; Storm et al., 2009). Accordingly, *olig 3* has a role in the development of both mossy and climbing fiber precerebellar nuclei as shown both by histochemical marker analysis of *olig3* null mutant mice (Liu et al., 2008) and Cre based genetic fate mapping (Storm et al., 2009). As pointed out by Ray and Dymecki (2009), *olig3* may represent the best and most inclusive LRL marker.

Further major insights came from fate mapping of cells depending on the bHLH factor MATH1, its encoding gene has been key to investigating rhombic lip and cerebellar development because of its exclusive expression in URL (and later EGL) and dorsal LRL (apart from anterior dorsal spinal cord, peripheral inner ear hair cells, and epidermal Merkel cells; Akazawa et al., 1995; Ben-Arie et al., 1997, 2000; Helms et al., 2000; Machold and Fishell, 2005; Wang et al., 2005). Using a *math1*-expression dependent Cre-recombinase strain in combination with a Cre-recombination mediated *lacZ* reporter line, the above discussed origin of cochlear nuclei (excitatory cells) and of mossy fiber precerebellar systems from the strongly *wnt1* expressing dorsal LRL (Landsberg et al., 2005), as well as the URL origin of the (excitatory) deep cerebellar nuclear cells and EGL of the cerebellum, was independently confirmed by determining the fate of *math1* expressing progeny (Machold and Fishell, 2005; Wang et al., 2005). These studies also demonstrated that IO formation is independent of *math1* expression. Beyond that, previously unknown *math1* expressing rhombic lip derivatives were revealed in three (auditory related) lateral lemniscal nuclei, in the superior vestibular nucleus, in the parabrachial nuclear and in an isthmic complex (the latter two related to arousal; see more below on isthmic complex). A later analysis showed that in addition excitatory neurons (mostly glutamatergic, never GABA-/glycinergic) of the (auditory) superior olive, spinal, and medial vestibular nuclei, as well as primary somatosensory nuclei (principal and spinal trigeminal, medial cuneate, and gracile nuclei) and some breathing (Kölliker-Fuse nucleus, pre-Bötzinger complex, rostral ventral respiratory group) and bladder-control related (Barrington's nucleus) medullary nuclei derive from *math1* expressing LRL (Rose et al., 2009). Although the vestibular nuclei also provide mossy fiber input to the cerebellum, they are not treated usually as precerebellar nuclei like the external cuneate and lateral reticular nucleus. The temporal succession of all subpopulations in each major migratory stream was also resolved, for example in the newly described rostral rhombic lip migratory stream (RLS) which forms the early subpial nuclear transition zone (E11,5) from which the isthmic and DN cells derive first before it subsequently gives rise to the EGL (E13,5) and internal granule cells. Further, somatosensory spinal cord interneurons, which provide also mossy fiber input to cerebellar granule cells (as the precerebellar systems do), derive from the spinal continuation of the rhombic lip *math1* expression domain.

An even finer temporal and anatomical analysis of the MATH1 dependent isthmic complex was obtained by using a inducible Cre-recombinase under the control of *math1* regulatory elements (Machold and Fishell, 2005). This study showed that the isthmic complex consists of the parabigeminal nucleus and the cholinergic pedunculopontine and laterodorsal tegmental nuclei, and further detailed the already described *math1* expressing progeny. Although not reported in that study, the mammalian parabigeminal and parabrachial nuclei also contain cholinergic cells (see discussion in Volkmann et al., 2010).

A normal expression study of *wnt1* and a cell fate mapping study of transgenically labeled *wnt1* expressing progeny in the mouse hindbrain (and midbrain) confirmed an LRL origin of cochlear nuclei and mossy fiber precerebellar systems, but not of the inferior olive (Nichols and Bruce, 2006). As discussed above, the IO was found to originate from the only weakly *wnt1* expressing ventral LRL (Landsberg et al., 2005). In addition, although *wnt1* expression was previously not noted prior to mouse E11,5 in URL/EGL cells (Echelard et al., 1994), Nichols and Bruce (2006) reported beginning of *wnt1* expression in URL cells from E10.5 onward and confirmed with *wnt1* expression mediated transgenic labeling the origin of the EGL (i.e., granule cells, deep cerebellar nuclei) from the URL. Interestingly, they described an anterior cellular migration (corresponding to the RLS of *math1* expressing progeny, see above) via URL and EGL into the basal anterior rhombencephalon to form there at least part of the parabrachial and laterodorsal tegmental nuclei, indicating that the cholinergic *math1* dependent groups (Machold and Fishell, 2005; see above) are also derivatives from *wnt1* expressing precursors.

Beyond MATH1, the role of additional proneural bHLH factors has only begun to be unraveled. An ISH analysis of mouse bHLH genes *ascl1* and *neurogenin 1/2* noted their expression in the developing VCP or close to it, but an absence of expression of those genes in the URL. Thus, there is no overlap of the expression of these three genes with cerebellar *math1* domains between E10 and E13,5 and no co-expression between *ngn1* and *ngn2*, but partial overlap of expression between *ngn1/2* with *ascl1* and *ptf1a* domains (Machold et al., 2007; Zordan et al., 2008). Thus, these bHLH factor-encoding genes were interpreted to be related to the development of different inhibitory cell types. Indeed, *ascl1* was recently shown to be co-expressed in VCP cells with *ptf1a*, with ASCL1 involved in Purkinje and inhibitory DN cell development (Kim et al., 2008). In contrast, *ptf1a/ngn1* co-expressing cells develop into Purkinje, Golgi and Lugaro cells (Lundell et al., 2009). In addition, *ngn2* expression was shown to be active downstream of *ptf1a*, but not of *ascl1*. The proneural factor coding gene *neuroD* which is well established to act downstream of Neurogenins in the forebrain (reviewed in Osório et al., 2010) is required in the developing cerebellum for granule cell differentiation as shown in a comparison of wild type mice with a non-functional NeuroD mutant line (Miyata et al., 1999).

RHOMBIC LIP DEFINITIONS

Eventually, the suggestion arose to re-define and equal the rhombic lip with the extent of the *math1* expression domain bordering the rhombic fossa, including its derivatives (Wang et al., 2005). Although convenient at first sight, such a definition hinders the understanding of this complex structure at the functional systems level. The *ptf1a/ngn1* expressing ventral part of the dorsal rim of the rhombic fossa and the dorsally adjacent *math1* domain have in common that they both are the source of long distance tangential cellular migrations leading to the formation of inferior olive/inhibitory cells of cochlear nuclei and mossy fiber precerebellar nuclei/excitatory cells of cochlear nuclei, respectively. Functionally not directly cerebellar/auditory-related systems, such as the locus coeruleus, do not arise from this ventral rhombic lip territory. Instead they originate more ventrally as shown with fate mapping studies using grafting (quail–chick) and mouse brain gene expression analysis visualizing noradrenergic cell markers (dopamine-ß-hydroxylase and transcription factors *Phox2a/b*; Aroca et al., 2006). This more ventral origin was confirmed in a study combining *wnt1* expression mediated transgenic labeling with tyrosine hydroxylase immunostaining (for catecholaminergic cells) where no cells in the mouse locus coeruleus were double-labeled (Nichols and Bruce, 2006). In contrast, Lin et al., 2001 claimed that the chick locus coeruleus originates from the EGL. Be that as it may, all amniote LRL derivatives share the functional context of being closely involved in cerebellar or auditory circuitry. We therefore use dorsal and ventral rhombic lip (dLRL/vLRL), respectively, for the *math1* and *ptf1a/ngn1* expressing portions of the LRL. The URL/EGL and the ventricular VCP are comparable to at least the anterior dorsal and ventral LRL, respectively, regarding inhibitory/excitatory cell production, with the additional contribution of the URL to the cholinergic isthmic groups just discussed. However, as explained above, the early separable VCP is terminologically treated as different from the URL (germinal trigone), as the VCP does not show the long distance migratory behavior of its descendant cells as the vLRL does.

ANAMNIOTE PATTERNS

STARTING POINTS

We will now discuss existing evidence and provide new insights into similar and dissimilar patterns of rhombic lip and cerebellar development in anamniotes, particularly in the zebrafish. A natural starting point is to establish whether adult structures known to develop from rhombic lip and ventral cerebellar proliferation (VCP) in amniotes are present in zebrafish. A cerebellum with a three-layered cortex, including the major inhibitory and excitatory (glutamatergic) cell types, is present in the zebrafish (Miyamura and Nakayasu, 2001; Mikami et al., 2004; Bae et al., 2009) as in all gnathostome vertebrates (but absent in lampreys and myxinoids, Wullimann and Vernier, 2007). Deep cerebellar nuclei in teleosts are represented by eurydendroid cells, which are large excitatory cells in the Purkinje cell layer (Lannoo et al., 1991; McFarland et al., 2008; Bae et al., 2009). Thus, teleostean eurydendroid cells apparently fail to migrate into the deep of the cerebellum. They receive (inhibitory) Purkinje cell input and form the axonal output of the cerebellum (for example in the goldfish; Ikenaga et al., 2005). In the zebrafish, cholinergic isthmic nuclei exist (i.e., nucleus isthmi, secondary gustatory, and superior reticular nucleus, refered to below as the teleostean cholinergic isthmic complex; Clemente et al., 2004; Mueller et al., 2004), which are homologous to parabigeminal, parabrachial, and pedunculopontine-laterodorsal tegmental nuclei. For lack of connectional information in the zebrafish, the closely related goldfish or carp may be mentioned for the presence of an inferior olive which represents the sole cerebellar climbing fiber origin (Xu et al., 2008) and of mossy fiber-type precerebellar nuclei (lateral reticular nucleus; lateral cuneate nucleus; Wullimann and Northcutt, 1988) as well as of hearing related primary sensory nuclei (McCormick and Braford, 1994; McCormick and Hernandez, 1996). In contrast, a pons does not exist in anamniotes, including teleosts. However, do the other mentioned structures share a rhombic lip/VCP origin in teleosts? An additional immediately interesting question is whether the primary central lateral line nucleus (medial octavolateralis nucleus, MON; New et al., 1996) is a rhombic lip derivative with excitatory cells derived from *atoh1* expressing progenitors similar to the amniote cochlear nuclei. All anamniotes – except for strictly terrestrial amphibians – have this additional sensory organ and the related central processing apparatus which is entirely lost in amniotes. However, LRL derived structures have not been revealed by genetic fate mapping in teleosts so far.

EMBRYONIC AND LARVAL GENE ACTIVITY IN ZEBRAFISH RHOMBIC LIP AND CEREBELLAR PLATE

As in amniotes, the dorsal edges of the zebrafish alar plate rhombencephalon are laterally displaced upon formation of the fourth ventricle and define in transverse view a V-shaped rhombic fossa only covered by the roof plate (see Distel et al., 2006; their Movie 4). Furthermore, the early cerebellar plate develops between 24 and 48 h in the most anterior dorsal rhombencephalon (rhombomere 1) as bilateral, elevated flaps which eventually will cover the ventricle (**Figures 2A,A′**). However, the anatomical resolution does not allow identifying a structure comparable to the amniote germinal trigone/URL at the posterior margin as different from the proper cerebellar plate (Mueller and Wullimann, 2005). How about diagnostic gene expression patterns? Because of an additional whole genome duplication in early ray-finned fish (actinopterygians), modern teleosts such as the zebrafish have three paralogous *atoh1* (*math1* homolog) genes, namely *atoh1a* (*atoh1.1*), *atoh1b* (*atoh1.2*), and *atoh1c* (Kim et al., 1997; Jászai et al., 2003; Adolf et al., 2004; Wang et al., 2009; Kani et al., 2010). The *atoh1a* and *atoh1b* (not shown) gene expression patterns (**Figures 2A′,B′ and 3B**) are very similar from 1 to 2.5 days: expression domains are seen in the fused dorsal neural tube of the anterior spinal cord and most posterior hindbrain, then outline in the more rostral hindbrain the shape of the laterally displaced medullary edges (lower rhombic lip) and form in the most anterior hindbrain, where the cerebellar plate develops, a transverse bridge of expression (Köster and Fraser, 2001a), defining a URL by molecular means (see Discussion below). In addition, a strong expression is seen in the developing valvula cerebelli, an anterior part of the midline cerebellum only present in ray-finned fish (**Figure 3B**). After 2.5 days, *atoh1a* and *atoh1b* expression are fastly downregulated in LRL and URL, with *atoh1b* expression persisting longer in the URL, and both gene expressions are upheld in the valvula (**Figure 3C**). In contrast *atoh1c* expression is never seen in the LRL, but starts late (at around 2 days) to be strongly expressed in the valvula and URL (Kani et al., 2010), where it remains active in the larva beyond 9 days (**Figures 2C–F and 3D**).

As in amniotes, zebrafish *wnt1* expression is not restricted to the URL and LRL, but it is expressed between 16 h postfertilization (hpf) and 2 days beyond the dorsal rhombencephalon in the most dorsal mesencephalon and in the MHB, with an initial gap in the region of the cerebellar plate (Elsen et al., 2008). However, around 30 hpf, *wnt1* expression also is seen in the cerebellar plate (Lekven et al., 2003; McFarland et al., 2008).

Expression of the zebrafish *pf1a* gene starts around 32 hpf and is seen at least up to 5 days, in dorsal whole mount views in locations superficially similar to the URL and LRL expression domains of the *atoh1a* gene (Kani et al., 2010). However, in sagittal sections, it becomes clear that *ptf1a* is restricted to the ventricular cerebellar proliferation (VCP) and extends later into the valvula, while *atoh1* gene expression is in a non-overlapping superficial/subpial position (Kani et al., 2010), already indicating that many *atoh1* expressing cells are in a comparable position of an amniote EGL (**Figure 1F**). The expression of *ptf1a* in the LRL is ventral to that of *atoh1a* (A. Babaryka, R. W. Köster, personal observation).

As discussed above, the first mouse *math1* and *wnt1* dependent URL cells that invade the cerebellar plate subpially will migrate via the RLS and form the cholinergic isthmic groups (PBGN/PBRN/PP-LDTN) and deep cerebellar nuclei (DN; see **Figure 1A**); this is followed by the establishment of the EGL/inner granule cells (Machold and Fishell, 2005; Wang et al., 2005; Nichols and Bruce, 2006). Confocal time-lapse imaging using embryos of a zebrafish transgenic *wnt1*-Gal4-GFP strain revealed that an early migration

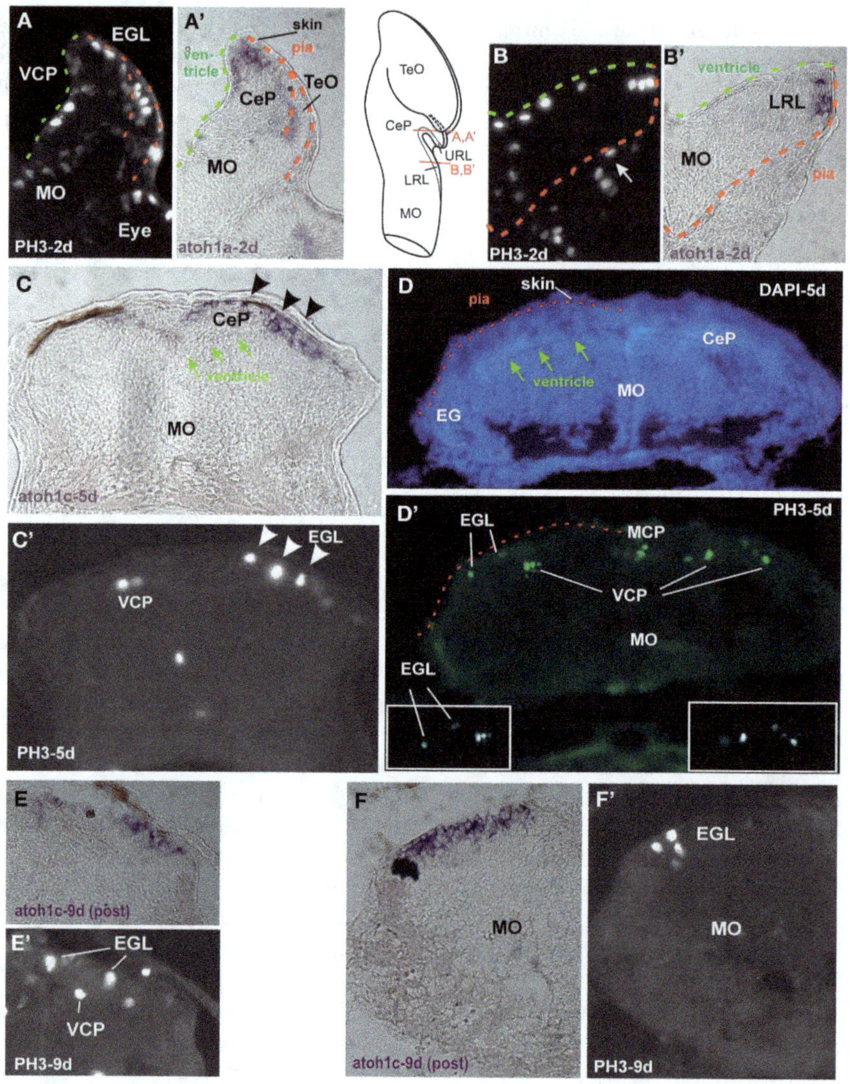

FIGURE 2 | Proliferation shown with phosphohistone 3-immunohistochemistry (PH3-IHC) and expression of bHLH genes *atoh1a* and *atoh1c* in zebrafish cerebellar plate (CeP; A,A′, C,C′, D,D′, E,E′, F,F′) and lower rhombic lip (LRL; B,B′) transverse sections. **(A)** PH3-IHC in CeP at 2 days. Note that proliferation in CeP is both on the ventricular (green dashed line) and pial (red dashed line) side. **(A′)** Identical section shows *atoh1a* ISH and overlap with both proliferative zones. **(B)** PH3-IHC in LRL at 2 days. Note that proliferation is only on ventricular side (green dashed line), not on pial side (red dashed line). More lateral PH3-positive cells are in connective tissue outside of brain (arrow). **(B′)** Identical section shows *atoh1a* ISH to overlap with PH3 cells at ventricle, and to extend more peripherally. **(C)** Expression of *atoh1c* at 5 days is mostly periphal (note arrows indicating ventricle) forming an EGL (arrowheads) and colocalizes with PH3 positive cells (shown in identical section in **(C′)**; arrowheads; left side shows PH3 positive cells in *atoh1c* negative ventral cerebellar proliferation). **(D)** DAPI stain and **(D′)** PH3-IHC stain (identical section) demonstrate that proliferative cells are present in ventricular cerebellar proliferation (VCP) and in external granular layer (EGL). Insets show PH3 positive cells in EGL ad VCP at a different focus. Dashed red line indicates pial surface of brain with skin above it. Arrows denote ventricle. **(E,E′)** and **(F,F′)** demonstrate that an EGL persists into later larval development, at least 9 days. Note in particular in **(F′)** how *atoh1c* expression is at the periphery of the cerebellar plate, that proliferative PH3 cells are restricted to most peripheral EGL and that proliferation is absent in the rest of the hindbrain at that stage. Methodological details will be provided elsewhere. CeP, cerebellar plate; EGL, external granular (or germinative) layer; IO, inferior olive; LRL, lower rhombic lip; MO, medulla oblongata; TeO, tectum opticum; VCP, ventral (or ventricular) cerebellar proliferation (ventricular germinal matrix).

between 24 and 48 hpf (Volkmann et al., 2010) precedes granule cell migration from the EGL, which only starts around 48 hpf (Volkmann et al., 2008). In particular, zygotes of this transgenic *wnt1*-reporter strain were injected with an UAS:mCherry construct to allow for precise visualization of this early migration. These *wnt1*-expressing cells co-express *atoh1a* and were shown to arise from proliferative cells (in an area indicated in **Figure 1F** with an X), move out into the subpial periphery of the cerebellar plate, before they migrate ventrally into the tegmentum of the most anterior rhombencephalon. Furthermore, this tegmental cluster exhibits expression of cholinergic and glutamatergic markers (Volkmann et al., 2010) and has differential and characteristic axonal projections to the optic tectum and the diencephalon indicating that this teleostean cholinergic isthmic complex includes the homologs of the cholinergic isthmic groups of mammals (Volkmann et al., 2010; summarized in **Figure 7**). It is also interesting that no *tbr1/tbr2* expressing cells

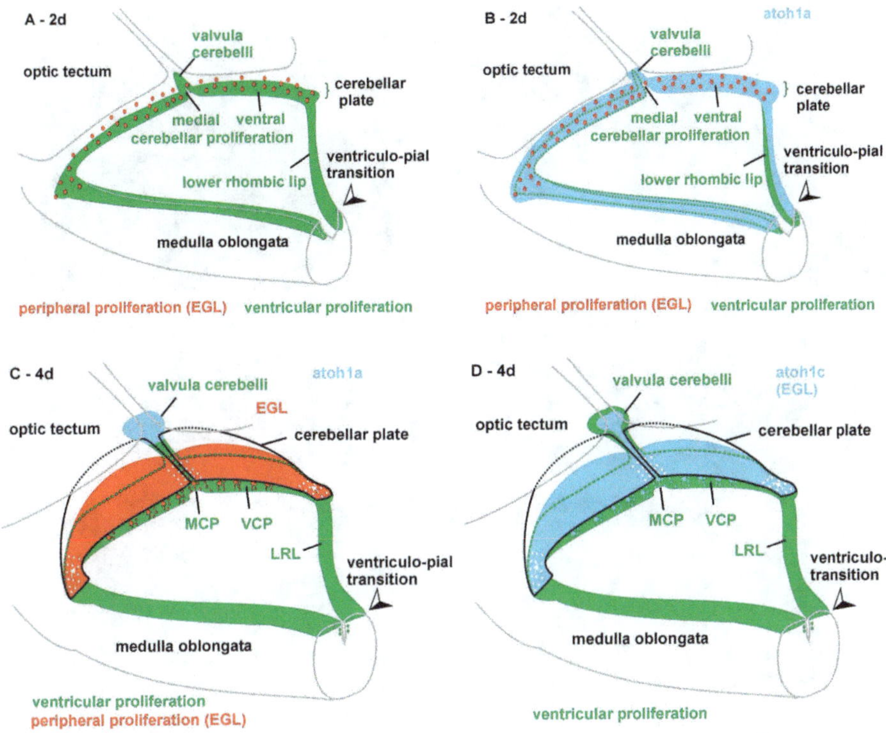

FIGURE 3 | Various 3D views of zebrafish cerebellar plate and lower rhombic lip (LRL) from a caudolateral angle at 2 days (A,B) and 4 days (C,D). (A) Ventricular proliferation in LRL, medial (MCP), and ventral cerebellar proliferation (VCP) and early valvula cerebelli is shown in green, peripheral proliferation in external granular layer (EGL) in red. Note ventriculo-pial boundary in LRL corresponding to meeting point of green and red dashed lines in **Figures 2B,B′**. **(B)** Same schema with expression of *atoh1a* added in light blue. **(C)** Ventricular proliferation in LRL, medial (MCP) and ventral cerebellar proliferation (VCP) and later in valvula cerebelli are shown in green, peripheral proliferation in EGL in red. Note that expression of *atoh1a* is now restricted to the valvula. Also, the ventriculo-pial boundary is in an everted position as shown in **Figures 4 F,G**. **(D)** Same schema with expression of *atoh1c* added in light blue. Note that in both **(C,D)** the exact position of little arrows indicating dorsal cell migrations for the formation of the EGL (but not its existence) is hypothetical. Synthesis of our data and those of Kani et al. (2010).

are seen in the migrating isthmic population (Volkmann et al., 2010), consistent with the fact that the eurydendroid cells, which are homologous to amniote DN, remain within the cerebellar cortex (Lannoo et al., 1991; McFarland et al., 2008; Bae et al., 2009).

THE ZEBRAFISH UPPER RHOMBIC LIP

Which region in the zebrafish brain corresponds to the amniote *atoh* positive cell producing URL (germinal trigone)? Köster and Fraser (2001a) have shown that *atoh1a* expression in the zebrafish is initiated at about 18 hpf in the cerebellar plate along the most dorsal ventricle (indicated by an X in **Figure 1F**) and then spreads into the subpial cerebellar plate periphery covering the entire cerebellar primordium up to the MHB by 20 hpf. This precedes by far the expression of *ptf1a*, which only starts around 32 hpf more ventrally (in the VCP), but directly adjacent to the *atoh1a* expression domain and this non-overlapping expression is maintained throughout development (A. Babaryka, R. W. Köster, personal observations; Kani et al., 2010). At the same time, *atoh1b* expressing cells and, in addition, from 2 days on into later larval life *atoh1c* expressing cells, are in the subpial periphery of the cerebellar plate with the *ptf1a* gene non-overlappingly expressed in the VCP (Kani et al., 2010, their **Figure 1**). In comparison to amniotes, these subpial *atoh1* cells correspond to an EGL and their ventricular point of origin as described above is in the caudal meeting point of ventral *ptf1a* positive zone and *atoh1*-positive subpial zone (the X in **Figure 1F**). This has been shown by *in vivo* time-lapse studies that observed *atoh1a* expressing cells proliferating at the dorsal cerebellar ventricle (Distel et al., 2010). Subsequently, *atoh1/wnt1* expressing URL cells move rostrally and migrate ventrally. Early URL emigrating cells give rise to neurons of tegmental hindbrain nuclei while later arising neurons will form the inner granular layer (Köster and Fraser, 2001b, 2006; Volkmann et al., 2008; Rieger et al., 2008; Kani et al., 2010; Volkmann et al., 2010).

THE ZEBRAFISH EXTERNAL GRANULAR LAYER

Thus, the subpial *atoh1* expressing cells in the zebrafish from 2 days on are in a position comparable to the amniote EGL and they originate from the most dorsal cerebellar plate ventricle (which corresponds to the amniote germinal trigone). For the recognition of an EGL, a critical issue is whether proliferation takes place during these developmental events not only at ventricular, but also on the subpial side of the zebrafish cerebellar plate. Phosphohistone 3 (PH3) immunohistology clearly shows that LRL and URL behave differently in this respect. Whereas the zebrafish LRL at 2 days shows PH3 positive cells only at the ventricular side (**Figure 2B**; note that pial and ventricular surface are indicated by stippled green and red lines, respectively, in all panels of this figure), with *atoh1a* positive cells extending radially out into the pial periphery (**Figure 2B′**),

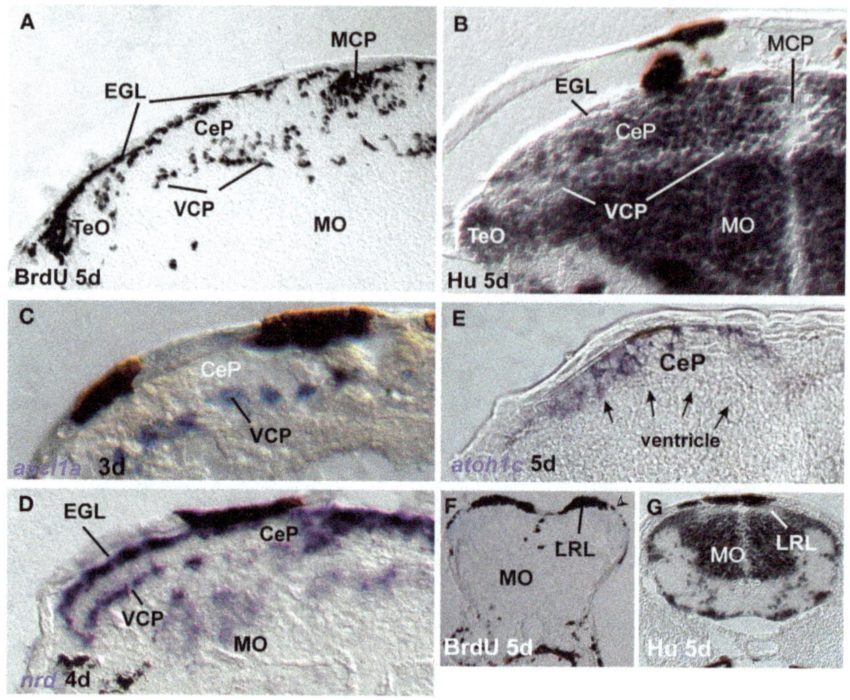

FIGURE 4 | Markers for proliferation and neurogenesis in zebrafish cerebellar plate (A–E) and [lower rhombic lip, LRL (G,F)] shown in transverse sections. **(A)** Proliferation in ventral and medial cerebellar proliferation and external granular layer shown with BrdU saturation labeling (see text). **(B)** Differentiation in cerebellar plate shown with Hu immunohistochemistry. Note complementarity of label to BrdU pattern. **(C)** Ventral cerebellar expression of proneural gene *ascl1a*. **(D)** Ventral and dorsal cerebellar expression domains of bHLH *neuroD*. Modified from Mueller and Wullimann (2002) and Wullimann and Mueller (2002). **(E)** Dorsal cerebellar expression of bHLH *atoh1c*. Note position of ventricle (arrows). **(F)** Proliferation at LRL level shown with BrdU saturation label. Note position of ventriculo-pial transition (arrowhead). **(G)** Differentiation at LRL level shown with Hu immunohistochemistry. Note Hu-free LRL. Both modified from Mueller and Wullimann (2005). CeP, cerebellar plate; EGL, external granular (or germinative) layer; IO, inferior olive; LRL, lower rhombic lip; MCP, middle cerebellar proliferation; MO, medulla oblongata; TeO, tectum opticum; VCP, ventral (or ventricular) cerebellar proliferation (ventricular germinal matrix).

the situation is different in the cerebellar plate. Here, proliferation is located both at the periventricular as well as at the subpial side (**Figure 2A**) and *atoh1a* extends from ventricularly located cells out into the pial periphery (**Figure 2A′**). In later larvae between 5 and 9 days *atoh1c* expression is seen to reach the periphery of the cerebellar plate and that some *atoh1c* positive cells at the pial periphery still do co-express PH3 (**Figures 2C,C′, E,E′, F,F′**). Of course, proliferation (PH3 reactivity) is also seen in the VCP (**Figures 2 D,D′, E,E′**). This shows that in the zebrafish cerebellar plate subpially migrated *atoh1* cells continue to proliferate into larval life, meeting one of the critical characteristics of an EGL. The LRL in later larval zebrafish brain development is more everted than at 2 days, but the ventriculo-pial transition point is still clearly identifiable (**Figures 3 and 4G,F**).

Previous studies of the early zebrafish cerebellar plate (3–5 days) development using proliferating cell nuclear antigen (PCNA) immunohistochemistry and BrdU had already provided evidence for distinct proliferative layers in the zebrafish VCP and in a subpial position (suggestive of an EGL) with postmitotic cells in between (Mueller and Wullimann, 2002; **Figures 4A,B and 5**). The latter were demonstrated with immunohistochemistry for Hu proteins (**Figures 4B and 5**) which mark early differentiated neuronal cells (Marusich et al., 1994). Further, expression of proneural bHLH genes *ascl1a* (Wullimann and Mueller, 2002) and *neuroD* (*nrd*; Mueller and Wullimann, 2002) supported this early cerebellar plate organization. Expression of *ascl1a*

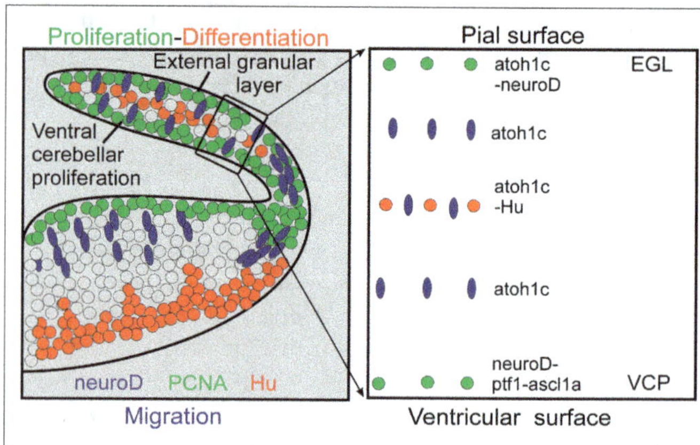

FIGURE 5 | Schema summarizes neurogenesis in zebrafish cerebellar plate. Left panel: Interpretative sketch based on localization of cellular marker in zebrafish cebellar plate as shown in **Figure 4**. GABA as shown in Mueller and Wullimann (2006). Right panel: summary of markers at various dorsoventral levels of zebrafish cerebellar plate. Data as shown in left panel and compiled from Kani et al., 2010 (*ptf1*).

is only seen in the zebrafish VCP (**Figures 4C and 5**), whereas *nrd* is present in both the VCP and EGL (or close to them, **Figures 4D and 5**), leaving the sandwiched Hu-positive cerebellar area in between

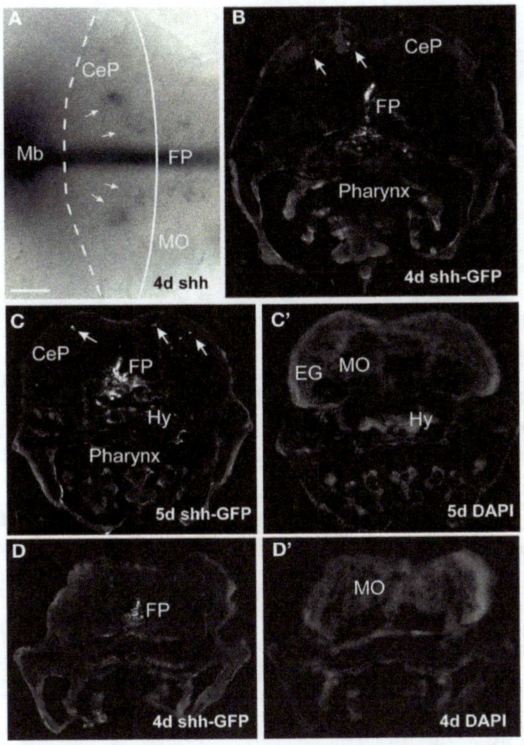

FIGURE 6 | Expression of *sonic hedgehog* in larval zebrafish cerebellar plate. (A) Whole mount shows midbrain and hindbrain expression of *shh* (ISH, performed as described in Volkmann et al., 2010). **(B–D)** Transverse sections at cerebellar plate **(B,C)** and medullary **(D)** levels from transgenic Tg(*2.4shha-ABC:GFP*)sb15 zebrafish (line originally published as Tg(*2.2shh:gfpABC#15*) by Shkumatava et al., 2004). Note GFP+ cells in floor plate and sparsely in cerebellar plate (arrows). **(C′,D′)** Identical sections in DAPI stain. Methodological details will be reported elsewhere. CeP, cerebellar plate; EG, eminentia granularis; FP, floor plate; Hy, hypothalamus; Mb, midbrain; MO, medulla oblongata.

free of expression. In contrast, *atoh1c* at that developmental time is expressed at the subpial side only (EGL plus additional cell layers ventrally, **Figures 4E and 5**). Since in the vertebrate forebrain *ascl1a* is involved with GABAergic and *nrd* with glutamatergic cell development, respectively (see discussion in Osório et al., 2010), these early studies already indicated the possibility that GABAergic cells are generated in the zebrafish VCP and glutamatergic cells in the EGL (Mueller and Wullimann, 2002; Wullimann and Mueller, 2002). GABA immunopositive cells are observed in the zebrafish cerebellar plate beginning with 3 days (Mueller et al., 2006). As discussed above, mouse *ascl* is indeed expressed downstream of *ptf1a* in VCP cells and involved in Purkinje cell development whereas mouse *neuroD* expression is involved in granule cell development. Intriguingly, zebrafish neurogenins (its two homologs *ngn1* and *ngn2* are apparently involved in GABAergic cell development in the mouse cerebellum, see above) were not observed to be expressed during zebrafish URL and LRL development so far (Mueller and Wullimann, 2003). Recent studies used transgenic zebrafish lines expressing reporter fluorescent proteins under the control of regulatory elements of proneural genes *ptf1a*, *wnt1*, *atoh1a*, and *olig2* (McFarland et al., 2008; Volkmann et al., 2008, 2010; Distel et al., 2010; Kani et al., 2010). This work established the fate of VCP and EGL zebrafish cerebellar plate cells showing essentially correspondence to the situation seen in the mammals (see above). During 2–5 days of zebrafish cerebellar plate development, *atoh1a*:EGFP cells give first rise to the tegmental cholinergic complex, followed by the formation of inner granule cells. These studies cleary demonstrate that the *atoh1a* expressing cells also begin to express the proneural gene *nrd* already close to the EGL and *nrd* positive cells later accumulate in the cerebellar inner granule layer, thus showing their subpial origin from *atoh1a* expressing progenitors (Volkmann et al., 2008). It was furthermore shown in a BrdU assay that proliferation does occur in the EGL during this developmental process (Kani et al., 2010). In contrast, *ptf1a*:EGFP cells are shown to originate in the VCP and migrate dorsally to form Purkinje cells

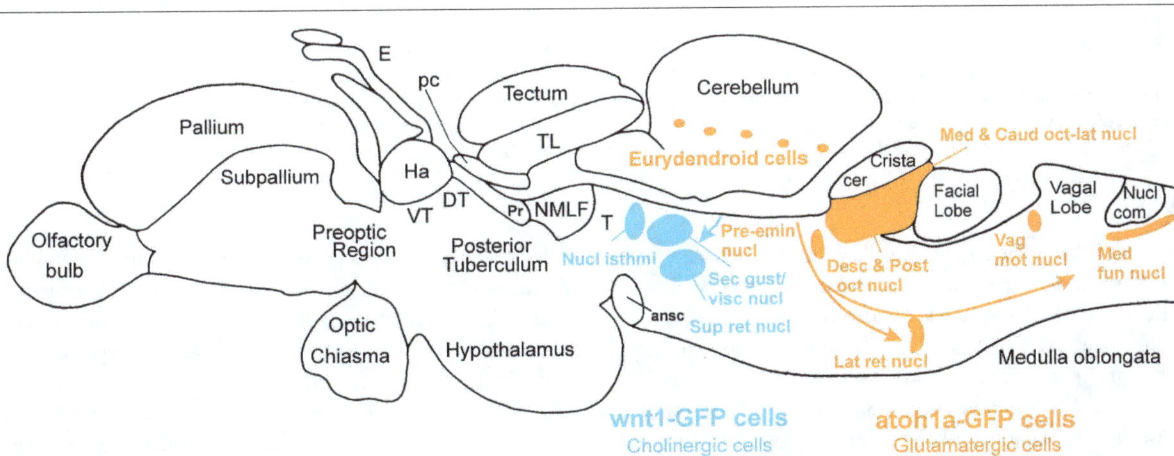

FIGURE 7 | Lateral view of adult zebrafish brain indicating major brain divisions and derivatives of *wnt1* expressing cerebellar plate/upper rhombic lip cells (blue) in rostral hindbrain (cholinergic nuclei) and hypothesized derivatives of *atoh1a* expressing cells (orange) from lower rhombic lip in posterior hindbrain. ansc, ansulate commissure; Crista cer, crista cerebellaris; Desc and Post oct nucl, descending/posterior octaval nuclei; DT, dorsal thalamus; E, epiphysis; Ha, habenula; Lat ret nucl, lateral reticular nucleus; Med fun nucl, medial funicular nucleus; NMLF, nucleus of medial longitudinal fascicle; Nucl com, nucleus commissuralis Cajal; Pc, posterior commissure; Pr, pretectum; Pre-emin nucl, pre-eminential nucleus; Sec gust/visc nucl, secondary gustatory/viscerosensory nuclei; Sup ret nucl, superior reticular nucleus; T mesencephalic, tegmentum; TL, torus longitudinalis; Vag mot nucl, vagal motor nucleus; VT, ventral thalalmus.

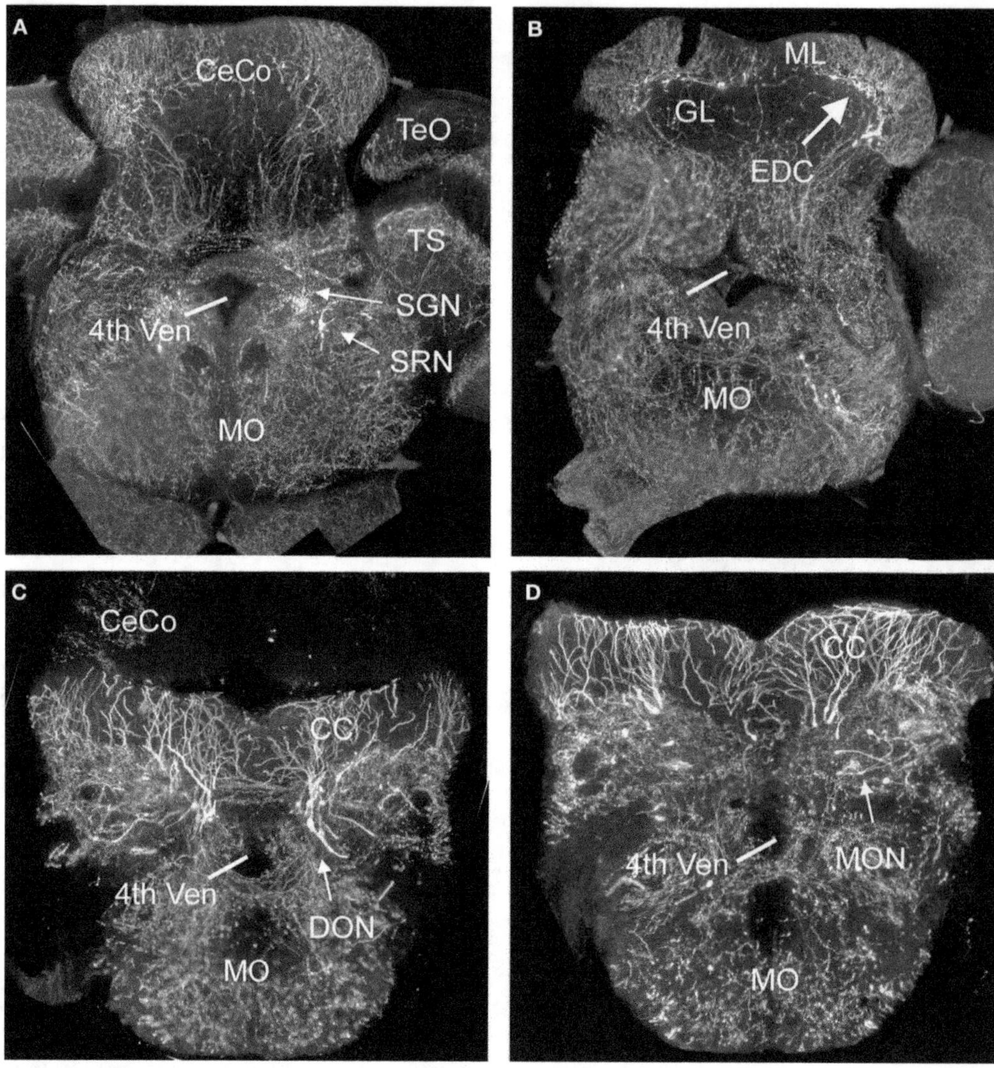

FIGURE 8 | Four transverse sections of the hindbrain from adult transgenic Tg(*atoh1a:Gal4TA4*)[hzm2] ×Tg(*4xUAS:GFP*)[hzm3] zebrafish from rostral (A) to caudal (D) showing various GFP expressing cells in nuclei known in amniotes (as far as present) to derive from lower rhombic lip. Note that most fluorescent label shows fibers, not somata. The generation of these transgenic strains has been described in detail in Distel et al., 2009, 2010). 4th ven, fourth ventricle; CC, crista cerebellaris; CeCo, cerebellar corpus; DON, descending octaval nucleus; EDC, eurydendroid cells; GL, granular layer; ML, molecular layer; MO, medulla oblongata; MON, medial octavolateralis nucleus; SGN, secondary gustatory nucleus; SRN, superior reticular nucleus; TS, torus semicircularis.

(and likely other inhibitory cerebellar cell types; Kani et al., 2010). A curious difference to the situation in the mouse was seen with respect to the origin of zebrafish eurydendroid cells, the homolog of the mammalian deep cerebellar nuclei. Early zebrafish cerebellar cells expressing the proneural factor-encoding *olig2* gene will give rise to eurydendroid cells (McFarland et al., 2008; Kani et al., 2010). Unlike in mammals, the vast majority of these (excitatory) cells does not derive from the *atoh1* expressing URL (although some do, Kani et al., 2010), but instead from the dorsal part of the *ptf1a* expressing VCP, immediately ventrally adjacent to the ventricular *atoh1a* expression domain. This fact may serve to explain why teleost eurydendroid cells behave like VCP derived Purkinje neurons. Future eurydendroid cells migrate only over short distances to populate the Purkinje cell layer rather than migrating over long distances into a deep cerebellar nuclear position like the *math1* expressing mammalian DN. A slight shift in *atoh1* or *ptf1a* expression could have modulated the migration behavior and final position of these DN homologous cells in teleosts. Correlated with this is an additional difference regarding the neurotransmitter type, as descendants of *ptf1a* expressing cells only give rise to GABAergic cells in mammals (see above), while in zebrafish *ptf1a* expressing cells also contribute to glutamatergic eurydendroid cells. Possibly the *nrd* expression in the zebrafish VCP (Mueller and Wullimann, 2002), which is not seen in the mouse, may be related to the production of these excitatory cells from the zebrafish VCP.

In contrast to the above reports, Chaplin et al. (2010) have argued that the zebrafish has no EGL comparable to amniotes because of absence of (1) subpial proliferation, (2) ventral migration of *atoh1* expressing cells, (3) complete subpial coverage of the cerebellar plate with *atoh1* cells in later larval stages, and most importantly, (4) absence of markers indicating the presence of transit amplification of the EGL proliferative activity via a SHH signal from Purkinje cells. The first claim is clearly refuted by data discussed above (Kani et al., 2010; data shown in **Figure 2**, summarized in **Figure 3**). In fact, Chaplin et al.'s (2010) own data (their **Figure 2G**) shows that both a VCP and EGL layer of PH3 positive cells is seen in the cerebellar plate. Similarly, the ventral migration of *atoh1a* cells has been amply documented (Köster and Fraser, 2001a, 2006; Volkmann et al., 2008; Kani et al., 2010). However, it is true that in later larval stages, the cerebellar plate is only covered caudally by proliferative *atoh1c* positive cells (only this paralog is relevant), which would be different from the ubiquitous subpial presence of an EGL in the postnatal mouse. However, a SHH mediated transit amplification of EGL proliferation in the zebrafish as seen in mammals during cerebellar development gains support by our finding of *shh* expression in the zebrafish cerebellar plate at 4–5 days using ISH or transgenic fish in which GFP expression is mediated by regulatory elements of *shh* (**Figure 6**). Thus, *atoh1* positive cells generated in the ventricular zone of the caudal URL invade the caudal cerebellar plate subpially, continue to proliferate there and give rise to cell migrations to the anteroventral tegmentum (cholinergic complex) and later inner granule cells, as seen in mammals. In conclusion, there is an EGL also in zebrafish.

THE ZEBRAFISH LOWER RHOMBIC LIP

Finally, we consider the zebrafish LRL and its potential derivatives. An immunohistochemical study on the distribution of PAX6 proteins in the zebrafish brain indicated that cerebellar and LRL domains are similar to the situation in the mouse (Wullimann and Rink, 2001). Importantly, a stream of PAX6 positive ventrally migrating cells was observed, indicative of a rhombic lip contribution to ventral medullary precerebellar nuclei. Detailed studies using transgenic zebrafish to show the fate of *atoh* or *wnt1* dependent cells are missing so far and no zebrafish hindbrain structure has been clearly shown to be derived from the LRL by fate mapping analysis. However, the use of a transgenic zebrafish Tg(*atoh1a:Gal4TA4*)^{hzm2} line to identify GFP expressing cells in the adult hindbrain produced some potentially exciting results. We found single GFP expressing cells in these brains in cerebellar eurydendroid cells (**Figures 8B and 7**), as well as in brain nuclei representing the cholinergic complex (**Figures 8A and 7**), in primary (descending and posterior) auditory nuclei (**Figures 8C and 7**), in the lateral reticular and in cells lateral to the medial funicular nucleus, the latter possibly corresponding to the lateral cuneate nucleus, which both project to the adult teleost cerebellum (Wullimann and Northcutt, 1988), in the lateral line primary mechanosensory (medial and caudal) octavolateralis nuclei (**Figures 8D and 7**), in the lateral line related pre-eminential nucleus and also in the vagal motor area (**Figure 7**). Since the location of most of these GFP labeled cells in the adult zebrafish brain is consistent with an origin from *atoh1a* expressing progenitors similar to the situation in amniotes, it is tempting to conclude that the label reflects their origin in embryonic/larval *atoh1a* expressing URL and LRL cells. In addition, the data indicate that structures of the lateral line system, which are functionally similar to the auditory system, do also derive from the LRL in anamiotes. However, these data have to be treated with caution, since it is highly likely that the GFP cells might alternatively represent descendants of adult *atoh1* expressing progenitors which still persist in the zebrafish cerebellum (Kani et al., 2010), likely due to ongoing hindbrain neurogenesis in the zebrafish (Zupanc et al., 2005; Adolf et al., 2006; Kaslin et al., 2009).

CONCLUSION

The morphogenesis of cerebellar cortex development is largely conserved between ray-finned fishes and amniotes. However, the eurydendroid cells, which represent the amniote deep cerebellar nuclei, are special because they are positioned within the Purkinje cell layer in adult ray-finned fishes and are not deep to the cerebellar cortex. Thus, the migratory behavior of eurydendroid cells appears to be evolutionarily truncated. Furthermore, the molecular regulation partially differs between these vertebrate groups (number of *atoh1* genes, origin of deep nuclear cells). The data reviewed and presented here speak for the presence of an EGL in early larval zebrafish, although it seems not ubiquitously present over the entire pial cerebellar surface as in amniotes. Furthermore, evidence for the existence of a simple EGL during cerebellar development has been provided for amphibians (Urey et al., 1987) and cartilaginous fishes (Rodríguez-Moldes et al., 2008). In contrast, a functional cerebellum is absent in jawless lampreys and hagfishes (Lannoo and Hawkes, 1997). Thus, since a lower and upper rhombic lip and ventral cerebellar proliferation with their major derivatives (deep cerebellar nuclei, external/internal granular layer, inhibitory cerebellar cells, precerebellar nuclei, cholinergic tegmental nuclei) occur both in anamniotes and amniotes, they likely are shared characters of gnathostomes. The situation in jawless fishes regarding the presence of a rhombic lip and the nature of its derivatives awaits future research.

ACKNOWLEDGMENTS

We thank Bea Stiening for preparing the *in situ* hybridized and immunohistological sections (unless otherwise stated) shown in the present paper and Enrico Kühn for various technical support. Furthermore, we thank Alena Shkumatava, Sabine Fischer, Ferenc Müller, Uwe Strähle, and Carl J. Neumann for sharing their *shh-GFP* line. The Munich Graduate School of Systemic Neurosciences (GSN) and the Deutsche Forschungsgemeinschaft (DFG, project Wu 211/2-1; Mario F. Wullimann), the Studienstiftung des deutschen Volkes (Martin Distel) and the Ministry of Education and Research (BMBF, BioFuture 0311889), and the Helmholtz Association (Reinhard W. Köster) are gratefully acknowledged for support.

REFERENCES

Acampora, D., Gulisano, M., Broccoli, V., and Simeone, A. (2001). Otx genes in brain morphogenesis. *Prog. Neurobiol.* 64, 69–95.

Adolf, B., Bellipanni, G., Huber, V., and Bally-Cuif, L. (2004). atoh1.2 und *beta*3.1 are two new bHLH-encoding genes expressed in selective precursor cells of the zebrafish anterior hindbrain. *Gene Expr. Patterns* 5, 35–41.

Adolf, B., Chapouton, P., Lam, C. S., Topp, S., Tannhäuser, B., Strähle, U., Götz, M., and Bally-Cuif, L. (2006). Conserved and acquired features of adult neurogenesis in the zebrafish telencephalon. *Dev. Biol.* 295, 278–293.

Akazawa, C., Ishibashi, M., Shimizu, C., Nakanishi, S., and Kageyama, R. (1995). A mammalian helix-loop-helix factor structurally related to the product of *Drosophila* proneural gene atonal1 is a positive transcriptional regulator expressed in the developing nervous system. *J. Biol. Chem.* 270, 8730–8738.

Alder, J., Cho, N. K., and Hatten, M. E. (1996). Embryonic precursor cells from the rhombic lip are specified to a cerebellar granule neuron identity. *Neuron* 17, 389–399.

Altman, J., and Bayer, S. A. (1985). Embryonic development of the rat cerebellum. I. Delineation of the cerebellar primordium and early cell movements. *J. Comp. Neurol.* 231, 1–26.

Altman, J., and Bayer, S. A. (1987a). Development of the precerebellar nuclei in the rat: I: the precerebellar neuroepithelium of the rhombencephalon. *J. Comp. Neurol.* 257, 477–489.

Altman, J., and Bayer, S. A. (1987b). Development of the precerebellar nuclei in the rat: II: The intramural olivary migratory stream and the neurogenetic organization of the inferior olive. *J. Comp. Neurol.* 257, 490–512.

Altman, J., and Bayer, S. A. (1987c). Development of the precerebellar nuclei in the rat: III: the posterior precerebellar extramural migratory stream and the lateral reticular and external cuneate nuclei. *J. Comp. Neurol.* 257, 513–528.

Altman, J., and Bayer, S. A. (1987d). Development of the precerebellar nuclei in the rat: IV: The anterior precerebellar extramural migratory stream and the nucleus reticularis tegmenti pontis and the basal pontine gray. *J. Comp. Neurol.* 257, 529–552.

Altman, J., and Bayer, S. A. (1987e). Prenatal development of the cerebellar system in the rat. I. Cytogenesis and histogenesis of the deep nuclei and the cortex of the cerebellum. *J. Comp. Neurol.* 179, 23–48.

Aroca, P., Lorente-Cánovas, B., Mateos, F. R., and Puelles, L. (2006). Locus coeruleus neurons originate in alar rhombomere 1 and migrate into the basal plate: studies in chick and mouse embryos. *J. Comp. Neurol.* 496, 802–818.

Bae, Y. K., Kani, S., Shimizu, T., Tanabe, K., Nojima, H., Kimura, Y., Higashijima, S., and Hibi, M. (2009). Anatomy of zebrafish cerebellum and screen for mutations affecting its development *Dev. Biol.* 330, 406–426.

Ben-Arie, N., Bellen, H. J., Armstrong, D. L., McCall, A. E., Gordadze, P. R., Guo, Q., Matzuk, M. M., and Zoghbi, H. Y. (1997). Math1 is essential for genesis of cerebellar granule neurons. *Nature* 390, 169–172.

Ben-Arie, N., Hassan, B. A., Bermingham, N. A., Malicki, D. M., Armstrong, Matzuk, M. M., Bellen, H. J., and Zoghbi, H. Y. (2000). Functional conservation of atonal and Math1 in the CNS and PNS. *Development* 127, 1039–1048.

Berrebi, A. S., Morgan, J. I., and Mugnaini, E. (1990). The Purkinje cell class may extend beyond the cerebellum. *J. Neurocytol.* 19, 643–654.

Bloch-Gallego, E., Ezan, F., Tessier-Lavigne, M., and Sotelo, C. (1999). Floor plate and Netrin-1 are involved in the migration and survival of inferior olivary neurons. *J. Neurosci.* 19, 4407–4420.

Book, K. J., and Morest, D. K. (1990). Migration of neuroblasts by perikaryal translocation: role of cellular elongation and axonal outgrowth in the acoustic nuclei of the chick embryo medulla. *J. Comp. Neurol.* 297, 55–76.

Bourrat, F., and Sotelo, C. (1988). Migratory pathways and neuritic differentiation of inferior olivary neurons in the rat embryo. Axonal tracing study using the in vitro slab technique. *Dev. Brain Res.* 39, 19–37.

Bourrat, F., and Sotelo, C. (1990). Migratory pathways and selective aggregation of the lateral reticular neurons in the rat embryo: A horseradish peroxidase in vitro study, with special reference to migration patterns of the precerebellar nuclei. *J. Comp. Neurol.* 294, 1–13.

Branda, C. S., and Dymecki, S. M. (2004). Talking about a revolution: the impact of site-specific recombinases on genetic analyses in mice. *Dev. Cell* 6, 7–28.

Cambronero, F., and Puelles, L. (2000). Rostrocaudal nuclear relationships in the avian medulla oblongata: a fate map with quail chick chimeras. *J. Comp. Neurol.* 427, 522–545.

Chaplin, N., Tendeng, C., and Wingate, R. J. T. (2010). Absence of an external granular layer in zebrafish and shark reveals a distinct, amniote ground plan of cerebellum development. *J. Neurosci.* 30, 3048–3057.

Chédotal, A. (2010). Should I stay or should I go? Becoming a granule cell. *Trends Neurosci.* 33, 163–172.

Chédotal, A., Bloch-Gallego, E., and Sotelo, C. (1997). The embryonic cerebellum contains topograhic cues that guide developing inferior olivary axons. *Development* 124, 861–870.

Clack, J. A. (1997). The evolution of tetrapod ears and the fossil record. *Brain Behav. Evol.* 50, 198–212.

Clemente, D., Porteros, A., Weruaga, E., Alonso, J. R., Arenzana, F. J., Aijon, J., and Arevalo, R. (2004). Cholinergic elements in the zebrafish central nervous system: histochemical and immunohistochemical analysis. *J. Comp. Neurol.* 474, 75–107.

Curran, T., and D'Arcangelo, G. (1998). Role of reelin in the control of brain development. *Brain Res. Rev.* 26, 285–294.

D'Arcangelo, G., and Curran, D. (1998). Reeler: new tales on an old mutnat mouse. *Bioessays* 20, 235–244.

Distel, M., Babaryka, A., and Köster, R. W. (2006). Multicolor in vivo time-lapse imaging at cellular resolution by stereomicroscopy. *Dev. Dyn.* 235, 843–845.

Distel, M., Hocking, J. C., Volkmann, K., and Köster, R. W. (2010). The centrosome neither persistently leads migration nor determines the site of axonogenesis in migrating neurons in vivo. *J. Cell Biol.* 15, 875–890.

Distel, M., Wullimann, M. F., and Köster, R. W. (2009). Optimized Gal4 genetics for permanent gene expression mapping in zebrafish. *Proc. Natl. Acad. Sci. U.S.A.* 106, 13365–13370.

Dubbeldam, J. L. (1998). "Birds," in *The Central Nervous System of Vertebrates*, eds R. Nieuwenhuys, H. J. Ten Donkelaar, C. Nicholson (Berlin: Springer), 1525–1636.

Echelard, Y., Vassileva, G., and McMahon, A. P. (1994). Cis-acting regulatory sequences governing Wnt-1 expression in the developing mouse CNS. *Development* 120, 2213–2224.

Elsen, G. E., Choi, L. Y., Millen, K. J., Grinblat, Y., and Prince, V. E. (2008). Zic1 and Zic4 regulate zebrafish roof plate specification and hindbrain ventricle morphogenesis. *Dev. Biol.* 314, 376–392.

Engelkamp, D., Rashbase, P., Seawright, A., and van Heyningen, V. (1999). Role of Pax6 in development of the cerebellar system. *Development* 126, 3585–3596.

Englund, C., Kowalcyk, T., Daza, R. A. M., Dagan, A., Lau, C., Rose, M. F., and Hevner, R. F. (2006). Unipolar brush cells of the cerebellum are produced in the rhombic lip and migrate through developing white matter. *J. Neurosci.* 26, 9184–9195.

Farago, A. F., Awatramani, R. B., and Dymecki, S. M. (2006). Assembly of the brainstem cochlear nuclear complex is revealed by intersectional and subtractive genetic fate maps. *Neuron* 50, 205–218.

Fink, A. J., Englund, C., Daza, R. A. M., Pham, D., Lau, C., Nivison, M., Kowalcyk, T., and Hevner, R. F. (2006). Development of the deep cerebellar nuclei: transcription factors and cell migration from the rhombic lip. *J. Neurosci.* 26, 3066–3076.

Fujiyama, T., Yamada, M., Terao, M., Terashima, T., Hioki, H., Inoue, Y. U., Inoue, T., Masuyama, N., Obata, K., Yanawaga, Y., Kawaguchi, Y., Nabeshima, Y., and Hoshino, M. (2009). Inhibitory and excitatory subtypes of cochlear nucleus neurons are defined by distinct bHLH transcription factors, Ptf1a and Atoh1. *Development* 136, 2049–2058.

Fujta, S. (1967). Quantitative analysis of cell proliferation and differentiation in the cortex of the postnatal mouse cerebellum. *J. Cell Biol.* 32, 277–287.

Gilthorpe, J. D., Papantoniou, E.-K., Chédotal, A., Lumsden, A., and Wingate, R. J. T. (2002). The migration of cerebellar rhombic lip derivatives. *Development* 129, 4719–4728.

Goldowitz, D., and Hamre, K. (1998). The cells and molecules that make a cerebellu. *Trends Neurosci.* 21, 375–382.

Grothe, B. (2003). New roles for synaptic inhibition in sound localization. *Nat. Rev. Neurosci.* 4, 1–11.

Grothe, B., Carr, C. E., Casseday, J. H., Fritzsch, B., and Köppl, C. (2004). "The evolution of central pathways and their neural processing patterns," in *Evolution of the Vertebrate Auditory System. Springer Handbook of Auditory Research*, eds G. A. Manley, A. N. Popper, and R. R. Fay (Springer: New York), 289–359.

Hanaway, J. (1967). Formation and differentiation of the external granular layer of the chick cerebellum. *J. Comp. Neurol.* 131, 1–14.

Harkmark, W. (1954). Cell migrations from the rhombic lip to the inferior olive, the nucleus raphe and the pons. A morphological and experimental investigation on chick embryos. *J. Comp. Neurol.* 100, 115–209.

Hatten, M. E. (1990). Riding the glial monorail: a common mechanism for glial-guided neuronal migratin in different regions of the developing mammalian brain. *Trends Neurosci.* 13, 179–184.

Hatten, M. E. (1999). Central nervous system neuronal migration. *Annu. Rev. Neurosci.* 22, 511–539.

Hatten, M. E., and Heintz, N. (1995). Mechanisms of neural patterning and specification in the developing cerebellum. *Annu. Rev. Neurosci.* 18, 385–408.

Hatten, M. E., Alder, J., Zimmermann, K., and Heintz, N. (1997). Genes involved in cerebellar cell differentiation specification and differentiation. *Curr. Opin. Neurobiol.* 7, 40–47.

Hatten, M. E., and Mason, C. A. (1990). Mechanisms of glial-guided neuronal migration in vitro and in vivo. *Experientia* 46, 907–916.

Helms, A. W., Abney, A. L., Ben-Arie, N., Zoghbi, H. Y., and Johnson, J. E. (2000). Autoregulation and multiple enhancers control Math1 expression in the developing nervous system. *Development* 127, 1185–1196.

Hoshino, M. (2006). Molecular machinery governing GABAergic neuron specification in the cerebellum. *Cerebellum* 5, 193–198.

Hoshino, M., Nakamura, S., Mori, K., Kawauchi, T., Terao, M., Nishimura, Y. V., Fukuda, A., Fuse, T., Matsuo, N., Sone, M., Watanabe, M., Bito, H., Terashima, T., Wright, C. V., Kawaguchi, Y., Nakao, K., and Nabeshima, Y. (2005). Ptf1a, a bHLH transcriptional gene, defines

GABAergic neuronal fates in cerebellum. *Neuron* 47, 201–213.

Huang, X., Ketova, T., Fleming, J. T., Wang, H., Dey, S. K., Litingtung, Y., and Chiang, C. (2009). Sonic hedgehog signaling regulates a novel epithelial progenitor domain of the hindbrain choroid plexus. *Development* 136, 2535–2543.

Ikenaga, T., Yoshida, M., and Uematsu, K. (2005). Morphology and immunohistochemistry of efferent neurons of the goldfish corpus cerebelli. *J. Comp. Neurol.* 487, 300–311.

Ito, M. (2006). Cerebellar circuitry as a neuronal machine. *Prog. Neurobiol.* 78, 272–303.

Ivanova, A., and Yuasa, S. (1998). Neuronal migration and differentiation in the development of the mouse dorsal cochlear nucleus. *Dev. Neurosci.* 20, 495–511.

Jászai, J., Reifers, F., Picker, A., Langenberg, T., and Brand, M. (2003). Isthmus-to-midbrain transformation in the absence of midbain-hindbrain organizer activity. *Development* 130, 6611–6623.

Kani, S., Bae, Y.-Y., Shimizu, T., Tanabe, K., Satou, C., Parsons, M. J., Scott, E., Higashijima, S., and Hibi, M. (2010). Proneural gene-linked neurogenesis in zebrafish cerebellum. *Dev. Biol.* 343, 1–17.

Kaslin, J., Ganz, J., Geffarth, M., Grandel, H., Hans, S., and Brand, M. (2009). Stem cells in the adult zebrafish cerebellum: initiation and maintenance of a novel stem cell niche. *J. Neurosci.* 29, 6142–6153.

Kim, C. H., Bae, Y. K., Yamanaka, Y., Yamashita, S., Shimizu, T., Fujii, R., Park, H. C., Yeo, S. Y., Huh, T. L., Hibi, M., and Hirano, T. (1997). Overexpression of neurogenin induces ectopic expression of HuC in zebrafish. *Neurosci. Lett.* 239, 113–116.

Kim, E. J., Battiste, J., Nakagawa, Y., and Johnson, J. E. (2008). Ascl1 (Mash1) lineage cells contribute to discrete cell populations in CNS architecture. *Mol. Cell. Neurosci.* 38, 595–606.

Komuro, H., and Rakic, P. (1998a). Distinct modes of neuronal migration in different domains of developing cerebellar cortex. *J. Neurosci.* 18, 1478–1490.

Komuro, H., and Rakic, P. (1998b). Orchestration of neuronal migration by activity of ion channels, neurotransmitter receptors, and intracellular Ca^{2+} fluctuations. *J. Neurobiol.* 37, 110–130.

Köster, R. W., and Fraser, S. E. (2001a). Direct imaging of in vivo neuronal migration in the developing cerebellum. *Curr. Biol.* 11, 1858–1863.

Köster, R. W., and Fraser, S. E. (2001b). Tracing transgene expression in living zebrafish embryos. *Dev. Biol.* 233, 329–346.

Köster, R. W., and Fraser, S. E. (2006). FGF signaling mediates regeneration of the differentiating cerebellum through repatterning of the anterior hindbrain and reinitiation of neuronal migration. *J. Neurosci.* 26, 7293–7304.

Kriegstein, A., and Alvarez-Buylla, A. (2009). The glial nature of embryonic and adult neural stem cells. *Annu. Rev. Neurosci.* 32, 149–184.

Landsberg, R. L., Awatrami, R. B., Hunter, N. L., Farago, A., DiPietrantonio, H. J., Rodriguez, C. I., and Dymecki, S. M. (2005). Hindbrain rhombic lip is comprised of discrete progenitor cell populations allocated by Pax6. *Neuron* 48, 933–947.

Lannoo, M. J., and Hawkes, R. (1997). A search for primitive Purkinje cells: zebrin II expression in sea lampreys (*Petromyzon marinus*). *Neurosci. Lett.* 237, 53–55.

Lannoo, M. J., Ross, L., Maler, L., and Hawkes, R. (1991). Development of the cerebellum and ist extracerebellar Purkinje cell projection in teleost fishes as determined by Zebrin-II immunocytochemistry. *Prog. Neurobiol.* 37, 329–363.

Lekven, A. C., Buckles, G. R., Kostakis, N., and Moon, R. T. (2003). wnt1 and wnt10b function redundantly at the zebrafish midbrain-hindbrain boundary. *Dev. Biol.* 254.172–187.

Leto, K., Calretti, B., Williams, I. M., Magrassi, L., and Rossi, F. (2006). Different types of cerebellar GABAergic interneurons originate from a common pool of multipotent progenitor cells. *J. Neurosci.* 26, 11682–11694.

Lin, J. C., Cai, L., and Cepko, C. L. (2001). The external granular layer of the developing chick cerebellum generates granule cells and cells of the isthmus and rostral hindbrain. *J. Neurosci.* 21, 159–168.

Liu, A., and Joyner, A. (2001). Early anterior/posterior patterning of the midbrain hindbrain and cerebellum. *Annu. Rev. Neurosci.* 24, 869–896.

Liu, Z., Li, H., Hu, X., Yu, L., Liu, H., Han, R., Colella, R., Mower, G. D., Chen, Y., and Qiu, M. (2008). Control of precerebellar neuron development by Olig3 bHLH transcription factor. *J. Neurosci.* 28, 10124–10133.

Lundell, T. G., Zhou, Q., and Doughty, M. L. (2009). Neurogenin1 expression in cell lineages of the cerebellar cortex in embryonic and postnatal mice. *Dev. Dyn.* 238, 3310–3325.

Machold, R., and Fishell, G. (2005). Math1 is expressed in temporally discrete pools of cerebellar rhombic-lip neural progenitors. *Neuron* 48, 17–24.

Machold, R. P., Jones-Kittel, D., and Fishell, G. J. (2007). Antagonism between Notch and bone morphogenetic protein receptor signaling regulates neurogenesis in the cerebellar rhombic lip. *Neural Dev.* 2, 1–13.

Marín, F., and Puelles, L. (1995). Morphological fate of rhombomeres in quail/chick chimeras: a segmental analysis of hindbrain nuclei. *Eur. J. Neurosci.* 7, 1714–1738.

Martí, E., and Bovolenta, P. (2002). Sonic hedgehog in CNS development: one signal, multiple outputs. *Trends Neurosci.* 25, 89–96.

Marusich, M. F., Furneaux, H. M., Henion, P. D., and Weston, J. A. (1994). Hu neuronal proteins are expressed in proliferating neurogenic cells. *J. Neurobiol.* 25,143–155.

McCormick, C. A., and Braford, M. R. Jr. (1994). Organization of inner ear endorgan projections in the goldfish, *Carassius auratus. Brain Behav. Evol.* 43, 189–205.

McCormick, C. A., and Hernandez, D. V. (1996). Connections of the octaval and lateral line nuclei of the medulla in the goldfish, including the cytoarchitecture of the secondary octaval population in goldfish and catfish. *Brain Behav. Evol.* 47, 113–138.

McFarland, K. A., Topczewska, J. M., Weidinger, G., Dorsky, R. I., and Appel, B. (2008). Hh and Wnt signaling regulate formation of olig2+ neurons in the zebrafish cerebellum. *Dev. Biol.* 318, 162–171.

Miale, I. L., and Sidman, R. L. (1961). An autoradiographic analysis of histogenesis in the mouse cerebellum. *Exp. Neurol.* 4, 277–296.

Mikami, Y., Yoshida, T., Matsuda, N., and Mishina, M. (2004). Expression of zebrafish glutamate receptor (2 in neurons with cerebellum-like wiring. *Biochem. Biophys. Res. Commun.* 322, 168–176.

Miyamura, Y., and Nakayasu, H. (2001). Zonal distribution of Purkinje cells in the zebrafish cerebellum: analysis by means of a specific monoclonal antibody. *Cell Tissue Res.* 305, 299–305.

Miyata, T., Maeda, T., and Lee, J. E. (1999). NeuroD is required for differentiation of the granule cells in the cerebellum and hippocampus. *Genes Dev.* 13, 1647–1652.

Mueller, T., Vernier, P., and Wullimann, M. F. (2004). The adult central nervous cholinergic system of a neurogenetic model animal, the zebrafish *Danio rerio*. *Brain Res.* 1011,156–169.

Mueller, T., Vernier, P., and Wullimann, M. F. (2006). A phylotypic stage in vertebrate brain development: GABA cell patterns in zebrafish compared with mouse. *J. Comp. Neurol.* 494, 620–634.

Mueller, T., and Wullimann, M. F. (2002). BrdU-, neuroD-(nrd) and Hu-studies show unusual non-ventricular neurogenesis in the postembryonic zebrafish forebrain. *Mech. Dev.* 117:, 123–135.

Mueller, T., and Wullimann, M. F. (2003). Anatomy of neurogenesis in the zebrafish brain. *Dev. Brain Res.* 140, 135–153.

Mueller, T., and Wullimann, M. F. (2005). *Atlas of Early Zebrafish Brain Development: A Tool for Molecular Neurogenetics*. Amsterdam: Elsevier.

New, J. G., Coombs, S., McCormick, C. A., and Oshel, P. E. (1996). Cytoarchitecture of the medial octavolateralis nucleus in the goldfish, *Carassius auratus*. *J. Comp. Neurol.* 366, 534–546.

Nichols, D. H., and Bruce, L. L. (2006). Migratory routes and fates of cells transcribing the Wnt-1 gene in the murine hindbrain. *Dev. Dyn.* 235, 285–300.

Nielsen, C. M., and Dymecki, S. M. (2010). Sonic hedgehog is required for vascular outgrowth in the hindbrain choroid plexus. *Dev. Biol.* 340, 430–437.

Nieuwenhuys, R. (1998). "Histogenesis," in *The Central Nervous System of Vertebrates*, eds R. Nieuwenhuys, H. J. Ten Donkelaar, and C. Nicholson (Berlin: Springer), 229–271.

Ono, K., and Kawamura, K. (1989). Migration of immature neurons along tangentially oriented fibers in the subpial part of the fetal mouse medulla oblongata. *Exp. Brain Res.* 78, 290–300.

Ono, K., and Kawamura, K. (1990). Mode of neuronal migration of the pontine stream in fetal mice. *Anat. Embryol.* 182, 11–19.

Ono, K., Yasui, Y., and Ikenaka, K. (2004). Lower rhombic lip-derived cells undergo transmedian tangential migration followed by radial migration in the chick embryo brainstem. *Eur. J. Neurosci.* 20, 914–922.

Osório, J., Mueller, T., Rétaux, S., Vernier, P., and Wullimann, M. F. (2010). Phylotypic expression of the bHLH genes Neurogenin2, NeuroD, and Mash1 in the mouse embryonic forebrain. *J. Comp. Neurol.* 518, 851–871.

Rakic, P. (1990). Principles of neural cell migration. *Experientia* 46, 882–891.

Ray, R. S., and Dymecki, S. M. (2009). Rautenlippe Redux – toward a unified view of the precerebellar rhombic lip. *Curr. Opin. Cell Biol.* 21, 741–747.

Redzic, Z. B., Preston, J. E., Duncan, J. A., Chodobski, A., and Szmydynger-Chodobska, J. (2005). The choroid plexus-cerebrospinal fluid system: from development to aging. *Curr. Top. Dev. Biol.* 71, 1–52.

Rieger, S., Volkmann, K., and Köster, R. W. (2008). Polysialyltransferase expression is linked to neuronal migration in the developing and adult zebrafish. *Dev. Dyn.* 237, 276–285.

Rodriguez, C. I., and Dymecki, S. M. (2000). Origin of thel precerebellar system. *Neuron* 27, 475–486.

Rodríguez-Moldes, I., Ferreiro-Galve, S., Carrera, I., Sueiro, C., Candal, E., Mazan, S., and Anadón, R. (2008). Development of the cerebellar body in sharks: spatiotemporal Pax6 expression, cell proliferation and differentiation. *Neurosci. Lett.* 432, 105–110.

Rose, M. F., Ahmad, K. A., Thaller, C., and Zoghbi, H. Y. (2009). Excitatory neurons of the proprioceptive, interoceptive, and arousal hindbrain networks share a developmental requirement for Math1. *Proc. Natl. Acad. Sci. U.S.A.* 106, 22462–22467.

Ryder, E. F., and Cepko, C. L. (1994). Migration patterns of clonally related granule cells and their progenitors in the developing chick cerebellum. *Neuron* 12, 1011–1029.

Saul, S. M., Brzezinski, J. A. IV, Altschuler, R. A., Shore, S. E., Rudolph, D. D., Kabara, L. L., Halsey, K. E., Hufnagel, R. B., Zhou, J., Dolan, D. F., and Glaser, T. (2008). Math5 expression and function in the central auditory system. *Mol. Cell. Neurosci.* 37, 153–169.

Sgaier, K. S., Millet, S., Villaneuva, M. P., Berenshteyn, F., Song, C., and Joyiner, A. L. (2005). Morphogenetic and cellular movements that shape the mouse cerebellum: insights form genetic fate mapping. *Neuron* 45, 27–40.

Sillitoe, R. V., and Joyner, A. L. (2007). Morphology, molecular codes, and circuitry produce the three-dimensional complexity of the cerebellum. *Annu. Rev. Cell Dev. Biol.* 23, 549–577.

Shkumatava, A., Fischer, S., Müller, F., Strahle, U., and Neumann, C. J. (2004). Sonic hedgehog, secreted by amacrine cells, acts as a short-range signal to direct differentiation and lamination in the zebrafish retina. *Development* 131, 3849–3858.

Sotelo, C. (2004). Cellular and genetic regulation of the development of the cerebellar system. *Prog. Neurobiol.* 72, 295–339.

Storm, R., Cholewa-Waclaw, J., Reuter, K., Bröhl, D., Sieber, M., Treier, M., Müller, T., and Birchmeier, C. (2009). The bHLH trancsription factor Olig3 marks the dorsal neuroepithelium of the hindbrain and is essential for the development of brainstem nuclei. *Development* 136, 295–305.

Taber-Pierce, E. (1966). Histogenesis of the nuclei griseum pontis, corporis pontobulbaris and reticularis tegmenti pontis (Bechterew) in the mouse. an autoradiographic study. *J. Comp. Neurol.* 126, 219–240.

Taber-Pierce, E. (1967). Histogenesis of the dorsal and ventral cochlear nuclei in the mouse. An autoradiographic study. *J. Comp. Neurol.* 131, 27–54.

Taber-Pierce, E. (1975). Histogenesis of the deep cerebellar nuclei in the mouse: an autoradiographic study. *Brain Res.* 95, 503–518.

Tan, K., and LeDouarin, N. M. (1991). Development of the nuclei and cell migration in the medulla oblongata. Application of the quail–chick chimera system. *Anat. Embryol.* 183, 321–343.

Traiffort, E., Charytoniuk, D., Watroba, L., Faure, H., Sales, N., and Ruat, M. (1999). Discrete localizations of hedgehog signalling components in the developing and adult rat nervous system. *Eur. J. Neurosci.* 11, 3199–3214.

Traiffort, E., Charytoniuk, D. A., Faure, H., and Ruat, M. (1998). Regional distribution of sonic hedgehog, patched, and smoothened mRNA in the adult rat brain. *J. Neurochem.* 70, 1327–1330.

Urey, N. J., Gona, A. G., and Hauser, K. F. (1987). Autoradiographic studies of cerebellar histogenesis in the prematomorphic bullfrog tadpole: I. Generation of the external granular layer. *J. Comp. Neurol.* 266, 234–246.

Volkmann, K., Chen, Y.-Y., Harris, M. P., Wullimann, M. F., and Köster, R. W. (2010). The zebrafish cerebellar upper rhombic lip generates tegmental hindbrain nuclei by long – distance migration in an evolutionary conserved manner. *J. Comp. Neurol.* 518, 2794–2817.

Volkmann, K., Rieger, S., Babaryka, A., and Köster, R. W. (2008). The zebrafish cerebellar rhombic lip is spatially patterned in producing granule cell populations of different functional compartments. *Dev. Biol.* 313, 167–180.

Voogd, J., and Glickstein, M. (1998). The anatomy of the cerebellum. *Trends Neurosci.* 21, 370–375.

Wang, V. Y., Rose, M. F., and Zoghbi, H. Y. (2005). Math1 expression redefines the rhombic lip derivatives and reveals novel lineages within the brainstem and cerebellum. *Neuron* 48, 31–43.

Wang, V. Y., and Zoghbi, J. Y. (2001). Genetic regulation of cerebellar development. *Nat. Rev. Neurosci.* 2, 484–491.

Wang, Y., Chen, K., Yao, Q., Zhengh, X., and Yang, Z. (2009). Phylogenetic analysis of zebrafish basic helix-loop-helix transcription factors. *J. Mol. Evol.* 68, 629–640.

Weisheit, G., Gliem, M., Endl, E., Pfeffer, P. L., Busslinger, M., and Schilling, K. (2006). Postnatal development of the murine cerebellar cortex: formation and early dispersal of basket, stellate and Golgi neurons. *Eur. J. Neurosci.* 24, 466–478.

Willard, F. H., and Martin, G. F. (1986). The development and migration of large multipolar neurons into the cochlear nucleus of the North American opossum. *J. Comp. Neurol.* 248, 119–132.

Wilson, L. J., and Wingate, R. J. T. (2006). Temporal identity transition in the avian cerebellar rhombic lip. *Dev. Biol.* 297, 508–521.

Wingate, R. J. T. (2001). The rhombic lip and early cerebellar development. *Curr. Opin. Neurobiol.* 11, 82–88.

Wingate, R. J. T., and Hatten, M. E. (1999). The role of the rhombic lip in avian cerebellum development. *Development* 126, 4395–4404.

Wullimann, M. F., and Mueller, T. (2002). Expression of Zash-1a in the postembryonic zebrafish brain allows comparison to mouse Mash1 domains. *Gene Expr. Patterns* 1, 187–192.

Wullimann, M. F., and Northcutt, R. G. (1988). Connections of the corpus cerebelli in the green sunfish and the common goldfish: a comparison of perciform and cypriniform teleosts. *Brain Behav. Evol.* 32, 293–316.

Wullimann, M. F., and Rink, E. (2001). Detailed immunohistology of Pax6 protein and tyrosine hydroxylase in the early zebrafish brain suggests role of Pax6 gene in development of dopaminergic diencephalic neurons. *Dev. Brain Res.* 131, 173–191.

Wullimann, M. F., and Vernier, P. (2007). "Evolution of the nervous system in fishes," in *Evolution of Nervous Systems 3: Evolution of Nervous Systems in Non-Mammalian Vertebrates*, ed. J. Kaas (Amsterdam: Elsevier), 39–60.

Wurst, W., and Bally-Cuif, L. (2001). Neural plate patterning: upstream and downstream ofl the isthmic organizer. *Nat. Rev. Neurosci.* 2, 99–108.

Xu, H. G., Yang, C.-Y., and Yamamoto, N. (2008). Afferent sources to the inferior olive an distribution of the olivocerebellar climbing fibers in cyprinids. *J. Comp. Neurol.* 507, 1409–1427.

Yamada, M., Terao, M., Terashima, T., Fujiyama, T., Kawaguchi, Y., Nabeshima, Y., and Hoshino, M. (2007). Origin of climbing fiber neurons and their developmental dependence on Ptf1a. *J. Neurosci.* 27, 10924–10934.

Zhang, L., and Goldman, J. E. (1996). Developmental fates and migratory pathways of dividing progenitors in the postnatal rat cerebellum. *J. Comp. Neurol.* 370, 536–550.

Zordan, P., Croci, L., Hawkes, R., and Consalez, G. G. (2008). Comparative analysis of proneural gene expression in the embryonic cerebellum. *Dev. Dyn.* 237, 1726–1735.

Zupanc, G. K., Hinsch, K., and Gage, F. H. (2005). Proliferation, migration, neuronal differentiation, and long-term survival of new cells in the adult zebrafish brain. *J. Comp. Neurol.* 488, 290–319.

Conflict of Interest Statement: The authors declare that the research was conducted in the absence of any commercial or financial relationships that could be construed as a potential conflict of interest.

17

The structural, functional, and molecular organization of the brainstem

Rudolf Nieuwenhuys*

Netherlands Institute for Neuroscience, Amsterdam, Netherlands

Edited by:
Luis Puelles, Universidad de Murcia, Spain

Reviewed by:
Jose L. Lanciego, University of Navarra, Spain
Luis Puelles, Universidad de Murcia, Spain
Fernando Martinez-Garcia, Universidad de Valencia, Spain

****Correspondence:***
Rudolf Nieuwenhuys, Papehof 25, 1391 BD Abcoude, Netherlands.
e-mail: rudolfn@planet.nl

According to His (1891, 1893) the brainstem consists of two longitudinal zones, the dorsal alar plate (sensory in nature) and the ventral basal plate (motor in nature). Johnston and Herrick indicated that both plates can be subdivided into separate somatic and visceral zones, distinguishing somatosensory and viscerosensory zones within the alar plate, and visceromotor and somatomotor zones within the basal plate. To test the validity of this "four-functional-zones" concept, I developed a topological procedure, surveying the spatial relationships of the various cell masses in the brainstem in a single figure. Brainstems of 16 different anamniote species were analyzed, and revealed that the brainstems are clearly divisible into four morphological zones, which correspond largely with the functional zones of Johnston and Herrick. Exceptions include (1) the magnocellular vestibular nucleus situated in the viscerosensory zone; (2) the basal plate containing a number of evidently non-motor centers (superior and inferior olives). Nevertheless the "functional zonal model" has explanatory value. Thus, it is possible to interpret certain brain specializations related to particular behavioral profiles, as "local hypertrophies" of one or two functional columns. Recent developmental molecular studies on brains of birds and mammals confirmed the presence of longitudinal zones, and also showed molecularly defined transverse bands or neuromeres throughout development. The intersecting boundaries of the longitudinal zones and the transverse bands appeared to delimit radially arranged histogenetic domains. Because neuromeres have been observed in embryonic and larval stages of numerous anamniote species, it may be hypothesized that the brainstems of all vertebrates share a basic organizational plan, in which intersecting longitudinal and transverse zones form fundamental histogenetic and genoarchitectonic units.

Keywords: brainstem, gene patterns, histogenesis, longitudinal zones, morphological units, morphotype, neuromeres, topological analysis

INTRODUCTION

The brainstem or truncus cerebri forms the intermediate part of the vertebrate central nervous system. Rostrally, it borders on the diencephalon and caudally, it grades into the spinal cord (**Figure 1**). It comprises derivatives of two of the three primary brain vesicles, the midbrain or mesencephalon and the hindbrain or rhombencephalon. The cerebellum, which develops

Abbreviations: Aoctl, area octavolateralis; caud, nucleus caudalis areae octavolateralis; cereb, cerebellum; cmsp, columna motoria spinalis; cnd, cornu dorsale; cnv, curnu ventrale; con, cochlear nuclei; crcb, crista cerebellaris; D, area dorsalis; dc, dorsal cell(s); desc, nucleus descendens of V; DL, area dorsolateralis; dors, nucleus dorsalis areae octavolateralis; effVIII, efferent octavus cells; egrl, eminentia granularis, pars lateralis; el org, electric organ; EW, nucleus of Edinger–Westphal; flm, fasciculus longitudinalis medialis; gc, griseum centrale; ic, inferior colliculus; int, nucleus intermedius areae octavolateralis; ip, nucleus interpeduncularis; is, nucleus isthmi; isth, isthmus rhombencephali c.q. isthmus neuromere; lc, locus coeruleus; lob el, lobus electricus; lob lin lat, lobus lineae lateralis; lob lin lat (el), electroreceptive part of lobus lineae lateralis; Lob lin lat (mech), mechanoreceptive part of lobus lineae lateralis; lobX, lobus vagi; lv, nucleus lateralis valvulae; mes, mesencephalic neuromere; meV, mesencephalic nucleus of V; mmpz, mesencephalic midventral proliferation zone; Mth, cell of Mauthner; Mü 1, 2 etc., cells of Müller; nucb, nucleus cerebelli; nuce, nucleus cuneatus externus; nucp, nucleus commissurae posterioris; nufl, nucleus funiculi lateralis; nuflm, nucleus of the fasciculus longitudinalis medialis; nufs, nucleus fasciculi solitarii; null, nucleus lemnisci lateralis; nuoma, nucleus octavomotorius anterior; nuomi, nucleus octavomotorius intermedius; nuomp, nucleus octavomotorius posterior; nurdV, nucleus of the radix descendens of V; nutegm, nucleus tegmentalis medialis; nVI, nervus ab du cens nX, nervus vagus; oli, oliva inferior; olsl, oliva superior, lateral nucleus; olsm, oliva superior, medial nucleus; pbn, parabrachial nuclei; pon, pontine nuclei; prom, nucleus profundus mesencephali; Q, nucleus Q; r1, r2 etc., rhombomeres; "r7," "r8" etc., cryptorhombomeres; rai, nucleus raphes inferior; ras, nucleus raphes superior; rhlip, rhombic lip; ri, nucleus reticularis inferior; rism, nucleus reticularis isthmi et mesencephali; rlt, recessus lateralis tecti; rm, nucleus reticularis medius; rmes, nucleus reticularis mesencephali; rub, nucleus ruber; rubm, nucleus ruber, pars magnocellularis; rs, nucleus reticularis superior; sa, sulcus a; sc, superior colliculus; sid, sulcus intermedius dorsalis; sis, sulcus isthmi; siv, sulcus intermedius ventralis; slH, sulcus limitans of His; slm, sulcus lateralis mesencephali; sm, somatomotor column; smi, sulcus medianus inferior; sms, sulcus medianus superior; snc, substantia nigra, pars compacta; sp1, first spinal neuromere; ss, somatosensory column; t, taenia; tect, tectum mesencephali; teg, tegmentum mesencephali; tegl, nucleus tegmentalis lateralis; tl, nucleus tori lateralis; tlong, torus longitudinalis; tsc, torus semicircularis; V, area ventralis; vem, nucleus vestibularis magnocellularis; vesn, vestibular nuclei; vm, visceromotor column; visc, nucleus visceralis secundarius; VL, area ventrolateralis; vs, viscerosensory column; zglmv, zona granularis marginalis, pars lateroventralis; III, nucleus nervi oculomotorii; IIIc, nucleus nervi oculomotorii, pars caudalis ; IIIl, nucleus nervi oculomotorii, pars lateralis; IIIm, nucleus nervi oculomotorii, pars medialis; IIIp, nucleus nervi oculomotorii, pars periventricularis; IIIs, nucleus nervi oculomotorii, pars superficialis; IV, nucleus nervi trochlearis; Vm, nucleus motorius nervi trigemini; Vpr, nucleus sensorius principalis nervi trigemini; VI, nucleus nervi abducentis; VIIm, nucleus motorius nervi facialis; VIIIa, nucleus anterior nervi octavi; VIIId, nucleus descendens nervi octavi; IX(m), nucleus motorius nervi glossopharyngei; X(m), nucleus motorius nervi vagi; Xmc, nucleus motorius nervi vagi caudalis; Xmr, nucleus motorius nervi vagi rostralis.

ontogenetically as a dorsal outgrowth of the most rostral part of the rhombencephalon, "emancipates" itself from the brainstem to become a principal brain part in its own right. The cell masses in the brainstem include (a) centers of origin and/or termination of all cranial nerves except for I, (b) a central core of loosely arranged cells, known as the reticular formation, and (c) numerous relay nuclei. Prominent among the latter are the so-called precerebellar nuclei, which are intercalated in ascending and descending projections terminating in the cerebellum.

According to the classical studies of His (1891, 1893), which were carried out mainly on human embryonic material, the lateral walls of the central nervous system consist throughout their extent of two longitudinal zones or plates: the ventrally situated basal plate and the dorsal alar plate. His pointed out that the former contains the primary motor centers, whereas the primary sensory centers are found in the latter. The boundary between these two entities was found to be marked by a distinct ventricular groove, which he named the sulcus limitans. Somewhat later, the noted American comparative neuroanatomists Herrick (1899) and Johnston (1902a,b,c) concluded that, at the level of the brainstem, the basal, and alar plates can both be divided into two functional columns. Thus, they distinguished a somatomotor ventral column and a visceromotor intermedioventral column within the basal plate, and a viscerosensory intermediodorsal column and a somatosensory dorsal column within the alar plate (**Figure 2A**). Although Herrick and Johnston confined their study of the functional columns to anamniote species, they were convinced that their analyses had revealed a *basic structural and functional plan*, prevailing throughout the vertebrate kingdom. Herrick (1913) was the first to apply this columnar scheme to the human brainstem, which has since been promulgated in practically every textbook of neuroanatomy (**Figure 2B**). However, a critical study of the relevant literature (reviewed in Nieuwenhuys, 1998a) revealed that many important questions regarding the structural and functional organization of the brain stem are still open. This is simply because cross sections as such, do not show the rostrocaudal extent of ventricular sulci and cell zones. Questions still awaiting a definitive answer include: (1) Is the brainstem really divisible into a motor basal plate and a sensory alar plate? (2) Are the centers contained within the basal plate and the alar plate arranged in a longitudinal zonal pattern? (3) If so, are the boundaries of these zones marked by ventricular sulci? (4) Do nuclei, that fall under common functional denominators, fit into a longitudinal zonal pattern? (5) Does the midbrain show a longitudinal zonal pattern, and if so, does this pattern correspond to that in the rhombencephalon? In order to tackle these and other related questions, I (Nieuwenhuys, 1972, 1974) developed a procedure, named topological analysis, which makes it possible to survey the entire ventricular surface of the brainstem, with its sulci, and the underlying cell masses in a single reconstruction. With the aid of this procedure, the brainstems of the following 16 anamniote species have been analyzed: the lamprey *Lampetra fluviatilis* (Nieuwenhuys, 1972; Nieuwenhuys and Nicholson, 1998), the cartilaginous fishes *Scyliorhinus canicula, Squalus acanthias, Raja clavata*, and *Hydrolagus colliei* (Smeets and Nieuwenhuys, 1976; Smeets et al., 1983), the actinopterygian fishes *Erpetoichthys calabaricus* (Nieuwenhuys and Oey, 1983), *Scaphirhynchus platorynchus* (Nieuwenhuys, 1998c), *Lepisosteus osseus* (Nieuwenhuys and Pouwels, 1983), *Amia calva* (Heijdra and Nieuwenhuys, 1994), the lungfishes *Lepidosiren paradoxa* (Thors and Nieuwenhuys, 1979) and *Neoceratodus forsteri* (Nieuwenhuys, unpublished), the coelacanth *Latimeria chalumnae* (Kremers and Nieuwenhuys, 1979; Nieuwenhuys, 1998d)), the urodele amphibian *Ambystoma mexicanum* (Opdam and Nieuwenhuys, 1976), and the anuran amphibians *Rana catesbeiana* and *Rana esculenta* (Opdam et al., 1976), and *Xenopus laevis* (Nikundiwe and Nieuwenhuys, 1983).

The present paper consists of seven parts. In the first, the procedure followed will be outlined. In the second part, topological maps of the brainstem of two representative species, namely the lamprey *L. fluviatilis*, and the shovelnose sturgeon *S. platorynchus*, will be presented. In the third part, the principal results of the

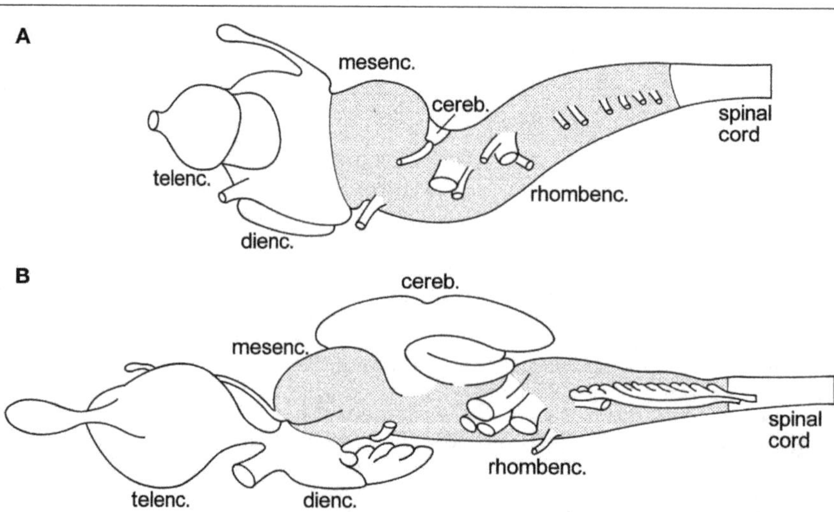

FIGURE 1 | Lateral views of the brains of the lamprey *Lampetra fluviatilis* (A), and the spiny dogfish *Squalus acanthias* (B). The brainstem, i.e., the mesencephalon plus the rhombencephalon minus the cerebellum, is stippled.

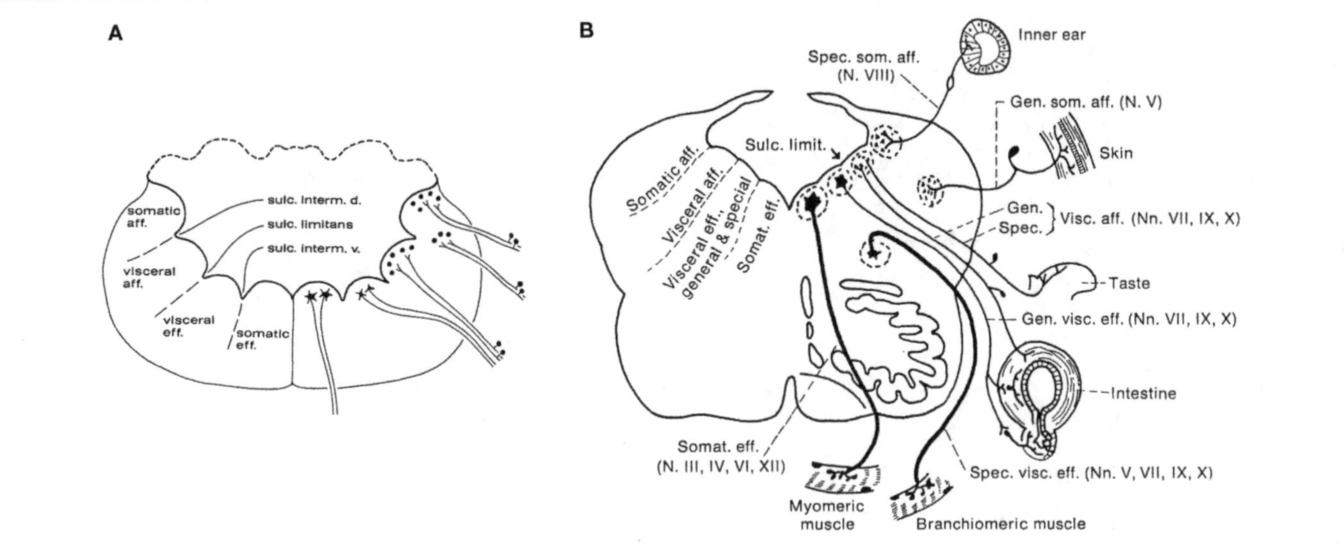

FIGURE 2 | Diagrammatic transverse sections through the rhombencephalon of an anamiote (A), and the human (B), to show the arrangement of the so-called functional columns.

project as a whole will be briefly discussed. In the fourth part, some functional correlations of the results of our topological analyses of the brainstem will be touched upon. In the fifth part, the significance of the topological approach for the study of the fundamental morphological pattern of the brainstem, as revealed by modern molecular studies, will be highlighted. In the sixth part, some general notes on the morphological interpretation of topological charts will be made, and in the seventh and final part, some perspectives for future research will be outlined.

TOPOLOGICAL ANALYSIS OF THE BRAINSTEM

The procedure followed is based on the observation that the central nervous system of vertebrates contains a built-in system of natural coordinates (Nieuwenhuys, 1998b). This natural coordinate system (NCS) includes: (a) two natural planes, i. e. the ventricular and meningeal surfaces of the neural tube, (b) a set of radially oriented curves, which connect these two surfaces, and (c) a set of tangential curves, which connect the floor and roof plates of the neural tube. The radial curves or *vectors* manifest themselves in the direction and orientation of: (i) the matrix cells, which during early development span the width of the walls of the neural tube, (ii) the radial glia cells, which are present during early neurogenesis in all vertebrates and throughout development in most anamniotes, and (iii) the blood vessels, which enter the walls of the neural tube radially across the meningeal surface. The tangential component of the NCS manifests itself in the course of "arcuate fibers," i. e. axonal processes which during early development, pass dorsoventrally, directly peripheral to the matrix layer. Numerous additional arcuate fibers are generated during further development. It is important to note that the processes of the radial glia cells and the arcuate fibers form important substrates for the radial and tangential migrations of neuroblasts that will come up in this and later sections of the present paper.

The material required for a topological analysis consists of one or more perfect, continuous series of transverse sections through the brainstem of the species to be studied, stained for neuronal perikarya (Nissl). The optimal thickness of the sections is 20 μm.

The procedure involves the following sequence of steps (**Figure 3**):

1. Forty equidistant sections are selected for a preliminary analysis. These sections are photographed and printed at a magnification of 30×.
2. The sections selected are analyzed as follows: (a) The deepest points of the ventricular sulci are marked. (b) The cell masses (and large individual cells) are delineated. These structures are projected on the ventricular surface with the aid of tangent radial curves. Because during ontogeny most cell masses in the central nervous system migrate radially outward from their respective matrix zones, it is reasonable to assume that, by the procedure followed, these entities are projected back to their *primary topological position.* (c) At the ventricular side the raphe corresponds to a distinct groove, the sulcus medianus inferior. In each section the deepest point of this sulcus is defined as the *zero point.* (d) With the use of a curvimeter, the distance from this zero point to the deepest points of other sulci and to the projections of the outlines of the cell masses are measured along the ventricular surface on either side. (e) All the distances measured in each individual section are now plotted on a line. *Thus, the end product of the analysis of each individual section is a straight line on which the deepest points of ventricular sulci and the projections of cell masses are plotted.*
3. A system of coordinates is introduced, consisting of a central vertical line, termed *the axis*, crossed by 40 equidistant horizontal lines. The distance of these horizontal lines depends on the total number of sections between the first and the last of the 40 selected sections, the thickness of the individual sections, and the magnification chosen.

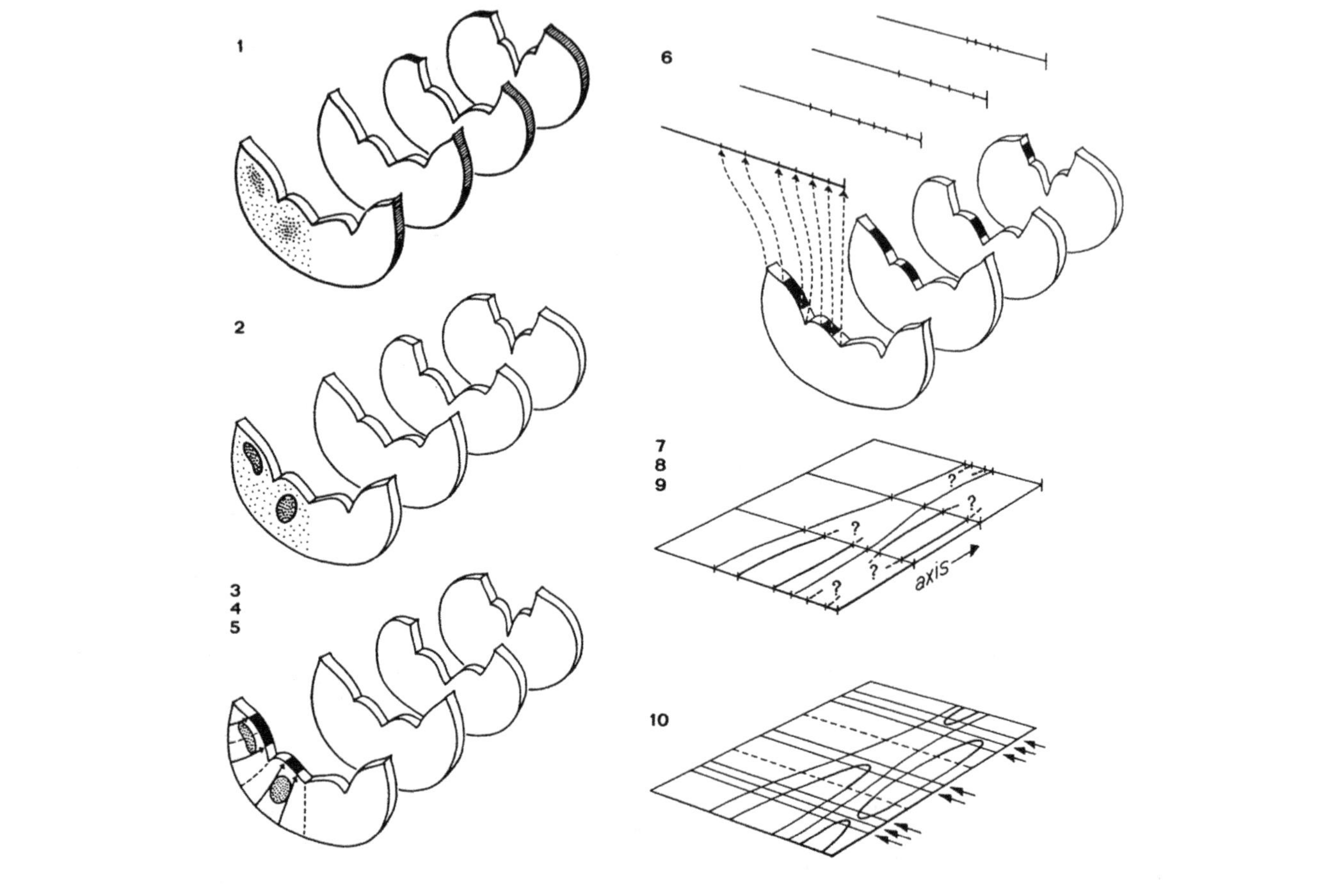

FIGURE 3 | Steps involved in the preparation of a topological reconstruction of the brainstem: (1) selection of sections; (2) drawing of sections and delineation of cell masses; (3) introduction of radial curves derived from the natural system of coordinates; (4) drawing of tangent curves; (5) projection of cell masses upon the ventricular surface; (6) transformation of the curvilinear profile of the ventricular surface into a straight line; (7) introduction of an orthogonal system of coordinates; (8) transfer of the lines representing the ventricular surfaces of the sections to the coordinate system; (9) connection of corresponding points; (10) collection of additional data concerning the beginning and the end of ventricular sulci and cell masses, and completion of the reconstruction.

4. The lines with the points of reference resulting from the analysis of the individual sections are consecutively transferred to the horizontal lines of the matrix, in such a fashion that their zero points coincide with the axis.
5. Corresponding points on the individual horizontal lines are connected, thus visualizing the course of the individual sulci and the contours of the various cell masses.
6. Quite often, the number of sections included in the preliminary analysis will appear to be insufficient to complete the reconstruction. In that case additional sections will have to be analyzed and interpolated.

The end product of the method described is a two-dimensional reconstruction, a chart enabling us to survey in one sweep a number of salient features of the brain stem analyzed (**Figures 4B** and **5B**). It will be clear that the essence of the method is that (i) the cell masses are projected upon the ventricular surface, and that (ii) this surface, with its sulci and the projections of the cell masses marked upon it, is flattened out, i.e., is subjected to a *one-to-one topological transformation.*

In the procedure described, the three-dimensional structure of a given brainstem is reduced to a two-dimensional chart; hence, one dimension, namely the thickness of the structure analyzed, had to be sacrificed. In order to compensate somewhat for this limitation, I have adopted the convention to allocate the cell masses to three categories: periventricular, intermediate, and submeningeal, and to indicate the nuclei of these categories by continuous-, dashed-, and dotted curves, respectively.

TOPOLOGICAL CHARTS OF TWO REPRESENTATIVE SPECIES

In this section, the results of the topological analyses of the brainstems of two representative species, the lamprey *L. fluviatilis*, and the shovelnose sturgeon *S. platorynchus*, will be presented first, and then the principal results of the project as a whole will be summarized.

Lampreys (and the related hagfishes) are the only extant jawless vertebrates (agnathans) and thus represent the sister group of gnathostome vertebrates (**Figure 4A**). Although these animals have a long independent phylogenetic history behind them, their small and simple brains form an optimal starting point for studies on the evolution of the vertebrate central nervous system

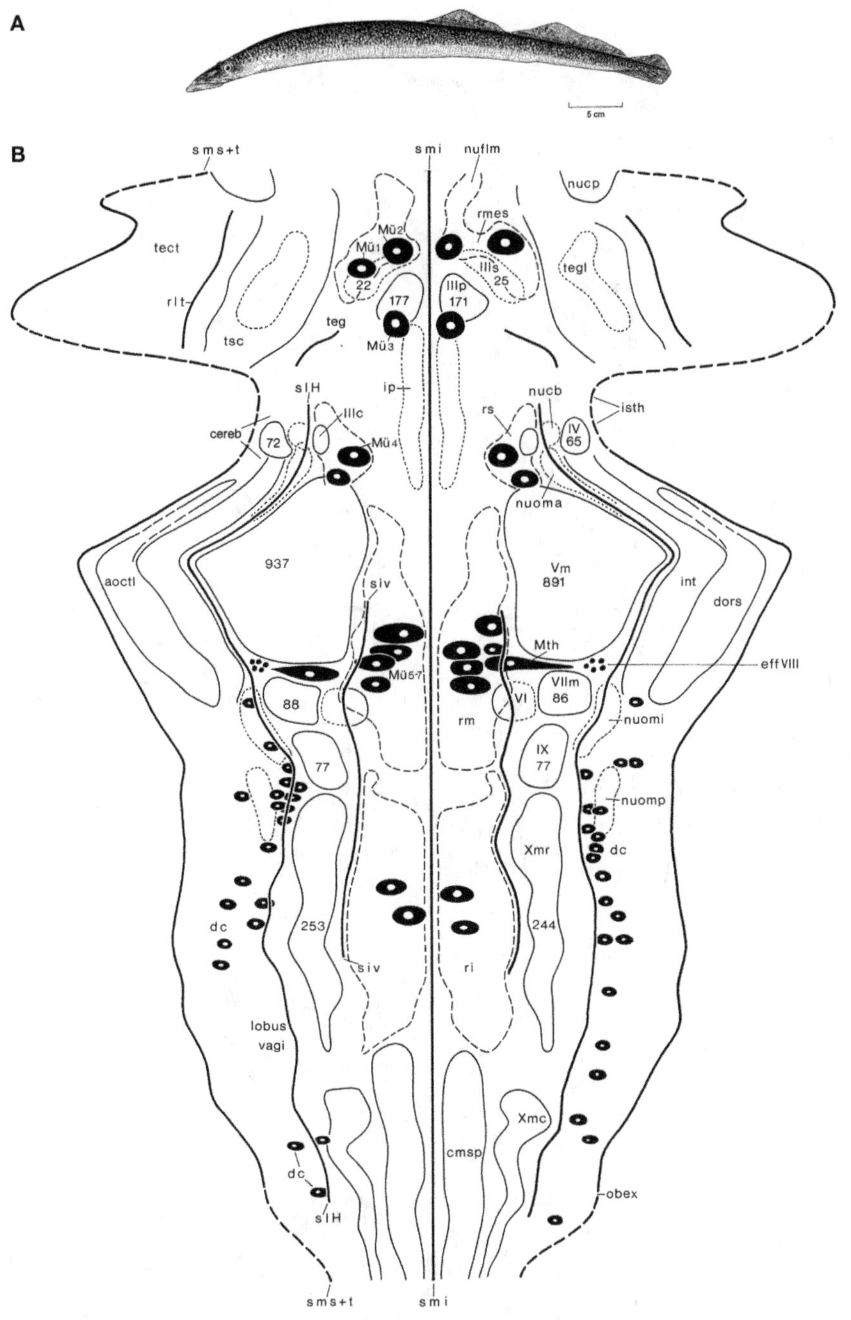

FIGURE 4 | The lamprey *Lampetra fluviatilis.* Holotype **(A)**, and topological chart of the brainstem **(B)**. The numbers of cells, present in some nuclei are, indicated by *numerals* enclosed within the outline of the structure. Modified from Nieuwenhuys and Nicholson (1998).

(**Figure 1A**). In our topological analyses of the brainstem of *L. fluviatilis* (Nieuwenhuys, 1972; Nieuwenhuys and Nicholson, 1998; **Figure 4B**), it appeared to be possible to map *the entire brainstem*, including the tiny cerebellar plate (**Figure 1A**) and the tectum mesencephali. The following six ventricular sulci could be mapped: sulcus medianus inferior, sulcus intermedius ventralis, sulcus limitans of His, a short unnamed, oblique sulcus in the isthmus region, recessus lateralis tecti, and the sulcus medianus superior. The lateral margin of the chart is formed by a curve, consisting of alternating dashed and continuous parts. The dashed parts represent the sulcus medianus superior, whereas the continuous parts represent the lines of attachment of the choroid roofs of the rhombencephalon and mesencephalon. The mesencephalic choroid roof is a unique feature of lampreys.

Some 20 different cell groups could be delineated and charted. Most of these represent primary afferent and primary efferent nuclei. A number of centers of higher order could also be distinguished. Prominent among these are the mesencephalic and

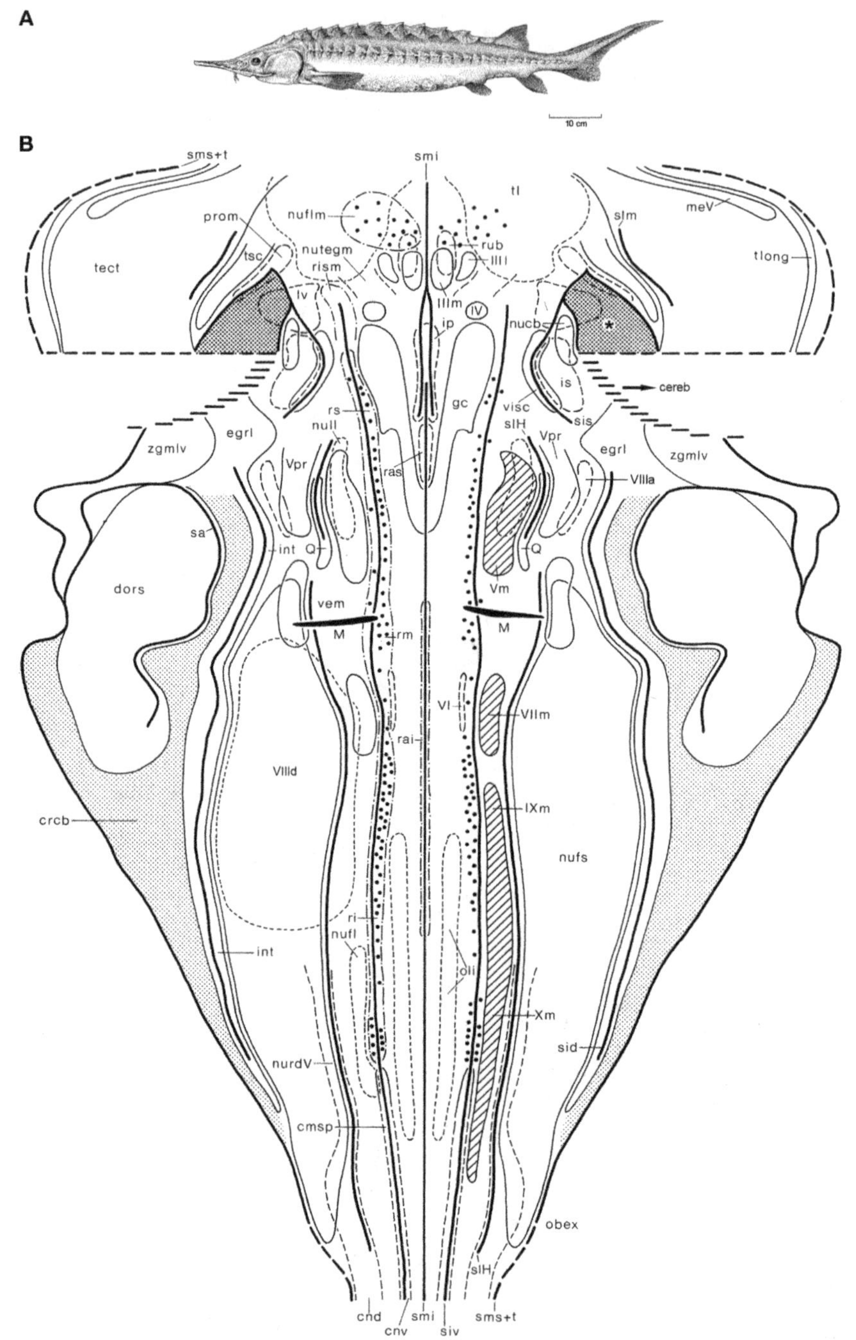

FIGURE 5 | The shovelnose sturgeon *Scaphirhynchus platorynchus*. Holotype **(A)**, and topological chart of the brainstem **(B)**. Modified from Nieuwenhuys (1998c).

rhombencephalic reticular nuclei, the nucleus tegmentalis lateralis, the interpeduncular nucleus, and nucleus cerebelli. Other relay nuclei, such as the nucleus funiculi lateralis and the inferior olive, which can be clearly distinguished in most gnathostomes, were not identified in the lamprey. It is remarkable that the trochlear nucleus lies far dorsally and is embedded in the alar plate rather than in the basal plate. This is another unique feature of lampreys. In addition to cell masses, a number of large neurons could be mapped individually. These include the cells of Mauthner (Mth), four groups of large reticular elements among which seven typical cells of Müller (Mü 1–7), and a number of primary somatosensory neurons. The latter are situated in the intermediate and caudal parts of the rhombencephalic alar plate and correspond to the spinal dorsal cells (dc). Another group of central primary somatosensory neurons, viz. the mesencephalic trigeminal nucleus, which is present in all gnathostomes, is lacking in lampreys.

The shovelnose sturgeon *S. platorynchus* (**Figure 5A**) is a member of the chondrosteans, a small group of ancient and rather primitive actinopterygian fishes. The structure of the brainstem of this fish is much more complex than that of the lamprey, as appears from the fact that some 40 cell masses, rather than only 27 found in the former, could be delineated (Nieuwenhuys, 1998c). The large cerebellum, which is partly invaginated into the fourth ventricle, was not included in our chart (**Figure 5B**), and the same holds true for the caudal part of the tectum. A rostral part of the cerebellum, i.e., the valvula cerebelli, invaginates into the mesencephalic ventricle. Laterally, the invaginated valvula is fused with part of the ventricular surface of the tegmentum mesencephali. The area of fusion of these two structures is indicated in the chart as a dotted field, marked by an asterisk. Throughout most of the rhombencephalon of the sturgeon, three distinct ventricular grooves bilaterally mark the boundaries of four longitudinal zones or columns. In the mesencephalon a zonal pattern is less clear. The Mauthner cells and the large elements in the reticular formation could be mapped individually. However, in order to avoid crowding, only every fifth large reticular element is included in the chart.

In the next section, reference will be frequently made to the two topological charts just shown. It should be kept in mind, however, that the synopsis of our principal results presented there, is based on topological analyses of the brainstems of 16, rather than two, anamniote species.

SYNOPSIS OF THE PROJECT AS A WHOLE

The principal results of the project as a whole can be summarized as follows:

1. The rhombencephalon can be divided into a basal plate and an alar plate. The boundary between these two entities is in all species studied marked by a sulcus limitans (**Figures 4B** and **5B**).
2. The designation of the alar plate as "sensory" and the basal plate as "motor" is correct insofar that all primary afferent centers are situated within the former and all primary efferent centers within the latter. A notable exception to this rule is that in lampreys, as already mentioned, the somatomotor trochlear nucleus is situated in the alar plate (**Figure 4B**).
3. The basal plate can be divided into a medial zone or column and an intermediomedial zone or column.
4. The boundary between the two morphological entities mentioned under 3 is in almost all species studied at least partially marked by a sulcus intermedius ventralis (**Figures 4B** and **5B**)
5. The medial zone can be characterized as somatomotor, because it harbors the motor nuclei of IV, VI and, where present, XII, as well as the rostral end of the spinal motor column.
6. The medial zone contains a number of cell masses, which can be designated as somatomotor coordinating centers. These include the superior, medius, and inferior reticular nuclei, and the superior and inferior raphe nuclei. Raphe nuclei could not be detected in the lamprey, however.
7. The medial zone contains a number of evidently non-somatomotor relay centers, including the interpeduncular nucleus and the inferior olive. The latter is, as already mentioned, lacking in the lamprey.
8. The functional designation of the intermedioventral zone as visceromotor is justified, because it contains in all species studied a conspicuous series of primary visceromotor cell masses, formed by the motor nuclei of V, VII, IX, and X (**Figures 4B** and **5B**).
9. However, the intermedioventral zone contains, just as the medial zone, a number of structures, which do not accord with its functional label. These include the Mauthner neuron, the efferent nucleus of the VIIIth nerve (**Figures 4B** and **5B**), the precerebellar nucleus of the funiculus lateralis, and the superior olive (in anurans) and the nucleus of the lateral lemniscus, two auditory (and, hence special somatosensory) relay nuclei.
10. The alar plate can be divided into an intermediodorsal zone or column and a dorsal zone or column.
11. The boundary between the two morphological entities mentioned under 10 is in many species at least partially marked by a sulcus intermedius dorsalis.
12. The caudal part of the intermediolateral zone contains a center known as lobus vagi (**Figure 4B**) or nucleus fasciculi solitarii (**Figure 5B**), which receives viscerosensory fibers via the VIIth, IXth, and Xth cranial nerves, whereas the most rostral part of the same zone harbors a cell mass which, as its name: nucleus visceralis secundarius indicates, represents a viscerosensory center of higher order (**Figure 5B**). It would be incorrect, however, to designate the entire intermediolateral zone as viscerosensory, because it contains several general somatosensory centers and special somatosensory centers as well. The general somatosensory centers include the very diffuse nucleus tractus descendens of the trigeminal nerve (**Figure 5B**), the nucleus princeps of the same nerve (**Figure 5B**) and, in lampreys, the primary somatosensory dorsal cells (**Figure 4B**). The special somatosensory component of the intermediodorsal zone is formed by a series of three to five cell masses extending from the level of the motor trigeminal nucleus to the level of entrance of the caudal roots of the vagus nerve. The names of these cell masses differ somewhat among the various anamniote groups. In *Scaphirhynchus* three of such cell masses, the anterior octavus nucleus, the magnocellular vestibular nucleus, and the descending octavus nucleus, could be delineated (**Figure 5B**). In *Lampetra*, the three octavomotor nuclei (**Figure 4B**) belong to the same functional category.
13. The dorsal zone of the rhombencephalon may be aptly designated as somatosensory, because it contains throughout most of its extent exclusively cell masses belonging in this functional category. These cell masses include: (1) the nucleus dorsalis areae octavolateralis, an electroreceptive lateral line center, occurring in lampreys, most groups of fish and all urodele amphibians (**Figures 4B** and **5B**); (2) the nucleus intermedius areae octavolateralis, a mechanoreceptive lateral line center, occurring in all groups of anamniotes, except for anuran amphibians (**Figures 4B** and **5B**), and (3), in anurans, the nucleus dorsalis nervi octavi. It is important to note, however, that the nucleus cerebelli and the nucleus isthmi, two cell masses situated in the most rostral part

of the rhombencephalic dorsal zone, cannot be classified as somatosensory centers.

14. The mesencephalon consists of the ventral tegmentum mesencephali and the dorsal tectum mesencephali. The rhombencephalic basal plate is rostrally continuous with the medial part of the tegmentum mesencephali, which has been designated on that account as the motor tegmentum. It contains the nuclei, the third cranial nerve, the nucleus of the fasciculus longitudinalis medialis and, in many species, the nucleus ruber (**Figure 5B**). The rhombencephalic alar plate passes over into the lateral part of the tegmentum and the tectum. Contrary to the statements of numerous previous authors, including Holmgren and van der Horst (1925), Gerlach (1933, 1947), Addens (1933) and Heier (1948), the sulcus limitans does not extend into the midbrain (**Figures 4B** and **5B**). The lateral part of the tegmentum and the tectum are both the recipients of important somatosensory pathways. The lateral tegmentum contains a large special somatosensory relay center, the torus semicircularis. The tectum mesencephali is to be considered as a general and special somatosensory correlation center of higher order. However, in all gnathostomes it also contains a primary somatosensory cell group: the nucleus mesencephalicus of V (**Figure 5B**).

Summarizing again: as indicated by Wilhelm His, the entire brainstem (i. e. the rhombencephalon plus the mesencephalon) can be divided into a primarily motor basal plate and a primarily sensory alar plate. A sulcus limitans, marking the boundary of the basal and alar plates on the ventricular side, is confined to the rhombencephalon. Within the rhombencephalon four morphological zones, which are designated here as area ventralis, area intermedioventralis, area intermediodorsalis, and area dorsalis, can be distinguished. The areae ventralis and intermedioventralis form together the rhombencephalic basal plate, whereas the areae intermedioventralis and dorsalis form together the rhombencephalic alar plate. The four morphological entities mentioned correspond largely, though not entirely, with the four functional zones or columns – somatomotor, visceromotor, viscerosensory, and somatosensory – of Herrick and Johnston (**Figure 2A**). This is so because all of the four morphological zones contain one or more cell masses, the functional significance of which do not mesh with the functional label of the pertinent zones.

FUNCTIONAL CORRELATIONS

Although the topological charts as such are representations of morphological data, many of the features shown by them refer directly to functional or behavioral aspects. Thus, the extraordinarily large size of the motor trigeminal nucleus in lampreys (**Figure 4B**) has to do with the fact that in these jawless animals the nerve in question innervates the musculature of the large sucking mouth, with which they attach themselves to and attack fish. The large size of the nucleus of the fasciculus solitarius in sturgeons (**Figure 5B**) is related to the strong development of the gustatory system. In these bottom-dwelling fishes, taste buds are not confined to the oral cavity, but also occur on the barbels and the tentacular fringes, that surround the mouth. These external taste organs play an important role in locating food. The large size of the nucleus dorsalis areae octavolateralis in sturgeons (**Figure 5B**) indicates that in these fishes the electroreceptive lateral line system is also well developed. Some further examples of such "central responses" to particular peripheral differentiations will now be discussed. In order to place these various "central responses" into perspective, the brains of the various specialized species to be discussed are in **Figure 6** compared with those of related, "more generalized" species. Thus, the brain of the electric ray *Torpedo ocellata* (**Figures 6D–F**) is compared to that of the spiny dogfish *S. acanthias* (**Figures 6A–C**), whereas the brains of three very specialized teleosts, viz. the cyprinid *Carassius carassius* (**Figures 6K–M**), the African notopterid *Xenomystus nigri* (**Figures 6N–P**), and the gymnotid *Eigenmannia virescens* (**Figures 6Q–S**) are compared to that of the holostean *A. calva* (**Figures 6G–H**).

1. In electric rays, such as *Torpedo*, the musculature of the expanded pectoral fins has been largely transformed into a pair of powerful electric organs (**Figure 6D**). These organs are innervated by branches of the VIIth, IXth, and Xth cranial nerves. Accordingly, the motor nuclei of these nerves, which constitute together the caudal portion of the rhombencephalic visceromotor column, consist mainly of large electromotor neurons and constitute collectively a pair of gigantic electric lobes (**Figures 6E,F**). In electric rays, the discharge of the electric organs is both a means of protection and a device for stunning prey.
2. In cyprinid teleosts, such as the common goldfish *Carassius* (**Figure 6K**), the gustatory system is well developed. Taste buds are scattered over the entire body, but the most specialized part of the gustatory system of these animals is the so-called palatal organ, which is situated in the roof of the mouth. This organ does not only bear an abundance of taste buds, but is also provided with a layer of muscle fibers. It is involved in the selection of food particles from substrate material (Sibbing 1984; Finger 1988; Ikenaga et al., 2009). The taste buds of the palatal organ are innervated by afferent fibers of the vagus nerve, and its musculature is supplied by efferent fibers of the same nerve. The computational aspects of the sophisticated food detection and selection just outlined, are carried out by the adjacent, vagal segments of the viscerosensory and visceromotor columns, which in cyprinids form together a pair of large and highly differentiated vagal lobes (**Figures 6L,M**).
3. A lateral line system is present in all anamniotes, except for adult anuran amphibians. The fibers, which carry the impulses from the lateral line organs centrally pass, by way of the anterior and posterior lateral line nerves to the most dorsal part of the rhombencephalic alar plate, where they terminate in an elongated intraventricular protrusion, known as the lateral line lobe. The lateral line receptor organs are of two kinds, mechanoreceptive and electroreceptive. The mechanoreceptive lateral line sense organs are hydrodynamic detectors, capable of detecting water movements. Most electroreceptive lateral line organs belong to a category known as ampullary organs. These organs respond to low frequency, low voltage signals, which surround

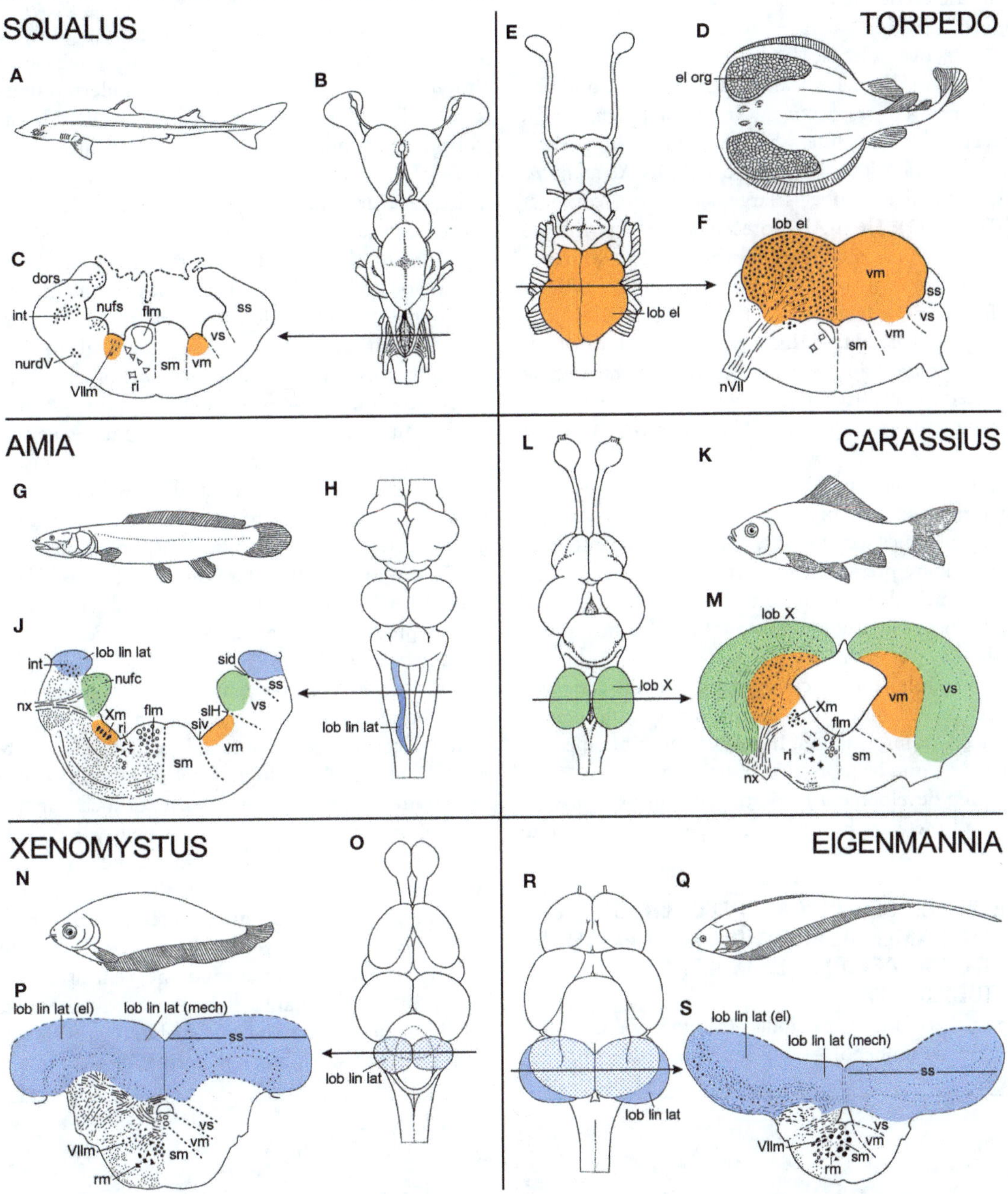

FIGURE 6 | Panels, showing holotypes, dorsal views of the brain, and transverse sections through the rhombencephalon of six different fishes, the spiny dogfish *Squalus acanthias* (A–C), the electric ray *Torpedo ocellata* (D–F), the holostean *Amia calva* (G–J), the cyprinid teleost *Carassius carassius* (K–M), the African notopterid teleost *Xenomystus nigri* (N–P), and the gymnotid teleost *Eigenmannia virescens* (Q–S). *Torpedo*, *Carassius*, *Xenomystus*, and *Eigenmannia* show functional specializations, which manifest themselves as local "hypertrophies" in their brains. In order to place these specializations into perspective, the brains of these four species are compared to those of two "less specialized" or "more generalized" fishes, viz. *Squalus* and *Amia*. For further explanation, see text.

many aquatic animals. By means of this receptor system, many fishes are able to detect the electric fields produced by prey fish and social partners. Fishes which possess only ampullary organs may be designated as "passive" electric fishes, which means that they are only able to detect electrical fields produced by other fish. However, two groups of teleosts with electroreceptors, the Gymnotidae and the Mormyridae, can be characterized as "active" electric fish, because they are able to detect signals which they emit themselves with an electric organ. They use their electric system for what may be called active electrolocation as well as for conspecific electrocommunication. The detection of the impulses, generated by the electric organs can be assigned to a special type of electric lateral line receptors, known as tuberous organs.

In **Figure 6**, "non-electric" bony fishes (i.e., fishes possessing only a mechanoreceptive lateral line system), "passive" electric bony fishes, and "active" electric bony fishes are represented by the bowfin *A. calva*, the false featherback *X. nigri*, and the glass knifefish *E. virescens*, respectively. In *Amia* (**Figure 6G**), the mechanoreceptive lateral line fibers terminate in a slender, elongated lateral line lobe (**Figures 6H,J**). In *Xenomystus* (**Figure 6N**), the lateral line lobe is larger and more compact than in *Amia* (**Figure 6O**). The mechanoreceptive fibers terminate in the smaller, medial part of this lobe, whereas the electroreceptive fibers terminate in its larger, lateral part (**Figure 6P**). In *Eigenmannia* (**Figure 6Q**), finally, the primary lateral line center is grown out to a huge, everted disk (**Figures 6R,S**), in which the afferents from the mechanoreceptive, "passive" electroreceptive, and "active" electroreceptive sense organs terminate in strictly separated compartments (see Meek and Nieuwenhuys, 1998, for details).

Summa summarum: the brainstem of anamniotes shows a distinct longitudinal zonal pattern. In the rhombencephalon four different morphological zones: ventral, intermedioventral, intermediodorsal, and dorsal are present, whereas in the mesencephalon three of such zones: medial tegmental, lateral tegmental, and tectal can be discerned. These longitudinal morphological zones correspond largely, though not entirely, with the functional columns of His, Herrick, and Johnston. Because of this parallelism, our topological charts do not only provide morphological information, but also functional information. In many anamniote species, local enlargements of one or more functional columns are coupled with the strong development of particular sense systems or effector organs, and these are in turn correlated with specialized behavioral profiles.

SIGNIFICANCE OF THE TOPOLOGICAL APPROACH FOR THE STUDY OF THE FUNDAMENTAL MORPHOLOGICAL PATTERN OF THE BRAINSTEM AS REVEALED BY MODERN MOLECULAR STUDIES

From the foregoing, it may be concluded that the brainstem of anamniotes contains a number of longitudinally oriented zones or columns, and the fact that these morphological entities are present in representatives of all major anamniote groups indicates that they form part of the fundamental morphological pattern or morphotype of the brainstem. The causal underpinning of this feature apparently relates to shared processes of dorsoventral patterning (columnar zonation), neurogenesis, and histogenesis. The question arises whether this longitudinal zonal pattern represents the entire structural plan, or whether other structural features, because of their constant occurrence, can also be incorporated in it. At the beginning of the twentieth century, it was well known that the central nervous system shows clear signs of segmentation during early development (Von Kupfer, 1906; **Figure 7**). Throughout most of the twentieth century, these neural segments or neuromeres were generally considered as transitory phenomena, which apparently had no relation whatsoever with the definitive structural and functional plan of the central nervous system. However, thanks to the pioneering work of the Swedish neuroembryologists Bergquist and Källen, and numerous recent studies, we know now that this view was wrong, and that neuromeres and their derivatives in the adult brains represent fundamental morphological entities that likewise bear upon functional peculiarities or specializations detected along the AP dimensions of the longitudinal columns.

Bergquist and Källén (numerous publications summarized in Bergquist and Källén (1954), and Nieuwenhuys (1998a)) systematically studied the ontogeny of the brain in representatives of all vertebrate groups. They found that neuromeres are present during a certain developmental period in all vertebrates. They coincide with bands of high mitotic rate and, hence with zones of proliferation. Three successive waves of such transversely oriented zones of proliferation pass over the embryonic neuraxis, forming proneuromeres, neuromeres, and postneuromeres or transverse bands, respectively. Shortly after the start of the third or postneuromeric wave, longitudinal zones of high mitotic activity are formed. Four of these zones, designated as the dorsal, the dorsolateral, the ventrolateral, and the ventral columns could be distinguished in the anlage of the rhombencephalon. The dorsal column appeared to be confined to the rhombencephalon, the ventral column was observed to extend into the mesencephalon,

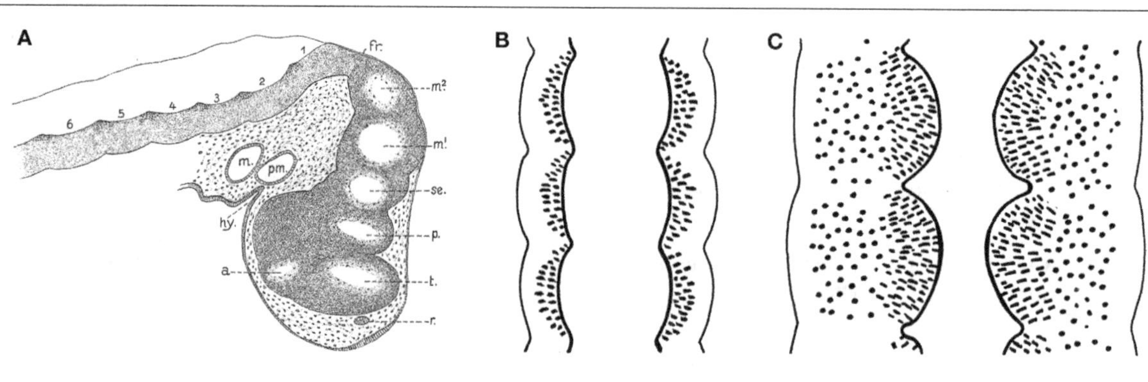

FIGURE 7 | Signs of segmentation in the brains of vertebrate embryos c.q. larvae. (A) Sagittal section through the brain of a 10-mm larva of the spiny dogfish *Squalus acanthias*. a, optic stalk; fr, fissura rhombo-mesencephalica; hy, hypophysis; m, mandibular cavity; m1, m2, mesomeres; p, parencephalon; pm, premandibular cavity; r, wall of olfactory groove; se, synencephalon; t, telencephalon; 1, 2 etc., rhombomeres. Reproduced from Von Kupfer (1906). **(B)** Diagrammatic horizontal section through the neuraxis of an early embryo. Each neural segment or neuromere is separated from its neighbors by external vertical constrictions, which correspond to internal sharp dorsoventral ridges. **(C)** Similar section through the neuraxis of a later developmental stage, in which the neuromeres present themselves as distinct and sharply separated intraventricular bulges.

whereas the remaining two columns could be traced into the forebrain. By intersection of the transverse bands and the longitudinal zones a chequered network develops, made up of squares with a high proliferative activity (**Figure 8A**). As far as the longitudinal columnar organization of the brainstem is concerned, the scheme of Bergquist and Källén closely resembles the pattern revealed by our topological analyses. It should be noted, however, that in the parcellation of Bergquist and Källën, the boundaries between the various columns are not marked by ventricular sulci, but rather by "incisures" in the mantle layer. Topological analyses of the brainstems of embryonic and larval vertebrate species are required to determine the precise relationships between the results of the two approaches.

Bergquist and Källén (1954) designated the squares with high proliferative activity as migration areas. They noted that these areas show a remarkable consistency in both number and pattern throughout the vertebrate kingdom. On that account, they considered the migration areas to be *fundamental morphological units*, providing a sound basis for the homologization of neural grisea. These units represent three-dimensional radial complexes, stretching from the ventricular to the meningeal surface, within the confines of which the principal histogenetic events, i.e., proliferation, migration, and differentiation, essentially take place (**Figure 8B**). It is important to note that the boundaries of the units, as well as the migration of neuroblasts within them, strictly adhere to the vectors of the natural system of coordinates, discussed in Section "Topological Analysis of the Brainstem" of the present paper. During the last decades, the remarkable results of the pioneering studies of Bergquist and Källén have been confirmed and extended by numerous publications, as may appear from the following synopsis.

1. *Segmental organization of early developing cells and cell groups.* It has been observed that in the brainstem of teleosts, early developing primary motoneurons, as well as reticulospinal neurons show a distinct segmental distribution (Metcalfe et al., 1986; Hanneman et al., 1988; Bass et al., 2008). A segment-related pattern of organization has also been observed in the embryonic

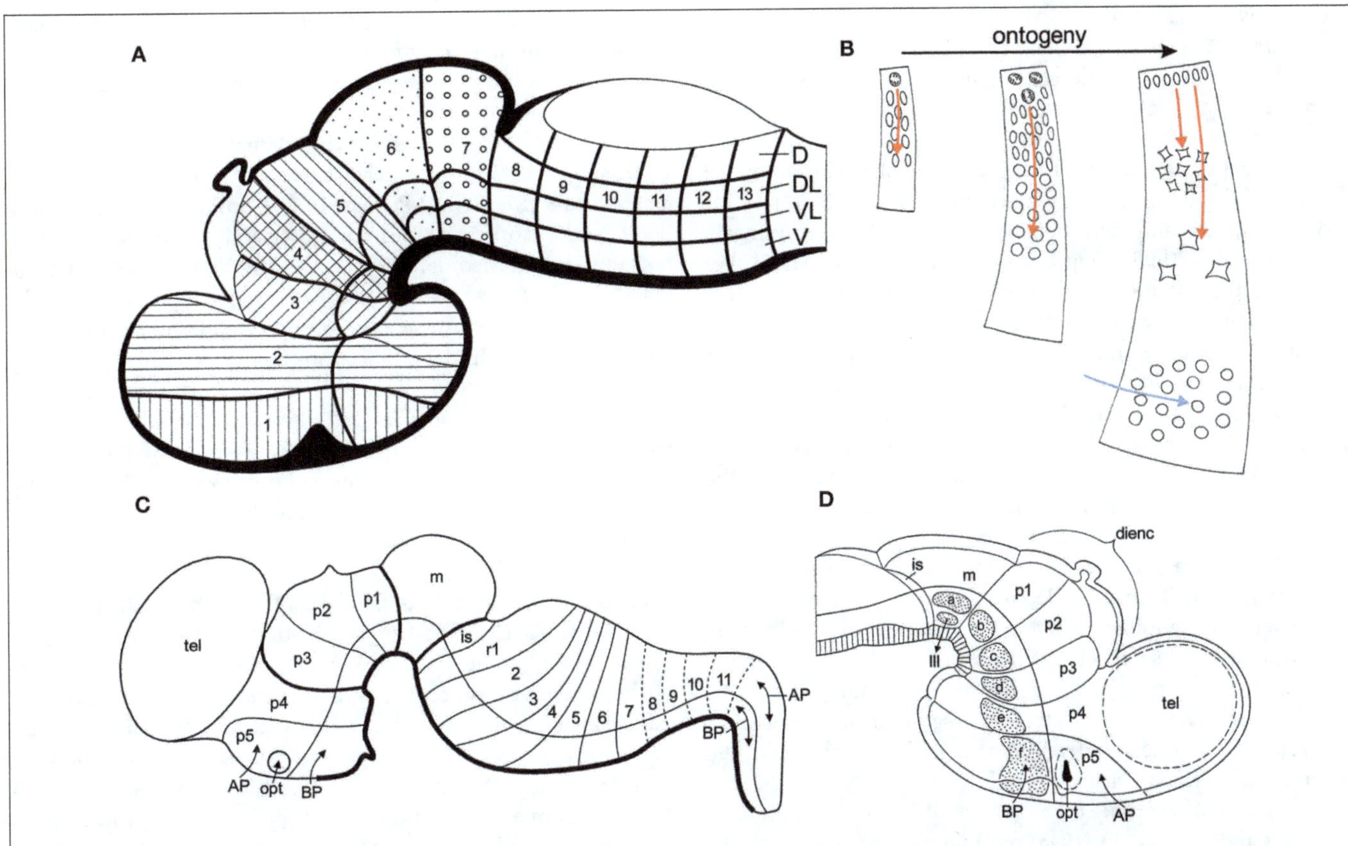

FIGURE 8 | Fundamental morphological units in the vertebrate brain. **(A)** Diagrammatic median section through a vertebrate embryo, showing that the boundaries of transverse bands (1, 2 etc.) and longitudinal zones of high mitotic rate (D, DL, VL, V), divide the wall of the developing brain into fundamental morphological units. These units represent three-dimensional radial complexes, stretching from the ventricular surface to the meningeal surface. Modified from Bergquist and Källén (1954). **(B)** Ontogeny of a fundamental morphological unit. The principal histogenetic events, i.e., proliferation, migration, and differentiation essentially take place within the confines of these units. The migration of neuroblasts is radially directed (red arrows). During later development, tangentially migrating neuroblasts, originating from other sources, may invade a given unit (blue arrow). **(C)** Schema of the brain of a mammalian embryo. The longitudinal and transverse delineations are primarily based on the expression patterns of a number of developmental regulatory genes. Based on Puelles et al. (2007). **(D)** Diagrammatic median section through the rostral part of the brain of a chick embryo. Distinct groups of early differentiating neuroblasts manifest themselves in the basal plate sections of the midbrain segment (m), and of the five prosomeres (p1–p5). Modified from Puelles et al. (1987).

chick brain, where early differentiating neuroblasts were found to appear as separate, distinct groups at the center of the basal plate portions of the mesencephalic and prosencephalic neuromeres (Puelles et al., 1987; **Figure 8D**). It is remarkable that these groups of early differentiating neurons fit into a transverse, neuromeric as well as in a longitudinal zonal pattern, and therewith in the organizational scheme of Bergquist and Källén (**Figure 8A**).

2. *Segmental cell lineage restrictions.* As early as 1887, Orr (1887), p. 335) presumed that "the cells of one neuromere do not extend into another neuromere." This presumption has been substantiated by cell-marking experiments on the rhombencephalon (Fraser et al., 1990), and diencephalon (Figdor and Stern, 1993) of chick embryos, which showed that the progeny of individually labeled matrix cells failed to cross interneuromeric borders. Marín and Puelles (1995) and Wingate and Lumsden (1996) used quail-chick grafting chimaeras to examine the fate of individual neuromeres. Fate mapping revealed that the progeny of individual rhombomeres form sharply delineated radially oriented compartments, which remained largely intact in late developmental stages.
3. *Fundamental morphological units and the development of fiber tracts.* In the embryonic central nervous system, the fibers growing out from the clusters of early differentiating neurons pass close to the border zones of the fundamental morphological units, together forming a discrete and stereotyped scaffold of transversely and longitudinally oriented axonal bundles (Wingate and Lumsden, 1996; Kimmel, 1993; Wingate and Lumsden, 1996; Wingate and Lumsden, 1996). Many fiber systems present in the brain of adult vertebrates, including the fasciculus longitudinalis medialis, the stria medullaris, the posterior commissure, and the fasciculus retroflexus, derive directly from the early embryonic axonal scaffold (Wingate and Lumsden, 1996; Puelles, 1995).
4. *Segmental expression of developmental regulatory genes.* The spectacular finding that the interneuromeric boundaries in the brain correspond with the limits of expression of a number of developmentally significant genes, and that each neuromere can thus be characterized by a specific set of gene expressions (conferring to them a "molecular identity"), has revolutionized neuromorphology. Whereas the longitudinal zonal model, advocated by Herrick (1910), Kuhlenbeck (1973) and many others, has dominated comparative neuroanatomy for almost a century, at present a complementary segmental morphological paradigm for understanding the structural organization of the vertebrate neuraxis, clearly prevails.
5. *Molecular underpinning of the concept of Bergquist and Källén.* Puelles and Rubenstein (1993) published a model of the mammalian brain, based on a diagrammatic medial view of the brain of a 12.5-day-old mouse embryo, in which the ventricular surface was subdivided by transverse lines into neuromeres, and by a curved horizontal line into a dorsal alar plate and a ventral basal plate. The expression domains of 45 different (putative) developmental regulatory genes were systematically plotted in this model. It appeared that these expressions consistently respected the proposed transverse and longitudinal boundaries. This model was revised in Puelles and Rubenstein (2003), and once again in Puelles et al. (2007); **Figure 8C**). The general conclusions drawn from these models were: (1) that the wall of the embryonic brain can be subdivided into a number of "rectangular" domains, each of which is characterized by the expression of a unique combination of developmental regulatory genes, and (2) that these molecularly defined domains represent radially oriented histogenetic units (Puelles and Medina, 2002; Puelles et al., 2004, 2007).

Parallel studies on genes involved functionally at the so-called "isthmic organizer" (review in Echevarria et al., 2003) have revealed special patterning effects restricted to midbrain and rostral hindbrain, including the cerebellum, which partly explains the columnar singularities detected at these levels.

This brief review of the recent literature may suffice to show that in future studies on the structural organization of the vertebrate brainstem, longitudinal zones as well as transverse bands or neuromeres should be taken into consideration, and that the search for radially arranged, fundamental histogenetic units will have to be placed central in such studies.

During the last decades, Luis Puelles and his collaborators have published a number of studies on the relationship between the localization of cell masses and the neuromeric organization in the brainstem of amniotes. Some of these studies were (largely) based on gene expression patterns (Aroca and Puelles, 2005; Puelles et al., 2007; Marín et al., 2008); others were based on quail-chick grafting experiments (Marín and Puelles, 1995; Cambronero and Puelles, 2000), and still others on the immunoreactivity of particular markers (Puelles and Medina, 1994; Puelles and Verney, 1998; Ju et al., 2004). In all of these studies, the results were summarized in tabular fate maps, one of which is reproduced in **Figure 9**. I used the data accumulated in the publications mentioned for the preparation of a provisional topological chart, in which the various cell masses are projected on a *natural* plane, viz. the ventricular surface of the brainstem (**Figure 10**). On the basis of this result, I encourage my friend Luis Puelles and other workers in this field, to present their future results in a topological, rather than in a tabular fashion.

NOTES ON THE MORPHOLOGICAL INTERPRETATION OF TOPOLOGICAL CHARTS OF THE BRAINSTEM

As expounded in the first section of the present paper, the essence of the topological procedure is that (i) the various cell masses in the brainstem, with the aid of radial vectors, are projected upon the ventricular surface, and that (ii) this surface, with the projections of the cell masses marked upon it, is transformed into a plane. This method has been designed, so that its product does not only yield information about the mutual positional relations of the various cell masses, but also about their presumptive neuroepithelial origin, and therewith about their *primary topological position.* We have seen that progenitor cells found at the ventricular surface of the brainstem can be divided into a number of "rectangular" fields, and that these fields are related to radially oriented, three-dimensional histogenetic units (**Figures 8A,C**). Because the postmitotic neurons of the various nuclei migrate radially outward within the confines of their respective histogenetic units (**Figure 8C**: red arrows), it may be expected that our projection

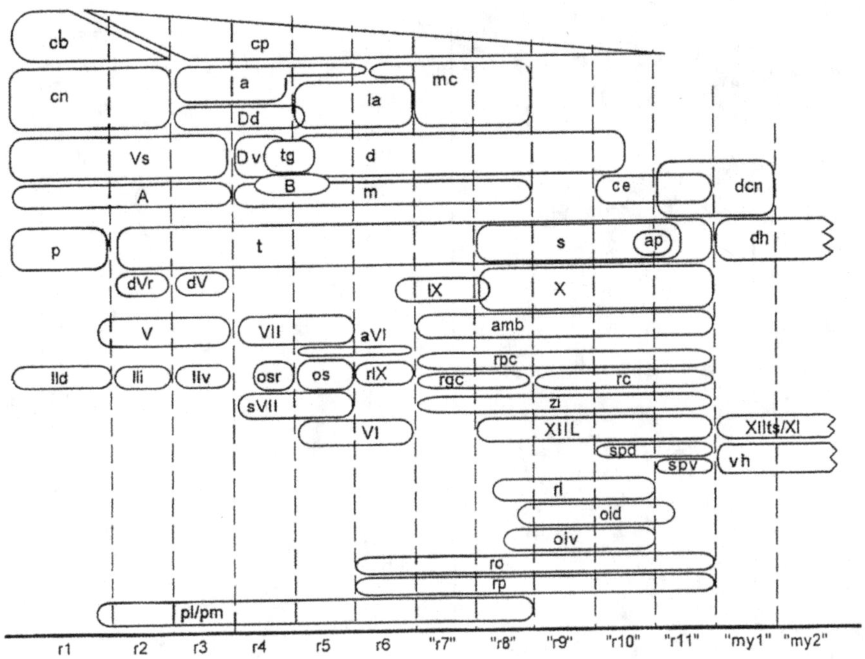

FIGURE 9 | Fate map of avian rhombomeric domains, summarizing data from Marín and Puelles (1995) for rhombomeres r1–r6, and from Cambronero and Puelles (2000) for cryptorhombomeres "r7"–"r11" and cryptomyelomeres "my1" and "my 2." The diagram shows the distribution of nuclei relative to the various segmental boundaries. The relative dorsoventral positions of the columns approximate that in the embryonic brain. Reproduced with permission from Cambronero and Puelles (2000).

method carries these nuclei back to their site of origin. Although this rule holds for many, if not most of the brainstem nuclei, it has some exceptions, the most important of which will be briefly discussed.

1. Populations of immature postmitotic neurons, stemming from different neuromeres and sharing given properties, may unite across the interrhombomeric limits to form bi- or plurisegmental complexes. Thus, the elements forming the abducens nucleus (**Figure 11**: 1), and those forming the motor trigeminal nucleus, originate both from two different, adjacent neuromeres, and many brainstem nuclei, exemplified here by the nucleus of the fasciculus solitarius (**Figure 11**: 2), are of plurisegmental origin. Moreover, some neuronal populations, such as those forming the catecholaminergic cell groups, constitute highly patterned, plurisegmental and plurizonal complexes (Cambronero and Puelles, 2000; Cambronero and Puelles, 2000). It is thought that such plurisegmental patterns represent a consequence of specific genetic effects shared across neighboring neuromeres (e.g., cell adhesion proteins and various differentiation traits), but nevertheless also imply subtle differences between the analogous populations inhabiting the individual neuromeric units, due to their differential primary segmental identities (i.e., differential constellations of early fate-specifying genes). Such minor differences turn up later in inner circuitry patterns, long-range connectivity patterns and specialized molecular traits related to specialized functional properties, such as the functional anteroposterior specializations observed along the adult cochlear, vestibular, trigeminal and visceral sensory columns.
2. The precursor cells of some brainstem nuclei shift laterally or caudally during ontogeny. As for lateral shift, Windle (1970) found that in human embryos, the neuroblasts, destined to form the branchiomotor nuclei (i.e., the motor nuclei of V, VII, IX, and X) originate close to the median plane of the brainstem, but shift later laterally, to attain their definitive position in the lateral part of the basal plate (**Figure 11**: 3). Ju et al. (2004), using a molecular definition of the alar–basal boundary and molecular markers, adduced evidence that in avian embryos, the branchiomotor nuclei even invade the rhombencephalic alar plate. The latter finding is hard to reconcile with the situation in adult anamniotes, implying that morphologic versus molecular delineation of the alar–basal limit is presently not consistent, representing a problem that has not yet been resolved. Some authors opted for not identifying either alar or basal territories, classifying structures more vaguely into "dorsal" and "ventral" elements. However, the concept of alar and basal plates, denoting "dorsalized" versus "ventralized" lateral brain wall regions apparently continues to have heuristic value. In the brainstems of all of the 16 different anamniote species investigated by us, the branchiomotor nuclei form a distinct column, occupying the intermediolateral zone of the rhombencephalic basal plate (**Figures 4B** and **5B**). As for caudal shift, it is well known that in mammals, the anlage of the main facial nucleus shifts from rhombomere 5 into rhombomere 6 (**Figure 11**: 4).

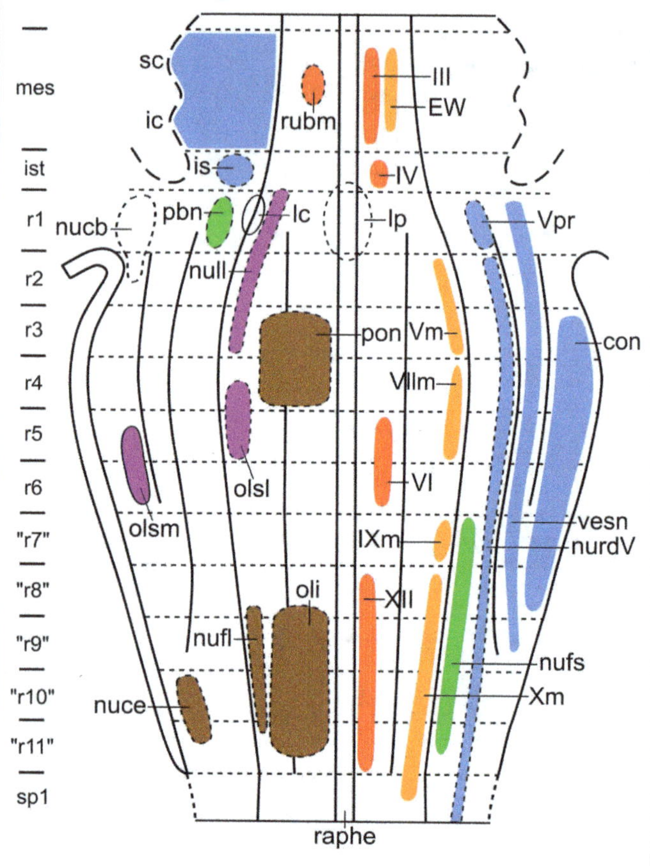

FIGURE 10 | Provisional topological chart of the brainstem of amniotes, showing the zonal and segmental allocation of cell masses, as determined by Puelles and collaborators. In order to avoid crowding, primary sensory and primary motor nuclei are shown to the right, whereas centers of higher order are shown to the left.

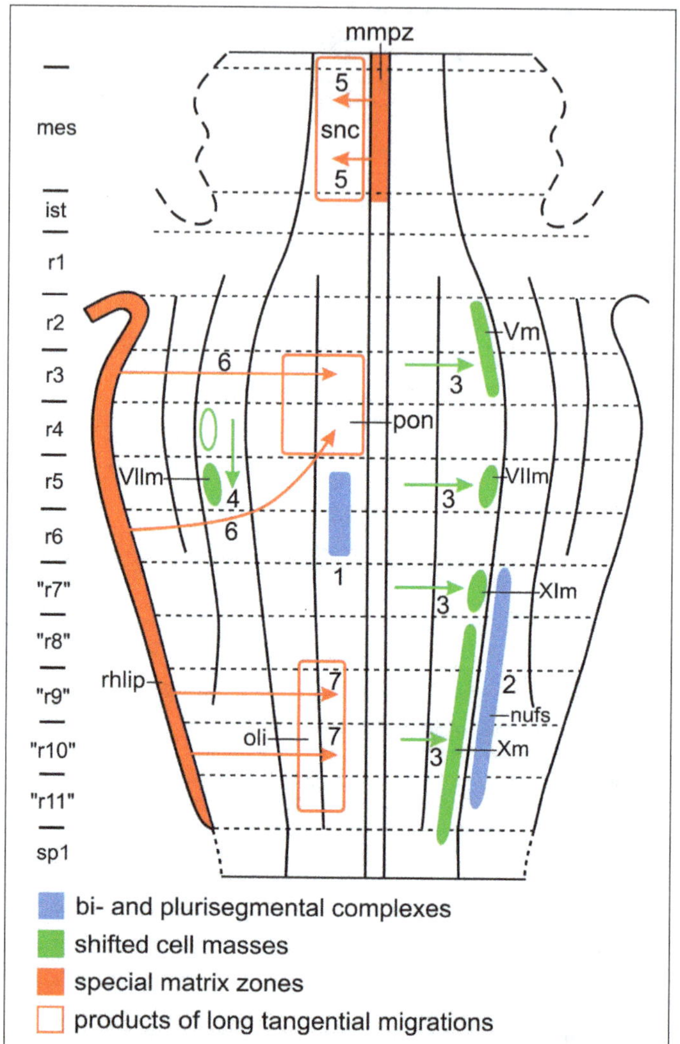

FIGURE 11 | Features which may complicate the morphological interpretation of topological charts. For explanation, see text.

3. Two special proliferation zones, the mesencephalic midventral proliferation zone and the rhombic lip, give rise to long tangential migrations in the brainstem. The proliferation zone first mentioned forms a conspicuous component of the mammalian mesencephalic floor plate. Neuroblasts originating from this zone migrate laterally through the marginal zone of the adjacent basal plate. The sheet of cells, resulting from this remarkable tangential migration, represents the dopaminergic, compact part of the substantia nigra (Verney et al., 2001; **Figure 11**: 5). The rhombic lip is a thickened proliferation zone in the rhombencephalic alar plate, situated directly adjacent to the attachment of the membranous roof of the fourth ventricle (**Figure 11**). Different sectors of the rhombic lip give rise to different structures (see Nieuwenhuys et al., 2008, for references and details). Thus, its most rostral sector provides the neuroblasts, destined to form the cerebellar granular layer. A rostral intermediate part of the rhombic lip gives rise to the cells of the cochlear nuclei, whereas a caudal intermediate portion produces a large stream of tangentially migrating neuroblasts, which invade the basal plate sector of rhombomeres 3 and 4, to form the pontine nuclei (**Figure 11**: 6). Several streams of tangentially migrating neuroblasts also arise from the caudal sector of the rhombic lip. The most prominent of these leads to the formation of the inferior olivary nucleus (**Figure 11**: 7). Other "precerebellar" nuclei, such as the nucleus cuneatus externus and the nucleus funiculi lateralis (**Figure 10**), arise from similar, though smaller streams.

The specific purpose of the brief exercitation just presented, is to show that topological maps, derived from the brainstems of adult specimens, have certain important limitations, irrespective of their overall explanatory power. The exceptions discussed, make plain that the topological procedure does not project all cell masses back to their sites of origin and therewith to their primary topological positions. Conversely, it is now clear that the preparation of a *topological supermap*, showing the genuine primary topological positions of all constituent nuclei in the brainstem of a given species, would require extensive neuroembryological studies involving, *inter alia*, the expression patterns of numerous developmental regulatory genes and the tracing of all tangential migrations.

LOOKING BACK, LOOKING FORWARD

At the time that the present author started this research program, comparative neuroanatomy was dominated by the doctrine that the central nervous system of vertebrates essentially consists of a number of homogeneous longitudinal zones or columns. The brainstem (i. e. the mesencephalon, plus the rhombencephalon, minus the cerebellum) was held to consist of four such zones, which represented, at the same time, structural *as well as* functional entities. These entities were designated by the noted North American neuroanatomists C. J. Herrick and J. B. Johnston as the somatosensory, viscerosensory, visceromotor, and somatomotor columns. In order to test the validity of this "four-structural/functional-zones" concept, I designed a topological procedure, which rendered it possible to survey the spatial relationships of the cell masses in the brainstem of a given specimen in a single figure. The brainstems of 16 different anamniote species were analyzed with the aid of this procedure. It appeared that the brainstem of anamniotes shows a distinct longitudinal zonal pattern. In the rhombencephalon four morphological zones: ventral, intermedioventral, intermediodorsal, and dorsal could be distinguished, whereas in the mesencephalon three of such zones: medial tegmental, lateral tegmental, and tectal appeared to be present. These morphological zones were found to correspond largely, though not entirely with the functional zones of Herrick and Johnston. This was so, because all of the four morphological zones appeared to contain one or some nuclei, the functional significance of which was not consistent with the functional label of the pertinent zones. In spite of these exceptions, the functional-brainstem-model has still a certain explanatory significance. Thus, it appeared to be possible to interpret certain brain specializations related to particular behavioral profiles, as local "hypertrophies" of one or two functional columns.

In the mean time, a dramatic paradigm shift occurred in neuromorphology. Different lines of research, and notably gene expression studies, led to the inescapable conclusion that neural segments or neuromeres, which up to that time were generally considered as early and transient embryonic epiphenomena, represent instead fundamental building blocks of the vertebrate neuraxis. In fact, this discovery, which can be positioned in the last decade of the twentieth century, was not entirely new. Forty years earlier, the Swedish neuroembryologists Bengt Källén and Harry Bergquist had already remarked upon the significance of neuromeres. These authors found that longitudinal zones and neuromeres both play a salient role in the development of the central nervous system. They demonstrated that, by intersection of the embryonic longitudinal and transverse zones, rectangular fields of high proliferation develop, whose derivatives in the mantle zone manifest themselves three-dimensionally as radially oriented areas, extending from the ventricular to the meningeal surface of the developing brain. According to Bergquist and Källén, the principal histogenetic events, i. e. proliferation, migration and differentiation, essentially take place within the confines of these areas. On that account, they considered the areas in question as *fundamental histogenetic units.* Because Bergquist and Källén considered these units as purely morphological entities, to which no functional significance was attributed momentarily, their findings where initially completely neglected. However, during the last two decades, numerous studies, using modern, molecular and neurophysiological techniques, have fully confirmed and substantiated the findings of Bergquist and Källén, indicating that the longitudinal columns have neuromeric subdivisions, whose functional specialties are increasingly becoming apparent in contemporaneous studies (see e. g., Straka et al., 2001, 2006).

The developments just outlined, have led to a complete renewal of the research program discussed. Within the frame of this new program, the following questions will be addressed:

1. What is the exact relationship between the longitudinal zones, as determined by Nieuwenhuys, Bergquist and Källén, and Puelles, respectively?
2. What is the exact number of neuromeres in the brain(stem) of a number of representative anamniotes?
3. Is it true that the brain(stems) of all vertebrates contain a fixed number of fundamental histogenetic units, as Bergquist and Källén surmised?
4. If so, what is the fate (i. e. the specific mode of differentiation) of a number of homologous units within the brain(stems) of some representative anamniotes?
5. Which processes may "disturb" or "complicate" the basic developmental events, occurring within the confines of certain fundamental histogenetic units?

These, and several other related questions will be tackled in the near future by an international research team, consisting of: Agustin González (Complutense, Spain), Michael Hofmann (Bonn, Germany), Ruth Morona (Complutense, Spain), Manuel Pombal (Vigo, Spain), Luis Puelles (Murcia, Spain), Isabel Rodríguez-Moldes (Santiago de Compostela, Spain), Hans Straka (Munich, Germany), Mario Wullimann (Munich, Germany), and myself (Amsterdam, the Netherlands).

ACKNOWLEDGMENTS

I am grateful to Luis Puelles for many stimulating discussions. Special thanks are due to Ton Put and Wil Maas for help with the illustrations, to Dr. Jenneke Kruisbrink for literature retrieval, and to Suzanne Bakker M Sc for moral support and reference management.

REFERENCES

Addens, J. L. (1933). The motor nuclei and roots of the cranial and first spinal nerves of vertebrates. Part I. Introduction and cyclostomes. *Z. Anat. Entwicklungsgesch. Gesch.* 101, 307–410.

Aroca, P., and Puelles, L. (2005). Postulated boundaries and differential fate in the developing rostral hindbrain. *Brain Res. Brain Res. Rev.* 49, 179–190.

Bass, A. H., Gilland, E. H., and Baker, R. (2008). Evolutionary origins for social vocalization in a vertebrate hindbrain-spinal compartment. *Science* 321, 417–421.

Bergquist, H., and Källén, B. (1954). Notes on the early histogenesis and morphogenesis of the central nervous system in vertebrates. *J. Comp. Neurol.* 100, 627–659.

Cambronero, F., and Puelles, L. (2000). Rostrocaudal nuclear relationships in the avian medulla oblongata: a fate map with quail chick chimeras. *J. Comp. Neurol.* 427, 522–545.

Echevarria, D., Vieira, C., Gimeno, L., and Martinez, S. (2003). Neuroepithelial secondary organizers and cell fate specification in the developing brain. *Brain Res. Brain Res. Rev.* 43, 179–191.

Figdor, M. C., and Stern, C. D. (1993). Segmental organization of embryonic diencephalon. *Nature* 363, 630–634.

Finger, T. E. (1988). Sensorimotor mapping and oropharyngeal reflexes in goldfish, *Carassius auratus. Brain Behav. Evol.* 31, 17–24.

Fraser, S., Keynes, R., and Lumsden, A. (1990). Segmentation in the chick embryo hindbrain is defined by cell lineage restrictions. *Nature* 344, 431–435.

Gerlach, J. (1933). Über das Gehirn von Protopterus annectens. *Anat. Anz.* 75, 310–316.

Gerlach, J. (1947). Beitrage zur vergleichenden Morphologie des Selachierhirnes. *Anat. Anz.* 96, 79–165.

Hanneman, E., Trevarrow, B., Metcalfe, W. K., Kimmel, C. B., and Westerfield, M. (1988). Segmental pattern of development of the hindbrain and spinal cord of the zebrafish embryo. *Development* 103, 49–58.

Heier, P. (1948). Fundamental principles in the structure of the brain: a study of the brain of *Petromyzon fluviatilis. Acta. Anat. Suppl. (Basel)* VI, 213.

Heijdra, Y. F., and Nieuwenhuys, R. (1994). Topological analysis of the brainstem of the bowfin, *Amia calva. J. Comp. Neurol.* 339, 12–26.

Herrick, C. J. (1899). The cranial and first spinal nerves of menidia; a contribution upon the nerve components of the bony fishes. Section 1. Introductory. *J. Comp. Neurol.* 9, 153–180.

Herrick, C. J. (1910). The morphology of the forebrain in amphibia and reptilia. *J. Comp. Neurol.* 20, 413–547.

Herrick, C. J. (1913) "Anatomy of the brain," in *The Reference Handbook of the Medical Sciences,* Vol. 2, (New York: Wood) 274–342.

His, W. (1891). Die Entwickelung des menschlichen Rautenhirns vom Ende des ersten bis zum Beginn des dritten Monats I. Verlängertes Mark. *Abh. Math. Phys. Kl. Kgl. Sächs. Ges. Wiss.* 17, 1–75.

His, W. (1893). Vorschläge zur Eintheilung des Gehirns. *Arch. Anat. Physiol. Anat. Abt.* 172–180.

Hjörth, J. T., and Key, B. (2001). Are pioneer axons guided by regulatory gene expression domains in the zebrafish forebrain? *Dev. Biol.* 229, 271–286.

Holmgren, N., and van der Horst, C. (1925). Contribution to the morphology of the brain of *Ceratodus. Acta Zool.* 6, 59–165.

Ikenaga, T., Ogura, T., and Finger, T. E. (2009). Vagal gustatory reflex circuits for intraoral food sorting behavior in the goldfish: cellular organization and neurotransmitters. *J. Comp. Neurol.* 516, 213–225.

Johnston, J. (1902a). The brain of Petromyzon. *J. Comp. Neurol.* 12, 1–86.

Johnston, J. (1902b). An attempt to define the primitive functional divisions of the central nervous system. *J. Comp. Neurol.* 12, 87–106.

Johnston, J. B. (1902c). The brain of *Acipenser. Zool. Jahrb. Abt. Anat. Ontogenie Tiere* 15, 59–260.

Ju, M. J., Aroca, P., Luo, J., Puelles, L., and Redies, C. (2004). Molecular profiling indicates avian branchiomotor nuclei invade the hindbrain alar plate. *Neuroscience* 128, 785–796.

Kimmel, C. B. (1993). Patterning the brain of the zebrafish embryo. *Annu. Rev. Neurosci.* 16, 707–732.

Kremers, J. W., and Nieuwenhuys, R. (1979). Topological analysis of the brain stem of the crossopterygian fish *Latimeria chalumnae. J. Comp. Neurol.* 187, 613–637.

Kuhlenbeck, H. (1973). *Central Nervous System of Vertebrates: Vol. 3 Pt. 2 Overall Morphologic Pattern.* Basel: Karger.

Lumsden, A., and Keynes, R. (1989). Segmental patterns of neuronal development in the chick hindbrain. *Nature* 337, 424–428.

Marín, F., Aroca, P., and Puelles, L. (2008). Hox gene colinear expression in the avian medulla oblongata is correlated with pseudorhombomeric domains. *Dev. Biol.* 323, 230–247.

Marín, F., and Puelles, L. (1995). Morphological fate of rhombomeres in quail/chick chimeras: a segmental analysis of hindbrain nuclei. *Eur. J. Neurosci.* 7, 1714–1738.

Meek, J., and Nieuwenhuys, R. (1998). "Holosteans and teleosts," in *The Central Nervous System of Vertebrates,* Vol. 2, eds R. Nieuwenhuys, H. J. ten Donkelaar, and C. Nicholson (Berlin: Springer), 759–937.

Metcalfe, W. K., Mendelson, B., and Kimmel, C. B. (1986). Segmental homologies among reticulospinal neurons in the hindbrain of the zebrafish larva. *J. Comp. Neurol.* 251, 147–159.

Nieuwenhuys, R. (1972). Topological analysis of the brain stem of the lamprey *Lampetra fluviatilis. J. Comp. Neurol.* 145, 165–177.

Nieuwenhuys, R. (1974). Topological analysis of the brain stem: a general introduction. *J. Comp. Neurol.* 156, 255–276.

Nieuwenhuys, R. (1998a) "Morphogenesis and general structure," in *The Central Nervous System of Vertebrates,* Vol. 1, eds R. Nieuwenhuys, H. J. ten Donkelaar, and C. Nicholson (Berlin: Springer), 158–228.

Nieuwenhuys, R. (1998b). "Histogenesis," in *The Central Nervous System of Vertebrates,* Vol. 1, eds R. Nieuwenhuys, H. J. ten Donkelaar, and C. Nicholson (Berlin: Springer), 229–272.

Nieuwenhuys, R. (1998c). "Chondrostean fishes," in *The Central Nervous System of Vertebrates,* Vol. 1, eds R. Nieuwenhuys, H. J. ten Donkelaar, and C. Nicholson (Berlin: Springer), 701–757.

Nieuwenhuys, R. (1998d). "The coelacanth, *Latimeria chalumnae*," in *The Central Nervous System of Vertebrates,* Vol. 2, eds R. Nieuwenhuys, H. J. ten Donkelaar, and C. Nicholson (Berlin: Springer), 1007–1043.

Nieuwenhuys, R., and Nicholson, C. (1998). "Lampreys, Petromyzontidae," in *The Central Nervous System of Vertebrates,* Vol. 1, eds R. Nieuwenhuys, H. J. ten Donkelaar, and C. Nicholson (Berlin: Springer), 397–496.

Nieuwenhuys, R., and Oey, P. L. (1983). Topological analysis of the brainstem of the reedfish, *Erpetoichthys calabaricus. J. Comp. Neurol.* 213, 220–232.

Nieuwenhuys, R., and Pouwels, E. (1983). The brain stem of actinopterygian fishes. *Fish Neurobiol.* 1, 25–87.

Nieuwenhuys, R., Voogd, J., and van Huijzen, C. (2008). *The Human Nervous System,* 4th revised edn. Heidelberg: Springer, 967.

Nikundiwe, A. M., and Nieuwenhuys, R. (1983). The cell masses in the brainstem of the South African clawed frog *Xenopus laevis*: a topographical and topological analysis. *J. Comp. Neurol.* 213, 199–219.

Opdam, P., and Nieuwenhuys, R. (1976). Topological analysis of the brain stem of the axolotl *Ambystoma mexicanum. J. Comp. Neurol.* 165, 285–306.

Opdam, R., Kemali, M., and Nieuwenhuys, R. (1976). Topological analysis of the brain stem of the frogs *Rana esculenta* and *Rana catesbeiana. J. Comp. Neurol.* 165, 307–332.

Orr, H. (1887). Contribution to the embryology of the lizard; with especial reference to the central nervous system and some organs of the head; together with observations on the origin of the vertebrates. *J. Morphol.* 1, 311–372.

Puelles, L. (1995). A segmental morphological paradigm for understanding vertebrate forebrains. *Brain Behav. Evol.* 46, 319–337.

Puelles, L., Amat, J. A., and Martinez-de-la-Torre, M. (1987). Segment-related, mosaic neurogenetic pattern in the forebrain and mesencephalon of early chick embryos: I. Topography of AChE-positive neuroblasts up to stage HH18. *J. Comp. Neurol.* 266, 247–268.

Puelles, L., Martinez-de-la-Torre, M., Paxinos, G., Watson, C., and Martinez, S. (2007). *The Chick Brain in Stereotaxic Coordinates.* San Diego: Academic Press.

Puelles, L., Martinez, S., Martinez-de-la-Torre, M., and Rubenstein, J. L. R. (2004). "Gene maps and related histogenetic domains in the forebrain and midbrain," in *The Rat Nervous System,* 3rd Edn, ed. G. Paxinos (San Diego: Academic Press), 3–25.

Puelles, L., and Medina, L. (1994). "Development of neurons expressing tyrosine hydroxylase and dopamine in the chicken brain: a comparative segmental analysis," in *Phylogeny and Development of Catecholamine Systems in the CNS of Vertebrates,* eds W. J. A. J. Smeets, and A. Reiner (Cambridge: Cambridge University Press), 135–181.

Puelles, L., and Medina, L. (2002). Field homology as a way to reconcile genetic and developmental variability with adult homology. *Brain Res. Bull.* 57, 243–255.

Puelles, L., and Rubenstein, J. L. (1993). Expression patterns of homeobox and other putative regulatory genes in the embryonic mouse forebrain suggest a neuromeric organization. *Trends Neurosci.* 16, 472–479.

Puelles, L., and Rubenstein, J. L. (2003). Forebrain gene expression domains and the evolving prosomeric model. *Trends Neurosci.* 26, 469–476.

Puelles, L., and Verney, C. (1998). Early neuromeric distribution of tyrosine-hydroxylase-immunoreactive neurons in human embryos. *J. Comp. Neurol.* 394, 283–308.

Sibbing, F. (1984). *Food handling and mastication in the carp (Cyprinus carpio L.).* Ph.D. thesis, University of Wageningen, Wageningen.

Smeets, W. J. A. J., and Nieuwenhuys, R. (1976). Topological analysis of the brain stem of the sharks *Squalus acanthias* and *Scyliorhinus canicula. J. Comp. Neurol.* 165, 333–368.

Smeets, W. J. A. J., Nieuwenhuys, R., and Roberts, B. L. (1983). *The Central Nervous System of Cartilaginous Fishes: Structural and Functional Correlations.* Heidelberg: Springer-Verlag.

Straka, H., Baker, R., and Gilland, E. (2006). Preservation of segmental hindbrain organization in adult frogs. *J. Comp. Neurol.* 494, 228–245.

Straka, H., Baker, R., and Gillard, E. (2001). Rhombomeric organization of vestibular pathways in larval frogs. *J. Comp. Neurol.* 437, 42–55.

Thors, F., and Nieuwenhuys, R. (1979). Topological analysis of the brain stem of the lungfish *Lepidosiren paradoxa*. *J. Comp. Neurol.* 187, 589–611.

Verney, C., Zecevic, N., and Puelles, L. (2001). Structure of longitudinal brain zones that provide the origin for the substantia nigra and ventral tegmental area in human embryos, as revealed by cytoarchitecture and tyrosine hydroxylase, calretinin, calbindin, and GABA immunoreactions. *J. Comp. Neurol.* 429, 22–44.

Von Kupfer, K. (1906). "Die Morphogenie des Centralnervensystems," in *Handbuch der Vergleichenden und experimentellen Entwicklungsgeschichte der Wirbeltiere*, ed. O. Von Hertwig (Jena: Ficher Verlag), 1–272.

Windle, W. F. (1970). Development of neural elements in human embryos of four to seven weeks gestation. *Exp. Neurol.* 28(Suppl.) 44–83.

Wingate, R. J., and Lumsden, A. (1996). Persistence of rhombomeric organisation in the postsegmental hindbrain. *Development* 122, 2143–2152.

Conflict of Interest Statement: The author declares that the research was conducted in the absence of any commercial or financial relationships that could be construed as a potential conflict of interest.

Permissions

All chapters in this book were first published in FN, by Frontiers Media SA; hereby published with permission under the Creative Commons Attribution License or equivalent. Every chapter published in this book has been scrutinized by our experts. Their significance has been extensively debated. The topics covered herein carry significant findings which will fuel the growth of the discipline. They may even be implemented as practical applications or may be referred to as a beginning point for another development.

The contributors of this book come from diverse backgrounds, making this book a truly international effort. This book will bring forth new frontiers with its revolutionizing research information and detailed analysis of the nascent developments around the world.

We would like to thank all the contributing authors for lending their expertise to make the book truly unique. They have played a crucial role in the development of this book. Without their invaluable contributions this book wouldn't have been possible. They have made vital efforts to compile up to date information on the varied aspects of this subject to make this book a valuable addition to the collection of many professionals and students.

This book was conceptualized with the vision of imparting up-to-date information and advanced data in this field. To ensure the same, a matchless editorial board was set up. Every individual on the board went through rigorous rounds of assessment to prove their worth. After which they invested a large part of their time researching and compiling the most relevant data for our readers.

The editorial board has been involved in producing this book since its inception. They have spent rigorous hours researching and exploring the diverse topics which have resulted in the successful publishing of this book. They have passed on their knowledge of decades through this book. To expedite this challenging task, the publisher supported the team at every step. A small team of assistant editors was also appointed to further simplify the editing procedure and attain best results for the readers.

Apart from the editorial board, the designing team has also invested a significant amount of their time in understanding the subject and creating the most relevant covers. They scrutinized every image to scout for the most suitable representation of the subject and create an appropriate cover for the book.

The publishing team has been an ardent support to the editorial, designing and production team. Their endless efforts to recruit the best for this project, has resulted in the accomplishment of this book. They are a veteran in the field of academics and their pool of knowledge is as vast as their experience in printing. Their expertise and guidance has proved useful at every step. Their uncompromising quality standards have made this book an exceptional effort. Their encouragement from time to time has been an inspiration for everyone.

The publisher and the editorial board hope that this book will prove to be a valuable piece of knowledge for researchers, students, practitioners and scholars across the globe.

List of Contributors

R. Glenn Northcutt
Laboratory of Comparative Neurobiology, Scripps Institution of Oceanography, University of California San Diego, La Jolla, CA, USA
Department of Neurosciences, School of Medicine, University of California San Diego, La Jolla, CA, USA

Agustín González
Department of Cell Biology, Faculty of Biology, University of Complutense of Madrid, Madrid, Spain

Nerea Moreno and Agustín González
Departamento de Biología Celular, Facultad de Biología, Universidad Complutense of Madrid, Madrid, Spain

James L. Goodson and Marcy A. Kingsbury
Department of Biology, Indiana University, Bloomington, IN, USA

Laura Domínguez, Agustín González and Nerea Moreno
Faculty of Biology, Department of Cell Biology, University Complutense of Madrid, Madrid, Spain

Christine J. Charvet
Department of Neurobiology and Behavior, Center for the Neurobiology of Learning and Memory, University of California, Irvine, CA, USA

Georg F. Striedter
Department of Neurobiology and Behavior, Center for the Neurobiology of Learning and Memory, University of California, Irvine, CA, USA
Department of Ecology and Evolutionary Biology, University of California, Irvine, CA, USA

Kei Yamamoto and Philippe Vernier
Neurobiology and Development (UPR3294), Institute of Neurobiology Alfred Fessard, CNRS, Gif-sur-Yvette, France

Nicanor Morales-Delgado
Department of Medical Sciences, School of Medicine, Regional Centre for Biomedical Research and Institute for Research in Neurological Disabilities, University of Castilla-La Mancha, Albacete, Spain
Department of Human Anatomy and Psychobiology, School of Medicine, University of Murcia, Murcia, Spain

Paloma Merchan, José L. Ferrán and Luis Puelles
Department of Human Anatomy and Psychobiology, School of Medicine, University of Murcia, Murcia, Spain

Sylvia M. Bardet
Department of Human Anatomy and Psychobiology, School of Medicine, University of Murcia, Murcia, Spain
UMR 1061, Unité de Génétique Moléculaire Animale, Institut National de la Recherche Agronomique, University of Limoges, Limoges, France

Carmen Díaz
Department of Medical Sciences, School of Medicine, Regional Centre for Biomedical Research and Institute for Research in Neurological Disabilities, University of Castilla-La Mancha, Albacete, Spain

Manuel A. Pombal, Rosa Álvarez-Otero, Juan Pérez-Fernández, Cristina Solveira and Manuel Megías
Neurolam Group, Department of Functional Biology and Health Sciences, Faculty of Biology, University of Vigo, Vigo, Spain

M. Angeles Luque, Julio Torres-Torrelo, Livia Carrascal, Blas Torres and Luis Herrero
Department of Physiology and Zoology, University of Seville, Seville, Spain

Amparo Novejarque and Fernando Martínez-García
Departament de Biologia Funcional i Antropologia Física, Facultat de Ciències Biològiques, Universitat de València, València, Spain

Nicolás Gutiérrez-Castellanos and Enrique Lanuza
Departament de Biologia Cellular, Facultat de Ciències Biològiques, Universitat de València, València, Spain

Guy N. Elston and Alejandra Elston
Centre for Cognitive Neuroscience, Sunshine Coast, QLD, Australia

Ruth Benavides-Piccione and Javier DeFelipe
Laboratorio de Circuitos Corticales (CTB), Universidad Politécnica de Madrid, Instituto Cajal (CSIC), Centro de Investigación Biomédica en Red sobre Enfermedades Neurodegenerativas (CIBERNED), Madrid, Spain

Paul R. Manger
School of Anatomical Sciences, Faculty of Health Sciences, University of the Witwatersrand, Johannesburg, South Africa

Isabel Rodríguez-Moldes, Ivan Carrera, Sol Pose-Méndez, Idoia Quintana-Urzainqui, Eva Candal, Ramón Anadón and Susana Ferreiro-Galve
Department of Cell Biology and Ecology, University of Santiago de Compostela, Santiago de Compostela, Spain

Sylvie Mazan
UMR 7150, Centre National de la Recherche Scientifique, Université Pierre et Marie Curie and Université Européene de Bretagne, Station Biologique de Roscoff, Roscoff, France

Isabel Ubeda-Bañon, Daniel Saiz-Sanchez, Carlos de la Rosa-Prieto and Alino Martinez-Marcos
Laboratorio de Neuroplasticidad y Neurodegeneración, Departamento de Ciencias Médicas, Centro Regional de Investigaciones Biomédicas, Facultad de Medicina de Ciudad Real, Universidad de Castilla-la Mancha, Ciudad Real, Spain

Palma Pro-Sistiaga
GIP Cyceron, Campus Jules Horowiz, Caen, France

Alicia Mohedano-Moriano
Laboratorio de Neuroanatomía Humana, Departamento de Ciencias Médicas, Centro Regional de Investigaciones Biomédicas, Facultad de Medicina de Albacete, Universidad de Castilla-La Mancha, Albacete, Spain

Nicolás Gutierrez-Castellanos, Enrique Lanuza and Fernando Martinez-Garcia
Laboratori de Neuroanatomia Funcional i Comparada, Departaments de Biologia Cellular i Biologia Funcional, Facultat de Ciències Biològiques, Universitat de Valencia, València, Spain

Gordon M. Shepherd
Department of Neurobiology, Yale University School of Medicine, New Haven, CT, USA

Paloma Merchán, Luis Puelles and José L. Ferran
Department of Human Anatomy and Psychobiology, Centre for Biomedical Research on Rare Diseases (CIBERER 736), School of Medicine, University of Murcia, Murcia, Spain

Sylvia M. Bardet
Unité de Génétique Moléculaire Animale, INRA UMR 1061, University of Limoges, Limoges, France

Mario F. Wullimann and Benedikt Grothe
Graduate School of Systemic Neurosciences and Department Biology II, Ludwig-Maximilians-Universität Munich, Planegg, Germany

Thomas Mueller
Department Developmental Biology, Institute of Biology I, University of Freiburg, Freiburg, Germany

Martin Distel, Andreas Babaryka and Reinhard W. Köster
Institute of Developmental Genetics, Helmholtz Zentrum München, German Research Center for Environmental Health, Neuherberg, Germany

Rudolf Nieuwenhuys
Netherlands Institute for Neuroscience, Amsterdam, Netherlands

Index

P

R

S

T

V

www.ingramcontent.com/pod-product-compliance
Lightning Source LLC
LaVergne TN
LVHW081032210926
848485LV00004B/1010